Nursing Now!

NURSING NOW!

Today's Issues, Tomorrow's Trends,

SIXTH EDITION

Learning Objectives

After completing this chapter, the reader will be able to:

- Discuss and analyze the difference between law and ethics.
- Define the key terms used in ethics.
- Discuss the important ethical concepts.
- Distinguish between the two most commonly used systems of ethical decision-making.
- Apply the steps in the ethical decision-making process.

Learning Objectives focus on the critical information in each chapter.

Key terms appear in bold type and are highlighted in yellow. *(Find a complete Glossary of Terms at the end of the book.)*

Autonomy is the right of self-determination, independence, and freedom. Autonomy refers to the client's right to make health-care decisions for himself or herself, even if the health-care provider does not agree with those decisions.

Evidence-based practice is emphasized throughout the book.

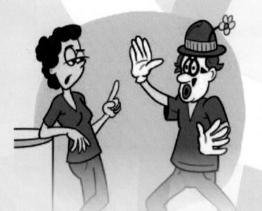

"YOU REALLY NEED TO WORK ON YOUR VERBAL SKILLS."

 Ethical theories do not provide recipes for resolution of ethical dilemmas. Instead, they provide a framework for decision-making that the nurse can apply to a particular ethical situation.

Insightful quotes and **colorful cartoons** make concepts easy to grasp.

Guidelines for Critiquing the Ethical Features of Research

1. Was the study approved by an institutional review board (IRB)?
2. Was informed consent obtained from every subject?
3. Is there information regarding anonymity or confidentiality?
4. Were vulnerable subjects used?
5. Does it appear that any coercion may have been used?
6. Is it evident that potential benefits of participation outweigh the possible risks?
7. Were participants invited to ask questions about the study and told how to contact the researcher, should the need arise?
8. Were participants informed how to obtain results of the study?

Case Study

When to Tell

A 48-year-old woman was scheduled for a below-the-knee amputation due to complications from diabetes. She was admitted to the preoperative area, signed a number of surgical permits, and was given her preoperative sedative medication. Because clients undergoing this type of surgery usually lose a significant amount of blood, several units of blood had been typed and cross-matched and placed on standby for her. After she was moved to the operating room and anesthetized, the nurse anesthetist rapidly administered the first unit of blood in preparation for the anticipated blood loss during surgery.

The circulating nurse was checking the paper work before the beginning of the operation and noticed that there was no consent signed for the administration of blood products. In examining the chart further, she noted that under the "Religion" section was listed "Jehovah's Witness." The Jehovah's Witness religion does not allow blood transfusions or transplantation of any tissue or organs. The circulating nurse told the nurse anesthetist about the client's religion, and his response was, "Holy cow—I can't believe this is happening!"

The family did not know about the blood transfusion, and obviously the client, who was under anesthesia, did not know she had received a unit of blood. The nurse anesthetist announced that it was not his fault because he was never told about the client's religion and was not going to tell the family or client about the mistake. The circulating nurse felt that because she did not administer the blood, she should not be the one to inform the family. The unit manager was called in, and the consensus was that she should be the one to reveal the information because she was ultimately responsible for what occurred in the surgical unit. Her feeling was that because no physical harm was done to the client, the whole incident should just be kept quiet.

Questions

1. Using the ethical decision-making model listed, work through the decision-making process for this ethical dilemma.
2. What are the key ethical principles involved in this dilemma?
3. What are the possible solutions to the dilemma and their consequences?
4. How would you resolve the dilemma? How would you defend your decision?

Critical Thinking Exercises

1. Ask the facility where you work or have clinical rotations what code of ethics they use. How does that differ from the ANA Code?
2. Ask your faculty what code of ethics is used for your evaluation.
3. Compare and contrast ethics with laws by delineating the purposes, scopes, and methods of enforcement of each.
4. Distinguish between the two types of obligations.
5. Compare the three categories of rights.
6. Analyze the following ethical dilemma case study using the ethical decision-making process:
   - What are the important data in relation to this situation?
   - State the ethical dilemma in a clear, simple statement.
   - What are the choices of action and how do they relate to specific ethical principles?
   - What are the consequences of these actions?
   - What decision can be made?

Critical Thinking Exercises ask you to apply what you've learned to think like a nurse.

Questions Interviewees Should Ask

- What are the responsibilities involved in the position?
- Who are the other staff or personnel working on this unit?
- What is the typical client-to-staff ratio for the unit?
- Are there any mandatory rotating shifts, weekend obligations, overtime, or floating?
- Does the hospital offer opportunities for continuing education, clinical ladder, advancement, or movement to other departments?
- Please describe the facility's policies for employee health and safety.

Practical advice prepares you for the real world.

FREE Online Resources at

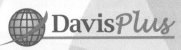

http://davisplus.fadavis.com
Keyword: **Catalano**

Annual Updates by the Author— Stay up to date on the issues and trends affecting nursing practice now… and in the future.

Resume Builder— Reference a sample and use a template to create a better resume.

Competencies— Understand what is expected of new graduates.

Web Links— Visit a variety of online resources to research and learn more about evidence-based practice.

Self-Assessment Tools— Complete these activities to develop your leadership, followership, and delegation skills.

Interactive Exercises— Practice with "Crossword Puzzle," "Guess the Term," and "Paragraph Match" exercises for each chapter.

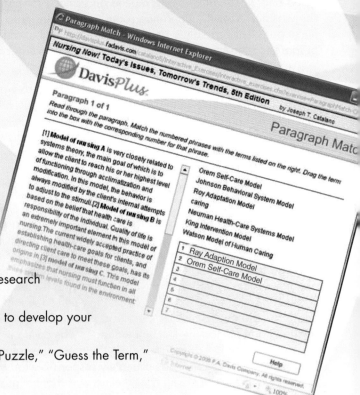

Nursing Now!
Today's Issues, Tomorrow's Trends

sixth edition

Joseph T. Catalano, PhD, RN
Program Consultant, Author
Ada, Oklahoma

F.A. Davis Company • Philadelphia

F. A. Davis Company
1915 Arch Street
Philadelphia, PA 19103
www.fadavis.com

Printed in the United States of America

Last digit indicates print number: 10 9 8 7 6 5 4 3 2

Acquisitions Editor: Joanne P. DaCunha, RN, MSN
Director of Content Development: Darlene D. Pedersen, MSN, APRN, BC
Project Editor: Elizabeth Hart
Illustration and Design Manager: Carolyn O'Brien

Library of Congress Cataloging-in-Publication Data

Catalano, Joseph T.
  Nursing now! : today's issues, tomorrow's trends / Joseph T. Catalano. — 6th ed.
     p. ; cm.
  Includes bibliographical references and index.
  ISBN-13: 978-0-8036-2763-5
  ISBN-10: 0-8036-2763-7
  I. Title.
  [DNLM: 1. Nursing—trends. WY 16.1]
  LC classification not assigned
  610.7306'9—dc23
                                                                                2011033259

Dedication

To all those nurses and students who believe that learning never stops and whose faith and courage will lead the nursing profession to its full potential.

Mind-boggling changes have occurred in health care since the last publication of this text. An African American president was elected and managed to get the biggest health-care reform bill passed in more than 50 years. As with all major changes, a vocal segment of the population stands in opposition. Nurses were at the table for the formulation of this bill and had significant input into its key elements. The nursing profession should wear this achievement as one of its shiniest merit badges!

The nation experienced one of the worst recessions in history and is finally on the road to recovery, however slow that may be. Although the nursing profession continues to be generally recession proof, in some areas of the country the economy was so bad that nurses were laid off. However, the future remains bright: estimates about the nursing shortage have remained the same or even increased slightly. Health-care reform is poised to bring in some 32 million newly insured clients over the next several years. Advanced practice nurses stand to provide a significant amount of the required primary and preventive care.

Nursing education has made major strides in increasing class sizes despite a political atmosphere of "cut taxes at all costs," as well as a continuous struggle with reduced funding and inability to attract qualified faculty because of low salaries. New advances in educational technology, changes in accreditation requirements, and calls for changes in curriculum structure and teaching methodologies have further challenged nursing educators.

Graduates from today's nursing programs have opportunities for professional practice and advancement that could only be dreamed about a few years ago. Yes, the demands are many, but the rewards are great. Today's nursing students must learn more, do more, and be more. Students entering nursing schools today come from diverse cultural, personal, and educational backgrounds. They must master a tremendous amount of information and learn a wide variety of skills so that they can pass the licensure exam and become highly skilled registered nurses.

The sixth edition of *Nursing Now! Today's Issues, Tomorrow's Trends* offers students a starting point to influence the future of health care in the United States. As with past editions, we listened to our readers and incorporated many of their suggestions. We are very excited about the revised text and believe its quality and content meet the high standards demanded by our readers.

Thanks to our readers' suggestions, we have added Chapter 15, "Incivility: The Antithesis of Caring." For a number of years, when I have met with nursing educators as well as a high percentage of nursing students, a recurring theme has been the fundamental lack of common courtesy and respect shown in nursing education, health-care facilities, and society in general. When I discussed this issue with my good friends at Southern University in Baton Rouge, they believed that the topic was important enough to merit its own chapter. The new chapter delves into the causes of incivility and offers suggestions for its prevention.

The chapter on the NCLEX exam was updated to reflect the recent changes by the National Council of State Boards of Nursing, including samples of the new alternative-format questions. All other chapters were revised with the addition of current content and resources. Health-care reform and its effect on nurses are discussed at length, and there is new material on transplantation issues, SBAR, QSEN, Six Sigma, and many other new developments in health care. Major revisions were made to the chapter on governance; the significant amount of new material includes a summary and discussion of the new Institute of Medicine report on the future of health care and nursing.

As in past editions, we have retained the interactive format of the text, in addition to the journal layout, current issues boxes, and integrated questions throughout. We deleted some of the older graphic illustrations and replaced them with new ones. We also added a number of new illustrations to increase the visual appeal of the book. The available website with interactive learning activities for students has been updated and expanded.

The book's primary purpose remains the same as in past editions. It presents an overview and synthesis of the important issues and trends that are basic to the development of professional nursing and that affect nursing both today and into the future. Our readers tell us that the book can be used both at the beginning of the student's educational process as an "Introduction to Nursing" course and also toward the end of the process as an "Issues and Trends" course. Some instructors even use it throughout their programs, incorporating chapters as the content is reflected in their course presentations. Nursing students remain the primary intended audience for *Nursing Now!* However, practicing nurses have reported a sufficiently wide range of current issues and topics covered in enough depth to be useful for their practice.

Another dichotomy that nurses face on a daily basis is the ability to hold onto key unchanging principles while working in a constantly changing environment. Simply stated, a nurse's ability to adapt to changes in the health-care system while remaining focused on providing high-quality care is the basis for successful professional practice. The only way that nurses will be able to effectively practice their profession in a demanding health-care system is to remain firmly rooted in those values and beliefs that have always served as their source of strength. Even more so than in the past, nurses need to look to each other for the inspiration and the strength that allow them to succeed. Professional organizations still serve as the single most powerful force for nurses, and membership in professional organizations is becoming increasingly important.

It is our belief that this book will help future nurses become familiar with the important issues and trends that affect the profession and health care. The nursing profession needs highly skilled nurses who can be civil, teach, do research, solve complicated client problems, provide highly skilled care, obtain advanced degrees, and influence the political realm that so affects all aspects of life. The leaders of the profession will come from those students who have a clear understanding of what it means to be a professional nurse and are willing to invest effort in attaining their goals.

Joseph T. Catalano, PhD, RN

Acknowledgments

I would like to express my thanks to my students and colleagues who have contributed their ideas and beliefs about the future of the nursing profession. I would also like to thank Pam, Sarah, Amanda, Dandy, and Pepper for their support and encouragement. And a special thank you to Anne-Adele, whose linguistic skills and perseverance are only matched by her creativity and sense of humor.

Heart, Hands and Ears

I lost a baby I wanted more than anything
    He was stillborn at 35 weeks
        You sat on the edge of my bed and listened
        to me sob when no one else would

I am only 8 and have leukemia
    The chemo shots hurt really really bad
        You sang a silly song with me while you
        gave the shot and made me laugh

I crashed my motorcycle and ripped open my leg
    It got a raging infection that required constant
    treatment
        You changed the dressing with skill and
        compassion

I had a stroke long before I should have
    My hands no longer work the way they used to
        You taught me how to use the fork with the
        big handle and now I can feed myself

I stood by my father's bedside while the machines he
was connected to went straight line
    He was sick for a long time but I loved him
    with every fiber of my being
        You stood quietly beside me and your
        strength gave me the courage to go on

I asked you one day "What does a nurse do?"
    I was wondering if it was something I too
    could do
        You answered:
        Nurses use their ears and compassion to
        listen
        Nurses use their hands and skills to heal
        Nurses use their hearts and souls to care
        Nurses take those who are at the crossroads
        of their lives,
        Who are battered and scarred with disease,
        and
        change their souls forever more with their
        hearts and their hands and their ears.

Joseph T. Catalano

Mary Abadie, RN, MSN, CPNP
Assistant Professor
Southern University and A&M College
School of Nursing
Baton Rouge, Louisiana

Tonia Aiken, RN, BSN, JD
President and CEO
Aiken Development Group
New Orleans, Louisiana

Sharon M. Bator, RN, MSN, CPE
Assistant Professor
Southern University and A&M College
School of Nursing
Baton Rouge, Louisiana

Barbara Bellfield, MS, RNP-C, RN
Family Nurse Practitioner
Ventura County Public Health
Loma Vista Road
Ventura, California

Cynthia Bienemy, RN, PhD
Director, Louisiana Center for Nursing
Louisiana State Board of Nursing
Baton Rouge, Louisiana

Doris Brown, Med, MS, RN, CNS
Public Health Executive Director
Robert Wood Johnson Nurse Fellow 2006–2009
Baton Rouge, Louisiana

Sandra Brown, RN, DNS, APRN, FNP-BC
Professor
Southern University and A&M College
School of Nursing
Baton Rouge, Louisiana

Joseph T. Catalano, PhD, RN
Program Consultant, Author
Ada, Oklahoma

Sarah T. Catalano
Public Relations Coordinator
Cothran Development Strategies
Ada, Oklahoma

Lydia DeSantis, RN, PhD, FAAN
University of Miami
School of Nursing
Miami, Florida

Joan Anny Ellis, RN, PhD
Director, Educational Services
Woman's Hospital
Baton Rouge, Louisiana
Associate Professor
Southern University and A&M College
School of Nursing
Baton Rouge, Louisiana

Mary Evans, JD, RN
316 N. Tejon
Colorado Springs, Colorado

Betty L. Fomby-White, RN, PhD
Southern University and A&M College
School of Nursing,
Baton Rouge, Louisiana
Associate Faculty
University of Phoenix Online

Edna Hull PhD, RN, CNE
Associate Professor & Program Director
Our Lady of the Lake College
Metropolitan New Orleans Center
New Orleans, Louisiana

Donna Gentile O'Donnell, RN, MSN
Deputy Health Commissioner (Retired)
Philadelphia, Pennsylvania

Anita H. Hansberry, RN, MS
Assistant Professor
Southern University and A&M College
School of Nursing
Baton Rouge, Louisiana

Nicole Harder, RN, BN, MPA
Coordinator, Learning Laboratories
Helen Glass Centre for Nursing
Faculty of Nursing
University of Manitoba
Winnipeg, Manitoba, Canada

Jacqueline J. Hill, RN, PhD
Associate Professor & Chair
Undergraduate Nursing Program
Southern University A&M College
Baton Rouge, Louisiana

Sharon W. Hutchinson, PhD, MN, RN, CNE
Associate Professor and Chair
Graduate Nursing Programs
Southern University School of Nursing
Southern University and A&M College
Baton Rouge, Louisiana

Joyce Miller, BSN, CPE, CCM
Clarity Hospice of Baton Rouge
Baton Rouge, Louisiana

Karen Mills, MSN, RN
Nurse Family Partnership State Nurse Consultant
Louisiana Office of Public Health
Baton Rouge, Louisiana

Roberta Mowdy, MS, RN
Instructor
Department of Nursing
East Central University
Ada, Oklahoma

Anyadie Onu, RN, MS
Assistant Professor
Southern University and A&M College
School of Nursing
Baton Rouge, Louisiana

Janet S. Rami, RN, PhD
Southern University and A&M College
School of Nursing
Baton Rouge, Louisiana

Mary Ann Remshardt, MS, EdD, RN
Nursing Recruitment & Retention Coordinator
Grayson College
Denison, Texas

Nancy C. Sharts-Hopko, RN, PhD, FAAN
Professor
Villanova University
Villanova, Pennsylvania

Enrica K. Singleton, RN, PhD
Professor
Southern University and A&M College
School of Nursing
Baton Rouge, Louisiana

Wanda Raby Spurlock, DNS, RN, BC, CNS, FNGNA
Associate Professor
Southern University and A&M College
School of Nursing
Baton Rouge, Louisiana

Melissa Stewart DNS, RN ,CPE
Assistant Professor
Our Lady of the Lake College
School of Nursing
Baton Rouge, Louisiana

Cheryl Taylor, PhD, RN
Associate Professor of Nursing
Director Office of Nursing Research
NLN Consultant to National Student Nurses
Association
Southern University and A&M College
School of Nursing
Baton Rouge, Louisiana

Karen Tomajan, MS, RN, NEA-BC
Clinical/Regulatory Consultant
INTEGRIS Baptist Medical Center
Oklahoma City, Oklahoma

Esperanza Villanueva-Joyce, EdD, CNS, RN
National Dean for Academics
Education Affiliates

Kathleen Mary Young, RN, C, MA
Instructor
Western Michigan University
Kalamazoo, Michigan

Contents

Part 1 The Growth of Nursing 1

    1   The Development of a Profession 3
    2   Historical Perspectives 22
    3   The Evolution of Licensure, Certification, and Nursing Organizations 37
    4   Theories and Models of Nursing 53
    5   The Process of Educating Nurses 84
    6   Critical Thinking 109

Part 2 Making the Transition to Professional 121

    7   Ethics in Nursing 123
    8   Bioethical Issues 142
    9   Nursing Law and Liability 169
    10 How to Take and Pass Tests 193
    11 NCLEX: What You Need to Know 209
    12 Reality Shock in the Workplace 230

Part 3 Leading and Managing 255

    13 Principles of Leadership and Management 257
    14 Communicating Successfully 274
    15 Incivility: The Antithesis of Caring 297
    16 Delegation in Nursing 310
    17 Governance and Collective Bargaining 322
    18 Health-Care Delivery Systems 343
    19 Nursing Informatics 336

Part 4 Issues in Delivering Care 387

    20 The Politically Active Nurse 389
    21 Spirituality and Health Care 411
    22 Cultural Diversity 430
    23 Developments in Current Nursing Practice 450
    24 Client Education: A Moral Imperative 467
    25 Nursing Research and Evidence-Based Practice 484
    26 Alternative and Complementary Healing Practices 505

Glossary 535
References 549
Bibliography 558
Index 567

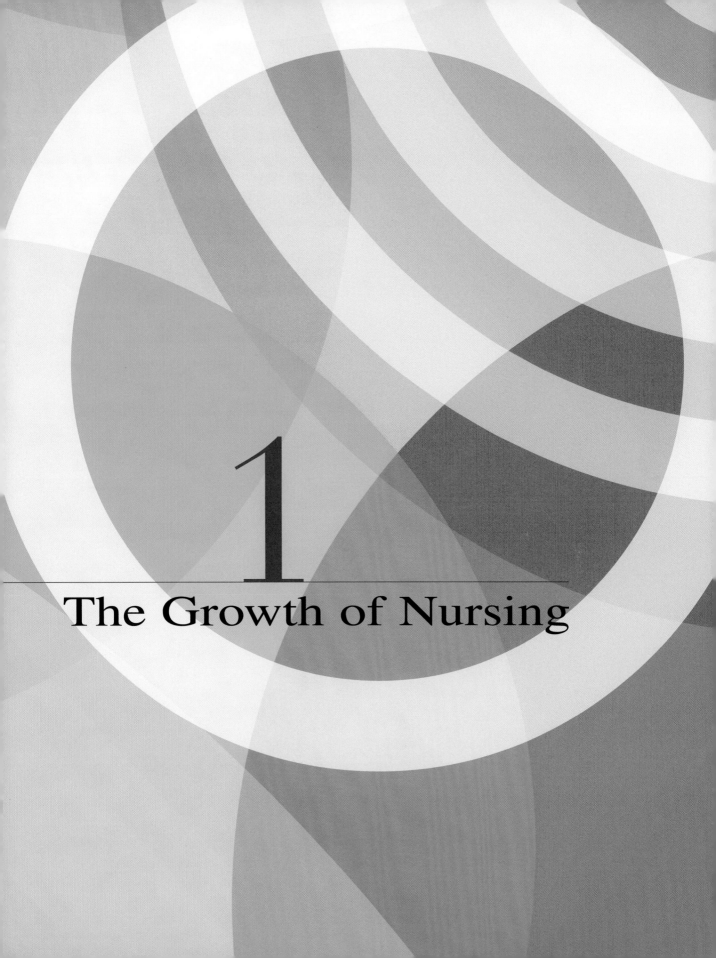

1

The Growth of Nursing

1

The Development of a Profession

Joseph T. Catalano

Learning Objectives

After completing this chapter, the reader will be able to:

- Define the terms *position, job, occupation,* and *profession.*
- Compare the three approaches to defining a profession.
- Analyze those traits defining a profession that nursing has attained.
- Evaluate why nursing has failed to attain some of the traits that define a profession.
- Correlate the concept of power with its important characteristics.

WHAT IS A PROFESSION?

Since the time of Florence Nightingale, each generation of nurses, in its own way, has fostered the movement to professionalize the image of nurses and nursing. The struggle to change the status of nurses from that of female domestic servants to one of high-level health-care providers who base their protocols on scientific principles has been a primary goal of nursing's leaders for many years. Yet some people, both inside and outside the profession of nursing, question whether the search for and attainment of professional status is worth the effort and price that must ultimately be paid.

At some levels in nursing, the question of **professionalism** takes on immense significance. However, to the busy **staff nurse**—who is trying to allocate client assignments for a shift; distribute the medications at 9 a.m. to 24 clients; and supervise two aides, a licensed practical nurse (LPN) or licensed vocational nurse (LVN), and a nursing student—the issue may not seem very significant at all.

Indeed, when nurses were first developing their identity separately from that of physicians, there was no thought about their being part of a **profession.** Over the years, as the scope of practice has expanded and the responsibilities have increased, nurses have increasingly begun to consider what they do as professional activities.

This chapter presents some of the current thoughts concerning professions and where nursing stands in relationship to these viewpoints.

APPROACHES TO DEFINING A PROFESSION

In common use, terms such as *position, job, occupation, profession, professional,* and *professionalism* often are used interchangeably and incorrectly. The following definitions will clarify what is meant by these terms within this text:

Position: A group of tasks assigned to one individual.

Job: A group of positions that are similar in nature and level of skill that can be carried out by one or more individuals.

Occupation: A group of jobs that are similar in type of work and that are usually found throughout an industry or work environment.

Profession: A type of occupation that meets certain criteria (discussed later in this chapter) that raise it to a level above that of an occupation.

Professional: A person who belongs to and practices a profession. (The term *professional* is probably the most misused of all these terms when describing people who are clearly involved in jobs or occupations, such as a "professional truck driver," "professional football player," or even "professional thief.")

Professionalism: The demonstration of high-level personal, ethical, and skill characteristics of a member of a profession.[1]

Experts in social science have been attempting to develop a "foolproof" approach to determine what constitutes a profession for almost 100 years, but with only minimal success. Three common models are the process approach; the power approach; and, most widely accepted, the trait approach.

Process Approach

The process approach views all occupations as points of development into a profession along a continuum ranging from position to profession:

Continuum of Professional Development:

Position   ◄————————►   Profession

Using this approach, the question becomes not whether nursing and truck driving are professions, but where they are located along the continuum. Occupations such as medicine, law, and the ministry are widely accepted by the public as being closest to the professional end of the continuum.[2] Other occupations may be less clearly defined.

The major difficulty with this approach is that it lacks criteria on which to base judgments. Final determination of the status of an occupation or profession depends almost completely on public perception of the activities of that occupation. Nursing has always had a rather poor public image when it comes to being viewed as a profession.

Power Approach

The power approach uses two criteria to define a profession:

1. How much independence of practice does this occupation have?
2. How much power does this occupation control?

> *Over the years, as the scope of practice has expanded and the responsibilities have increased, nurses have increasingly begun to consider what they do to be professional activities.*

The concept of power is discussed later in this chapter, but in this context, it refers to political power and the amount of money that the person in that occupation earns.[3]

Using this determinant, occupations such as medicine, law, and **politics** clearly would be considered professions. The members of these occupations earn high incomes, practice their skills with a great deal of independence, and exercise significant power over individuals, the public, and the political community, both individually and in organized groups. The ministry is generally perceived as having power and influence. However, most people in this group, except for a few individuals, such as television evangelists, have relatively low income levels. Nursing, of course, with its relatively lower salaries, low membership in professional organizations, and perceived lack of political power, would clearly not meet the power criteria for a profession.

The question that comes to mind is whether power, independence of practice, and high income are the only elements that determine professional status. Although those three factors confer status in our culture, other elements can be considered significant in how a profession is viewed. For example, to many people, members of the clergy have a great deal of power when they act as counselors, speakers of the truth, and community leaders.

Trait Approach

Of the many researchers and theorists who have attempted to identify the traits that define a profession, Abraham Flexner, Elizabeth Bixler, and Eliza Pavalko are most widely accepted as the leaders in the field. These three social scientists have determined that the following common characteristics are important:

- High intellectual level
- High level of individual responsibility and **accountability**
- Specialized body of knowledge
- Knowledge that can be learned in institutions of higher education
- Public service and altruistic activities
- Public service valued over financial gain
- Relatively high degree of **autonomy** and independence of practice
- Need for a well-organized and strong organization representing the members of the profession and controlling the quality of practice
- A **code of ethics** that guides the members of the profession in their practice
- Strong professional identity and commitment to the development of the profession
- Demonstration of professional competency and possession of a legally recognized license[4]

NURSING AS A PROFESSION

How does nursing compare with other professions when measured against these widely accepted professional traits? The profession of nursing meets most of the criteria but falls short in a few areas.

High Intellectual Level of Functioning

In the early stages of the development of nursing practice, this criterion did not apply. Florence Nightingale raised the bar for education, and graduates of her school were considered to be highly educated in comparison with other women of that time. However, most of the tasks performed by these early nurses are generally considered by today's standards to be menial and routine.

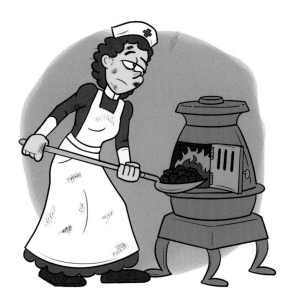

On the other hand, as health care has advanced and made great strides in technology, pharmacology, and all branches of the physical sciences, a high level of intellectual functioning is required for even relatively simple nursing tasks, such as taking a client's temperature or blood pressure using automated equipment. Nurses use **assessment** skills and knowledge, have the ability to reason, and make routine judgments based on clients' conditions daily. Without a doubt, professional nurses must and do function at a high intellectual level.

High Level of Individual Responsibility and Accountability

Not too long ago, a nurse was rarely, if ever, named as a **defendant** in a malpractice suit. The public, in general, did not view nurses as having enough knowledge to be held accountable for errors that were made in client care. This is not the case in the health-care system today. Nurses are often the primary, and frequently the only, defendants named when errors are made that result in injury to the client. Nurses must be accountable and demonstrate a high level of individual responsibility for the care and services they provide.[5]

The concept of accountability has legal, ethical, and professional implications that include accepting responsibility for actions taken to provide **client** care, as well as accepting responsibility for the consequences of actions that are not performed. Nurses can no longer state that "the physician told me to do it" as a method of avoiding responsibility for their actions.

Specialized Body of Knowledge

Most early nursing skills were based either on traditional ways of doing things or on the intuitive knowledge of the individual nurse. As nursing developed into an identifiable, separate discipline, a specialized body of knowledge called "nursing science" was compiled through the research efforts of nurses with advanced educational degrees.[6] As the body of specialized nursing knowledge continues to grow, it forms a theoretical basis for the practice of nursing today. As more nurses obtain advanced degrees, conduct research, and develop philosophies and theories about nursing, this body of knowledge will increase in scope and quantity.

Evidence-Based Practice

In professional nursing today, there is an increasing emphasis on evidence-based practice. Almost all the currently used nursing theories address this issue in some way. Simply stated, evidence-based practice is the practice of nursing in which interventions are based on data from research that demonstrates that they are appropriate and successful. It involves a systematic process of uncovering, evaluating, and using information from research as the basis for deciding about and providing client care.[7] Many nursing practices and interventions of the past were performed merely because they had always been done that way (accustomed practice) or because of deductions from physiological or pathophysiological information. Clients are now more sophisticated and knowledgeable about health-care issues and demand a higher level of knowledge and skill from their health-care providers.

The development of information technology has made evidence-based practice in nursing a reality. In the past, nurses relied primarily on units within their own facilities for information about the success of treatments, decisions about health care, and outcomes for clients. Nursing education now requires nursing students to perform Web-based research for papers and projects, so that by the time of gradua-

> *Evidence-based practice is the practice of nursing in which interventions are based on data from research that demonstrates that they are appropriate and successful.*

tion, they feel comfortable accessing a wide range of the best and most current information through electronic sources. Of course, one of the key limiting factors of evidence-based practice is the quality of the information on which the practice is based. Evaluating the quality of information on the Web can be difficult at times.

The first step in developing an evidence-based practice is to identify exactly what the intervention is supposed to accomplish. Once the goal or client outcome is identified, the nurse needs to evaluate current practices to determine whether or not they are achieving the desired client outcomes. If they are unsuccessful, or if the nurse feels they can be more efficient with fewer complications, research sources need to be collected. These can be from published journal articles (either electronic or hard copy) and from presentations at research or practice conferences, which often present the most current information. Then a plan should be developed to implement the new findings. This process can be applied to changing policy and procedures or developing training programs for facility staff. Research data should always be used when initiating new practices or modifying old ones (see Chapter 25).

Public Service and Altruistic Activities

Almost all major nursing theorists, when defining nursing, include a statement that refers to a goal of helping clients adapt to illness and achieve their highest level of functioning. The public (variously referred to as consumers, patients, clients, individuals, or humans) is the focal point of all nursing models and nursing practice. The public service function of nursing has always been recognized and acknowledged by society's willingness to continue to educate nurses in public, tax-supported institutions as well as in private schools. In addition, nursing has been viewed universally as an altruistic profession composed of selfless individuals who place the lives and well-being of their clients above their personal safety. In the earliest days, dedicated nurses provided care for victims of deadly plagues with little regard for their own welfare. Today, nurses are found in remote and often hostile areas, providing care for the sick

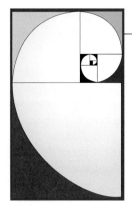

Issues Now

Web Sites: Friend or Foe?

Have a paper or report to do for class? Need information on pheochromocytoma, Smith-Strang disease, Kawasaki disease? No problem, look it up on the Web, right? Well, yes and no. Without any question, there is a tremendous amount of information about almost any subject available just a few mouse clicks away. But the bigger question is: how good is that information? The truth of the matter is that anyone can post almost anything online these days, and there are no organizations or agencies that oversee or review the information for quality, accuracy, or objectivity. So how are you supposed to know what is good and what is not? Although there is no foolproof method for determining the quality of any given Web site, some telltale markers can point you in the right direction when you are rating the quality of the information you seek.

Marker 1: Peer Review

All major professional journals have a peer review process that requires any manuscripts submitted to be reviewed by two or three professionals who are considered experts, or at least knowledgeable in the subject matter. Peer review is one of the key elements in ensuring the accuracy of the information in the manuscript. When considering a Web source, look for a clear statement of the source of the information and how that information is reviewed. If the information is from an established source, such as a recognized professional journal, it has been peer reviewed and has a higher degree of accuracy. Examine the format and writing style of the document. If it seems to be very choppy, or if the style, tone, or person the article is written in changes throughout the article, it is an indication that it was not well edited and probably not peer reviewed. Use the information with caution.

Marker 2: Author Credentials

The name of the author and his or her titles and credentials should be listed. Be cautious if no author or publisher is listed. Of course, anyone can use another person's name as the author, but it is relatively easy to cross-check authors' names through other databases, such as those found in libraries. Before accepting the information as gospel, it is probably worth looking up the author and seeing what other articles or books he or she has written. Another key to establishing author credentials is to establish to whom the website belongs. In general, personal website pages are less likely to contain authoritative information. You can also look at the last three letters in the website address. The ones that end in ".gov," ".org," or ".edu" will tend to have higher-quality information. Also, see whether the information has a copyright. If the information is copyrighted, the person felt strongly enough about what he or she was posting to go to the effort of making sure no one else could use it as their original information.

Marker 3: Prejudice and Bias

Although there is almost always a small degree of prejudice and bias in all written material, most legitimate authors strive to be as objective as possible. Many times, if you read a document with a critical eye, you can discern obvious prejudicial

(continued)

Issues Now continued

viewpoints. See if the author has a vested interest in the content of the document. You can be pretty sure that an article about the effects of tobacco use on the respiratory system written by a scientist who was hired by the R. J. Reynolds Company would have a decidedly different viewpoint than an article written by a scientist who was employed by the National Health Information Center. See if contact information is provided by the author and who the sponsor or publisher of the document is. If these are not provided, be suspicious about the information.

Marker 4: Timeliness

Of course, all of us want the most recent information we can find and sometimes mistakenly make the assumption that because it is on the Web, it is new. In reality, professional journals that post their partial-text or full-text articles on their websites usually take anywhere from 6 to 9 months to do so. If you want absolutely the most current information, the hard-copy journal texts found in the library still are your best bet. Some forms of the Web have been around for as long as 10 years now, so some of the material can be very outdated. See if you can determine when the site was last updated and how extensively the information was revised. It is also a good practice to look to other sources (Web, journals, books, etc.) to compare the material for currency. Many websites have links where you can access other related information. If those links have messages such as "Page discontinued" or "Link no longer available," be extremely cautious with the information. Good links should connect you to other reliable sites.

Marker 5: Presentation

Although the old saying is that "you can't tell a book by its cover," experienced Web surfers can often tell a lot about a website by its presentation. Some look well developed and professional, and others look very amateurish. There is no guarantee that the slick-looking websites are better, but it is one factor to consider in the overall evaluation of the information you are seeking. Take a look at the graphics. They should be balanced with the text and help explain or demonstrate information in the text. If the graphics seem to be just decorative, it should raise a red flag about the content of the site. Some sites use a compressed format that requires special programs such as Adobe Acrobat to view them. If you do not have access to these programs, the information in the site is unusable. Move on to the next site.

In summary, the Internet can be a valuable source of information about a wide variety of subjects. However, each source needs to be evaluated carefully. Following the five markers discussed here will place you on the path to deciding the quality of the information presented in any website.

Sources: Carlson EA: What to look for when evaluating Web sites. Orthopaedic Nursing 28(4):199–202, 2009.

Fetter MS: Graduating nurses' self-evaluation of information technology competencies. Journal of Nursing Education 48(2):86-90, 2009.

McGough G: Webwise. Nursing Standard 24(25):30, 2010.

Spector ND; Matz PS; Levine LJ; Gargiulo KA; McDonald MB 3rd; McGregor RS: e-Professionalism: Challenges in the age of information. Journal of Pediatrics 156(3):345–346, 2010.

and dying, working 12-hour shifts, being "on call," and working rotating shifts.

Few individuals enter nursing to become rich and famous. It is likely that those who do so for these reasons quickly become disappointed. Although the pay scale has increased tremendously since the 1990s, nursing is, at best, a middle-income occupation. Surveys among students entering nursing programs continue to indicate that the primary reason for wishing to become a nurse is to "help others" or "make a difference" in someone's life and to have "job security." Rarely do these beginning students include "to make a lot of money" as their motivation.[7]

Well-Organized and Strong Representation

Professional organizations represent the members of the profession and control the quality of professional practice. The National League for Nursing (NLN) and the American Nurses Association (ANA) are the two major national organizations that represent nursing in today's health-care system. The NLN is primarily responsible for regulating the quality of the educational programs that prepare nurses for the practice of nursing, whereas the ANA is more concerned with the quality of nursing practice in the daily health-care setting. These and other organizations are discussed in more detail in Chapter 3.

Both these groups are well organized, but neither can be considered powerful when compared with other professional organizations, such as the American Hospital Association, the American Medical Association (AMA), or the American Bar Association (ABA). One reason for their lack of strength is that fewer than 10 percent of all nurses in the United States are members of any professional organization at the national level.[3] Many nurses do belong to specialty organizations that represent a specific area of practice, but these lack sufficient political power to produce changes in health-care laws and policies at the national level.

Nurses' Code of Ethics

Nursing has several codes of ethics that are used to guide nursing practice. The ANA Code of Ethics for Nurses, the most widely used in the United States, was first published in 1971, updated in 1985, and last updated in 2001. The current ANA Code of Ethics, while maintaining the integrity found in earlier versions, is now more relevant to current health-care and nursing practices. This code of ethics is recognized by other professions as a standard with which others are compared. The nurses' code of ethics and its implications are discussed in greater detail in Chapter 7.

Competency and Professional License

Nurses must pass a national licensure examination to demonstrate that they are qualified to practice nursing. Only after passing this examination are nurses allowed to practice. The granting of a nursing **license** is a legal activity conducted by the individual state under the **regulations** contained in that state's nurse practice act.

WHEN NURSING FALLS SHORT OF THE CRITERIA

Before Florence Nightingale practiced nursing, people considered it to be unnecessary, if not outright dangerous, to educate nurses through independent nursing programs in publicly supported educational institutions. As nursing has developed, particularly in the United States, the recognition of the intellectual nature of the practice, as well as the vast amount of knowledge required for the job, has led to a belief by some nursing leaders that college education for nurses is now a necessity.

Nursing is the only major discipline that does not require its members to hold at least a baccalaureate degree in order to obtain licensure. Although the number of diploma programs in nursing has decreased tremendously since 1990, associate degree programs continue to maintain high enrollment and graduate large numbers of individuals. Whether a baccalaureate degree nursing program should be the minimum requirement for entry-level nurses remains a hotly debated issue.[1,6,7–10]

Autonomy and Independence of Practice

Historically, the handmaiden or servant relationship of the nurse to the physician was widely accepted. It was based on several factors, including social norms. For example, women became nurses, whereas men became physicians; women were subservient to men, the nature of the work being such that nurses cleaned and physicians cured. In terms of the relative levels of education of the two groups, the average nursing program lasted for 1 year, whereas physician education lasted for 6 to 8 years.

Unfortunately, despite efforts to expand nursing practice into more independent areas through updated nurse practice legislation, nursing retains much of its subservient image. In reality, nursing is both an independent and interdependent discipline. Nurses in all health-care settings must work closely with physicians, hospital administrators, pharmacists, and other groups in the provision of care. In some cases, nurses in **advanced practice** roles, such as **nurse practitioners,** can and do establish their own independent practices. Most state **nurse practice acts** allow nurses more independence in their practice than they realize. To be considered a true profession, nursing will need to be recognized by other disciplines as having practitioners who practice nursing independently.

Professional Identity and Development

The issue of job versus career is in question here. A job is a group of positions, similar in nature and level of skill, that can be carried out by one or more individuals. There is relatively little commitment to a job, and many individuals move from one job to another with little regard to the long-term outcomes. A career, in contrast, is usually viewed as a person's major lifework, which progresses and develops as the person grows older. Careers and professions have many of the same characteristics, including a formal education, full-time employment, requirement for lifelong learning, and a dedication to what is being achieved. Although an increasing number of nurses view nursing as their life's work, many still treat nursing more as a job.

The problem becomes circular. The reason nurses lack a strong professional identity and do not consider nursing a lifelong career is that nursing does not have full status as a profession. Until nurses are fully committed to the profession of nursing, identify with it as a profession, and are dedicated to its future development, nursing will probably not achieve professional status.

MEMBERS OF THE HEALTH-CARE TEAM

The health-care delivery system employs large numbers of diagnosticians, technicians, direct care providers, administrators, and support staff (Table 1.1). It is estimated that more than 300 job titles are used to describe health-care workers. Among these are nurses, physicians, physician assistants, social workers, physical therapists, occupational therapists, respiratory therapists, clinical

psychologists, and pharmacists. All these individuals provide services that are essential to daily operation of the health-care delivery system in this country.

Of particular importance among this array of health-care workers are various types of nurses: registered nurses, licensed practical (vocational) nurses, nurse practitioners, case managers, and clinical nurse specialists. Each of these requires a different type of educational background, clinical expertise, and, sometimes, professional credentialing. In general, all nurses make valuable contributions within the health-care delivery system. There has been an increased demand for nurses who are educated to deliver care in the community setting and in long-term health-care settings rather than in the hospital. There has also been a need for nurse case managers who are prepared to coordinate care for vulnerable populations requiring costly services over extended periods. Nursing education programs are attempting to meet these needs by preparing individuals who can practice independently and autonomously, network, collaborate, and coordinate services. These programs also offer more clinical experiences in rehabilitation, nursing home, and community settings.

What Do You Think?

List and rate several of your recent experiences with the health-care system. In what roles did you observe registered nurses functioning?

Registered Nurses, Licensed Practical Nurses, and Unlicensed Assistive Personnel

Registered nurses (RNs) who have been educated at the associate, diploma, or baccalaureate level have traditionally been considered the cornerstone of the current health-care delivery system. In the past, most RNs worked within hospital settings and provided direct client care and nursing administration functions within these facilities. Owing to past trends in health-care funding, there were fewer hospital admissions, which temporarily decreased the demand for RNs in acute care facilities and increased the need for well-prepared nurses who could function autonomously within the community. However, current trends in population and health care have demonstrated a need for RNs in both acute care and community settings. The need still remains within institutional settings for licensed practical nurses (LPNs) and unlicensed assistive personnel

Table 1.1 Other Key Health-Care Team Members

Title	Credential	Practice
Physician (MD)	License—Medical	Medical—limited only by specialization Some serve as primary care providers
Physician (DO)	License—Osteopath	Medical, with focus on body movement and holistic health—similar to MD Can serve as primary care providers
Physician (DC)	License—Chiropractor	Limited—focus on spinal column and nervous system Unable to prescribe medications
Physician (DPM)	License—Podiatry	Limited—foot problems Can prescribe medications, perform foot surgery
Physician Assistant	Certification—no individual license	Practices on physician's license Practice limited by medical practice act and wishes of supervising physician
Social Worker	License	Increasingly important as health care becomes more complex Resolves financial, housing, psychosocial, and employment problems; does discharge planning and assists clients in transfer between facilities May serve in case management roles to coordinate services
Physical Therapist	License	Focuses on helping clients maintain or regain the highest level of function possible after strokes, spinal cord injury, arthritis, or residual effects of traumatic accidents Helps prevent physical decline and regain the ability to groom, eat, and walk through individualized range of motion and exercise programs Therapy occurs in hospitals, clinics, or the community
Respiratory Therapist	License	Strives to restore normal or as near to normal pulmonary functioning as possible by conducting diagnostic tests and administering treatments that have been prescribed by a physician
Clinical Psychologist	License	Helps clients to manage mental health problems Private practice, clinics
Pharmacist	License	Distributes prescribed and over-the-counter medications, educates clients, monitors appropriate medication selections, detects interactions and untoward responses in community pharmacies and institutional settings Valuable resource for nurses

(UAPs) who work under the supervision of an RN. This pattern of care is particularly evident in nursing homes and other long-term care facilities.[2]

Advanced Practice Nurses

For individuals who are unfamiliar with the health-care delivery system, it is sometimes difficult to understand the similarities and differences between nursing titles and roles. This confusion is particularly evident in the case of clinical nurse specialists (CNSs) and nurse practitioners (NPs), who are sometimes collectively referred to as advanced practice registered nurses (APRNs).[4]

The Nurse Practitioner

In general, NPs are prepared to provide direct client care in primary care settings, focusing on health promotion, illness prevention, early diagnosis, and treatment of common health problems. Their educational preparation varies, but in most cases individuals successfully complete a graduate nurse practitioner program and are certified by the American Nurses Credentialing Center (ANCC) or an appropriate professional nursing organization. Depending on the individual state nurse practice act, NPs have a range of responsibilities for diagnosing diseases and prescribing both treatments and medications. A growing number of states now grant NPs direct third-party reimbursement for their services without a physician.

The Clinical Nurse Specialist

Clinical nurse specialists usually practice in secondary or tertiary care settings and focus on care of individuals who are experiencing an acute illness or an exacerbation of a chronic condition. In general, they are prepared at the graduate level and are ANCC certified. These highly skilled practitioners are comfortable working in high-tech environments with seriously ill individuals and their families. Because of the nature of their work, they are excellent health-care educators and physician collaborators.

> *Depending on the individual state nurse practice act, NPs have a range of responsibilities for diagnosing diseases and prescribing both treatments and medications.*

Attempts have been made to combine the roles of the CNS and NP so that the best qualities of both roles are preserved. The goal of this combination is to provide high-quality care to individuals in a wide array of health-care settings who have a wide range of health problems. Advocates of this movement include the NLN, the American Association of Colleges of Nursing (AACN), and the ANA. Titling for this new blended role is unconfirmed, and state legislatures may make the final decisions through their licensing laws. As such, titling, educational preparation, and practice privileges will probably vary from one state to another.

Case Managers

One argument for the blended NP–CNS role is the need for case managers who possess the expertise of both levels of preparation. Case managers coordinate services for clients with high-risk or long-term health problems who have access to the full continuum of health-care services. Case managers provide services in various settings, such as acute care facilities, rehabilitation centers, and community agencies. They also work for managed care companies, insurance companies, and private case management agencies. Their roles vary according to the circumstances of their employment; however, their overall goal is to coordinate the use of health-care services in the most efficient and cost-effective manner possible.

Case management is the glue that holds health-care services together across practitioners, agencies, funding sources, locations, and time. Titling, educational preparation, and certification of nurse case managers are now available. The ANCC has developed certification eligibility criteria for nurse case managers, and an examination is available. At this time, case managers can be physicians, social workers, registered nurses, and even well-intentioned laypersons with little health-care education.

EMPOWERMENT IN NURSING

One concern that has plagued nursing, almost from its development as a separate health-care specialty, is the relatively large amount of personal responsibility shouldered by nurses combined with a relatively small amount of control over their practice. Even in the more enlightened atmosphere of today's society, with its concerns about equal opportunity, equal pay, and collegial relationships, many nurses still seem uncomfortable with the concepts of power and control in their practice. Their discomfort may arise from the belief that nursing is a helping and caring profession whose goals are separate from issues of power.

Historically, nurses have never had much power, and previous attempts at gaining power and control over their practice have been met with much resistance from groups who benefit from keeping nurses powerless. Nevertheless, all nurses use power in their daily practice, even if they do not realize it. Until nurses understand the sources of their power, how to increase it, and how to use it in providing client care, they will be relegated to a subservient position in the health-care system.

The Nature of Power

The term *power* has many meanings. From the standpoint of nursing, power is probably best defined as the ability or capacity to exert influence over another person or group of persons. In other words, power is the ability to get other people to do things even when they do not want to do them. Although power in itself is neither good nor bad, it can be used to produce either good or bad results.

Power is always a two-way street. By its very definition, when power is exerted by one person, another person is affected; that is, the use of power by one person requires that another person give up some of his or her power. Individuals are always in a state of change, either increasing their power or losing some; the balance of power rarely remains static. **Empowerment** refers to the increased amount of power that an individual or group is either given or gains.

Origins of Power

If power is such an important part of nursing and the practice of nurses, where does it come from? Although there are many sources, some of them would be inappropriate or unacceptable for those in a helping and caring profession. The following list includes some of the more accessible and acceptable sources of power that nurses should consider using in their practice.[3,8,9] These sources are:

• Referent
• Expert
• Reward
• Coercive
• Legitimate
• Collective

Referent Power

The referent source of power depends on establishing and maintaining a close personal relationship with someone. In any close personal relationship, one individual often will do something he or she would really rather not do because of the relationship. This ability to change the actions of another is an exercise of power.

Nurses often obtain power from this source when they establish and maintain good therapeutic relationships with their clients. Clients take medications, tolerate uncomfortable treatments, and participate in demanding activities that they would clearly prefer to avoid because the nurse has good relationships with them. Likewise, nurses who have good collegial relationships with other nurses, departments, and physicians are often able to obtain what they want from these individuals or groups in providing care to clients.

Expert Power

The expert source of power derives from the amount of knowledge, skill, or expertise that an individual or group has. This power source is exercised by the individual or group when knowledge, skills, or expertise is either used or withheld in order to influence the behavior of others. Nurses should have at least a minimal amount of this type of power because of their education and experience. It follows logically that increasing the level of nurses' education will, or should, increase this expert power. As nurses attain and remain in positions of power longer, the increased experience will also aid the use of expert power. Nurses in advanced practice roles are good examples of those who have expert power. Their additional education and experience provide these nurses with the ability to practice skills at a higher level than nurses prepared at the basic education level.

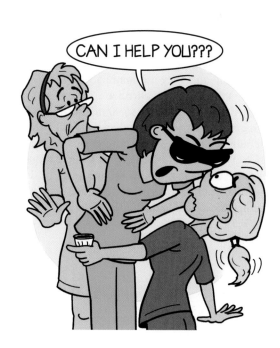

By demonstrating their knowledge of the client's condition, recent laboratory tests, and other elements that are vital in the client's recovery, nurses demonstrate their expert power. This knowledge may increase the amount of respect they are given by physicians. Nurses access this expert source of power when they use their knowledge to teach, counsel, or motivate clients to follow a plan of care. Nurses can also use expert power when dealing with physicians.

Power of Rewards

The reward source of power depends on the ability of one person to grant another some type of reward for specific behaviors or changes in behavior. The rewards can take on many different forms, including personal favors, promotions, money, expanded privileges, and eradication of punishments. Nurses, in their daily provision of care, can use this source of power to influence client behavior. For example, a nurse can give a client extra praise for completing the prescribed range-of-motion exercises. There are many aspects of the daily care of clients over which nurses have a substantial amount of reward power. This reward source of power is also the underlying principle in the process of behavior modification.

Coercive Power

The coercive source of power is the flip side of the reward source. The ability to punish, withhold rewards, and threaten punishment is the key element underlying the coercive source of power. Although nurses do have access to this source of power, it is probably one that they use minimally, if at all. Not only does the use of the coercive source of power destroy therapeutic and personal relationships, but it can also be considered unethical and even illegal in certain situations. Threatening clients with an injection if they do not take their oral medications may motivate them to take those medications, but it is generally not considered to be a good example of a therapeutic communication technique.

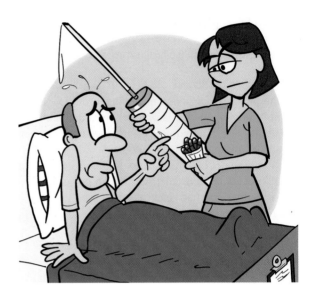

Legitimate Power

The legitimate source of power depends on a legislative or legal act that gives the individual or organization a right to make decisions that they might not otherwise have the authority to make. Most obviously, political figures and **legislators** have this source of power. This power can also be disseminated and delegated to others through legislative acts. In nursing, the state board of nursing has access to the legitimate source of power because of its establishment under the nurse practice act of that state. Similarly, nurses have access to the legitimate source of power when they are licensed by the state under the provisions in the nurse practice act or when they are appointed to positions within a health-care agency. Nursing decisions made about client care can come only from individuals who have a legitimate source of power to make those decisions—that is, licensed nurses.

Collective Power

The collective source of power is often used in a broader context than individual client care and is

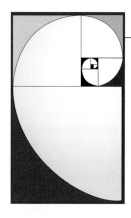

Issues in Practice

Kasey is an RN who has worked on the busy surgical unit of a large city hospital for the past 6 years. As one of three RNs on the unit's day shift, she often serves as the charge nurse when the assigned charge nurse has a day off. She is hard working, caring, and well organized and provides high-quality care for the often very unstable postoperative clients they receive on a daily basis.

About 2 weeks ago, Kasey's mother was admitted for a high-risk surgical removal of a brain tumor that was not responding to chemotherapy or radiation therapy. The surgery did not go well, and Kasey's mother was admitted to the surgical unit after the procedure. During the past 2 weeks, she has shown a gradual but steady decline in condition and is no longer able to recognize her family, speak, or do any self-care. It is believed she will probably not live more than a week longer.

Per hospital policy, Kasey is not assigned to care for her mother; however, during her shifts, Kasey is spending more and more time with her mother, sometimes to the detriment of her assigned clients. She is also beginning to make more demands on the unit nursing staff, often overseeing their care and requesting that only certain nurses care for her mother. One of the other nurses on the unit suggested that Kasey's mother be moved to a less specialized unit. When Kasey heard about the suggestion, she became livid and loudly scolded the nurse for her insensitivity in the middle of the nurses' station.

QUESTIONS FOR THOUGHT

1. Is the practice of not allowing nurses to provide care for their relatives evidence-based or accustomed practice?

2. Identify the steps in making this policy evidence based.

3. Do you think nurses should be allowed to care for relatives? Why? Why not?

the underlying source for many other sources of power. When a large group of individuals who have similar beliefs, desires, or needs become organized, a collective source of power exists.[6] For individuals who belong to professions, the professional organization is the focal point for this source of power. The main goal of any organization is to influence policies that affect the members of the organization. This influence is usually in the form of political activities carried out by politicians and **lobbyists.**

Professional organizations that can deliver large numbers of votes have a powerful means of influencing politicians. The use of the collective source of power contains elements of reward, coercive, expert, and even referent sources. Each source may come into play at one time or another.

How to Increase Power in Nursing

Despite some feelings of powerlessness, nurses really do have access to some important, and rather substantial, sources of power. What can nurses, either as individuals or as a group, do to increase their power?

Professional Unity

Probably the first, and certainly the most important, way in which nurses can gain power in all areas is through professional unity. The most powerful groups are those that are best organized and most united. The power that a professional organization has is directly related to the size of its membership. According to the ANA, there are approximately 2.7 million nurses in the United States. It is not difficult to imagine the power that the ANA could have to influence legislators and legislation if all of those nurses were members of the organization rather than the 250,000 who actually do belong. This point—that nurses need to belong to their national nursing organization—cannot be emphasized too much.

Political Activity

A second way in which nurses can gain power is by becoming involved in **political action.** Although this produces discomfort in many, nurses must realize that they are affected by politics and political decisions in every phase of their daily nursing activities.

The simple truth is that, if nurses do not become involved in politics and participate in important legislation that influences their practice, someone other than nurses will be making those decisions for them. Nurses need to become involved in political activities from local to national levels. The average legislator knows little about issues such as clients' rights, national health insurance, quality of nursing care, third-party reimbursement for nurses, and expanded practice roles for nurses, yet they make decisions about these issues almost daily. It would seem logical that more informed and better decisions could be made if nurses took an active part in the legislative process.

> *By demonstrating their knowledge of the client's condition, recent laboratory tests, and other elements that are vital in the client's recovery, nurses demonstrate their expert power. This knowledge may increase the amount of respect that they are given by physicians.*

Accountability and Professionalism

A third method of increasing power is by demonstrating the characteristics of accountability and professionalism. Nursing has made great strides in these two areas in recent years. Nurses, through professional organizations, have been working hard to establish standards for high-quality client care. More important, nurses are now concerned with demonstrating competence and delivering high-quality client care through processes such as peer review and evaluation. By accepting responsibility for the care that they provide and by setting the standards to guide that care, nurses are taking the power to govern nursing away from non-nursing groups.

Networking

Finally, nurses can gain power through establishing a nurse support network. It is common knowledge that the "old boy" system remains alive and well in many segments of our seemingly enlightened 21st century society. The old boy system, which is found in most large organizations ranging from universities to businesses and governmental agencies, provides individuals, usually men, with the encouragement, support, and nurturing that allow them to move up quickly through the ranks in the organization to achieve high administrative positions. An important element in making this system work involves never criticizing another "old boy" in public, even though there may be major differences of opinion in private. Presentation of a united front is extremely important in maintaining power within this system. Nursing and nursing organizations have never had this type of system for the advancement of nurses.

Part of the difficulty in establishing a nurse support network arises from the fact that nurses have not been in high-level positions for very long. The framework for a support system for nurses is now in place; with some commitment to the concept and some activity, it can grow into a well-developed network to allow the brightest, best, and most ambitious people in the profession to achieve high-level positions.

> " *Probably the first, and certainly the most important, way in which nurses can gain power in all areas is through professional unity. The most powerful groups are those that are best organized and most united.* "

Future Trends in the Nursing Profession

Clearly, it would be difficult to make an airtight case for nursing as a profession. Yet nursing does meet many of the criteria proposed for a profession. Although it would probably be most accurate to call nursing a developing or aspiring profession, for the purposes of this book, nursing will be referred to as a profession. Only when nurses begin to think of nursing as a profession, work toward raising the educational standards for entry level, and begin practicing independently as professionals will the status of profession become a reality for nursing. The movement of any discipline from the status of occupation to one of profession is a dynamic and ongoing process with many considerations.

All the experts now predict a severe shortage of professional nurses, ranging from 200,000 to 800,000, by the year 2020. In the past, the way that nursing shortages were handled was to use a quick-fix method of producing more nurses in a shorter period of time by reducing the educational requirements. The current nursing education system is producing approximately 40,000 graduates from diploma and associate degree programs every year.[10] Although this number may help alleviate the nursing shortage, the more critical question to ask is whether this level of education is going to prepare nurses to meet the challenges of a rapidly changing and demanding health-care system into the 21st century.

As the national employment picture continues to evolve for registered nurses from bedside caregivers to coordinators of care, and as financial resources become stressed, perhaps more nurses will begin to look on what they do as a lifelong commitment. Professional commitment is a complicated issue, but little doubt exists that nurses will not have increased independence of practice until they begin to demonstrate that they are professionals committed to the field of nursing.

Conclusion

Ongoing changes in the health-care system will have a major impact on how and where nursing is practiced, and even on who practices it. Unless nurses become involved in decisions about the direction in which health care is going, band together as a profession, and exert some of their tremendous potential power, politicians, physicians, hospital administrators, and insurance companies will ultimately be shaping their future. The move toward mandated staffing ratios is one way that nurses are demonstrating their power to achieve a goal when they band together and exert power as a group.

Nursing has taken great strides forward in achieving professional status in the health-care system. Currently, many nurses accept the premise that nursing is a profession and therefore are not very concerned about furthering the process. Even as nursing has matured and evolved into a field of study with an identifiable body of knowledge, the questions and problems that have plagued this profession persist. In addition, advances in technology, management, and society have raised new questions about the nature and role of nursing in the health-care system. Only by understanding and exploring the issues of professionalism will nurses be prepared to practice effectively in the present and meet the complex challenges of the future.

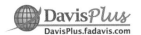
DavisPlus.fadavis.com

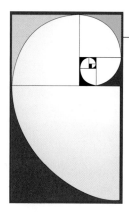

Issues in Practice

Mandatory Staffing Ratios: Pros and Cons

California was the first state that approved laws that mandate nurse-to-client staffing ratios. Guidelines were developed in January 2002 and went into effect in January 2004. Other states have since adopted various forms of mandatory staffing and requirements to report staffing ratios, but none are as prescriptive as California's laws.

Follow-up studies of the effects of the mandatory staffing ratios in California and other states have produced somewhat mixed results. Many studies disproved the claim that mandatory staffing would be too costly and cause the closing of hospital units, if not entire institutions. The overall effect was only marginal for hospitals' bottom lines, neither improving nor decreasing the profit margin.

The unknown effects of mandatory staffing ratios in the era of health-care reform have renewed the debate. Many who initially believed that mandatory staffing ratios would raise hospital costs, decrease the quality of nursing care, and put smaller hospitals out of business have proclaimed that these negative aspects would only be amplified under new health-care regulations. They point to the relatively small number of studies that demonstrate improved client care and decreased costs to hospitals as proof of their assertions. Other negatives that may result from mandatory staffing ratios in the era of health-care reform include worsening of the nursing shortage, decreased public and private sector support for nurses, and an across-the-board decrease in nursing morale. The opponents of mandatory staffing ratios also point to nursing's possible loss of flexibility in responding to the many changes that might result from health-care reform. Although there will probably be some requirements for nurses to take on new management and client advocate roles in the coming years, the overall effects of health-care reform are still several years in the future. The debate is guaranteed to continue.

On the positive side, several nursing groups point to recent studies showing that better staffing ratios produce better client care, which in turn reduces costs for insurance and settlements from malpractice law suits. Others believe that hospitals, in meeting the mandatory staffing levels, are using fewer of the very expensive agency nurses. All groups seem to agree that increased staffing levels increase nurses' morale and, as a result, reduce turnover rates.

A growing body of research demonstrates the connection between staffing levels and positive or negative health-care outcomes for hospitalized clients. Nursing associations and consumer groups feel that the quality of care is increased, along with client safety, with higher levels of RNs in the health-care setting. There is no research that demonstrates that mandatory staffing levels increase the shortage of nurses. Logically, it seems that increased staffing will help reduce the nursing shortage by addressing one of the leading causes of attrition among nurses—burnout from poor working conditions. If the health-care industry can keep more nurses in health care rather than having them leave for less stressful work settings, a major contribution will have been made to address the nursing shortage.

(continued)

Issues in Practice continued

QUESTIONS FOR THOUGHT

1. Do you think the proposed staffing ratios are a good thing? Why or why not? How would they affect health care in your town?

2. Does your state have any proposed legislation regarding mandatory staffing ratios? If so, obtain copies of the bills, read them, and discuss them with your class.

3. Do you know who your legislator is? Have you contacted him or her about how you feel about mandatory staffing ratios? If not, call him or her today!

4. How will health-care reform affect mandatory staffing?

Sources: Buerhaus PI: What is the harm in imposing mandatory hospital nurse staffing regulations? Nursing Economic$ 28(2):87-93, 2010.

Buerhaus PI: It's time to stop the regulation of hospital nurse staffing dead in its tracks. Nursing Economic$ 28(2):110-113, 2010.

Chernew M, Sabik L, Chandra A, Newhouse J: Ensuring the fiscal sustainability of health care reform. New England Journal of Medicine 362(1):1-3, 2010.

Nickitas DM: Re-evaluating nurse-patient ratios: Beyond the numbers and the law. Nursing Economic$ 28(2):73, 93, 2010.

Patton DM: Staffing ratios debate hasn't changed. Nursing Spectrum 22(12):10, 2010.

Upenieks V: Assessing nursing staffing ratios: Variability in workload intensity. Policy, Politics & Nursing Practice 8(1):7–19, 2007.

Critical Thinking Exercises

- Distinguish between an occupation and a profession.
- Is nursing a profession? Defend your position.
- Discuss four ways in which nursing can improve its professional status.
- Name the three sources of power to which nurses have the most access. Discuss how nurses can best use these sources of power to improve nursing, nursing care, and the health-care system.

2

Historical Perspectives

Joseph T. Catalano

Learning Objectives

After completing this chapter, the reader will be able to:

- Explain why studying the history of health care and nursing is important to the nursing profession.
- Name three "historical threads" found in the study of nursing history and discuss why they are important.
- Discuss Christian influences on health care and nursing.
- Discuss the influences of the Renaissance and Reformation on health care and nursing.
- Describe the major changes in health care and nursing that occurred during and immediately after World War II.

UNDERSTANDING OUR HISTORY

Knowledge about the profession's past can help us understand how nursing developed and even suggest solutions to problems that face the profession today. Several threads run throughout the history of nursing, including society's beliefs about the causes of illness, the value placed on individual life, and the role of women in society. The wars of modern history have also had a significant impact on nursing, particularly in influencing the development of technology and guiding the direction of health care. This chapter is not a treatise on the history of health care and nursing but presents some key historical milestones that helped to form the foundations of health and nursing care.

ORIGINS OF NURSING

Before Nursing

Current nursing practice is a relatively recent development. The major concern of most early civilizations was the survival of the group, and because illness and injury threatened this survival, many primitive health-care practices grew from processes of trial and error. In prehistoric times, women tended to care for the ill and injured. Evil spirits were thought to be the cause of illness, and the medicine men and women who practiced witchcraft were considered religious figures.

Driving Out Demons

In ancient Eastern civilizations, starting from about 3500 B.C., health care was intertwined with religion. Taoism emphasized balance and the driving of demons out of the ailing body. Acupuncture developed over the next several thousands of years, and medicinal herbs were used in preventive health care.

In Southeast Asia, Hinduism emphasized the need for good hygiene, and written records would soon chronicle a number of surgical procedures. This was also the first culture to document medical treatment outside the home, although women were prohibited from working. The rise of Buddhism around 530 B.C. caused a surge in health care, with public hospitals and high standards for doctors and other hospital workers and an emphasis on hygiene and prevention of disease. The development of medical knowledge was hindered to a degree by the refusal of the physicians to come in contact with blood and infectious body secretions and the prohibition against dissection of the human body.

Ancient Sciences

During the same period, the ancient Egyptians' belief that all disease was caused by evil spirits and punishing gods was changing. Health-care providers from that time showed a well-developed understanding of the basis of disease. Writings from 1500 B.C. refer to surgical procedures, the role of the midwife, bandaging, preventive care, and even birth control. Women enjoyed a higher status in Egyptian society and even worked in hospitals.[1] Physicians, however, were still men, who served in multiple roles as surgeons, priests, architects, and politicians.

> *The major concern of most early civilizations was the survival of the group, and because illness and injury threatened this survival, many primitive health-care practices grew from processes of trial and error.*

The Babylonian Empire, united in 2100 B.C., was a civilization that focused on astrology. Its health-care practices included special diets, massage therapy, and rest to drive evil spirits from a body. People would go to the marketplace to seek advice on how to treat their ailments. During the height of the Empire, strict guidelines governed doctors' fees and responsibilities in medical practice. There is also evidence from this period of child care and treatment of some diseases, but most care still took place in the home.

By 1900 B.C., the Hebrews had formed a nation along the Mediterranean and adopted many of the health practices of their neighbors. They integrated elements of the Egyptian sanitary laws to form the Mosaic Code that, as in many other cultures, mixed religion and medicine. Caring for widows, orphans, and other strangers in need was part of daily life. Hebrews had good knowledge of anatomy and physiology, especially the circulatory system. Physician-priests routinely performed operations such as cesarean sections (named later by the Romans), amputations, and circumcisions. They also enforced rules of purification, performed sacrifices, and conducted rituals related to food preparation.

What Do You Think?

Is the study of history really necessary for nursing students? Why or why not?

The Father of Medicine

Ancient Greece was a culture that focused on appeasing the gods, and its medical practice was no exception. The god Apollo was devoted to medicine and good health. The Greeks performed sacrifices to appease the gods and practiced abortion and infanticide in an attempt to control the population. People took hot baths at spas to improve health, but the sick and injured were cared for at clinics. Although women were held in high esteem, they were not permitted to provide any health care outside the home.

Around 400 B.C., the writings of Hippocrates began to change medical practice in Greece. One of a roving group of physician-priests, Hippocrates was called "the father of medicine." His beliefs focused on harmony with the natural law instead of on appeasing the gods. He emphasized treating the whole client—mind, body, spirit, and environment—and making diagnoses on the basis of symptoms rather than on an isolated idea of a disease. He was also concerned with ethical standards for physicians, expressed in the now-famous Hippocratic oath.

Health Care in the Roman Empire

Ancient Romans clung to superstitions and polytheism as the foundations for medical as well as religious practices. The dominant Roman Empire ruled from around 290 B.C.. and absorbed useful elements of whatever culture it conquered—including the Greeks and Hebrews—into its own. The Romans developed a quite advanced system of medicine and a pharmacology that included more than 600 medications derived from herbs and plants. Roman physicians were eventually able to distinguish among various conditions and performed many surgeries. They also did physical therapy for athletes; diagnosed symptoms of infections; identified job-related dangers of lead, mercury, and asbestos; and published medical textbooks.

The Romans' advances in creating an unlimited supply of clean water through aqueducts were critical in maintaining the good health of the citizens, as were central heating, spas and baths, and more advanced systems for sewage disposal. Because the great Roman armies were so crucial to the Empire, they developed early hospitals to care for sick and injured soldiers. These were mobile and were staffed by female as well as male attendants, who performed duties that would today be thought of as nursing care: cleaning and bandaging wounds, feeding and cleaning clients, and providing comfort to the wounded and dying. In many ways, women enjoyed an equal place in society, and they provided home health care as well as midwifery.

Early Efforts at Nursing
The Sanctity of Life

The rise of Christianity, starting from 30 A.D., brought with it a strong belief in the sanctity of all human life. Christians considered practices such as human sacrifice, infanticide, and abortion—which had been common in Roman society—to be murder. Following the teachings of Jesus meant that caring for the sick, poor, and disadvantaged was of primary importance, and groups of believers soon organized to offer care for those in need.

Early writings of the Christian period record women's important role in ministering to the sick and providing food and care for the poor and homeless. Wealthy Roman women who had converted to Christianity established hospital-like institutions and residences for these caregivers in their homes. The term *nurse* is thought to have originated in this period, from the Latin word *nutrire,* meaning to nourish, nurture, or suckle a child. The majority of care was still provided by a family member in the home. Most early Christian hospitals were roadside houses for the sick, poor, or

destitute, who were cared for by male and female attendants alike. The attendants learned from a process of trial and error and by observing others.

A Time of Disease

The Dark Ages, from roughly 500 to 1000 A.D., were marked by widespread poverty, illness, and death. Plagues and other diseases such as smallpox, leprosy, and diphtheria ravaged the known world and killed large segments of populations. Health care at this time was almost nonexistent.

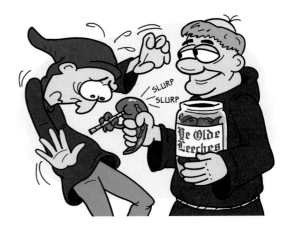

However, the strong beliefs of the Catholic Church, which was based in Rome, produced monasteries and convents that became centers for the care of the poor and the sick. By 500 A.D., there were several religious nursing orders in what is today England, France, and Italy. Men and women worked there and also traveled to rural areas where they were needed, combining religious rituals with home remedies as well as treatments such as bandaging, cautery, bloodletting, enemas, and leeching. The biggest contribution to health care in this period may have been the insistence on cleanliness and hygiene, which lessened the spread of infections. Medieval nurses did not have any formal schooling but learned through apprenticeships with older monks or nuns. Eventually hospitals came to be built outside of monastery grounds. Secular orders were also established, which could provide a wider range of services to the sick because they were not limited by religious restrictions and obligations.

Early Military Hospitals

At the end of the Dark Ages, there were a series of holy wars and invasions, including the Crusades, which produced many sick and injured who were far from home. Military nursing orders developed to care for the soldiers, but these were made up exclusively of men who wore suits of armor to protect themselves and their hospitals against attacks. These orders, with the emblem of the red cross, were extremely well organized and dedicated, and they existed well into the Renaissance.

Development of the Modern Nurse
Health Care in the Renaissance

In the intellectual reawakening of the Renaissance in Europe, starting in about 1350, nursing emerged in a recognizable form, although it did not grow steadily as a profession during this period. Inventions from this time include the microscope and thermometer, but the use of more modern diagnoses and treatment was viewed with skepticism. Monastic hospitals still regarded the restoration of health as secondary to the salvation of the soul. Major political changes initiated by the Protestant Reformation in 1517 had the greatest effect on the health care of the period. In Catholic nation-states, including Italy, France, and Spain, health care remained generally unchanged from that of the Middle Ages, although the number of male nursing orders gradually decreased. By 1500, the majority of health care was provided by female religious orders.

> *The term* nurse *is thought to have originated in this period, from the Latin word* nutrire, *meaning to nourish, nurture, or suckle a child.*

What Do You Think?

Imagine yourself living in one of the historical periods discussed in this chapter. Given your or your family's health-care problems, how would your lives be different?

A Nursing Hierarchy

In the nation-states that broke away from the Catholic Church, such as England, Germany, and the Netherlands, health care soon degenerated to a condition even worse than that of the Middle Ages. The role of women was reduced under Protestant leadership, and the male nurse all but disappeared. Secular nursing orders gradually took over the duties of the

many substandard hospitals that had been established in metropolitan areas. The most famous of these was the Sisters of Charity, established in 1600.

These orders were the first to establish a nursing hierarchy. Primary nurses were called sisters and those assisting them were called helpers and watchers. It is at this time that people began to recognize the benefit of skilled nursing care. The first nursing textbooks appeared, and the use of midwives became widespread. Although hospitals were gaining importance, most clients still received health care at home.

The Industrial Revolution (1850–1950) caused a flood of people from rural areas throughout Europe into cities, and cramped living situations caused very bad health conditions and the spread of disease and plagues. Factory owners supported some forms of health care to keep their workers on the job, and this led to an early form of community health nursing. The Sisters of Charity expanded their care to include home care. Only a few male nursing orders survived the Protestant Reformation and Industrial Revolution, and several non-Catholic nursing orders were founded, including the famous Quaker Society of Protestant Sisters of Charity, which provided care primarily for prisoners and children.

NURSING IN THE UNITED STATES

Five hospitals existed in America before the Revolutionary War, housing the homeless and the poor and including rudimentary infirmaries. However, there were no identifiable groups of nurses for these infirmaries.[2] Health care in America at this time reflected that of the European countries the settlers had come from. Infant mortality rates were very high, ranging between 50 and 75 percent. One of the first schools of nursing was established in 1640 by the Sisters of St. Ursula in Quebec, and Spanish and French religious orders would establish hospital-based training schools in the New World over the next 100 years.

In Colonial Times

During the Revolutionary War, there was no organized medical or nursing corps, but small groups of untrained volunteers cared for the wounded and sick in their homes or in churches or barns. Benjamin Franklin founded Pennsylvania Hospital, the first U.S. hospital dedicated to treating the sick, in 1751.

Between the Revolutionary and Civil Wars, health care in the United States increased markedly with the influx of religious nursing orders from Europe. More early schools of nursing developed at this time. Despite the rapid increase in the number of hospitals, most nursing care was still given at home by family members. Hospitals were considered a last resort and still had very high mortality rates.

When the States Went to War

The Civil War caused more death and injury than any war in the history of the United States, and the demand for nurses increased dramatically. Women volunteers (as many as 6000 for the North and 1000 for the South) began to follow the armies to the battlefields to provide basic nursing care, although many of them were untrained. Navy Nurses, the American Red Cross, and the Army Nurse Corps all date from this period. Large numbers of women came out of their homes to work in the hospitals, and a number of African American volunteers in the North paved the way for others to enter the health-care field in the future.

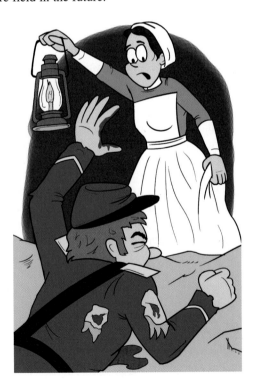

Technological developments in the 19th century included medications such as morphine and codeine for pain and quinine to treat malaria. The arrival of 30 million immigrants in this century meant that the need for health care increased accordingly. Hospitals sprang up, and many instituted their own schools of nursing. Still, home care was the preferred type of nursing.

After 1914
Untrained Nurses

At the beginning of World War I, there were only about 400 nurses in the Army Nurse Corps, but by 1917, that number swelled to 21,000. Because many hospitals were recruiting untrained women to provide basic care, a committee on nursing was formed to establish standards, and eventually the Red Cross began a training program for nurse's aides. This was supported by physicians but opposed by many nursing leaders, who were concerned that it relegated nursing to "women's work," which would be seen as something anyone could do with minimal training. Because nurse's aides were a cheap source of labor, they began to replace more trained nurses in hospitals. Unfortunately, this also resulted in a lower quality of care.

Between Wars

After the war, a segment of the nursing profession began to focus intensely on improving the educational standards of nursing care. At this time, 90 percent of nursing care was still given at home, but nurses began to practice in industry and in branches of government outside of the military. The standards of nursing care were low, and external quality controls were nonexistent.

The Great Depression took its toll on health care and nursing, as jobs became scarce and many nursing schools closed. At this time, the federal government became one of the largest employers of nurses. The newly organized Joint Committee on Nursing recommended that jobs go to more qualified nurses and that the work day be reduced from 12 to 8 hours, although these measures were not widely implemented. During this period, hospitals became the primary source of health care, supported by hospital insurance programs. As the size of hospitals increased, more nursing jobs became available.

Establishing Standards

World War II produced another nursing shortage, and in response, Congress passed the Bolton Nurse Training Act, which shortened hospital-based training programs from 36 to 30 months. The new Cadet Nurse Corps established minimum educational standards for nursing programs and forbade discrimination on the basis of race, creed, or sex.[2] Many schools revised and improved their curricula to meet these new standards.

To encourage more nurses to enter the military, the U.S. government granted women full commissioned status and gave them the same pay as men with the same rank. By the end of the war, African American and male nurses were also admitted to the armed services.

Modern Times: Emerging Specialties
A Team of Nurses

The advancements in health care made during World War II required that nurses receive more highly specialized education to meet clients' unique needs. After the war, many nurses left the profession to raise families, and the spaces were filled by graduates of new programs that trained licensed practical nurses (LPNs) and licensed vocational nurses (LVNs) in just 1 year. At this time, the concept of team nursing came to be widely accepted, although it removed the registered nurses (RNs) from direct client care, requiring them to serve as team leaders.

A Growing Need

Technical nursing programs, which granted associate degrees (associate degree nurse [ADN]) at 2-year community colleges, were developed to help with the nursing shortage. With the baby boom, the need for nurses continued to grow, and what had been a quick-fix solution began to take a stronger hold. By the mid-1960s, ADNs outnumbered the nurses with baccalaureate degrees (BSN) and the technical LPNs. Also, ADNs won the right to take the same licensing examinations as RN graduates from diploma and BSN programs.

Still, as the health-care system became increasingly complicated, some nursing leaders questioned whether 1- or 2-year LPN and ADN programs were adequate to meet the needs of the profession. Slowly the number of BSN programs and graduate-level programs began to increase.

Vietnam: Traveling Hospitals

The mobile army surgical hospital (MASH) units that had been developed during the Korean War were replaced during the Vietnam War with medical unit, self-contained transportable (MUST) hospitals, which were staffed by nurses as well as physicians. Some 5000 nurses served in this war, and for the first time, graduates of 2-year ADN programs were commissioned into the armed services. Several Navy nurses were injured in the line of duty, and one Army nurse was killed. The efforts of these and other women who served are recognized at the Vietnam Women's War Memorial in Washington, dedicated in 1993.

THE EVOLUTION OF SYMBOLS IN NURSING

> *Medieval nurses did not have any formal schooling but learned through apprenticeships with older monks or nuns.*

The Lamp
Pushing Back Darkness

The significance of the lamp is really the significance of light. Its origins can be traced back to the first attempts of human beings to control fire and use it as a tool of survival. These early humans soon found that fire was a source of warmth on cold nights, kept wild animals from attacking, and was useful for cooking.

Light, first in the form of torches and candles, and later in the form of the oil lamp, has been used by human beings for literally thousands of years to push back the darkness of night. It dispelled fear and allowed people to pursue learning long after the sun went down.

The lamp has long been used as a religious symbol. It often represents the eternal flame that dispels darkness and evil. Commonly found in Christian symbolism is the "Lady of Light," often depicted as radiant and glowing brightly and filled with goodness, purity, and wisdom. The lamp can also represent the flame of life, eventually extinguished by death.

As schools and universities developed during the Middle Ages, many adopted the lamp as a symbol of learning. The burning of the lamp signified the continual seeking of knowledge. It also symbolizes the enlightenment that accompanies knowledge. The coats-of-arms or logos used by many universities contain the image of a lamp.

A Sign of Caring

The lamp was first introduced as a symbol for the nursing profession at the time of Florence Nightingale. In addition to her fame as an early health-care reformer and pioneer, she became well known for her role in caring for injured soldiers during the Crimean War. She made history when she took her 38 nurses to Turkey to try to improve the squalid, filthy conditions she found in the primitive British field hospitals. As Nightingale and her nurses made their night rounds, caring for the wounded in unlit wards, they carried oil lamps to light the way. For the wounded and suffering, these lamps became signs of caring, comfort, and often the difference between life and death.

Nightingale's lamp was not the often-depicted "genie" or "Aladdin's" lamp. Rather, Nightingale would have used one of the many lamps in circulation around the wards, picking up whichever was closest at hand—an ordinary camp lamp or a Turkish candle lantern. She later became immortalized as the "Lady with the Lamp" in a poem written by Longfellow. In our modern society, oil lamps are sometimes used for atmosphere or nostalgic reminders of the past, although when the power goes out, they can be very handy. However, for graduate nurses, the lamp, or its close cousin the candle, retains its significance as a symbol of the ideals and selfless devotion of Florence Nightingale. It also signifies the knowledge and learning that the graduates have attained during their years in the nursing program. Even though the nursing graduates may not physically carry an oil lamp during pinning ceremonies, they symbolically carry the brightly burning lamp of their care and devotion as they minister to the sick and injured in their nursing practice.

The Nursing Pin

Unlikely as it may seem, the modern nursing pin can trace its origins to the heavy protective war shields

Large numbers of women came out of their homes to work in the hospitals, and a number of African American volunteers in the North paved the way for others to enter the health-care field in the future.

used by soldiers as far back as the Greek and Roman Empires. The primary purpose of these shields was to protect the warriors from the spears, swords, and arrows of the opposing army. These ancient war shields, adorned with the emblems of the country the soldier was from and his particular unit in the army, also served as a quick way to distinguish friend from foe.

During the Crusades, the Knights Hospitallers of St. John of Jerusalem were formed to provide medical care for the wounded and sick. The Knights wore black tunics over their armor, carried no weapons, and wore a white Maltese cross on chains around their necks. Those wearing this cross became known for their skills in treating the injured and healing the wounded. Since that time, the Maltese cross has been recognized as a symbol of those who care for the sick. Although large by today's standards, the Maltese cross is often considered the first true nursing pin.

The shields of some medieval knights were painted with the coats-of-arms of the kings they were defending. Only the best knights, recognized for their skills in battle, strength, honesty, and dedication to the service of the king, were permitted to use the king's coat-of-arms on their shields. The coat-of-arms displayed to the world the characteristics by which the king wished to be known. A classic example is the symbol of the lion, found on the shields of the knights who served King Richard the Lion-Hearted, that indicated the King's fearlessness and power.

Similarly, during the Middle Ages when most of the population was illiterate, tradesmen and craft guilds began adopting symbols as pictorial representations of their services, skills, and crafts. Modern companies use trademarks and brand names in the same way today. Medieval schools and universities also began using symbols to represent their values and goals. The modern practice of "branding the university," or adopting an official symbol or logo for the school, can be traced back to these early practices. These symbols were embossed on clothing, buttons, badges, and pins that were worn by members of the group. Also traceable to this time in history are the "shields" and badges worn by fire-fighters and law enforcement officers. Although these shields offer little in the way of protection from arrows and spears, they symbolize official authority and identify the wearer as belonging to a unique, specially trained group.

The first modern nursing pin is attributed to Florence Nightingale. After receiving the medal of the Red Cross of St. George from Queen Victoria for her selfless service to the injured and dying in the Crimean War, Nightingale chose to extend the honor she had received to her most outstanding graduate nurses by awarding each of them a "badge of excellence." The badge or pin she designed for her school is a deep-blue Maltese cross. In the center of the cross is a relief image of Nightingale's head. As the number of nursing schools increased, each program designed a unique pin to represent its own particular values, philosophy, beliefs, and goals.

The pinning ceremony is part of a long tradition that acknowledges nursing graduates as belonging to a unique group and identifies them as new members of the health-care community. The historical origins of the pin remind nursing professionals of what it symbolizes. Like the badge worn by law enforcement officers, it is also a sign of their legal authority as licensed professionals. Nursing graduates wear their pins proudly in the work setting as evidence of their successful completion of the nursing program.

> " *The Civil War caused more death and injury than any war in the history of the United States, and the demand for nurses increased dramatically.* "

QUESTION

Obtain a picture of your nursing school's pin. What do the various symbols on the pin signify?

The Cap
A Symbol of Service

It is rare to see a nurse wearing the traditional "nursing cap" in today's modern hospitals. However, the cap has a long, rich history. Although it may seem sexist by today's standards, throughout much of history, women were required to keep their heads covered with some type of garment. This practice was prevalent in the early Hebrew, Greek, and Roman cultures that served as the roots for modern Western society and the current profession of nursing.

The origins of what we identify as modern nursing can be traced back to an early Christian era group of women, called "deaconesses." Deaconesses were set apart from other women of the period by their white head covering, which indicated that their primary service was to care for the sick. During the early centuries of Christianity, groups of deaconesses banded together and formed what later became the religious orders that were so prevalent in the Holy Roman Empire. The former deaconesses, now recognized as religious order nuns, remained the primary providers of care for the sick throughout the Middle Ages. The traditional garb of nuns, the long-robed habit with the wimple or veil, can be considered the first official nurse's uniform. Each religious order had its own unique style of habit and wimple. The order the nun belonged to could be easily identified from the habit or veil she was wearing.

Religious orders continued to be the primary source of care for the sick well into the 19th century. However, as the Industrial Revolution gained speed and the concept of the modern hospital developed, the care of the sick moved away from religious orders to care by lay people who did not wear the nun's robe and veil.

By the time Florence Nightingale trained in the Institute of Protestant Deaconesses in Germany, the veil had evolved into a white cap that signified "service to others." However, Florence Nightingale lived and practiced nursing during the Victorian era, which required "proper" women to keep their heads covered. The nursing cap Florence Nightingale wore was similar to the head garb worn by cleaning ladies of the day. It was hood shaped with a ruffle around the face and tied under the chin. This early cap served multiple purposes. It met the requirements of the times for women to keep their heads covered; it kept the nurse's long hair, which was fashionable during the Victorian era, up and off her face; and it kept the hair from becoming soiled.

A Cap for Every School

In the United States, the first standardized nursing cap is generally attributed to Bellevue Training School in New York City around 1874. The cap's primary purpose was to keep the nurse's long hair from getting in the way, but it also identified nurses who had graduated from Bellevue. The Bellevue cap covered the whole head to just above the ears and resembled a modern knitted ski hat, except for being white linen with a rolled fringe at the bottom.

As the number of nursing schools increased, there was a corresponding increase in the need for unique caps. Each nursing school designed its own cap. Nursing caps became very frilly, elaborate, and sometimes large and unwieldy. Some caps adopted the upside-down ice cream cone shape, similar to the cloth cone through which ether was given as an anesthetic. By looking at the cap, a person could still determine the school from which the nurse had graduated.

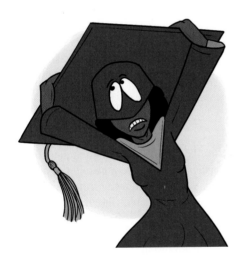

Traditionally, in the 3-year hospital-based schools of nursing, there were two separate ceremonies, one for capping and one for pinning. The capping ceremony usually took place after the student completed the initial 6 months of classroom education, which was considered the probationary period of the program. Capping indicated that the student was now off probation and that she had earned the right to wear the cap during clinical rotations in the hospital.

During nursing school, the cap was also used as a sign of rank and status. In the 3-year hospital-based nursing schools, first-year students wore plain white caps with no black bands anywhere. Second-year students had a vertical black band added to the edge of the cap, and third-year students were given a second vertical black band. When the student graduated, the vertical black bands were removed, and a horizontal black band was placed across the front of the cap.

Unchanging Values

As shorter hair became an acceptable style for women in the 20th century, the nursing cap lost its function of controlling long hair. However, it continued as a status symbol and a source of pride and identity for the graduates of nursing schools into the 1970s. As technology increased in the health-care work environment, the traditional nursing cap became more of an obstacle for nurses in the practice setting. Also, research demonstrated that the cap, rather than protecting clients from infection by organisms from the nurse's hair, actually helped to colonize organisms. By the 1980s, health-care facilities no longer required nurses to wear caps as part of the uniform, and nursing schools eliminated the cap as a mandatory item of students' uniforms.

Most nursing programs have eliminated the capping ceremony as a throwback to an era that was repressive to women. However, the nursing cap connects graduates to a rich and long history. It retains its significance, from the time of Florence Nightingale, as a sign that the primary goal of nursing is "service to those in need." The nursing cap is a reminder of the unchanging values of wisdom, faith, honesty, trust, and dedication. These values are as important in today's modern, technology-filled hospitals as they were in the era when washing floors was a required basic nursing skill.

QUESTION

Does your nursing school have a unique nursing cap that was used in the past? What is the symbolism of the cap's design?

NURSING LEADERS

The nursing profession as it is practiced today owes a great deal to a number of outstanding nurses who had a vision for the future. The few discussed here are representative of the great drive and dedication of the many individuals who created change and influenced the development of the nursing profession, even to this day.

Florence Nightingale (1820–1910)

Universally regarded as the founder of modern nursing, Florence Nightingale dedicated her long life to improving health care and nursing standards. Raised in England, Nightingale was considered highly educated for her time. Through travels with her family, she became aware of the substandard health care in many countries in Europe. In 1851, she attended a 3-month nurses' training program at the church-run hospital in Kaiserwerth, Germany. She was impressed with the program but came to believe that this brief training was insufficient. She later ran a private nursing home and realized that the only way to improve health care was to educate women to be reliable, high-quality nurses.

Volunteering Under Fire

Plans to develop a school of nursing in England were interrupted in 1854 by a cholera epidemic. Nightingale volunteered her services and learned a great deal about how to prevent the spread of disease. When the Crimean War broke out that same year, she obtained permission to take a group of 37 volunteer nurses into the battlefield area. British medical officers initially refused their assistance, but as conditions worsened, the nurses were admitted to the hospital.

After just 6 months of the nurses cleaning and bandaging wounds, cooking, and cleaning the wards, the mortality rate dropped from 42 to 2 percent.[3] Nightingale expanded her reform to include supplies, a military post office, convalescent camps for long-term recovery, and residences for soldiers' families. She also began to help with the care given at the front lines. At the height of her work in the war, Nightingale supervised 125 nurses in several large hospitals, and her accomplishments were recognized by the Queen of England with an Order of Merit, the highest award given to English civilians.

What Do You Think?

What would current nursing practice and nursing education be like without the influences of Florence Nightingale?

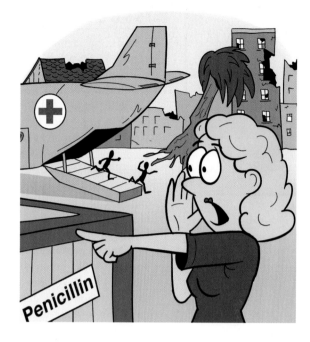

A Health-Care Reformer

The war experience strengthened Nightingale's convictions that nursing education required major reform. Believing that nursing schools should be run by nurses and be independent of hospitals and physicians, she advocated a program of at least 1 year that included basic biological science, techniques to improve nursing care, and supervised practice. She regarded nursing as a lifelong endeavor and felt that nurses should be in direct contact with clients rather than doing menial jobs such as cooking and cleaning. She worked tirelessly for the reform of health care and nursing and was appointed to many related committees and commissions. A prolific writer, she wrote extensively about improving hospital conditions, sanitation, nursing education, and health care in general.

Her famous Nightingale Training School for Nurses opened in 1860 and began to train nurses, who were in great demand throughout Europe and the United States. At this school, Nightingale advocated health maintenance and the concept that nursing was both an art and a science. She taught that each person should be treated as an individual and that nurses should meet the needs of clients, not the demands of physicians.

The school flourished, although it faced strong opposition from physicians who felt that nurses were already overtrained. Many early graduates went on to become important nursing leaders.

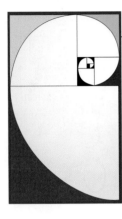

Issues Now

Travel Nursing as a Career

As a nursing student, you may have heard of *travel nursing* or *traveling nurses,* but not really know what they are or if it might be something you would be interested in as a career. Much like the recruitment posters for the armed services, "See the World" seems to be an attractive slogan for those looking for new experiences and adventure. However, there may be some drawbacks to travel nursing.

Generally, travel nurse staffing companies require a BSN or higher degree. This standard allows the nurses to meet any staffing requirements of individual facilities, and research has demonstrated good client outcomes. Travel nurses differ from agency nurses in several ways. Travel nurses are usually committed to working for a facility for a predetermined length of time, usually about 3 months. To allow preparation for travel to the facility, they are scheduled for their time about 2 months before their start date. Agency nurses generally work on a per diem (by the day) basis and live near the facility. They work a few days at a time to meet a short-term staffing need. Travel nurses provide more continuity of care and fill in for long-term needs, such as extended illness, maternity leave, or even sabbatical leave.

Travel nurses can select where they want to work and the time period of the work schedule. They usually follow the schedule required by the facility but have scheduled days off like any other nurses. Their salaries tend to be higher, and, depending on the company, the benefits may range from "bare bones" to what regular staffers would receive at a large health-care facility. The staffing agency also pays for the nurse's license and housing costs. Staffing agencies also have a group of employees who support the nurse and act as liaisons with the facilities to resolve any problems that may arise.

A nurse must be careful when selecting a travel nurse staffing company. The nurse should investigate the company carefully, talk to other nurses it employs, and examine the benefits closely. Generally, the larger the firm, the more locations it serves, and the better the benefits and support services. Some nurses use travel nurse employment to research locations in which they may be interned, and then permanently relocate when they find the ideal location.

So, if you want to be a travel nurse, the opportunities are out there. Travel nursing certainly provides a high degree of autonomy and control of your schedule and career. One of the key elements reported by nurses for career satisfaction is quality of life. The freedom of choice provided by travel nursing would certainly fulfill that need.

Sources: Johnson L: Professionalism: Tips for traveling nurses. RN 27-8, 2009.

Shaffer F: Travel nursing: Is it right for you? American Nurse Today 2(2):52–53, 2007.

Spotlight on travel nursing. Nursing 36(11):72, 2006.

Nightingale's ideas were somewhat diluted during the first half of the 20th century, but they have since resurfaced and are now evaluated in the light of a rapidly changing health-care system.

Isabel Adams Hampton Robb (1860–1910)

Isabel Adams Hampton Robb started out as a teacher in her home province of Ontario, Canada, but in 1881 she went to New York City to train to be a nurse. After graduation, she moved to Rome and became a superintendent of a hospital there. She had always focused on the academic rather than the clinical side of nursing, but in Italy her conviction grew that nurses needed a solid theoretical education—a belief that was not well accepted by the medical community of the time. From that point on, she dedicated her life to raising the standards of nursing education in the United States, first as director of the Illinois Training School for Nurses, a school that was unique for its time in that it was university based and emphasized academic learning. She later headed the new Johns Hopkins Training School for Nurses and would implement her ideas there as well.

Hampton Robb brought together leaders from key nursing schools to form the American Society of Superintendents of Training Schools for Nurses, and she served as its chairman. The group was the precursor to the National League for Nursing, which was dedicated to improving the standards for nursing education. In 1896, Hampton Robb became the first president of a group for staff nurses in active practice, called the Nurses Associated Alumnae of the United States and Canada, which would later become the American Nurses Association (ANA), dedicated to the improvement of clinical practice. She later helped develop the *American Journal of Nursing,* the first professional journal dedicated to the improvement of nursing, which is still the official journal of the ANA.

Lillian Wald (1867–1940)

Lillian Wald was raised in Ohio and graduated from the New York Hospital School of Nursing in 1901. After working as a hospital nurse, she entered medical

> *The war experience strengthened Nightingale's convictions that nursing education required major reform. Believing that nursing schools should be run by nurses and be independent of hospitals and physicians, she advocated a program of at least 1 year that included basic biological science, techniques to improve nursing care, and supervised practice.*

school, but encounters with New York's poor and sick caused her to change direction. She instead opened the Henry Street Settlement, a storefront health clinic in one of the poorest sections of the city, which organized nurses to make home visits, focusing on sanitary conditions and children's health. Wald became a dedicated social reformer, an efficient fundraiser, and an eloquent speaker. Although women still did not have the right to vote, her political influence was felt worldwide.

Under Wald's auspices, Columbia University developed courses to prepare nurses for careers in public health. Wald also advocated wellness education, which the medical community did not value at the time. The Metropolitan Life Insurance Company saw the value in her beliefs, however, and asked her to organize its nursing branch. She is also credited with founding the American Red Cross's Town and Country Nursing Service and with initiating the concept of school nursing. In 1912, she founded and became the first president of the National Organization of Public Health Nursing. Many child health and wellness programs in use today are based on her efforts. Current proposals for health-care reform often include her ideas about public health nursing, independent clinics, and health maintenance.

What Do You Think?

Who is your favorite historical nursing leader? What are some of that person's characteristics that attracted you? Is there a current nurse or nurse educator who provides you with a role model? What are some of that person's characteristics that attract you?

Lavinia Lloyd Dock (1858–1956)

Lavinia Lloyd Dock left her home in Pennsylvania to attend New York's Bellevue Training School for Nurses in 1885. She noticed that many of her fellow students struggled to learn about all the medications that were becoming available, and she would later write the first medication textbook for nurses. She worked alongside Lillian Wald at the Henry Street Settlement and Isabel Hampton Robb at Johns Hopkins Hospital.

Like Wald, Dock believed that poverty and squalor contributed to poor health, and she dedicated herself to social reform to address these problems. However, she soon learned that she was limited in her influence because she was a woman, and she spent most of her career dedicated to the pursuit of equal rights. For 20 years she lobbied legislators at all levels about women's right to vote, believing that this was the only way to influence social reform and health care. An excellent example of the diverse ways that nurses can help achieve higher-quality health care, she is considered one of the most influential leaders in the early 20th century.

Annie W. Goodrich (1866–1954)

Annie Goodrich provided nursing care at Lillian Wald's Henry Street Settlement in New York after receiving her nursing degree. She was known as an outstanding nursing educator and ran a number of nursing schools in New York. In 1910, she was appointed a state inspector of nursing schools, a position that up to that time had been held only by physicians. After the U.S. Army asked her to survey its hospital nursing departments, Goodrich proposed that it organize its own nursing school. The school opened later that year, with her as its dean, and this school would serve as the model for others established at Army hospitals during World War I.

To respond to the need for nurses in the war, Goodrich also established a nursing training program at Vassar College, and after the war other colleges and universities slowly began to develop their own nursing programs. Goodrich had demonstrated that teaching theoretical information in a classroom was just as important in training highly skilled nurses as clinical practice. When the war was over, Goodrich returned to the Henry Street Settlement and then became a nursing educator, eventually serving as dean at the Yale University School of Nursing. Her many writings about nursing education and her experiences with military nursing have been a great contribution to the nursing profession.[4]

Conclusion

Many of the problems and difficulties with today's health-care system, and those of nursing in particular, are based in the historical development of the profession. Knowledge of these historical roots can help us understand why the profession of nursing is the way it is and even suggest solutions to problems that may seem unsolvable. For example, nursing today appears to be a profession with a high level of responsibility but a low level of power.

How did this situation develop? What can be done about it? A great deal of confusion exists about the education of nurses, unlike the situation in other health-care professions. Why does nursing have this problem, and how can this confusion be addressed? Those who belong to the nursing profession have a responsibility not only to learn how these and other conditions developed but also to relate that knowledge to nursing's possibility for growth in the future.

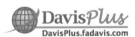

DavisPlus
DavisPlus.fadavis.com

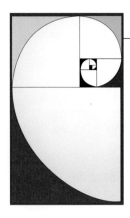

Issues in Practice

Case Study

Mrs. Lee, a 56-year-old high school teacher, had been "feeling something in her eye" for 3 days. She visited the retail optometry store where she had purchased her last pair of glasses. The optometrist at the store examined her and did not find any foreign objects in her eye or scratches on her cornea. However, he felt that the symptoms were serious enough to have Mrs. Lee visit the emergency department (ED) at a local hospital.

At the hospital, the ED triage nurse assessed Mrs. Lee's vital signs, which were normal, and also gave her a basic eye examination for visual acuity. The exam revealed 20/200 vision in the right eye and 20/30 vision in the left eye (20/20 is normal).

The triage nurse had a second-year ophthalmology resident from the hospital's outpatient vision clinic examine Mrs. Lee. The resident examined both eyes but extensively examined the right eye, which had the worse vision. He could find no irregularities and sent Mrs. Lee home with eye drops and an appointment to see an ophthalmologist the next day. The ophthalmologist ordered a computed tomography (CT) scan, which was taken the same day. He also sent Mrs. Lee home with an appointment to see a neurologist the next day.

Mrs. Lee went home after the CT scan. She collapsed and died from a ruptured cerebral aneurysm before the scan was read by the hospital radiology department and before she could see the neurologist. The family filed a malpractice law suit against the triage nurse, the physicians, and the hospital.

Case Outcome

After a lengthy trial, the jury in the Supreme Court of Kings County, New York, concluded that ED personnel committed negligence by failing to have the client examined by a neurologist at admission to the ED. Expert witness testimony convinced the jury that the great disparity in the vision between the two eyes was a primary indicator of some type of brain problem. This should have been recognized immediately by the nurse and ED staff, and a neurologist should have been part of the team from the beginning. The jury awarded $2.15 million to the family.

Source: Collazo v. NY Eye and Ear Infirmary, 2009 WL 1199357. Superior County Kings Court, New York, March 18, 2009.

Critical Thinking Questions

1. Do you think there was any malpractice involved in this case? If yes, what is its nature?

2. Should the triage nurse have noticed any abnormalities that might suggest the condition was worse than an eye problem?

3. What would you have done differently in this case if you were the triage nurse?

3

The Evolution of Licensure, Certification, and Nursing Organizations

Joseph T. Catalano

Learning Objectives

After completing this chapter, the reader will be able to:

- Identify the purposes and needs for nurse licensure.
- Distinguish between permissive and mandatory licensure.
- Explain why institutional licensure is unacceptable in today's health-care system.
- Evaluate the importance of nurse practice acts.
- Analyze the significance of professional certification.

MEETING EXPECTATIONS

Almost from the inception of nursing, societal needs and expectations have been the driving forces behind the establishment of the standards that guide the profession. In the early days of nursing, when health care was relatively primitive and society's expectations of nurses were low, there was little demand for regulations or controls over and within the profession. However, as technology and health care have advanced and become more complex, there has been a corresponding increase in societal expectations for nurses. All nurses now accept **licensure** and **certification** examinations as a given in today's health-care system. Where did these examinations come from, and what do they mean to the profession? This chapter explores the answers to these questions.

Rather than looking on the advent of sophisticated telecommunications, growing information technologies, redesigned health-care organizations, and increasing **health-care consumer** demands with fear and trepidation, nurses should consider this an exciting time of growth and opportunity. In today's health-care system, nurses have an almost unlimited number of ways to provide new and creative nursing care for clients in all settings. As society's needs and expectations change, so will the regulations and standards that help define nursing practice. Through their professional nursing organizations, nurses can help shape health-care regulations that establish the most freedom to provide effective care while maintaining the goal of protecting the public. It is likely that in the future state boards of nursing will look very different, just as the profession of nursing will differ from that of its past.

THE DEVELOPMENT OF NURSE PRACTICE ACTS

A nurse practice act is state legislation regulating the practice of nurses that protects the public, defines the scope of practice, and makes nurses accountable for their actions. Nurse practice acts establish state boards of nursing (SBNs) and define specific SBN powers regarding the practice of nursing within the state. Rules and regulations written by the SBNs become **statutory laws** under the powers delegated by the state **legislature.**

Regulatory Powers

Although nurse practice acts differ from one state to another, the SBNs have many powers in common. All SBNs have the power to grant licenses, to approve nursing programs, to establish standards for nursing schools, and to write specific regulations for nurses and nursing practice in general in that state.

Of particular importance is the SBNs' power to deny or revoke nurse licenses (Box 3.1).[1] Other functions of nurse practice acts include defining nursing and the scope of practice, ruling on who can use the titles registered nurse (RN) and licensed practical nurse/licensed vocational nurse (LPN/LVN), setting up an application procedure for licensure in the state, determining fees for licensure, establishing requirements for renewal of licensure, and determining responsibility for any regulations governing expanded practice for nurses in that particular state.

The Need for Licensure

Imagine what the quality of health care would be if anyone could walk into a hospital, claim to know how to care for clients, and be given a job as a nurse. This situation might sound impossible in today's health-care system, but in the past, it was the norm rather than the exception.

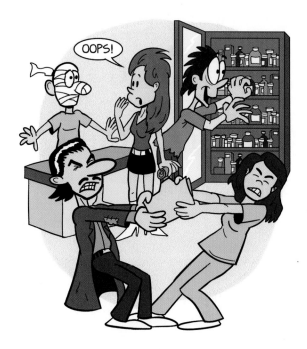

Throughout the last half of the 19th century and the first half of the 20th century, rapid growth in health-care technology led to the increasing use of hospitals as the primary source of health care. Individuals who were qualified to provide this care, however, were in short supply. There were wide variations both in the abilities of those who claimed to be nurses and in the quality of the care they provided. Paradoxically, nursing leaders who had always advocated some type of **credentialing** for nurses to ensure competency found that their attempts to initiate

Box 3.1

Reasons the State Boards of Nursing May Revoke a Nursing License

- Conviction for a serious crime
- Demonstration of gross negligence or unethical conduct in the practice of nursing
- Failure to renew a nursing license while still continuing to practice nursing
- Use of illegal drugs or alcohol during the provision of care for clients or use that carries over and affects clients' care
- Willful violation of the state's nurse practice act

registration or licensure met with strong opposition from physician groups, hospital administrators, and practicing nurses themselves.

Early Attempts at Licensure

Although the idea of registering nurses had been in existence for some time, Florence Nightingale was the first to establish a formal list, or register, for graduates of her nursing school. In the United States and Canada, there was widespread recognition of the need for some type of credentialing of nurses as far back as the mid-1800s. The first organized attempt to establish a credentialing system was initiated in 1896 by the Nurses Associated Alumnae of the United States and Canada (later to become the American Nurses Association [ANA]). As with other early attempts at licensure, it was met with resistance and eventually failed.[2]

Several early American nursing leaders, including Lillian Wald and Annie Goodrich, recognized the inconsistent quality of nursing care and the need for licensure to protect the public. In 1901, after an extensive and lengthy campaign to educate the public, physicians, hospital administrators, and nurses themselves about the need for licensure, the International Council of Nurses passed a resolution that required each state to establish a licensure and examination procedure for nurses. It took 3 more years before the state of New York, through the New York Nurses Association, developed a licensure bill that passed the legislature (Box 3.2). Other states that followed New York's lead were North Carolina, New Jersey, and Virginia. Although these states had bills that were weaker than New York's nurse practice act, passage of such legislation was considered a major accomplishment for several reasons. Women did not even have the right to vote in general elections at the time these bills were passed. In addition, few licensure requirements and regulations of any type existed during this period in the history of the United States, even for the medical profession.

The Importance of Licensure Examinations

The thought of having to take an examination that can determine whether or not one can practice nursing can make even the best student anxious. Adding to the tension is the fact that the examination is given outside of the academic setting, by computer, and is created by individuals other than the students' teachers. (See Chapters 10 and 11 for a detailed discussion of NCLEX-RN, CAT.)

A Measure of Competency

Some type of objective method, however, is necessary to prove that the individual is qualified to practice nursing safety; otherwise the public is not protected from unqualified practitioners. Early attempts at creating licensure examinations for nurses were met with strong resistance. Although all states had some form of licensure examination by 1923, the format and length of the examinations varied widely. Some states required both written and practical examinations to demonstrate safety of practice; others added an oral examination.

Although licensure was and is a state-controlled activity, the major nursing organizations in the United States eventually realized that, to achieve consistency of quality across the country, all nurses needed to pass a uniform examination. The ANA Council of State Boards of Nursing was

Box 3.2

Key Points in the New York State Licensure Bill (1904)

- Established minimum educational standards
- Established the minimum length of basic nursing programs at 2 years
- Required all nursing schools to be registered with the state board of regents (who oversee all higher education)
- Established a state board of nursing (SBN) with five nurses as members
- Formulated rules for the examination of nurses
- Formulated regulations for nurses that, if violated, could lead to the revocation of licensure

Source: Hirsh IL: Statement on nursing's scope describes how two levels of nurses practice. American Nurse 20:13, 1988.

organized in 1945 to oversee development of a uniform examination for nurses that could be used by all state boards of nursing.

The NCLEX-RN, CAT

The National League for Nursing Testing Division developed a test that was implemented in 1950. Originally the test was simply called the State Board Examination, but it was renamed the National Council Licensure Examination (NCLEX) in 1987. In 1994, the computerized version of the examination was implemented—the National Council Licensure Examination Computerized Adaptive Testing, for Registered Nurses (NCLEX-RN, CAT).

Licensure for nurses has undergone a major change. States are currently in the process of implementing the Mutual Recognition Model for Nursing Licensure, which will allow nurses licensed in one state to practice nursing in other states that belong to their regional agreement. The eventual goal is to have a "universal" nursing license that will allow nurses to practice in all states without having to become relicensed each time they cross a state border.

REGISTRATION VERSUS LICENSURE

The terms *registration* and *licensure* are often used interchangeably, although they are not synonymous. They serve a similar purpose, but some technical differences exist.

Registration

Registration is the listing, or registering, of names on an official roster after certain pre-established criteria have been met. Before mandatory licensure by the states became the norm, the only way a health-care institution could find out whether an applicant had met the standards for the position was by calling the applicant's school to see if the person had graduated or passed an examination. The school would tell the institution whether the applicant's name appeared on the official roster or register—hence the origin of the term *registered nurse*. With the advent of state board examinations, an institution merely has to contact the

SBN to find out whether the individual is registered or licensed.

Licensure

Licensure is an activity conducted by the state through the enforcement powers of its regulatory boards to protect the public's health, safety, and welfare by establishing professional standards. Licensure for nurses, as for other professionals who deal with the public, is necessary to ensure that everyone who claims to be a nurse can function at a minimal level of competency and safety. There are several different types of licensure.

Permissive Licensure

Permissive licensure allows individuals to practice nursing as long as they do not use the letters "RN" after their names. Basically, permissive licensure only protects the "registered nurse" title but not the practice of nursing itself. Under a permissive licensure law, anyone could carry out the functions of an RN, regardless of educational level, without having to pass an examination indicating competency.

Health-care administrators seem to support the concept of permissive licensure because it allows them to employ less-educated and lower-paid employees rather than the more highly educated and better-paid RNs. However, they also recognize that the quality of care decreases when the education level of health-care providers is lower. Although most early licensure laws were permissive, all states now have mandatory licensure.

> *Through their professional nursing organizations, nurses can help shape health-care regulations that establish the most freedom to provide effective care while maintaining the goal of protecting the public.*

What Do You Think?

Should permissive licensure be re-established because it will help reduce the cost of health care? Why? Why not?

Mandatory Licensure

Mandatory licensure requires anyone who wishes to practice nursing to pass a licensure examination and become registered by the SBN. Because different levels of nursing practice exist, different levels of licensure are necessary. At the technical level, the individual must take and pass the LPN/LVN examination; at the professional level, the individual must take and pass the RN examination.

Mandatory licensure forced SBNs to distinguish between the activities that nurses at different levels could legally perform. The scope of practice defines the boundaries for each of the levels: advanced practice nurse (APN), RN, and LPN/LVN. As more levels of nursing education (e.g., the associate degree in nursing [ADN]) have been added, however, lines dividing the different scopes of practice have become blurred. In the current health-care system, it is not unusual to find LPNs/LVNs performing activities that are generally considered professional.

A particularly confusing element in today's health-care system is the use of unlicensed individuals to provide health care. The advent of certified nursing assistants (CNAs) and unlicensed assistive personnel (UAP) has led to widespread use of such individuals in all health-care settings. Although they must be supervised by an RN or LPN/LVN, these individuals are sometimes illegally assigned nursing tasks much more advanced than their levels of training. (See Chapter 14 for a more detailed discussion of delegation.) Even though permissive licensure is no longer legal, CNAs and UAP appear to fall under an unofficial type of permissive licensure.

Institutional Licensure
Cut Corners, Cut Costs

Although universally rejected by every major nursing organization, **institutional licensure** has become a reality for many other types of health-care workers, such as respiratory therapists and physical therapists. In some state legislatures, bills have been introduced to allow **foreign graduate nurses** and nurses who are licensed in foreign countries to work in specific institutions without taking the U.S. licensure examination. Up to this point, these bills have been stopped by the state nursing organizations before they could become law. Institutional licensure has been proposed periodically over the years as an alternative to governmental licensure.

Institutional licensure allows individual health-care institutions to determine which individuals are qualified to practice nursing within general guidelines established by an outside board. Although

this type of licensure appeals to hospitals and nursing homes because it would allow them to hire individuals with less education at a reduced cost, some serious difficulties are associated with it.

A Lack of External Control

Probably the most critical problem is the lack of any external control to determine a minimal level of competency. The designations of RN and LPN/LVN would be virtually meaningless under institutional licensure. These nurses would not be under the control of a state licensing board and thus would not be held to the same standards of practice as nurses who were licensed by the states.

A second problem is that nurses who wished to move to a new place of employment would have to undergo whatever licensure procedure the new institution had established before being allowed to work there. Currently, nurses who move from one state to another can obtain licensure by endorsement by having the state recognize their nursing license from the original state of licensure. This process is generally referred to as *reciprocity*.

CERTIFICATION

At first glance, it may appear that there is not much difference between certification and licensure. Strictly defined, licensure can be considered a type of legal certification. In the more widely accepted use of the term, however, certification is a granting of credentials to indicate that an individual has achieved a level of ability higher than the minimal level of competency indicated by licensure.[3] As technology increases and the health-care environment becomes more complex and demanding, nurses are finding a need to increase their knowledge and skill levels beyond the essentials taught in their basic nursing courses.

Certification acknowledges the attainment of increased knowledge and skills and provides nurses with a means to validate their own self-worth and competence. Some certification also carries with it a legal status, similar to licensure; but in many cases, certification merely indicates a specific professional status. The public, employers, and even nurses themselves have difficulty understanding what certification means.

Another element that adds confusion to the understanding of the process of certification is that a large number of groups can offer certification. These are usually professional specialty groups like the National Association of Pediatric Nurse Associates and Practitioners (NAPNAP) and the American Association of Critical-Care Nurses (AACN), but they can also be national organizations like the National League for Nursing (NLN) or the ANA.

Individual Certification

The most common type of certification is called individual certification. When a nurse has demonstrated that he or she has attained a certain level of ability above and beyond the basic level required for licensure in a defined area of practice, that nurse can become certified. Usually some type of written and practical examination is required to demonstrate this advanced level of skill.

The ANA has its own certifying organization, the American Nurses Credentialing Center (ANCC), that offers widely recognized certifications in more than 40 areas. Almost all nurses with individual certification are required to maintain their skills and competencies through continuing education and a specified number of continuing education units (CEUs). Recertification may be achieved through CEUs or retaking of the certification examination.

Organizational Certification

Organizational certification is the certification of a group or health-care institution by some external agency. It is usually referred to as *accreditation* and indicates that the institution has met standards established either by the government or by a nongovernmental agency. Often the ability of the institution to collect money from insurance companies or the federal government depends on whether or not the institution is certified by a recognized agency. Most hospitals are accredited by The Joint Commission (formerly The Joint Commission on Accreditation of Healthcare Organizations, or JCAHO) as a minimum level of accreditation. In most states, the State Health Department certifies health-care institutions, particularly nursing homes and extended care facilities.

Advanced Practice

Some state governments may either award or recognize certification granted to nurses in areas of advanced practice. In these cases, the certification becomes a legal requirement for practice at the APN level. Depending on the individual state's nurse practice act, nurses thus certified fall under regulations in the state's practice act that control the type of activities nurses may legally carry out when they perform advanced roles.[4]

For example, many states recognize the position of **nurse midwife** as an advanced practice role for nurses. In these states, a nurse midwife may practice those skills allowed under the nurse practice act of that state after obtaining certification. Generally nurse midwives are allowed to conduct prenatal examinations, do prenatal teaching, and deliver babies vaginally in uncomplicated pregnancies. They are not usually allowed to perform cesarean sections.

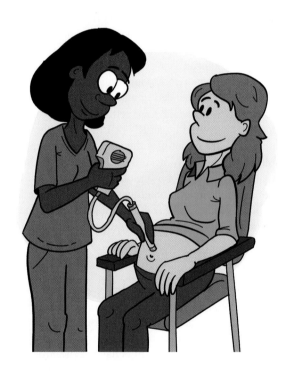

Varying Standards

An independent certification center was proposed in 1978 to establish uniform criteria and standards and to oversee all certification activities. Although it would eliminate much of the current confusion about certification and would help with the legal recognition of APNs, this proposal has not yet been acted on because of opposition from physician and health-care administration groups.

Unfortunately, there is no uniformity among states in the recognition of certification of APNs.

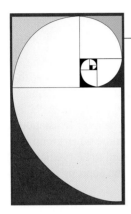

Issues Now

Health-Care Reform and Advanced Practice Nurses—Who's Driving the Bus?

Those who favor health-care reform see it as a giant step toward increasing health-care coverage for the some 56 million Americans who either don't have coverage or have only limited coverage. Those who oppose it see it as giant step toward socialization and an era of big government control. Either way, it is here, and one of the many issues that need to be worked out is the role of APNs and how they will be regulated in the future.

Although nursing as a profession has consistently been ranked number one among the most trusted professions, the public still seems to have a very narrow view of what nurses can really do and the contributions they can make to health care. The role of APN is even more obscure to the public, except for people who receive their care. For many years, APNs have been quietly asserting their role as autonomous practitioners amid a swamp filled with confusing state regulations, multiple certifications, licensure issues, and political squabbling. Health-care reform will only fill the swamp with more alligators.

The American Medical Association (AMA) has always viewed APNs as a threat to their scope of practice and even their livelihood, although study after study has shown this to be untrue. Their main concern on paper is the educational preparation of APNs, and they have devoted significant research funds to comparing the education of APNs to the education of MDs. Of course, it is the obligation of all professions to examine their preparation techniques and reflect on their growth and scope of practice. However, it seems strange that the medical profession is so concerned with how nursing educates its nurses. Nurses certainly do not expend the same amount of (if any) energy and resources to examining physician preparation.

Unfortunately, several major physician organizations see health-care reform as a back-door way to exert more influence over nursing practice, if not to control the regulation process of the nursing profession outright. The AMA has long held the belief that diagnosing, prescribing, and performing high-level clinical skills is the exclusive domain of physicians. APNs, who graduate from accredited institutions of higher education and are certified by national organizations and licensed by their states, have shown that they too can successfully and safely carry out formerly exclusive physician practice areas, and usually more economically.

A more basic question is, who gave physicians the right to control the boundaries of the nursing profession? Anyone with a rudimentary sense of justice and a minimal ethical compass can see that professional groups such as nurses need to establish their own regulations to promote and achieve the outcomes of their profession. All nurses, not just APNs, need to control their own scope of practice and make their own decisions on how best to provide care for those in need. As health-care reform is fully implemented over the next several years, more and more clients will be seeing health-care providers for the first time. This situation is particularly suited for the skill set that ANPs bring to the table.

So are physicians the enemies of nurses? The answer is no. Both nurses and physicians will need the educational and skills preparation to be able to work together to deal with the large influx of new clients in the near future. Will there

(continued)

Issues Now

be tensions between the two groups at the legislative and professional level? Without a doubt there will be. However, the nursing profession must stand its ground and vigorously guard against allowing other groups to regulate and define APN practice. The ANA and most of the state organizations closely monitor legislation that deals with nursing practice and send out the alarm when some other group is trying to change the scope of practice for nurses. All nurses need to be politically tuned in to these attempts and quickly respond by contacting the appropriate legislators.

Sources: Rashid C: Benefits and limitations of nurses taking on aspects of the clinical role of doctors in primary care: Integrative literature review. Journal of Advanced Nursing 66(8):1658–1670, 2010.

Traynor M, Boland M, Buus N: Autonomy, evidence and intuition: Nurses and decision-making. Journal of Advanced Nursing 66(7):1584–1589, 2010.

Ulrich CM: Who defines advanced nursing practice in an era of health care reform? Clinical Scholars Review 3(1):5–7, 2010.

Some states recognize almost all certifications and have provisions in their nurse practice acts to help guide these practices. Other states have very little legal recognition of certification levels and thus few guidelines for practice. This confusion may result from so many organizations offering certification in different areas. In some advanced practice specialties, such as nurse practitioner, two or more organizations may offer certification for the same title. The certification standards vary from organization to organization, and the method of determining certification may also be different.

A More Significant Role

It is expected that advanced practice nurses will play a larger role in the rapidly evolving health-care system of the future. What that role will be depends on how well governmental organizations and the public understand the contributions practitioners can make as **primary care nurses.** Without a uniform definition of this specialty, such nurses will not be utilized to their full potential.

Licensure and certification are both methods of granting credentials to demonstrate that an individual is qualified to provide safe care to the public. Without proof of competency, the profession of nursing would become chaotic, disorganized, and even dangerous. It is important for nurses to keep a watchful eye on pending legislation and practices that health-care institutions are initiating. Many of these proposals and practices are covert ways of reintroducing permissive and institutional licensure.

NURSING ORGANIZATIONS AND THEIR IMPORTANCE

Strength in Numbers

The establishment of a professional organization is one of the most important defining characteristics of a profession. Many professions have a single major professional organization to which most of its members belong and several specialized suborganizations that members may also join. Professions with just one major organization generally have a great deal of political power.

Nurses need and use power in every aspect of their professional lives, ranging from supervising unlicensed personnel to negotiating with the administration for increased independence of practice. Clearly, an individual nurse probably does not have much power; but for nurses as a group, the potential is increased exponentially by the organization. The dedication to high-quality nursing standards and improved methods of practice by the major nursing organizations has led to improved care and increased benefits to the public as a whole.[5]

Speaking With One Voice

National nursing organizations need the participation and membership of all nurses in order to claim that they are truly representative of the profession. A large membership allows the organization to speak with one voice when making its values about health-care issues known to politicians, physicians' groups, and the public in general.

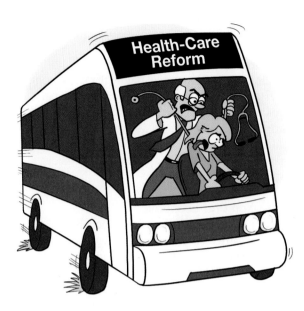

The National League for Nursing
Purposes
The primary purpose of the National League for Nursing (NLN) is to maintain and improve the standards of nursing education. The NLN is also a strong force in community health nursing, occupational health nursing, and nursing service activities. Its bylaws state that its purpose is to foster the development and improvement of hospital, industrial, public health, and other organized nursing services and of nursing education through the coordinated action of nurses, allied professional groups, citizens, agencies, and schools so that the nursing needs of the people will be met.

Membership
Although membership is open to individual nurses, the primary membership of the NLN comes in the form of agency membership, usually through schools of nursing. One of the major functions of this organization, through the National League for Nursing Accrediting Commission (NLNAC), is to accredit schools of nursing through a self-study process. The schools are given a set of criteria, or **essentials for accreditation,** and are then required to evaluate their programs against these criteria. After the evaluation report is written and sent to the NLNAC, site representatives visit the school to verify the information in the report and see whether the school has met the criteria. If the school meets the evaluation criteria, it is accredited for up to 8 years.

Accreditation of a school of nursing by the NLNAC indicates that the school meets national standards. In some work settings, a nurse must be a graduate of an NLNAC-accredited school of nursing before the nurse can be hired or accepted into many master's level nursing programs.

Other services and activities that the NLN carries out include testing; evaluating new graduate nurses; supplying career information, continuing education workshops, and conferences for all levels of nursing; publishing a wide range of literature and videotapes covering current issues in health care; and compiling statistics about nursing, nurses, and nursing education.

The American Association of Colleges of Nursing
Purposes
The American Association of Colleges of Nursing (AACN) was established to help colleges with schools of nursing work together to improve the standards for higher education for professional nursing. The AACN, through the Commission on Collegiate Nursing Education (CCNE), has developed standards for the accreditation of baccalaureate schools of nursing and is poised to become a major accreditation agency, competing with the NLNAC. The AACN has developed and published a set of guidelines for the education of professional nursing students that is widely used as the theoretical basis for baccalaureate curricula.

Membership
Only deans and directors of programs that offer baccalaureate or higher degrees in nursing with an upper-division nursing major are permitted membership in the AACN.

The American Nurses Association
Purposes
The ANA grew out of a concern for the quality of nursing practice and the care that nurses were providing. The major purposes for the existence of the ANA, as stated in its bylaws, include improvement of the standards of health and access to health-care services for everyone, improvement and maintenance of high standards for nursing practice, and promotion of the professional growth and development of all nurses, including economic issues, working conditions, and independence of practice.[6]

The AACN was established to help colleges with schools of nursing work together to improve the standards for higher education for professional nursing.

Membership

Membership in the ANA is limited to 52 constituents: 50 state organizations, Washington, DC, and Puerto Rico. An individual joins a state organization and through the state organization indirectly is a member of the ANA. Certain discounts in membership are offered for new members and new graduate nurses. Various levels of membership are available for nurses who work part-time or those who are retired. The ANA makes every effort to encourage individual nurses to join the organization. Unfortunately, most nurses do not belong to this potentially powerful, politically active, and very influential organization.

Each state has the opportunity to determine what is needed from each member to run the state association; the amount of the dues that is sent to ANA is predetermined. Although dues are not inexpensive (they change a little from year to year, but are about $200 per year), the ANA offers various plans for payment, such as three equal payments over the course of a year or monthly payroll deductions. Because of the efforts of the ANA, nurses' salaries have risen to a point at which this sum is affordable.

Other Services

When nurses pursue advanced education and levels of practice, as many are doing today, the ANA ANCC is essential for testing and certification of many of these practice levels. Although other organizations offer advanced practice certification, without the ANCC, there would be even less standardization for and less recognition of these practitioners by the public, physicians, or lawmakers.

Entry Into Practice

Another important issue that the ANA has been involved in is the entry-level education requirement for professional nurses. The ANA has supported the baccalaureate degree as the minimum educational requirement for nurses for the past 30 years. The ANA is in the forefront of the debate over

> *Clearly, an individual nurse probably does not have much power; but for nurses as a group, the potential is increased exponentially by the organization.*

entry into practice, which has continued into the 21st century.

Standards of Practice

Additional functions carried out by the ANA include the establishment and continual updating of standards of nursing practice. These standards are the yardstick against which nurses are measured and held accountable by courts of law. The ANA also established the official code of ethics that guides professional practice.

Legislation and Economics

Many of the political and economic activities of the ANA are carried out in the halls of legislatures and offices of legislators. The ANA Political Action Committee (ANA-PAC) is one of the most powerful in Washington, DC. (See Chapter 20 for a more detailed discussion.) Such activities have a profound effect on the role that nurses play and will continue to play in health care well into the 21st century.

Successful PAC activities require money and the power of a large, unified membership. The ANA-PAC seeks to influence legislation about nurses, nursing, and health care in general. It has been and will be a strong voice in the formulation of current national health-care reform.

Another important function of the ANA is economic. In many states, the ANA is the official **bargaining agent** for nurses in the negotiation of **contracts** with hospitals, nursing homes, and other health-care agencies that employ nurses. However, **collective bargaining** is done on a state-to-state basis—some states are **collective bargaining units,** and others are not. (See Chapter 17 for a more detailed discussion.) Professional organizations represent professional groups better than a labor union that has little knowledge of professional activities or needs.

The National Student Nurses' Association
Purposes

The National Student Nurses' Association (NSNA) is an independent legal corporation established in 1953 to represent the needs of nursing students. Working closely with the ANA, which offers services, an official publication, and close communication, the NSNA consists of state chapters that represent student nurses in those particular states.

The main purpose of the NSNA is to help maintain high standards of education in schools of nursing, with the ultimate goal of educating high-quality nurses who will provide excellent health care. Students' ideas, concerns, and needs are extremely important to nursing educators. Most nursing programs have committees in which students are asked to participate, including curriculum development and evaluation techniques. It is important that students belong to these committees and actively participate in the committees' activities.

Membership

Membership consists of all nursing students in registered nurse programs. Students can join at the local, state, or national level or at all levels if desired. Dues are low, with a discount for the first year's membership.

Other Services

Additionally, the NSNA is concerned with developing and providing workshops, seminars, and conferences that deal with current issues in nursing and health care, with a wide range of subjects, from ethical and legal concerns to recent developments in pharmacology, test-taking skills, and professional growth. Student nurses who belong to the NSNA and who take an active part in its functions are much more likely to join the ANA after they graduate. Professional identity and professional behavior are learned. By beginning the process during the formal school years, student nurses develop professional attitudes and behaviors that they will maintain for the rest of their lives.

Benefits for Students

Many benefits exist for student nurses who belong to the NSNA. A number of scholarships are available through this organization to members of the NSNA. Members receive the official publication of the organization, *Imprint,* and the *NSNA News,* which keep the student nurse current on recent developments in health care and nursing.

The student member also has political representation on issues that may affect the student now or in the future. Some of these issues include educational standards for practice, standards of pro-

fessional practice, and health insurance. The NSNA is also concerned with the difficulty that many nursing students from minority groups experience in the educational process. The Breakthrough Project is an attempt by the NSNA to help such students enter the profession of nursing.

Practicing Professionalism

Student nurses who join the NSNA experience first-hand the operation, activities, and benefits of a professional organization. In schools with active memberships, the NSNA can be a very exciting and useful organization for students.

Many NSNA chapters are involved in community activities that provide services at a local level and allow the student to practice "real" nursing. These services include providing community health screening programs for hypertension, lead poisoning, vision, hearing, and birth defects; setting up information and education programs; giving immunizations; and working with groups concerned with drug abuse, child abuse, drunken driving, and teen pregnancy. All nursing students should be encouraged to belong to this organization.

The International Council of Nurses

Membership in the International Council of Nurses (ICN) consists of national nursing organizations, and the ICN serves as the international organization for professional nursing. The ANA is one member among 104 nursing associations around the world. Each member nation sends delegates and participates in the international convention held every 4 years. The quadrennial conventions, or congresses, are open to all nurses and delegates from all nations.

The goal of the ICN is to improve health and nursing care throughout the world. The ICN coordinates its efforts with the United Nations and other international organizations when appropriate in the pursuit of its goals.

Some issues that have been the focus of concern of the ICN are the social and economic welfare of nurses, the changing role of nurses in the present health-care environment, the challenges being faced by the various national nursing organizations, and how government and politics affect the nursing profession and health care. Overseeing the ICN is the Council of National Representatives. This body meets every 2 years and serves as the governing organization. ICN headquarters is located in Geneva, Switzerland.

Sigma Theta Tau

Sigma Theta Tau is an honors organization that was established in colleges and universities to recognize individuals who have demonstrated leadership or made important contributions to professional nursing. It is international, and candidates are selected from among senior nursing students or graduate or practicing nurses.

The organization has its headquarters in Indianapolis, where it has a large library open to members to use for scholarly activities and research. It also boasts the first online nursing journal, which can be accessed by any nurse with a computer anywhere in the world. Local chapters of Sigma Theta Tau collect and distribute funds to nurses who are conducting nursing research. The organization also holds educational conferences and recognizes those who have made contributions to nursing.

Grassroots Organizations

A growing trend in contemporary nursing has been the formation of grassroots nursing organizations. In reality, all nursing organizations start as the grassroots efforts of local nursing groups that are trying to solve a particular problem. Over time, these small grassroots organizations become more structured, larger, and eventually national or international when they spread to other areas across the country or around the world. Unfortunately, the large organizations tend to lose sight of the fundamental issues they were originally formed to solve, or they are unable to deal effectively with local problems.

> *In reality, all nursing organizations start as the grassroots efforts of local nursing groups that are trying to solve a particular problem.*

Working to Bring About Change

Grassroots organizations usually have relatively small memberships; are localized to a town, city, or sometimes a state; and attempt to solve a problem or deal with an issue that the members feel is not being adequately handled by a large national organization. They may be created as a completely new and separate organization, or they may break away from a larger, established group. Because all the members of grassroots organizations are passionately concerned about only one or two issues at a time that affect them directly, they tend to work hard to effect change and can bring a great deal of concentrated power to bear on people, such as legislators, who make the decisions about the issues.

Grassroots groups use a number of techniques that are often frowned on by the more established organizations to attain their goals. In addition to the traditional techniques of writing letters, sending e-mail, and calling legislators, members of grassroots groups actively seek media attention, march on capitol buildings and state houses, introduce resolutions, and testify before committee hearings. Their success varies from issue to issue and location to location.

Successful Grassroots Efforts

Two examples of successful grassroots efforts are found in California and Pennsylvania. The California Nurses Association decided to break away from the ANA because it was not addressing some key state issues such as length of hospital stays, reduction in professional nursing staffs, and **managed care's** preoccupation with profit. The grassroots group in Pennsylvania formed a completely new organization, the Nurses of Pennsylvania (NPA), and focused their energies on the trend to replace licensed registered nurses with unlicensed technicians, sometimes called "downskilling."

Special-Interest Organizations
Why Do They Exist?

The historical origins of special-interest organizations in nursing are even older than those of the main national organizations. For example, the Red Cross, established in 1864, is one of the oldest special-interest organizations that nurses have been involved with. Like the Red Cross, most specialty organizations in nursing were founded when a group of nurses with similar concerns sought professional and individual support. These organizations usually start out small and informal, then increase in size, structure, and membership over a number of years. There were relatively few of these organizations until 1965, when an explosion in specialty organizations in nursing took place. During the next 20 years, almost 100 new organizations were formed, with the associated effect of diminishing membership levels in the ANA.

Clinical Practice

Specialty organizations are usually organized according to clinical practice area. Organizations exist for almost every clinical specialty and subspecialty known in nursing, such as obstetrics/gynecology, critical care, operating room, emergency department, and occupational health, as well as less known areas such as flight nursing, urology, and cosmetic surgery.

Education and Culture

Another focal area for these organizations is education and ethics. Organizations such as the AACN and the Western Interstate Commission for Higher Education fall into this category. Often organizations focus on the common **ethnic group,** cultural, or religious backgrounds of nurses. The National Association of Hispanic Nurses and the National Black Nurses Association represent this type of specialty organization.

Education and Standards

Although many of these organizations promote the personal and professional growth of their membership, they also carry out many other activities. Particularly important among these activities is establishing the standards of practice for the particular specialty area. Much as the ANA establishes overall standards of practice for nursing in general, the specialty organizations establish standards for their particular clinical areas. Providing educational services for their members is another important activity of specialty organizations. Conferences, workshops, and seminars in the clinical area represented are important venues for nurses to keep current on new developments and to maintain high standards of practice.[7]

Should They Matter to You?

How many of these specialty nursing organizations are there? No one really knows. Many such organizations are informal and run by volunteers. Organizations are continually being formed, and others are being disbanded.

Should nurses belong to these organizations? The answer is yes, but only after they belong to the ANA. Many of the larger specialty organizations have recognized this fact and have established close ties with the ANA. The ANA, in its turn, is well aware of the membership bleed-off from the specialty organizations and has initiated efforts to become more involved in the specialty nursing areas.

Before nurses join a specialty organization, they should determine whether its purposes are at odds with those of the ANA. Many of the large specialty organizations have their own lobbyists in both state and national legislatures. Because the legislators really do not know the differences between the various nursing organizations, they can easily become confused over health-care issues if they are receiving pressure from two nursing groups representing opposing sides of the same issue. At this point, legislators may simply surmise that nurses really do not know what they want and vote on an important issue without regard to nurses and nursing.

The tendency toward specialization has led to an ever-increasing number of nursing organizations, each focusing on a particular practice field within the profession. This trend has diluted the unity and ultimately lessened the power that nursing as a profession can exert in health-care issues. Although it is important to recognize the complexity of today's health-care system and the pluralism inherent in nursing, unity of opinion on major issues is essential if nursing is to have any influence on the future of the profession.

The challenge for nurses in the future is to use the diversity in the profession as a positive force and to unite as a group on important issues. Awareness of earlier development of nursing organizations provides a perspective for the current situation and can act as a framework for planning the future.

What Do You Think?

What type of power does the individual nurse have? Cite examples of individual nurses who have used their power to effect changes in health care and nursing.

Conclusion

Nursing, in its journey toward professionalism, has been propelled and shaped by its nursing organizations, which were the main vehicles for the development of educational and practice standards, initiation of licensure, promotion of advanced practice, and general improvement in the level of care nurses provided. From their beginnings, nursing organizations have served as channels of communication among nurses, consumers of health care, and other health-care professionals. In many cases, the nursing organizations have served as a focus of power for the profession to influence those important health policies that affect the whole nation. That continued unity is essential for the survival of nursing.

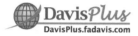
DavisPlus.fadavis.com

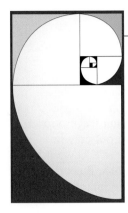

Issues in Practice

Juanita R, an RN at a large inner-city hospital, has been working on her off-hours as a volunteer in a storefront clinic to treat the indigent and underserved population of that part of the city. The clinic clientele is primarily Mexican American, as are the majority of the 20 nurses working at the clinic. Because all the nurses, including a family nurse practitioner, volunteer their time and receive no pay, the small private grant that Juanita had managed to secure was adequate to cover the cost for rental of the building, basic supplies for the clinic, and a few medications. However, the grant is about to run out and is nonrenewable.

Juanita first tried to obtain money from the hospital to keep the clinic going, but she was told that the hospital was having its own financial problems because of managed care demands and could not spare any money. At a staff meeting of the nurses from the clinic, the nurses decided to band together and form a grassroots organization called the Storefront Clinic Nurses to focus their efforts on obtaining funds to keep the clinic open. They printed and passed out flyers, called local and city politicians, encouraged the patrons of the clinic to talk to people they knew, and even called the local television station for an interview about their plight.

Although most of the nurses' effort went unrewarded, a large pharmaceutical company became aware of their plight and wanted to provide a sizable financial stipend to the clinic, in addition to supplying free medications, for a period of at least 5 years. In addition to their philanthropic interests, the pharmaceutical company also wanted to gather long-term data about a newly developed antihypertensive medication. The company would provide the medication free to the clients at the clinic, the majority of whom had some degree of hypertension, and all the nurses would have to do is take and record the clients' blood pressure readings and complete "reported side effects" forms on each client. Client identifier codes, rather than names, would be used to maintain confidentiality. Juanita, as the group's coordinator, would be responsible for coordinating and preserving the data.

Although Juanita saw it as an answer to her prayers, she was concerned about the medication project. The pharmaceutical company said that no research consent forms were needed because the medication had already been through clinical trials and had received approval by the Food and Drug Administration. Juanita called another meeting of her nurses to discuss the issue. Without the grant, the clinic would close, but if they accepted the grant, they would have to participate in a medication research project that made Juanita feel uncomfortable.

1. What are the main issues in this case study?
2. What ethical principles are being violated? What is the ethical dilemma that Juanita is facing?
3. Are there any other solutions to this problem?

Critical Thinking Exercises

- Develop a strategy for increasing the membership of the ANA.
- A labor union is attempting to organize the nurses at your hospital. Is it better for the professional nursing organization to represent the nurses? Why?
- A new graduate nurse is working in the intensive care unit (ICU) of a large hospital. She wants to join a nursing organization but only has a limited amount of money to spend. Her coworkers in the ICU want her to join the AACN, but she would also like to join the ANA. Basing her decision on economic and professional issues, which organization should she join?
- Compare and contrast certification and licensure. Should certification be legally recognized? Justify your answer.

4

Theories and Models of Nursing

Joseph T. Catalano

Learning Objectives

After completing this chapter, the reader will be able to:

- Explain why theories and models are important to the profession of nursing.
- Analyze the four key concepts found in nursing theories and models.
- Interrelate systems theory as an important element in understanding nursing theories and models.
- Evaluate how the four parts of all systems interact.
- Synthesize three nursing theories, identifying how the different nursing theorists define the key concepts in their theories.

CARING FOR REAL PEOPLE

For many nurses, and for most nursing students, the terms *theory* and *model* evoke images of textbooks filled with abstract, obscure words and convoluted sentences. The visceral response is often, "Why is this important? I want to take care of real people!" The simple answer is that understanding and using nursing theories or models will help you be a better nurse and provide better care to real people.

DIFFERENCES BETWEEN THEORIES AND MODELS

What Is a Theory?

Although the terms *theory* and *model* are not synonymous, in nursing practice they are often used interchangeably. Strictly speaking, a theory refers to a speculative statement involving some element of reality that has not been proved. For example, the theory of relativity has never been proved, although the results have often been observed.

The nursing profession tends to use the term *theory* when attempting to explain apparent relationships between observed behaviors and their effects on a client's health. In this nursing context, the goal of a theory is to describe and explain a particular nursing action to make a **hypothesis,** which predicts the effect on a client's outcome, such as improved health or recovery from illness. For example, the action of turning an unresponsive client from side to side every 2 hours should help prevent skin breakdown and improve respiratory function.

In recent years, nursing has been moving toward using research findings to guide nursing practice. This approach, called evidence-based practice, is an important element in improving nursing care and proving many of the long-standing theories that the nursing profession has developed over the years.[1]

What Is a Model?

A model is a hypothetical representation of something that exists in reality. The purpose of a model is to explain a complex reality in a systematic and organized manner. For example, a hospital organizational chart is a model that attempts to demonstrate the interrelationships of the various levels of the hospital's administration.

What Do You Think?

Do you consider yourself to be healthy? What factors make you healthy? What factors are indicators of illness?

What Do Nurses Do?

Although a model tends to be more concrete than a theory, they both help explain and direct nursing actions. This ability, using a systematic and structured approach, is one of the key elements that raises nursing from a task-oriented job to the level of a profession that uses judgment and knowledge to make informed decisions about client care. With the use of a **conceptual model,** nurses can provide intelligent and thoughtful answers to the question, "What do nurses do?" Consider this scenario:

> Mr. X had surgery for intestinal cancer 4 days ago. He has a colostomy and needs to learn how to take care of it at home because he is going to be discharged from the hospital in 2 days. When the nurses attempt to teach him colostomy care, he looks away, makes sarcastic personal comments about the nurses, and generally displays a belligerent and hostile attitude.

Without an understanding of the underlying dynamics involved, the nurses' reactions to this client's behavior might be to become sarcastic and scold the client about his behavior or simply to minimize the amount of contact with him. This type of response will not improve Mr. X's health status. If, however, the nurses knew about and understood the dynamics of the grief theory, they would realize that Mr. X was probably in the anger stage of the grief process. This understanding would direct the nurses to allow, or even to encourage, Mr. X to express his anger and **aggressiveness** without condemnation and to help him deal with his feelings in a constructive manner. Once Mr. X gets past the anger stage, he can move on to taking a more active part in his care and thus improve his health status. The **client goals** would then be achieved.

If a researcher were to stop 10 people at random on the street and ask the question, "What do nurses do?" he or she would likely get 10 different answers, but the confusion about nurses' activities extends far beyond the public at large. What if the researcher asked 10 hospital administrators, 10 physicians, or even 10 nurses the same question? It could be anticipated that the answers would vary almost as much as the answers from laypersons.

The need to increase client satisfaction and achieve successful outcomes of nursing care is a key element in the Health Care Reform Act, passed in 2010. Even more than in the past, these elements will be a basis of reimbursement for health-care providers.

The Iowa Project
A Classification System

In an attempt to identify what exactly it is that nurses do, J. C. McCloskey and G. M. Bulechek, two nurse researchers at the University of Iowa, have been conducting a research project since 1990 to develop a **taxonomy** of the **interventions** that nurses use in their practice (Box 4.1). This research has been called Nursing Interventions Classification (NIC), the Iowa Interventions Project, or simply the Iowa Project.[2–5]

The first results, published in 1994, categorized and ranked 336 interventions that nurses use when they provide care to clients. A follow-up study was conducted about 2 years after the original study categorized and ranked 433 interventions used by nurses. McCloskey and Bulechek[6] also investigated what nursing interventions were commonly used by nurses in specialty settings. Forty specialty areas responded, and the researchers were able to develop a table that lists what core skills are used by each organization. In 2008 the list was

Box 4.1
What Constitutes Care?

At first glance, it would seem that everybody knows that nurses take care of clients. But what constitutes care? A study conducted by the faculty of the University of Iowa, called the Nursing Interventions Classification (NIC) or simply the Iowa Project, has identified 336 tasks or interventions that nurses are responsible for in their care of patients. Not all nurses carry out all 336 of these tasks all the time, but during an average career, a nurse would likely be involved in the majority of these tasks. Although this project was undertaken in the mid-1990s, it remains the benchmark study. Since the original study, several additional studies have been conducted that reaffirm the findings of the Iowa Project, and several researchers have undertaken projects to use the data generated by the Iowa Project in actual client care situations.

This project is an excellent example of how a nursing theory led to a research project that developed information that can be used by nurses in their daily practice. On the principle that nursing interventions are specific actions that a nurse can perform to bring about the resolution of a potential or actual health-care problem, the NIC attempted to identify and classify nursing interventions. It also attempted to rank those interventions according to the number of times a nurse was likely to perform one during a working day. The goal of the project was to develop a nursing information system that could be incorporated into the current information systems of all clinical facilities. By using the NIC system, hospital administrators, physicians, nurses, and even the public should be better able to recognize and evaluate the multiple interventions that nurses are responsible for in their daily work.

It is a generally acknowledged fact that nurses, as the largest single group of health-care providers, are essential to the welfare and care of most clients. Yet, in an age of health-care reform, nurses are finding it increasingly difficult to delineate the specific contributions they make to health care. If nurses are unable to define the care they provide, how are the reformers, politicians, and public going to be able to identify the unique contribution made by nursing?

Unfortunately, many of the contributions that nurses make to health care are currently invisible because there is no method of classification for them in the computerized database systems now in use. Commonly used nursing interventions such as active listening, emotional support, touch, skin surveillance, and even family support cannot be measured and quantified by most current information systems.

The large number of interventions used daily by nurses demonstrates the complex and demanding nature of the profession. The breadth and depth of knowledge and skills demanded of nurses on a daily basis are much greater than are found in many other health-care professions. One study found that nurses working in general medical-surgical units during a 6-month period were likely to care for 500 clients with more than 600 individual diagnoses (many clients have multiple diagnoses). These researchers also found that the physical demands of the work were actually less difficult and tiring than dealing with the emotional and technical demands of handling the huge amounts of information generated by the care given.

Sources: Bulechek GM, Butcher HK, Dochterman JM: Nursing Interventions Classification (NIC) (5th ed). St. Louis, MO: Mosby Elsevier, 2008.

Scherb CA, Weydt AP: Work complexity assessment, nursing interventions classification, and nursing outcomes classification: Making connections. Creative Nursing 15(1):16–22, 2009.

Moorhead S, et al: Nursing Outcomes Classification (NOC): Iowa Outcomes Project (3rd ed). St. Louis, Mosby, 2004.

again updated. It now contains 542 interventions within a taxonomy of seven domains (physiological: basic; physiological: complex; behavioral; safety; family; health systems; and community) and 30 classes of interventions.

Research into nursing intervention classification systems is ongoing and has served as the foundation of new methods to define nursing practice and measure the outcomes of client care. The need to increase client satisfaction and achieve successful outcomes of nursing care is a key element in the Health Care Reform Act, passed in 2010. Even more than in the past, these elements will be the basis of reimbursement for health-care providers.

Using the NIC as a starting point, Work Complexity Assessment (WCA) was developed so that nurses are now able to identify specific interventions they routinely perform for various client populations. Taking the process one step further, the Nursing Outcomes Classification system closes the loop by providing a means for nurses to evaluate whether or not the outcomes were achieved.[2]

Although initially used primarily to help nurses with the delegation of duties to unlicensed personnel by linking skills with performance requirements, WCA is now an important tool in the improvement of the quality of nursing care. When nurses analyze the care they provide and actually look at the various interventions they use, they increase their understanding of both the methods and rationales for care. WCA also fits nicely into the use of evidence-based practice when nurses share what they have learned about improving care with other nurses.

This type of research helps identify the important contributions made by nursing to the health and well-being of clients. It also demonstrates the complex and demanding nature of the nursing profession. Much of the public, and even many physicians and nurses themselves, do not really understand what nurses do for clients on a daily basis. Using classification systems aids in clarifying what nurses bring to client care, makes what they do measurable, and validates the importance of the profession of nursing.

Nursing Competencies
One way in which the nursing profession identifies what nurses do is by looking at **competencies.** In nursing, the word *competence* is often defined as the combination of skills, knowledge, attitudes, values, and abilities that support the safe and effec-

tive practice of the nurse. A nurse practices competently when he or she has mastered a range of skills and decision-making processes demonstrated in the care of clients. All the major nursing organizations have developed list of competencies for nurses. These are usually general, broad statements rather than catalogues of specific skills. (See Issues Now: Looking to the Future in this chapter.)

More recently, nursing researchers have attempted to develop specific lists of skills based on the general competency statements from the various nursing organizations. These skills lists help differentiate the various levels of nursing practice. One such list of skills is presented in Table 4.2 at the end of this chapter.

KEY CONCEPTS COMMON TO NURSING MODELS

Although nursing models vary in terminology and approach to health care, four concepts are common to almost all of them: client or patient (individual or collective), health, environment, and nursing. Each nursing model has its own specific definition of these terms, but the underlying definitions of the concepts are similar.

Client
The concept of client (or patient) is central to all nursing models because it is the client who is the primary recipient of nursing care. Although the term *client* is usually used to refer to a single individual, it can also refer to small groups or to a large collective of individuals (for community health nurses, the community is the client).

A Complex Relationship
The concept of client has changed over the years as knowledge and understanding of human nature have developed and increased. A client constitutes more than a person who simply needs **restorative care** and comes to a health-care facility with a **disease** to be cured. Clients are now seen as complex entities affected by various interrelating factors, such as the mind and body, the individual and the **environment,** and the person and the person's family. When nurses talk about clients, the term *biopsychosocial* is often used to express the complex relationship between the body, mind, and

environment. These elements are at the heart of preventative care that has been an emphasis of professional nursing since the time of Florence Nightingale. The prevention of disease and promotion of health are key provisions in the health-care reform bill passed in 2010 and open the door for nurses to practice what have always been a part of their educational history.

Modeling a Healthy Client

A client, in many of the nursing models, does not have to have an illness to be the central element of the model (this explains the preference for using the term *client* over the term *patient*). This is also one of the clearest distinctions between medical models and nursing models. Medical models tend to be restrictive and reactive, focusing almost exclusively on curing diseases and restoring health after the client becomes ill. Nursing models tend to be proactive and **holistic.** Nursing models, like medical models, are certainly concerned with curing disease and restoring a client's health, but they also focus on prevention of disease and maintenance of health. A healthy person is just as important to many nursing models as the person with a disease.

> *Although nursing models vary in terminology and approach to health care, there are four concepts that are common to almost all of them: client or patient (individual or collective), health, environment, and nursing.*

Health

Like the concept of client, the concept of health has undergone much development and change over the years as knowledge has increased. Traditionally, health was originally thought of as an absence of disease. A more current realistic view is that of health as a continuum, ranging from a completely healthy state, in which there is no disease, to a completely unhealthy state, which results in death. At any given time in their lives, all people are located somewhere along the health continuum and may move closer to one side or the other depending on circumstances and health status.[7]

Health is difficult to define because it varies so much from one individual to another. For example, a 22-year-old bodybuilder who has no chronic diseases perceives health differently than an 85-year-old who has diabetes, congestive heart failure, and vision problems. The perception of health also varies from one culture to another and at different historical periods within the same culture. In some past cultures, a sign of health was pure white skin, whereas in the modern American culture, a dark bronze suntan has been more desirable as a sign of health—although research has shown how harmful ultraviolet light is to the skin.

Environment

The concept of environment is another element in most current nursing models. Nursing models often broaden the concept of environment from the simple physical environment to include elements such as living conditions, public sanitation, and air and water quality. Factors such as interpersonal relationships and social interactions are also included.

Some internal environmental factors that affect health include personal psychological processes, religious beliefs, sexual orientation, personality, and emotional responses. It has long been known that individuals who are highly self-motivated and internally goal directed (i.e., type A personality) tend to develop ulcers and have myocardial infarctions at a higher rate than the general population. Medical models, which are primarily illness oriented, although acknowledging this factor, may not consider it to be treatable. Nursing models that consider personality as one of the environmental factors affecting health are more likely to attempt to modify the individual's behavior (internal environment) to decrease the risk for disease.

Like the other key concepts found in nursing models, the concept of environment is used so that it is consistent within a particular model's overall context. Nursing models try to show how various aspects of environment interrelate and how they affect the client's health status. In addition, nursing models treat environment as an active element in the overall health-care system and assert that positive alterations in the environment will improve the client's health status.

Nursing
The Concept of Nursing

The culminating concept in all the various nursing models is nursing itself. After consideration of what it means to be a client, what it means to be healthy, and how the environment influences the client's health status either positively or negatively, the concept of nursing delineates the function and role of nurses in their relationships with clients that affects the clients' health.

Historically, the profession of nursing has been interested in providing basic physical care (i.e., hygiene, activity, and nourishment), psychological support, and relief of discomfort. Modern nursing, although still including these basic elements of client care, has expanded into areas of health care that were only imagined a generation ago.

Client as Partner

In the modern nurse–client relationship, the client is no longer the passive recipient of nursing care. The relationship has been expanded to include clients as key partners in curing and in the health maintenance process. In conjunction with the nurse, clients set goals for care and recovery, take an active part in achieving those goals, and help in evaluating whether or not those actions have achieved the goals.[8]

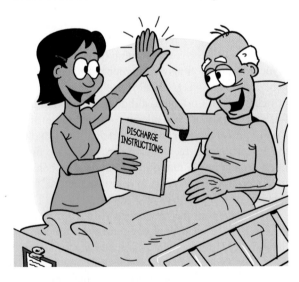

What Do You Think?

How do you define nursing? What activities are important for the nurse to carry out?

Because of the broadened understanding of environment, several nursing models include manipulation of environmental elements that affect health as an important part of the nurse's role. The environment may be directly altered by the nurse with little or no input from the client, or the client may be taught by the nurse to alter the environment in ways that will contribute to curing disease, increasing comfort, or improving the client's health status.[9]

Four Key Concepts

To analyze and understand any nursing model, it is important to look for these four key concepts: client, health, environment, and nursing. These concepts should be clearly defined, closely interrelated, and mutually supportive. Depending on the particular nursing model, one element may be emphasized more than another. The resultant role and function of the nurse depend on which element is given greater emphasis.

GENERAL SYSTEMS THEORY

A widely accepted method for conceptualizing and understanding the world and what is in it derives from a systems viewpoint. Generally understood as an organized unit with a set of components that interact and affect each other, a system acts as a whole because of the interdependence of its parts.[10] As a result, when part of the system malfunctions or fails, it interrupts the function of the whole system rather than affecting merely one part. Humans, plants, cars, governments, the health-care system, the profession of nursing, and almost anything that exists can be viewed as a system. The terminology and principles of systems theory pervade U.S. society.

A Basis in Thought
Manageable Fragments

Although general systems theory in its pure form is rarely, if ever, used as a nursing model, its process and much of its terminology underlie many nursing models. Elements of general systems theory in one form or another have found their way into many textbooks and much of the professional literature. General systems theory often acts as the unacknowledged **conceptual framework** for many educational programs. An understanding of the mechanisms and terminology of general systems theory is helpful in providing an orientation to understanding nursing models.

General systems theory, sometimes referred to simply as **systems theory,** is an outgrowth of an innate intellectual process. The human mind has difficulty comprehending a large, complex entity as a single unit. As a result, the mind automatically divides that entity into smaller, more manageable fragments and then examines each fragment separately. This is similar to the process of deductive reasoning, in which a single complex thought or theory is broken down into smaller, interrelated pieces. All scientific disciplines, from physics to biology and the social sciences (e.g., sociology and psychology), use this method of analysis.

Reassembling the Fragments

Systems theory takes the process a step further. After analyzing or breaking down the entity, systems theory attempts to put it back together by showing how the parts work individually and together within the system. This interrelationship of the parts makes the system function as a unit. Often, particularly when the system involves biological or sociological entities, the system that results is greater than the sum of its parts.

For example, a human can be considered to be a complex, biosocial system. Humans are made up of a large number of smaller systems such as the endocrine system, neurological system, gastrointestinal system, urinary system, and so forth. Although each of these systems is important, in and of themselves they do not make a human. Many animals have the same systems, yet the human is more than the animal and more than the sum of the systems.

A Set of Interacting Parts

Although the early roots of general systems theory can be traced as far back as the 1930s,

von Bertalanffy is usually credited with the formal development and publication of general systems theory around 1950.[11] His major achievement was to standardize the definitions of the terms used in systems theory and make the concept useful to a wide range of disciplines. Systems theory is so widely applicable because it reflects the reality that underlies basic human thought processes.

Very simply, a system is defined as a set of interacting parts. The parts that compose a system may be similar or may vary a great deal from each other, but they all have the common function of making the system work well to achieve its overall purpose.

A school is a good example of how the dynamics and interrelatedness of a system work. A school as a system consists of a large number of units, including buildings, administrators, teachers, students, and various other individuals (e.g., counselors, financial aid personnel, bookkeepers, and maintenance persons). Each of these individuals has a unique job but also contributes to the overall goal of the school, which is to provide an education for the students and to further the development of knowledge through research.

> *The culminating concept in all the various nursing models is nursing itself. After consideration of what it means to be a client, what it means to be healthy, and how the environment influences the client's health status either positively or negatively, the concept of nursing delineates the function and role of nurses in their relationships with clients that affects the clients' health.*

All systems consist of four key parts: the system itself (i.e., whether it is open or closed), input and output, throughput, and a feedback loop.

Open and Closed Systems

A system is categorized as being either open or closed. Very few systems are completely open or completely closed. Rather, they are usually a combination of both open and closed systems.

Open Systems

Open systems are those in which relatively free movement of information, matter, and **energy** into and out of the system exists. In a completely open system, there would be no restrictions on what moves in and out of the system, thus making its boundaries difficult to identify. Most systems have some control over the movement of information, energy, and matter around them. This control is maintained through the semipermeable nature of their boundaries, which allows some things in and keeps some things out, as well as allowing some out while keeping others in. This control of input and output leads to the dynamic equilibrium found in most well-functioning systems.

Closed Systems

Theoretically, a **closed system** prevents any movement into and out of the system. In this case, the system would be totally static and unchanging. Probably no absolutely closed systems exist in the real world, although some systems may tend to be closed to outside elements. A stone, for example, considered as a system, seems to be almost perfectly closed. It does not take anything in or put anything out. It does not change very much over long periods. In reality, though, it is affected by a number of elements in nature. It absorbs moisture when it is damp, freezes when cold, and becomes hot in the summer. Over long periods, these factors may cause the stone to crack, break down, and eventually become topsoil.

Systems that nurses deal with frequently are relatively open. Primarily, the client can be categorized as a highly open system that requires certain input elements and has output elements also. Other systems that nurses commonly work with (e.g., hospital administrators and physicians) are generally considered to be open systems, although their degree of openness may vary widely.

Input and Output

The processes by which a system interacts with elements in its environment are called *input* and *output.* Input is defined as any type of information, energy, or material that enters the system from the environment through its boundaries. Conversely, output is defined as any information, energy, or material that leaves the system and enters the environment through the system's boundaries. The end product of a system is a type of output that is not reusable as input. Open systems require relatively large amounts of input and output.

Throughput

A third term sometimes used in relationship to the system's dynamic exchange with the environment is *throughput.* Throughput is a process that allows the input to be changed so that it is useful to the system.

For example, most automobiles operate on some form of liquid fossil fuel (input) such as gasoline or diesel fuel. However, going to the gas station and pouring liquid fuel on the roof of the car will not produce the desired effects. If the fuel is put into the gas tank, it can be transformed by the carburetor or fuel injection system into a fine mist, which when mixed with air and ignited by a spark plug burns rapidly to produce the force necessary to propel the car. Without this internal process (throughput), liquid fuel is not a useful form of energy.

Feedback Loop

The fourth key element of a system is the *feedback loop.* The feedback loop allows the system to monitor its internal functioning so that it can either restrict or increase its input and its output and maintain the highest level of functioning.

Positive Feedback

Two basic types of feedback exist. Positive feedback leads to change within the system, with the goal of improving the system. Students in the classroom, for example, receive feedback from the teacher in several ways; it may be through direct verbal statements such as "Good work on this assignment" or through examination and homework grades. Feedback is considered positive if it produces a change in a student's behavior, such as motivating him or her to study more, spend more time on assignments, or prepare more thoroughly for class.

Negative Feedback

Negative feedback maintains stability; that is, it does not produce change. Negative feedback is not necessarily

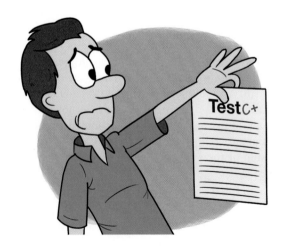

bad for a system. Rather, when a system has reached its peak level of functioning, negative feedback helps it maintain that level. For example, if a person on a weight loss regime has reached the target weight, he or she knows what type of diet and exercise is needed to stay at the ideal weight. Negative feedback—in the form of numbers on the bathroom scale—indicates that no changes in diet or exercise patterns are required.

The feedback loop is an important element in systems theory. It makes the process circular and links the various elements of the system together. Without a feedback loop, it is virtually impossible for the system to have any meaningful control over its input and output.

Feedback loops are used at all levels in a hospital. Nurses get feedback about the care they provide both from clients and from their supervisors. The hospital administration gets feedback from clients and accrediting agencies. Physicians get feedback from clients, nurses, and the hospital administration. Systems theory is present, if sometimes unseen, in almost all health-care settings. Professional nurses need to be able to understand and identify the components of systems theory when they are encountered to improve their nursing practice and quality of care.

> *The feedback loop is an important element in systems theory. It makes the process circular and links the various elements of the system together.*

MAJOR NURSING THEORIES AND MODELS

At least 15 published nursing models (or theories) have been used to direct nursing education and nursing care.[12] The six nursing models discussed here (Table 4.1) have been selected because they are the most widely accepted and are good examples of how the concepts of client, health, environment, and nursing are used to explain and guide nursing actions. Discussion of these theories is not intended to be exhaustive, but rather to provide an overview of the main concepts of the nurse theorist. It is important to understand the terms used in the theories as defined by their authors and to see the interrelationship between the elements in each theory as well as the similarities and differences among the various different models.

The Roy Adaptation Model

As developed by Sister Callista Roy, the Roy Adaptation Model of nursing is very closely related to systems theory.[13] The main goal of this model is to allow the client to reach his or her highest level of functioning through adaptation.

Client

The central element in the Roy Adaptation Model is man (a generic term referring to humans in general, or the client in particular, collectively or individually). Man is viewed as a dynamic entity with both input and output. As derived from the context of the four modes in the Roy Adaptation Model, the client is defined as a biopsychosocial being who is affected by various stimuli and displays behaviors to help adapt to the stimuli. Because the client is constantly being affected by stimuli, adaptation is a continual process.[13]

Inputs are called stimuli and include internal stimuli that arise from within the client's environment as well as stimuli coming from external environmental factors such as physical surroundings, family, and society. The output in the Roy Adaptation Model is the behavior that the client demonstrates as a result of stimuli that are affecting him or her.

Output, or behavior, is a very important element in the Roy Adaptation Model because it provides the **baseline data** about the client that the nurse obtains through assessment techniques. In this model, the output (behavior) is always modified by the client's internal attempts to adapt to the input, or stimuli. Roy has identified four internal adaptational activities that clients use and has called them the four adaptation modes:

1. The physiological mode (using internal physiological process)
2. The self-concept mode (developed throughout life by experience)
3. The role function mode (dependent on the client's relative place in society)
4. The interdependence mode (indicating how the client relates to others)

Table 4.1 Comparison of Selected Nursing Models

Nursing Theory	Client	Health	Environment	Nursing
Roy Adaptation Model	Human being—a dynamic system with input and output	A continuum with the ability to adapt successfully to illness	Both internal and external stimuli that affect behaviors	Multistep process that helps the client adapt and reach the highest level of functioning
Orem Self-Care Model	Human being—biological, psychological, social being with the ability for self-care	Able to live life to the fullest through self-care	The medium through which the client moves	Assistance in self-care activities to help the client achieve health
King Model of Goal Attainment	Person—exchanges energy and information with the environment to meet needs	Dynamic process to achieve the highest level of functioning	Personal, interpersonal, and social systems and the external physical world	Dynamic process that identifies and meets the client's health-care needs
Watson Model of Human Caring	Individual—has needs, grows, and develops to reach a state of inner harmony	Dynamic state of growth and development leading to full potential as a human being	The client must overcome certain factors to achieve health	Science of caring that helps clients reach their greatest potential
Johnson Behavioral System Model	Person—a behavioral system; an organized, integrated whole composed of seven subsystems	A behavioral system able to achieve a balanced, steady state	All the internal and external elements that affect client behavior	Activities that manipulate the environment and help clients achieve the balanced state of health
Neuman Health-Care Systems Model	An open system that constantly interacts with internal and external environment	An individual with relatively stable internal functioning of a high state of wellness (stability)	Internal and external stressors that produce change in the client	Identifies boundary disruption and helps clients in activities to restore stability

Health

In the Roy Adaptation Model, the concept of health is defined as the location of the client along a continuum between perfect health and complete illness. Health, in this model, is rarely an absolute. Rather, "a person's ability to adapt to stimuli, such as injury, disease, or even psychological stress, determines the level of that person's health status."[13] For example, a client who was in an automobile accident, had a broken neck, and was paralyzed but who eventually went back to college, obtained a law degree, and became a practicing lawyer would, in the Roy Adaptation Model, be considered to have a high degree of health because of the ability to adapt to the stimuli imposed.

Environment

The Roy Adaptation Model's definition of environment is synonymous with the concept of stimuli. The environment consists of all those factors that influence the client's behavior, either internally or externally. This model categorizes these environmental elements, or stimuli, into three groups: (1) focal, (2) contextual, and (3) residual.

Focal stimuli are environmental factors that most directly affect the client's behavior and require most of his or her attention. Contextual stimuli form the general physical, social, and psychological environment from which the client emerges. Residual stimuli are factors in the client's past, such as personality characteristics, past experiences, religious beliefs, and social norms, that have an indirect effect on the client's health status. Residual stimuli are often very difficult to identify because they may remain hidden in the person's past memory or may be an integral part of the client's personality.

Nursing

Assessment

In the Roy Adaptation Model, nursing becomes a multistep process, similar to the nursing process, to aid and support the client's attempt to adapt to stimuli in one or more of the four adaptive modes. To determine what type of help is required to promote adaptation, the nurse must first assess the client.

The primary nursing assessments are of the client's behavior (output). Basically, the nurse should try to determine whether the client's behavior is adaptive or maladaptive in each of the four

adaptational modes previously defined. Some first-level assessments of the pneumonia client might include a temperature of 104°F, a cough productive of thick green sputum, chest pain on inspiration, and signs of weakness or physical debility, such as the inability to bring in wood for the fireplace or to visit friends.

A second-level assessment should also be made to determine what type of stimuli (input) is affecting the client's health-care status. In the case of the client with pneumonia, this might include a culture and sensitivity test of the sputum to identify the invasive bacteria, assessment of the client's clothes to determine whether they were adequate for the weather outside, and an investigation to find out whether any neighbors could help the client when he or she is discharged from the hospital.

Analysis

After performing the assessment, the nurse analyzes the data and arranges them in such a way as to be able to make a statement about the client's adaptive or maladaptive behaviors; that is, the nurse identifies the problem. In current terminology, this identification of the problem is called a **nursing diagnosis.** The problem statement is the first part of the three-part PES (problem–etiology–signs and symptoms) formulation that completes the nursing diagnosis (Fig. 4.1).

Setting Goals

After the problem has been identified, goals for optimal adaptation are established. Ideally, these goals should be a collaborative effort between the nurse and the client. A determination of the actions needed to achieve the goals is the next step in the process. The focus should be on manipulation of the stimuli to promote optimal adaptation. Finally, an evaluation is made of the whole process to determine whether the goals have been met. If the goals have not been met, the nurse must determine why, not how, the activities should be modified to achieve the goals.[11]

The Orem Self-Care Model

Dorothea E. Orem's model of nursing is based on the belief that health care is each individual's own responsibility. The model is aimed at helping clients direct and carry out activities that either help maintain or improve their health.[14]

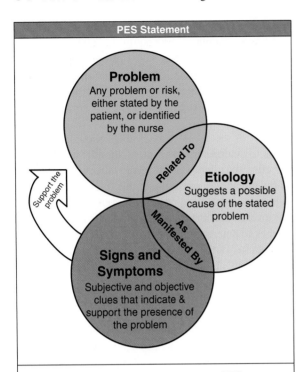

PES Statement

Problem
Any problem or risk, either stated by the patient, or identified by the nurse

Related To

Etiology
Suggests a possible cause of the stated problem

Support the problem

As Manifested By

Signs and Symptoms
Subjective and objective clues that indicate & support the presence of the problem

Together, these components make up the *PES* (**P**roblem, **E**tiology, **S**igns/symptoms) statement, which is demonstrated below

Pain, acute, may be *related to surgical wound, as manifested by facial grimacing, increased heart rate* and *verbal complaints* of pain at the incision site

Figure 4.1 Together, these components make up the **PES** (**p**roblem–**e**tiology–**s**igns and **s**ymptoms) statement: *Pain,* acute, may be related to *surgical wound,* as manifested by *facial grimacing, increased heart rate,* and *verbal complaints* of pain at the incision site.

Client

As with most other nursing models, the central element of the Orem model is the client, who is a biological, psychological, and social being with the capacity for self-care. Self-care is defined as the practice of activities that individuals initiate and perform on their own behalf to maintain life, health, and well-being. Self-care is a requirement both for maintenance of life and for optimal functioning.

Health

In the Orem Self-Care Model, health is defined as the person's ability to live fully within a particular physical, biological, and social environment, achiev-

ing a higher level of functioning that distinguishes the person from lower life forms.

Quality of life is an extremely important element in this model of nursing. A person who is healthy is living life to the fullest and has the capacity to maintain that life through self-care. An unhealthy person is an individual who has a self-care deficit. This group of unhealthy individuals also includes adults with diseases and injuries, young and dependent children, elderly people, and disabled people. This deficit is indicated by the inability to carry out one or more of the key health-care activities. These activities have been categorized into six groups:

• Air, water, and food
• Excretion of waste
• Activity and rest
• Solitude and social interactions
• Avoiding hazards to life and well-being
• Being normal mentally under universal self-care

Self-Care

In the Orem model, self-care is a two-part concept. The first type of self-care is called universal self-care and includes those elements commonly found in everyday life that support and encourage normal human growth, development, and functioning. Persons who are healthy, according to the Orem model, carry out the activities listed in order to maintain a state of health. To some degree, all these elements are necessary activities in maintaining health through self-care.[15]

The second type of self-care comes into play when the individual is unable to conduct one or more of the six self-care activities. This second type of self-care is called health deviation self-care. Health deviation self-care includes those activities carried out by individuals who have diseases, injuries, physiological or psychological stress, or other health-care concerns. Activities such as seeking health care at an emergency department or clinic, entering a drug **rehabilitation** unit, joining a health club or weight control program, or going to a physician's office fall into this category.

Environment

Environment, in the self-care model, is the medium through which clients move as they conduct their daily activities. Although less emphasized in this model, the environment is generally viewed as a negative factor in a person's health status because many environmental factors detract from the ability to provide self-care. Environment includes social interactions with others, situations that must be resolved, and physical elements that affect health.

Nursing

The primary goal of nursing in the Orem model is to help the client conduct self-care activities in such a way as to reach the highest level of human functioning. Because there is a range of levels of self-care ability, three distinct levels, or systems, of nursing care are delineated, based on the individual's ability to undertake self-care activities. As clients become less able to care for themselves, their nursing care needs increase.

Wholly Compensated Care

A person who is able to carry out few or no self-care activities falls into the wholly compensated nursing care category, in which the nurse must provide for most or all of the client's self-care needs. Examples of clients who require this level of care include comatose and ventilator-dependent clients in an intensive care unit, clients in surgery and the immediate recovery period, women in the labor and delivery phases of childbirth, and clients with emotional and psychological problems so severe as to render them unable to conduct normal activities of daily living.

Partially Compensated Care

Clients in the partially compensated category of nursing care can meet some to most of their self-care needs but still have certain self-care deficits that require nursing intervention. The nurse's role becomes one of identifying these needs and carrying out activities to meet them until the client reaches a state of health and is able to meet the needs personally. Examples of this level of nursing care include postoperative clients who can feed themselves and do basic activities of daily living (ADL) but are unable to care for a catheter and dressing, and clients with newly diagnosed diabetes

who have not yet learned the technique of self-administered insulin injections.

Supportive Developmental Care

Clients who are able to meet all of their basic self-care needs require very few or no nursing interventions. These clients fall in the supportive developmental category of nursing care, in which the nurse's main functions are to teach the client how to maintain or improve health and to offer guidance in self-care activities and provide emotional support and encouragement.

What Do You Think?

Based on your experiences with the health-care system, write your own definition of client (patient). What factors led you to this definition?

> *The primary goal of nursing in the Orem model is to help the client conduct self-care activities in such a way as to reach the highest level of human functioning.*

Also, the nurse may adjust the environment to support the client's growth and development toward self-care or may identify community resources to help in the self-care process.[15] Conducting prenatal classes, arranging for discharge planning, providing child screening programs through a community health agency, and organizing aerobic exercise classes for postcoronary clients all are nursing actions that belong in the supportive developmental category of care.

A Three-Step Process

Nursing care is carried out through a three-step process in the Orem model. Step 1 determines whether nursing care is needed. This step includes a basic assessment of the client and identification of self-care problems and needs. Step 2 determines the appropriate nursing care system category and plans nursing care according to that category. Step 3 provides the indicated nursing care or actions to meet the client's self-care needs.

Five Methods

In the Orem model, step 3—the provision of nursing care (implementation phase)—is carried out by helping the client through one or a combination of five nursing methods:[12]

• Acting for or doing for another person
• Guiding another person
• Supporting another person (physically or psychologically)
• Providing an environment that promotes personal development
• Teaching another person

The King Model of Goal Attainment

The current widely accepted practice of establishing health-care goals for clients, and directing client care to meet these goals, has its origins in the King Model of Goal Attainment developed by Imogene M. King. It is also called the King Intervention Model.[16]

The King model also noted that nursing must function in all three system levels found in the environment: personal, interactional, and social. The primary function of nursing is at the personal systems level, where care of the individual is the main focus. However, nurses can effectively provide care at the interactional systems level, at which they deal with small to moderate-sized groups in activities such as group therapy and in health promotion classes. Finally, nurses can provide care at the social systems level through activities such as programs in community health. In addition, the role of nursing at the social systems level can be expanded to include involvement in policy decisions that have an effect on the health-care system as a whole.

Client

As in other nursing models, the focal point of care in the King model is the person or client. The client is viewed as an open system that exchanges energy and information with the environment—a personal system with physical, emotional, and intellectual needs that change and grow during the course of life. Because these needs cannot be met completely by the client alone, interpersonal systems are developed through interactions with others depending on the client's perceptions of reality, communications with others, and transactions to reduce stress and tension in the environment.

Environment

Environment is an important concept in the King model and encompasses a number of interrelated elements. The personal and interpersonal systems or groups are central to King's conception of environment. They are formed at various levels according to internal goals established by the client.

Personal Systems

At the most basic level are the personal systems, where an interchange takes place between two individuals who share similar goals. An example of such a personal system is a client–nurse relationship.

Interpersonal Systems

At the intermediate level are the interpersonal systems that involve relatively small groups of individuals who share like goals, for example, a formal weight-loss program in which the members have the common goal of losing weight. Human interactions, communications, role delineation, and stress reduction are essential factors at this level.

Social Systems

At the highest level are social systems, which include the large, relatively homogeneous elements of society. The health-care system, government, and society in general are some important social systems. These social systems have as their common goals organization, authority, power, status, and decision. Although the client may not be in direct interaction with the social systems, these systems are important because the personal and interpersonal systems necessarily function within larger social systems.

Invoking the principle of nonsummativity,* whenever one part of an open system is changed, all the other parts of the system feel the effect. For example, a decision made at the governmental level to reduce Medicare or Medicaid payments may affect when and how often a client can use health-care services such as doctor's office visits, group therapy, or emergency department care. The King model also includes the external physical environment that affects a person's health and well-being. As the person moves through the world, the physical setting interacts with the personal system to either improve or degrade the client's health-care status.

---

*Nonsummativity is the degree of interrelatedness among the systems parts. The higher the degree of nonsummativity, the greater the interdependence of parts.

Health

Viewed as a dynamic process that involves a range of human life experiences, health exists in people when they can achieve their highest level of functioning. Health is the primary goal of the client in the King model. It is achieved by continually adjusting to environmental stressors, maximizing the use of available resources, and setting and achieving goals for one's role in life. Anything that disrupts or interferes with people's ability to function normally in their chosen roles is considered to be a state of illness.

Nursing

The King model considers nursing to be a dynamic process and a type of personal system based on interactions between the nurse and the client. During these interactions, the nurse and the client jointly evaluate and identify the health-care needs, set goals for fulfillment of the needs, and consider actions to take in achieving those goals. Nursing is a multifaceted process that includes a range of activities such as the promotion and maintenance of health through education, the restoration of health through care of the sick and injured, and preparation for death through care of the dying.[11]

The process of nursing in the King model includes five key elements considered central to all human interactions:

- Action
- Reaction
- Interaction
- Transaction
- Feedback

The Watson Model of Human Caring

Although the concept of caring has always been an important, if somewhat obscure, element in the practice of nursing, the Watson Model of Human Caring defines caring in a detailed and systematic manner. In the development of her model, Jean Watson used a philosophical approach rather than the systems theory approach seen in many other nursing models. Her main concern in the development of this model was to balance the impersonal aspects of nursing care that are found in the technological and scientific aspects of practice with the personal and interpersonal elements of care that grow from a humanistic belief in life. Watson is also one of the very few theorists who openly recognize the client's and family's spirituality and spiritual beliefs as an essential element of health.[17]

Client

The concept of client or person in the Watson model is not well developed as separate from the concept of nursing. The individuality of the client is a key concern. The Watson model views the client as someone who has needs, who grows and develops throughout life, and who eventually reaches a state of internal harmony.

The client is also seen as a gestalt, or whole, who has value because of inherent goodness and capacity to develop. This gestalt, or holistic, view of the human being is a recurring theme in the Watson model; it emphasizes that the total person is more important to nursing care than the individual injury or disease process that produced the need for care. "The Watson model views the client as someone who has needs, who grows and develops throughout life, and who eventually reaches a state of internal harmony."

Environment

Environment in the Watson model is a concept that is also closely intertwined with the concept of nursing. Viewed primarily as a negative element in the health-care process, the environment consists of those factors that the client must overcome to achieve a state of health. The environment can be both external (physical and social elements) and internal (psychological reactions that affect health).

Health

To be healthy according to the Watson model, the individual must be in a dynamic state of growth and development that leads to reaching full potential as a human. As with other nursing models, health is viewed as a continuum along which a person at any point may tend more toward health or more toward illness.

Illness, in the Watson model, is the client's inability to integrate life experiences and the failure to achieve full potential or inner harmony. In this model, the state of illness is not necessarily synonymous with the disease process. If the person reacts to the disease process in such a way as to find meaning, that response is considered to be healthy. A failure to find meaning in the disease experience leads to a state of illness.

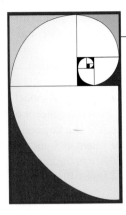

Issues Now

Looking to the Future: The Pew Commission Final Report

Projected estimates of the nursing shortage based on data collected by the U.S. Bureau of the Census Current Population Survey, Division of Nursing, the Pew Commission, and the Buerhaus and Staiger data collection agency in 1998 are now considered woefully inadequate. Current projections of the nursing shortage range from 400,000 to as many as 1,000,000 by the year 2015. The Pew Commission's final report addressed the competencies that nurses in the future will need:

Twenty-One Competencies for the 21st Century

1. Embrace a personal ethic of social responsibility and service.
2. Exhibit ethical behavior in all professional activities.
3. Provide evidence-based, clinically competent care.
4. Incorporate the multiple determinants of health in clinical care.
5. Apply knowledge of the new sciences.
6. Demonstrate critical thinking, reflection, and problem-solving skills.
7. Understand the role of primary care.
8. Rigorously practice preventive health care.
9. Integrate population-based care and services into practice.
10. Improve access to health care for those with unmet health needs.
11. Practice relationship-centered care with individuals and families.
12. Provide culturally sensitive care to a diverse society.
13. Partner with communities in health-care decisions.
14. Use communication and information technology effectively and appropriately.
15. Work in interdisciplinary teams.
16. Ensure care that balances individual, professional, system, and social needs.
17. Practice leadership.
18. Take responsibility for quality of care and health outcomes at all levels.
19. Contribute to continuous improvement of the health-care system.
20. Advocate for public policy that promotes and protects the health of the public.
21. Continue to learn and help others to learn.

The Pew Commission also went on to identify five key areas for professional education:

1. Change professional training to meet the demands of the new health-care system.
2. Ensure that the health professions workforce reflects the diversity of the nation's population.
3. Require interdisciplinary competence in all health professionals.
4. Continue to move education into ambulatory practice.
5. Encourage public service of all health professional students and graduates.

The changes that will occur over the next decade may threaten some health-care professionals, but they will also open up a vista of opportunities for those willing to look creatively into the future. Nursing has to recognize that it will

Issues Now continued

grow only to the extent that it is able to contribute to the needs of an evolving health-care system. These needs will change with time. The Pew Report, although broad in scope, provides the nursing profession with a blueprint for dealing with these changes as they occur. It is a call to action that nurses and the nursing profession need to hear.

Sources Bellack JP, O'Neil EH: Recreating nursing practice for a new century:
Recommendations of the Pew Health Professions Commission's Final Report. Nursing and Health Care Perspectives 21(1):14–21, 2000.
Brady M, et al: A proposed framework for differentiating the 21 Pew Competencies by level of nursing education. Nursing and Health Care Perspectives 22(1):30–36, 2001.
Pontious M: Where have all the nurses gone? Oklahoma Nurse 47(1):1, 18, 2002.
More than one million new nurses needed by 2010. American Nurse 34(1):5, 2002.
Critical Challenges: Revitalizing the Health Professions for the 21st Century. Pew Health Professions Commission, San Francisco, 1995.

Nursing

Watson makes a clear distinction between the science of nursing and the practice of curing (medicine).[12] She defined nursing as the science of caring in which the primary goal is to assist the client to reach the greatest level of personal potential. The practice of curing involves the conduct of activities that have the goal of treatment and elimination of disease.

The process of nursing in the Watson model is based on the systematic use of the scientific problem-solving method for decision making. To best understand nursing as a science of caring, the nurse should hold certain beliefs and be able to initiate certain caring activities.

Values

Basic to the beliefs necessary for the successful practice of nursing in the Watson model is the formation of a humanistic, altruistic system of values based on the tenet that all people are inherently valuable because they are human. In addition, the nurse should have a strong sense of faith and hope in people and their condition because of the human potential for development.

Caring

A number of activities are important in the practice of nursing according to Watson's caring way. These activities include establishing a relationship of help and trust between the nurse and the client; encouraging the client to express both positive and negative feelings with acceptance; manipulating the environment to make it more supportive, protective, or corrective for the client with any type of disease process; and assisting in whatever way is deemed appropriate to meet the basic human needs of the client.

The Johnson Behavioral System Model

By integrating systems theory with behavioral theory, Dorothy E. Johnson has developed a model of nursing that considers client behavior to be the key to preventing illness and to restoring health when illness occurs. Johnson holds that human behavior is really a type of system in itself that is influenced by input factors from the environment and has output that in its turn affects the environment.[12]

Client

Drawing directly on the terminology of systems theory, the Johnson model describes the person, or client, as a behavioral system that is an organized and integrated whole. The whole is greater than the sum of its parts because of the integration and functioning of its subsystems. In the Johnson model, the client as a behavioral system is composed of seven distinct behavioral subsystems. In turn, each of these seven behavioral subsystems contains four structural elements that guide and shape the subsystem.

Security

The first behavioral subsystem is the attachment, or affiliate, subsystem, which has security as its driving force. The type of activity that this subsystem undertakes is, for the most part, inclusion in social functions, and the behavior that is observed from this subsystem is social interaction.

Dependency

The second behavioral subsystem is the dependency subsystem, which has as its initiating force the goal of helping others. The primary type of activity involved is nurturing and promoting self-image. The observable behaviors that are a result of this activity include approval, attention, and physical assistance of the person.

Taking In

The third behavioral subsystem is called the ingestive subsystem, which has as its driving force the meeting of the body's basic physiological needs of food and nutrient intake. Correspondingly, its primary activity is seeking and eating food.

Eliminative Behavior

The fourth behavioral subsystem is the eliminative; its goal is removal of waste products from the system. Its primary activity is means of elimination, which is observed as the behavior of expelling waste products.

Sexual Behavior

The fifth behavioral subsystem is sexual behavior, which is found in the Johnson model's description of the person. The sexual subsystem has gratification and procreation of the species as its goals. It involves the complex activities of identifying gender roles, sexual development, and actual biological sexual activity. It manifests itself in courting and mating behaviors.

Self-Protection

The sixth behavioral subsystem is called the aggressive subsystem, and its driving force is the goal of self-preservation. All the actions that individuals undertake to protect themselves from harm, either internal or external, derive from this subsystem and are shown in actions toward others and the environment in general.

Achievement

The seventh, and final, behavioral subsystem is identified as achievement. Achievement has as its driving force the broad goal of exploration and manipulation of the environment. Gaining mastery and control over the environment is the primary activity of this subsystem; it can be demonstrated externally when the individual shows that learning has occurred and higher-level accomplishments are being produced.[18]

As with all open systems, the behavioral system that makes up the person seeks to maintain a dynamic balance by regulating input and output. This regulation process takes the form of adapting to the environment and responding to others. However, the Johnson model sees human behavior as being goal directed, which leads the person to constant growth and development beyond the maintenance of a mere steady state.

Health

A state of health exists, according to the Johnson model, when balance and steady state exist within the behavioral systems of the client. Under normal circumstances, the human system has enough inherent flexibility to maintain this balance without external intervention. At times, however, the system's balance may be disturbed to such a degree by physical disease, injury, or emotional crisis as to require external assistance. This out-of-balance state is the state of illness.

> *The Johnson model sees human behavior as being goal directed, which leads the person to constant growth and development beyond the maintenance of a mere steady state.*

Environment

In the Johnson model, the environment is defined as all those internal and external elements that have an effect on the behavioral system. These environmental elements include obvious external factors, such as air temperature and relative humidity; sociological factors, such as family, neighborhood, and society in general; and the internal environment, such as bodily processes, psychological states, religious beliefs, and political orientation.

All seven behavioral subsystems are involved with the client's relationship to the environment through the regulation of input and output. The client is continually interacting with the environment in the attempt to remain healthy by maintaining an internal dynamic balance.

Nursing

In the Johnson model, nursing is an activity that helps the individual achieve and maintain an optimal level of behavior (state of health) through the manipulation and regulation of the environment.[11] Nursing has functions in both health and illness. Nursing interventions to either maintain or restore health involve four activities in the regulation of the environment:

• Restricting harmful environmental factors
• Defending the client from negative environmental influences
• Inhibiting adverse elements from occurring
• Facilitating positive internal environmental factors in the recovery process

As a professional, the nurse in the Johnson model provides direct services to the client. By interacting with, and sometimes intervening in, the multiple subsystems that are found in the client's environment, the nurse acts as an external regulatory force. The goal of nursing is to promote the highest level of functioning and development in the client at all times.

Nursing actions include helping the client act in a socially acceptable manner, monitoring and aiding with biological processes necessary for maintenance of a dynamic balance, demonstrating support for medical care and treatment during illness, and taking actions to prevent illness from recurring. In this model, nursing makes its own unique contribution to the health and well-being of individuals and provides a service complementary to that provided by other health-care professionals.

The Neuman Health-Care Systems Model

As envisioned by Betty Neuman, the Health-Care Systems Model focuses on the individual and his or her environment and is applicable to a variety of health-care disciplines apart from nursing. Drawing from systems theory, the Neuman model also includes elements from stress theory with an overall holistic view of humanity and health care.[16]

Client

In this model, the client is viewed as an open system that interacts constantly with internal and external environments through the system's boundaries. The client-system's boundaries are called lines of defense and resistance in the Neuman model and may be represented graphically as a series of concentric circles that surround the basic core of the individual. The goal of these boundaries is to keep the basic core system stable by controlling system input and output.

Neuman classifies these defensive boundaries according to their various functions. The internal lines of resistance are the boundaries that are closest to the basic core and thus protect the basic internal structure of the system. The normal lines of defense are outside the internal lines of resistance; they protect the system from common, everyday environmental stressors. The flexible line of defense surrounds the normal line of defense and protects it from extreme environmental stressors. The general goal of all these protective boundaries is to maintain the internal stability of the client.

Health

Health, then, in the Neuman model is defined as the relatively stable internal functioning of the client. Optimal health exists when the client is maintained in a high state of wellness or stability.

As in other nursing models, health is not considered an absolute state, but rather a continuum that reflects the client's internal stability while moving from wellness to illness and back. It takes a considerable amount of physical and psychological energy to maintain the stability of the person who is in good health.

The opposite of a healthy state, illness exists when the client's core structure becomes unstable through the effects of environmental factors that overwhelm and defeat the lines of defense and resistance. These environmental factors, whether internal or external, are called stressors in this model.

Environment

The environment is composed of internal and external forces, or stressors, that produce change or response in the client. Stressors may be helpful or harmful, strong or weak.

Stressors are also classified according to their relationship to the basic core of the client-system. Stressors that are completely outside the basic core are termed extrapersonal stressors and are either physical, such as atmospheric temperature, or sociological, such as living in either a rural or an urban setting. Interpersonal stressors arise from interactions with other human beings. Marital relationships, career expectations, and friendships are included in this group of interpersonal stressors. Those stressors that occur within the client are called intrapersonal and include involuntary physiological responses, psychological reactions, and internal thought processes.

Nursing
Identifying Stressors
The nurse's role in the Neuman model is to identify at what level or in which boundary a disruption in the client's internal stability has taken place and then to aid the client in activities that strengthen or restore the integrity of that particular boundary. The Neuman model expands the concept of client from the individual to include families, small groups, the community, or even society in general.

Nursing's main concern in this model is either to identify stressors that will disrupt a defensive boundary in the future (prevention) or to identify a stressor that has already disrupted a defensive boundary, thereby producing instability (illness).[16] The Neuman model is based on the nursing process and identifies three levels of intervention: primary, secondary, and tertiary.

Types of Intervention
A **primary intervention** has as its main goal the prevention of possible symptoms that could be caused by environmental stressors. Teaching clients about stress management, giving immunizations, and encouraging aerobic exercise to prevent heart disease are examples of primary interventions.

A **secondary intervention** is aimed at treating symptoms that have already been produced by stressors. Many of the actions that nurses perform in the hospital or clinic (e.g., giving pain medications or teaching a client with cardiac disease about the benefits of a low-sodium diet) fall into this secondary intervention category.

Tertiary care actions seek to restore the client's system to an optimal state of balance by adapting to negative environmental stressors.

> " *In the Johnson model, nursing is an activity that helps the individual achieve and maintain an optimal level of behavior (state of health) through the manipulation and regulation of the environment.* "

Teaching a client how to care for a colostomy at home after discharge from the hospital is an example of nursing activities at the tertiary level.

TRENDS FOR THE FUTURE IN NURSING THEORY

Although the search for the perfect nursing model continues, the emphasis in recent years has shifted from developing new theories to applying existing theories to nursing practice. Also, the new theorists seem to be more interested in expanding existing nursing theories by including such concepts as cultural diversity, spirituality, family, and social change rather than starting all over again from the beginning. A good example of this trend is the cultural meaning–centered theory that was published by Mendyka and Bloom.[19] This theory expands the King model by adding a cultural perspective.

A More Recent Theory
One of the more recent of the established nursing theories is the Man-Living-Health Model proposed by Rosemary Rizzo Parse. Although her original work started in 1981, a more developed form of her theory was published in 1987.[20–22] Parse's theory stresses the elements of experience, personal **values,** and lifestyle choices in the maintenance of health.

A Matter of Choice
In this theory, the client can be any person or family who is concerned with the quality of their life situation. The client is viewed as an open, whole being who is influenced by past and present life experiences. The ability to make free choices is essential in this theory. The client, through choices he or she makes, interacts with the environment to influence health either positively or negatively.

Health, for Parse, is an ongoing process. Because clients make free choices, their health status is continually unfolding. In addition, health is determined by lived experiences, synthesis of values, and the way the client lives.[23]

Finding Meaning

The main role of nursing in the Parse model is to guide clients in finding and understanding the meaning of their lives. Once the client chooses a healthy life situation, the nurse can further increase the quality of the client's life and improve his or her health status. The ability to change the client's health-related values is an important skill for nurses to master in this model.

Parse never really defines the concept of environment in relationship to her theory. Specifically, it seems to be any health-related setting, but it can also be expanded to include past and present experiences.

New Challenges to Nursing Theory

As with any developing science, nursing will continue to change and respond to the dynamic trends of society. Older nursing models will be either replaced by new ones or modified to include developing concepts. Indeed, one of the hallmarks of a sound nursing theory or model is its flexibility and ability to adapt to new discoveries.

The increasing number of **independent nurse practitioners** and other advanced practice nurses are testing nursing theories as they have never been tested before. The theories that are flexible, realistic, and usable in practice will survive and remain as the pillars of professional nursing.[23] Those that are too theoretical or rigid will fall by the wayside and become mere footnotes in nursing texts.

(text continues on page 82)

Table 4.2 Competencies for Nursing Skills

Associate Degree RN	Baccalaureate Degree RN
Administering Blood Products	
Obtain and document baseline vital signs according to agency policies and procedures.	Same
Obtain blood transfusion history. Initiate administration of blood products according to agency policies and procedures.	Same
Evaluate and document client response to administration of blood products.	Same
Admission, Transfer, Discharge	
Admit client to a health-care facility following facility's policies and procedures.	Same
Transfer client within a health-care facility following facility's policies and procedures.	Same
Assist client to exit a health-care facility following facility's policies and guidelines.	Same
Assess client to determine readiness for discharge.	Manage the discharge planning process.
Facilitate the continuity of care within and across health-care settings.	Same
Assessment of Vital Signs	
Monitor and assess oral, rectal, and axillary temperature.	Same
Measure and record temperature using an electronic or tympanic thermometer.	Same
Monitor and assess peripheral pulses.	Same
Monitor and assess apical pulse.	Same
Monitor and assess apical-radial pulse.	Same
Monitor and assess blood pressure.	Same
Monitor and assess respiratory rate and character.	Same

(continued)

Table 4.2 Competencies for Nursing Skills (continued)

Associate Degree RN	Baccalaureate Degree RN
Bowel Elimination	
Document characteristics of feces.	Same
Perform test for occult blood.	Same
Administer enemas for cleansing or retention.	Same
Remove a fecal impaction.	Same
Provide and teach colostomy and ileostomy care.	Same
Administer a rectal suppository.	Same
Administer a rectal tube.	Same
Develop client's bowel retraining protocol.	Same
Care of the Dying Client	
During dying process, provide measures to decrease client's physical and emotional discomfort.	Same
Evaluate final progress note on client's chart to determine completeness of information.	Same
Notify appropriate people and departments according to agency's policies and procedures.	Same
Evaluate family's response to client's death and make referrals as appropriate.	Develop services that support dying clients and their families.
Provide care for body after client's death according to agency's policies and procedures.	Same
Circulatory Maintenance	
Evaluate fetal heart rate pattern.	Same
Apply antiembolism stockings.	Same
Obtain cardiopulmonary resuscitation certification.	Same
Client Teaching	
Assess and document client's and/or family member's knowledge of specific procedure or health problem.	Assesses client's readiness to learn.
Assess client and significant support person(s) for learning strengths, capabilities, barriers, and educational needs.	Develop materials to provide client and/or family member with information concerning procedure or health problem.
Develop an individualized teaching plan based on assessed needs.	Same
Modify teaching plan based on evaluation of progress toward meeting identified learning outcomes.	Same
Provide client and significant support person(s) with the information to make choices regarding health.	Same
Teach client and significant support person(s) the information and skills needed to achieve desired learning outcomes.	Same
Evaluate progress of client and significant support person(s) toward achievement of identified learning outcomes.	Using multiple teaching strategies, teach heterogeneous groups of clients, accounting for individual differences.
Implement teaching plan using individualized teaching and learning strategies with clients and/or groups in structured settings.	Implement teaching plan using individualized teaching and learning strategies with clients and/or groups in unstructured settings.

Associate Degree RN	Baccalaureate Degree RN
Communication	
Effectively use communication skills during assessment, intervention, evaluation, and teaching.	Same
Express oneself effectively using a variety of media in different contexts.	Same
Adapt communication methods to clients with special needs (e.g., sensory or psychological disabilities).	Same
Produce clear, accurate, and relevant writing.	Same
Use therapeutic communication within the nurse–client relationship.	Same
Maintain confidentiality of nurse–client interactions.	Same
Appropriately, accurately, and effectively communicate with diverse groups and disciplines using a variety of strategies.	Evaluate effectiveness of communication patterns.
Elicit and clarify client preferences and values.	Same
Evaluate dynamics of family interactions.	Same
Evaluate data concerning coping mechanisms of client/family/support system.	Same
Provide emotional support to client/family/support system.	Same
Evaluate strengths of client and family/significant other.	Same
Evaluate need for alternative methods of communicating with client.	Same
Use assertive communication skills in interactions with clients and other health-care providers.	Teach assertive communication skills to clients, unlicensed assistive nursing personnel, and other licensed nurses.
Communicate data concerning client to appropriate members of the health-care team.	Same
Communicate the need for consultation/referral to interdisciplinary care team.	Identify and plan for services to assure continuity in meeting health-care needs during transition from one setting to another.
Collaborate with other health-care team members to provide nursing care.	Collaborate with community members in planning care for the community.
Critical Thinking	
Within acquired knowledge base, create alternative courses of action, develop reasonable hypotheses, and develop new solutions to problems.	Same
Develop an awareness of personal values and feelings and examine basis for them.	Same
Evaluate credibility of sources used to justify beliefs.	Same
Examine assumptions that underlie thoughts and behaviors.	Same
Seek out evidence and give rationale when questioned.	Use critical thinking to further develop working hypotheses, using patterns and inconsistencies in data.
Delegation and Supervision	
Provide assistive personnel with relevant instruction to support achievement of client outcomes.	Specify aspects of nursing care that can appropriately be delegated to unlicensed health-care providers and assistive personnel.

(continued)

Table 4.2 Competencies for Nursing Skills (continued)

Associate Degree RN	Baccalaureate Degree RN
Coordinate the implementation of an individualized plan of care for clients and significant support person(s).	Coordinate and/or implement plan of care for clients with multiple nursing diagnoses, especially both physiological and psychosocial diagnoses.
Delegate aspects of client care to qualified assistive personnel.	Delegate performance of nursing interventions.
Supervise and evaluate activities of assistive personnel.	Delegate nursing care given by others while retaining accountability for the quality of care given to the client.
	Supervise performance of nursing interventions.
	Supervise nursing care given by others while retaining accountability for the quality of care given to the client.
	Manage community-based care for a group of clients.
	Direct care for clients whose conditions are changing.
	Direct care for clients in situations with a potential for variation in client condition.
	Supervise implementation of a comprehensive client teaching plan.
Documentation	
Maintain privacy of client's record.	Same
Accurately document data according to agency's policies and procedures.	Same
Use common abbreviations and nomenclature for recording information in the client's record.	Same
	Establish a reporting and recording system to provide for continuity and accountability of programs in designated structured and unstructured settings (e.g., school health, occupational health, community).
Health Assessment	
Using a systematic process, perform a head-to-toe assessment.	Perform a holistic assessment of the individual across the life span.
Assess physical, cognitive, and psychosocial abilities of individuals in all developmental stages.	
Assess family structure, roles of family members, and family's strengths and weaknesses.	Perform a risk assessment of the individual and family, including lifestyle, family and genetic history, and other risk factors.

Associate Degree RN	Baccalaureate Degree RN
Evaluate an individual's capacity to assume responsibilities for self-care.	Same
	Perform assessment of using a family genogram.
Assess community resources to determine possible referral sources.	Perform a community assessment for diverse populations.
	Perform an assessment of the environment in which health care is being provided.
	Establish processes to identify health risks in designated structured and unstructured settings (e.g., school health, occupational health, community).
	Integrate data from client, other health-care personnel, and other systems to which client is linked (e.g., work, church, neighborhood).
	Modify data collection tools to make them appropriate to client's situation (e.g., language and culture, literacy level, sensory deficit).
Use assessment findings to diagnose and evaluate quality of care and to deliver high-quality care.	Perform family assessment.
Evaluate family's emotional reaction to client's illness (e.g., chronic disorder, terminal illness).	Same
Evaluate client's emotional response to treatment.	Same
Evaluate adequacy of client's support systems.	Same
Assist in diagnostic procedures used to determine client's health status.	Same
Health Promotion	
Facilitate parental attachment with newborn.	Same
Determine the need for a health promotion program.	Develop and implement a health promotion program.
Evaluate risk factors related to client's potential for accident/injury/disease.	Same
Evaluate client's knowledge of disease prevention.	Same
Evaluate client's knowledge of lifestyle choices (e.g., smoking, diet, exercise).	Same
Heat and Cold Therapy	
Evaluate client's response to heat therapy.	Same
Evaluate client's response to cold therapy.	Same
Evaluate client's response to sitz bath.	Same
Monitor and evaluate client's response to hypothermia blanket.	Same
Monitor and evaluate infant's response to radiant warmer.	Same
Home Care Management	
Evaluate ability of family/support system to provide care for client.	Same

(continued)

Table 4.2 Competencies for Nursing Skills (continued)

Associate Degree RN	Baccalaureate Degree RN
Evaluate client's home environment for self-care modifications (e.g., doorway width, accessibility for wheelchair, safety bars).	Develop criteria to evaluate client's home environment for self-care modifications (e.g., doorway width, accessibility for wheelchair, safety bars).
Infection Control	
Use aseptic practices: hand washing, donning and removing a face mask, gowning, donning and removing disposable gloves, bagging articles, managing equipment use for isolation clients, assessing vital signs.	Same
Use universal precautions.	Same
Use body substances isolation procedures.	Same
Evaluate client's immunization status.	Same
Use surgical aseptic practices: hand scrub, donning and removing a sterile gown, donning and removing sterile gloves, preparing and maintaining a sterile field.	Same
Assist with a sterile procedure.	Same
Information and Health-Care Technology	
Use technology, analyze information, and select resources effectively.	Use technology, synthesize information, and select resources effectively.
Demonstrate competence with current technologies.	Same
Use computers for record keeping and documentation in health-care facilities.	Same
	Use data management system to evaluate a comprehensive program for monitoring health of populations in designated structured and unstructured settings (e.g., school health, occupational health, community).
Intravenous Therapy	
Perform venipuncture to obtain blood specimens.	Same
Perform venipuncture with an over-the-needle device.	Same
Prime tubing and hang IV fluids.	Same
Load and discontinue a PCA pump.	Same
Administer and document IV piggyback medications.	Same
Administer and document IV push medications.	Same
Calculate IV flow rates.	Same
Document medications administered through IV.	Same
Discontinue an IV and document procedure.	Same
Monitor and maintain an IV site and infusion.	Same
Change IV tubing and container.	Same
Prime tubing and hang IV fluids.	Same
Determine amount of IV fluid infused and left-to-count each shift.	Same
Assess implanted infusion devices.	Same
Maintain implanted infusion devices.	Same

Associate Degree RN	Baccalaureate Degree RN
Medication Administration	
Assess family members' knowledge of medication therapy: reasons for taking medication, daily dosages, side effects.	Same
Instruct clients and their families in the proper administration of medications.	Same
Accurately calculate medication dosages.	Same
Gather information pertinent to the medication(s) ordered: actions, purpose, normal dosage and route, common side effects, time of onset and peak action, nursing implications.	Same
Administer and document administration of enteral and parenteral medications per order.	Same
Administer and document administration of topical medications per order.	Same
Evaluate client's response to medication.	Same
Perform eye and/or ear irrigation according to agency guidelines.	Same
Meeting Mobility Needs	
Evaluate client's need for range-of-motion exercises.	Same
Evaluate client's level of mobility.	Same
Manage care of client who uses assistive devices.	Same
Provide client or family member with list of resources to contact when mobility or body alignment is impaired.	Evaluate client's need for range-of-motion exercises.
Evaluate client and/or family members' ability to perform range-of-motion exercises.	Evaluate client's level of mobility.
	Manage care of client who uses assistive devices.
	Provide client or family member with list of resources to contact when mobility or body alignment is impaired.
	Evaluate client and/or family members' ability to perform range-of-motion exercises.
Nursing Process	
Analyze collected data to establish a database for client.	Perform comprehensive assessment to determine client's ability to manage self-care, including physiological, psychosocial, developmental, and cognitive factors and their interaction with each other.
Identify client health-care needs to select nursing diagnostic statements.	Formulate individualized nursing diagnoses, based on a synthesis of knowledge from nursing, biological and behavioral sciences, and humanities, that reflect a health problem and its etiology.
	Consider complex interactions of actual and potential nursing diagnoses (e.g., two or more physiological and/or psychosocial nursing diagnoses).

(continued)

Table 4.2 Competencies for Nursing Skills (continued)

Associate Degree RN	Baccalaureate Degree RN
Consider complex interactions of actual and potential nursing diagnoses.	Same
Identify client goals and appropriate nursing interventions.	Same
Develop and communicate nursing care plan.	Develop comprehensive plan of care in collaboration with client.
Implement and document planned nursing interventions.	Same
	Implement a care plan for individuals, families, and communities with complex health problems that have unpredictable outcomes.
	Use preventive, supportive, and restorative measures to promote client comfort, optimum physiological functioning, and emotional well-being.
	Base care planning on knowledge of primary, secondary, and tertiary levels of prevention.
Establish priorities for nursing care needs of clients.	Same
Evaluate and document the extent to which goals of nursing care have been achieved.	Participate in obtaining collective data concerning client outcomes.
	Deliver care that reflects an understanding of interactions among potentially conflicting nursing interventions.
	Initiate a comprehensive plan for discharge of client at time of admission.
	Care for clients in an environment that may not have established protocols.
	Care for clients in situations requiring independent decision making (e.g., community-based practice settings).
Pain Management	
Evaluate data from comprehensive pain history.	Same
Evaluate and document client's response to pharmacological and nonpharmacological interventions.	Same
Document client's response to interventions used to prevent or reduce pain.	Same
Assess client when pain is not relieved through ordered pharmacological and nonpharmacological methods.	Collaborate with other members of health-care team to identify alternative interventions.
Evaluate appropriateness of any pain medication taken by clients.	Same
Educate clients on correct use of medications.	Same
Manage and monitor client receiving epidural analgesia.	Same
Teach client to use a PCA device.	Same

Associate Degree RN	Baccalaureate Degree RN
Perioperative Care	
Preoperatively, assess client's risk for postoperative respiratory complications.	Same
Postoperatively, assess client's ability to perform respiratory exercises.	Same
Preoperatively, assess client's risk for postoperative thrombus formation.	Same
Postoperatively, assess client's ability to perform passive range-of-motion exercises.	Same
Preoperatively, assess client's willingness and capability to learn exercises.	Same
Preoperatively, assess family members' willingness to learn and to support client postoperatively.	Same
Postoperatively, assess client's condition during operative procedure, including range of vital signs, blood volume or fluid loss, fluid replacement, type of anesthesia, type of airway, and size and extent of surgical wound.	Same
Personal Hygiene of Clients	
Provide or assist with personal hygiene on developmental and/or chronological age basis.	Same
Provide or assist with personal hygiene needs as determined by physical limitations and/or diagnosis.	Same
Provide or assist with personal hygiene needs with respect to client's culture and/or religious values.	Same
Provide or assist with personal hygiene care in hospital, nursing home, or client's home.	Same
Assess and maintain chest tubes.	Same
Safety and Comfort	
Implement measures to protect the immunosuppressed client.	Same
Protect the client from injury.	Same
Verify identity of the client.	Same
Implement agency policies and procedures in the event of client injury.	Same
Follow policies and procedures for agency fires and safety measures.	Same
Follow procedures for handling biohazardous materials.	Same
Assess need for restraints or other safety devices.	Develop protocols for use of restraints or other safety devices.
Implement nursing measures to reduce the risk for falls, poisoning, and electrical hazards.	Same
Prepare for internal and external disasters.	Same
Develop a plan for reducing environmental stressors (e.g., noise, temperature, pollution).	Same
Evaluate client's orientation to reality.	Same
Evaluate need for measures to maintain client's skin integrity.	Same
Vascular Access Devices	
Assist with insertion of central venous catheters.	Same
Change a central venous catheter dressing.	Same
Monitor administration of medications/nutrients via a vascular access device.	Same

(continued)

Table 4.2 Competencies for Nursing Skills (continued)

Associate Degree RN	Baccalaureate Degree RN
Measure and monitor central venous pressure.	Same
Maintain central vein infusions in adults and children.	Same
Change parenteral hyperalimentation dressing and tubing.	Same
Wound Care and Dressings	
Assess and manage wounds, including irrigation, application of dressings, and suture/staple removal.	Same

PCA = patient-controlled analgesia.

Sources: Cowan DT: Competence in nursing practice: A controversial concept—a focused review of literature. Accident & Emergency Nursing 151(1):20–26, 2007.

Dickey C, et al: Nursing Skills Identified as Required Competencies. Helene Fuld Educational Mobility Grant. Oklahoma Nursing Articulation Consortium, Kramer School of Nursing, Oklahoma City University.

Levett-Jones TL: Facilitating reflective practice and self-assessment of competence through the use of narratives. Nurse Education in Practice 7(2):112–119, 2007.

Conclusion

As nursing takes its rightful place among the other helping professions, nursing theory will take on additional importance. Nursing theory and models are the systematic conceptualizations of nursing practice and how it fits into the health-care system. Nursing theories help describe, explain, predict, and control nursing activities to achieve the goals of client care. By understanding and using nursing theory, nurses will be better able to incorporate theoretical information into their practice to provide new ways of approaching nursing care and improving nursing practice.

The development of nursing theory and models indicates a maturing of the profession. As the knowledge associated with the profession increases and becomes unique, more complex, and better organized, the general body of nursing science knowledge also increases. Only when nursing has a well-developed body of specialized knowledge will it be fully recognized as a separate scientific discipline and a true profession.

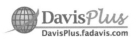

DavisPlus.fadavis.com

Critical Thinking Exercises

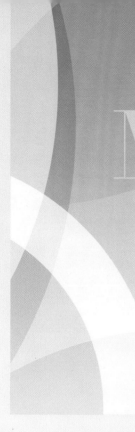

rs. M, an 88-year-old woman, has been a resident of St. Martin's Village, a lifetime care community, since her husband died 8 years ago. Her health status is fair. She has adult-onset diabetes controlled by oral medication and a scar from a tumor behind her left ear that was removed surgically. The wound from this tumor removal has never healed completely, and it has continuously oozed a serous fluid requiring a dressing.

At St. Martin's Village, Mrs. M has her own apartment; which she maintains with minimal assistance; receives one hot meal each day in a common dining room, and has access to a full range of services such as a beauty shop, recreational facilities, and a chapel. She is generally happy in this setting. She has no immediate family nearby, and the cost of the facility was covered by a large, one-time gift from her now deceased husband. Recently, she has become much weaker and has had difficulty walking; attending activities, including meals; and changing the dressing on her ear. The nurse at St. Martin's Village is sent to evaluate this client.

- Select two nursing models and apply their principles to this case study. Make sure you include the concepts of client, health, environment, and nursing.

5

The Process of Educating Nurses

Joseph T. Catalano

Learning Objectives

After completing this chapter, the reader will be able to:

- Compare the major differences among the diploma, associate degree nursing, and bachelor of science in nursing educational programs.
- Discuss at least three types of advanced nursing degrees.
- Distinguish between the different types of doctoral degrees available to nurses.
- Explain the concept of advanced practice for nurses.

EDUCATIONAL PATHWAYS

Unlike many other professions, nursing has several related, but unique, educational pathways that lead to licensure and professional status. Indeed, the current system of nursing education creates a great deal of confusion about nursing not only among the public but also among nurses themselves. Perhaps the belief that "a nurse is a nurse is a nurse" developed because, even though registered nurses may be prepared in educational programs that vary in length, orientation, and content, the graduates all take the same licensing examination and, superficially, all seem to be able to provide the same level of care. The licensure examination measures knowledge at the minimal level of safe practice. The workplace, in general, has not provided pay differences to distinguish levels of education despite studies showing performance differences.

PARADIGM SHIFTING

As in times past, the current profession of nursing faces many difficult challenges and extraordinary opportunities. Future trends in health care are being driven by a number of powerful societal forces that are producing an inevitable reshaping of health-care delivery. Traditionally somewhat insulated from the forces of change, nursing educators have been forced to recognize that graduates need to be prepared with knowledge and skills that are in tune with a rapidly evolving health-care system (Box 5.1). The most powerful of these forces of change are:

- Health-care reform that will increase the availability of health care to increasing numbers of clients and ethnic groups who previously were shut out of the health-care market

Box 5.1
New Administration = New $$$$ for Nursing Students!

If you are a nursing student, you know first-hand how expensive nursing school can be. The good news is that there is now significantly more money available through federal grants and loans than there has been in more than the previous 8 years. Barack Obama has been a champion for nurses since his time in the Illinois state senate, when he served on the Public Health Committee. As a U.S. Senator, he sponsored the Safe Nursing and Patient Care Act of 2007, which limits mandatory overtime for nurses except in major emergencies. He recognizes the value of nurses in the health-care system and the key role they will play in the recently passed Health Care Reform Act. He is also well aware of the nursing shortage and its effect on quality of care and the safety of clients.

In 2009, shortly after taking office, President Obama wrote an executive order that reversed the reduction in funds for nursing students implemented by the previous administration in a misguided attempt to cut spending. In 2009, he signed into law a $15 million increase for nursing grants and scholarships, bringing the total to $171 million, the highest amount since 2000.

Some grants and loans available through the Title VII Workforce Development Program include:
- *Workforce Diversity Grants.* These grants are aimed specifically at individuals who come from a disadvantaged background. They benefit students with very low incomes, ethnic and racial minorities, and groups that are under-represented in the nursing profession. These are outright grants directly to the student and do not need to be repaid.
- *Nurse Education, Practice, and Retention Grants.* These grants go to schools of nursing and other entities that educate nurses or work to improve the quality of health care. Students benefit from these grants indirectly with better facilities, additional faculty, and improved learning. For example, some schools have received money to purchase PDAs or iPads for all their students to enhance electronic learning.
- *Nurse Student Service Corps.* These grants go directly to nursing students to repay loans after they graduate if they decide to work in a designated shortage area for 2 years after graduation. They generally will pay off 60% to 85% of any loans used during nursing school.
- *Comprehensive Geriatric Education Grants.* These grants go directly to nursing students who make a commitment to care for elderly clients after graduation. The grants can also be obtained by faculty who wish to increase their knowledge of working with elderly clients and to schools of nursing that provided continuing education in elder care.

This is only a partial list of funds that have become available since 2009. As with all government-related funding, considerable forms and paperwork need to be completed. However, the effort of spending an hour or so filling out forms can reap great rewards.

Sources: Conant R: President Obama signs omnibus ... includes $15 million of Nursing Workforce Development Programs. 2009. Retrieved August 2010 from http://www.rnnation.org.
Ebner AL: What nurses need to know about health care reform. Nursing Economic$ 28(3):191–194, 2010.
Three easy steps to finding a nursing scholarship ... plus five great scholarships to get you started. American Nurse Today 5(6), 2010.

- The wider use of capitated managed care for financing coverage and a market-driven system
- The increasing age and diversity of the U.S. population
- A shortage of registered nurses
- A shortage of qualified nursing faculty
- The rapid leaps forward in health-care and information technology

Since the year 2000, about 60 percent of nurses have been employed in acute care hospitals.[1] Hospitals have attempted to slow the drain to other employment settings by seeking Magnet Status certification, which identifies the facility as being "nurse friendly" and a place where nurse turnover rate is low.[2] The other 40% of nurses are employed in a wide variety of settings, including private practice, public health agencies, home health care, primary nursing school–operated nursing centers, **ambulatory care centers,** insurance and managed-care companies, education, and health-care research. There is also an ever-growing group of **emerging health occupations** that have not yet been officially recognized by professional organizations.

What Do You Think?

Does an individual prepared in a technical course of study have enough knowledge to be a provider of professional nursing care in today's more complex health-care system? Do you think that the American Nurses Association (ANA) position statement on nursing education advocates a valid position? If yes, what can be done to bring nursing education into line with it?

What Nursing School Graduates Must Know and Be Able to Do

It has always been a challenge for nursing educators to decide what nursing students need to learn before they graduate. Some of the curricular content is dictated by the licensure examination, but high-quality nursing programs recognize that this test knowledge is the minimum required for safe practice at an entry level. The health-care marketplace demands more than the minimum. In this regard, the consumers of the products of nursing education, that is, the health-care entities that hire nursing school graduates, have had an important if somewhat unstructured role in determining curricular content.

In an attempt to structure the input from the facilities, a study was conducted to survey administrators who worked at hospitals, home health-care agencies, and nursing homes. They were asked to rank 45 skills or knowledge-based competencies they expected to see in the baccalaureate-level graduate nurses they hired. The results showed a mix of skills and knowledge competencies that

were most sought after. Those that ranked the highest included:

- Teaching clients health promotion and prevention
- Teaching clients about how lifestyle affects health
- Effective supervision of less educated staff
- Effective delegation and monitoring of staff
- Efficient organization of routine daily tasks
- Safe administration of medications
- Competence in the use of computer databases and charting
- Ability to organize nursing care for 6 to 10 clients at the same time

Overall, the expectations for new graduates cluster around the ability to initiate and adapt to change, use critical thinking in problem-solving, attain a basic level of skills, and be able to communicate with both clients and staff. It is interesting to note that the basic competencies have not changed much since Nightingale organized her first nursing school. Like her students, current students still need to master basic skills and learn to communicate effectively. Current leaders in nursing education have built on these principles and developed the Quality and Safety Education for Nurses (QSEN) competencies to help guide what is being taught in nursing curricula. (See Issues Now: QSEN Competencies Guide Nursing Curriculum, later in this chapter.)

Health-care technology has advanced so rapidly in recent years, however, that it has put a strain on both the faculty teaching nursing students and students attempting to master it.

The Pew Report

The Pew Health Professions Commission Report, sometimes referred to as the Pew Report, was published in the late 1990s. However, its recommendations for nursing education reform ring as true today as they did when the report was first issued.[3] Its 21 recommendations for all schools preparing health-care professionals are comprehensive and include:

- Expanding the scientific basis of the programs
- Promoting interdisciplinary education
- Developing cultural sensitivity
- Establishing new alliances with managed-care companies and government
- Increasing the use of computer technology and interactive software

The Pew Report also recommends a differentiated practice structure to simplify and consolidate the titles that are used for the different practitioner levels so that there is just one title for each level.

Nursing educators are continually challenged to evaluate whether the graduates of their programs are adequately prepared to meet the demands of all areas of care. Nursing educators also need to evaluate whether their own educational and skill preparation is sufficient to meet the needs of diverse health-care settings.

NURSES OF THE FUTURE

Nurses of the future will need to practice with self-reliance, independence, and flexibility. They will be required to have well-developed decision-making skills on the basis of critical thinking ability, a working knowledge of community resources, and computer and technical competencies. Just as important, they will need to deliver high-quality client education and care while working within the constraints of a managed-care system with tight cost-control measures.

Will nursing education ever be able to prepare a graduate who fulfills all the qualities required of nurses of the future? Nursing education responds with a "yes," but only with curricular revisions that provide graduates with the tools to continue to learn as they advance in their careers.

Hospital Skills and More
Hospital-based acute care nursing practice will always have an important place in any health-care system. Highly skilled acute care nurses will always find a place to practice. It is generally accepted that the older population requires more health care of all types—acute, chronic, and community based. Although the current system experienced a decrease in the use of acute care beds, a gradual reverse in this trend is beginning as the "baby boomers" become the senior citizens who require more care for acute problems.

Paradigm shifting in nursing education does not need to be an either/or proposition. It is sometimes felt that nursing education is either acute care focused or community focused. Nursing education needs to combine the two so that the graduate can practice with competence in either or both settings. The skills are similar, but the emphasis may be different. Although some hospital skills are being done by non-nurses at a cheaper cost, nursing education must still teach such important skills as critical think-ing, therapeutic relationship, **primary care,** and **case management,** as well as how to be comfortable with a consumer-driven health-care system.

Critical Thinking
Critical thinking has been an important element in nursing practice for many years. It is generally recognized as the ability to use basic core knowledge and decision-making skills in resolving situations with a relatively small amount of data and a high degree of risk and ambiguity. It is the basis for clinical judgment used by nurses in making decisions about client care and a key part of the nursing licensure examination. Although it has not always been called critical thinking, nursing has long been concerned with the ability to make good judgments and decisions about client care. (See Chapter 6 for a fuller discussion of critical thinking.)

At a fundamental level, the nursing process is a type of critical thinking. Unfortunately, in the health-care system of the future, a nurse's critical thinking skills will have to go far beyond those of the basic nursing process. Nursing education will need to prepare students for more advanced critical thinking by exposing them to real-life situations that require the use of creativity, intuition, analysis, and deductive and inductive reasoning. These situations are introduced in the classroom as case studies and are reinforced in the clinical setting through guided experiences and mentoring.

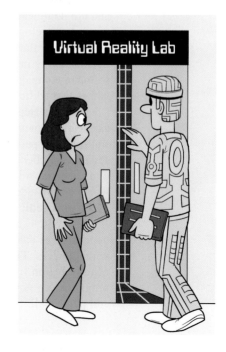

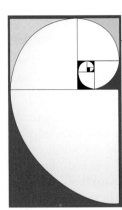

Issues Now

Here to Stay: e-Nursing Education

As everyone is now aware, there is a nursing shortage, projected to get worse over the next 10 to 20 years. Compounding the nursing shortage is a shortage of nursing faculty qualified to educate new nurses. One current trend viewed by some as a possible solution to the lack of nursing faculty is e-nursing education.

Almost all schools of nursing have been gradually incorporating more and more computer technology into their programs. However, full immersion into e-nursing education requires not only a total acceptance of technology but also a shift in fundamental thought processes that go beyond what is currently accepted for the age of information. As a general rule, nurses find change difficult, and nursing faculty like change even less. Fortunately, the changes in technology have come in small doses, which are much more palatable than major upheavals in knowledge.

Both nursing students and nursing instructors can look forward to several key technologies in the not-too-distant future. "Intelligent" assistive health-care devices have spurred the growth of new industries that did not exist even 10 years ago. Artificial limbs that respond to computer-mediated signals from the brain are being used by the victims of the violence in the Middle East. Elderly people and those with mobility problems are being helped by intelligent walkers not only to ambulate but also aid to change position from sitting to standing and back. Nursing education will need to keep pace with these developments by teaching students how to use these devices and educate clients in their use.

All nursing faculty are aware that current nursing students are not like students of the past, even the recent past. Referred to as "Generation E" or "Millennials" and raised with computers and cell phones, these students do not respond well to sitting in lecture classes. They like to be more interactive and adapt readily to new technologies. They are masters at electronic multitasking and are nonlinear in their thought processes. The challenge for nursing educators is to develop and use technologies that keep these students engaged while ensuring that they master the vast amount of material required to practice nursing safely in today's complex health-care environment. Several educational software companies are beginning to develop simulators and electronic learning games that address this need.

One step beyond simulation learning is virtual reality. Still in its infancy as a learning methodology, it has great potential for education. It would allow students total participation in health-care scenarios, ranging from counseling sessions for clients with psychiatric disorders to advanced life support resuscitation of a client in cardiac arrest. Combined with simulation technology, virtual reality would allow students to use the equipment that they can expect to be familiar with in the work setting.

Wireless technology also has the potential to provide new learning opportunities and techniques. Access to the Internet is no longer tied to hard-wired devices. Through the cellular networks, anyone can access a whole world of information from e-mail to video streaming. Students enrolled in online programs can now access them from almost any place where they can make a cell phone call. Some publishing companies have begun offering textbooks in

ISSUES NOW continued

electronic form (e-texts). Incorporated into these books are interactive exercises, videos, and simulation activities. Students can now "read" their textbooks anywhere they can take their wireless computers.

What will the nursing classroom of the future look like? It is a sure bet that the whole experience will be different. In reality, there may be no centrally located classrooms at all. Classroom lectures and interactive discussions will be conducted electronically over wireless devices. The way students learn will not be as important as what they learn, and learning will be measured through outcome testing. Nursing education will be asynchronous and available to anyone anywhere. In the far distant future, there may be only one nursing school for the whole country.

Sources: Connors H: HIT plants SEEDS in healthcare education . . . Health Information Technology . . . Simulated E-eEalth Delivery System. Nursing Administration Quarterly 31(2):129–133, 2007.

Newman L: Creating new futures in nursing education: Envisioning the evolution of e-nursing education. Nursing Education Perspectives 27(1):12–15, 2006.

Ornes LL: Computer competencies in a BSN program. Journal of Nursing Education 46(2):75–78, 2007.

Spalla TL: Technology. You've got mail: A new tool to help Millennials prepare for the National Council Licensure Examination. Nurse Educator 32(2):52–54, 2007.

The Therapeutic Relationship
Trust Is Essential

Therapeutic relationship skills have been long stressed by mental health nursing faculty as a key element in the treatment of psychiatric problems. In reality, therapeutic relationship skills are essential for all nurses to fulfill their roles as health-care providers and healers. Although these skills are currently being taught in a limited and focused way in most schools of nursing, they need to be expanded to involve directed services and relationship-centered nursing care.

Relationship-centered nursing care is client focused and revolves around the client's trust in, value of, and understanding of the nurse's skills and role in the healing process. The client must be able to feel comfortable with the nurse and share his or her understanding of both illness and health.

Follow-up Care

Currently, in many licensed practical nurse and licensed vocational nurse (LPN/LVN) programs and schools offering the associate degree in nursing, clinical experiences consist of one-time, 8-hour provision of care for an acute or chronically ill client. Little time is spent in follow-up care. However, many bachelors of nursing science (BSN) programs and some associate degree nursing (ADN) programs have expanded clinical experiences to include **discharge planning** and follow-up home health-care experiences.

To meet the demands of the future health-care system, all nursing education programs must be able to develop learning experiences for students that involve care for selected individuals or families over extended periods of time, perhaps ranging from several weeks to several semesters.

Case Management
A Growing Need

Care management is a general term that refers to a method of coordinating care either with an individual client or on a system-wide basis. **Case management,** in a health-care system driven by the demand for cost-effective care, usually is associated with coordinating care for an individual client as he or she moves from one level to another through the health-care system. Case management is now a certified specialty; however, there is an identified lack of qualified nurses trained in case management. Almost all the proposals for revisions in the health-care system include the **case manager** as an important element in the overall management of care.

Currently, case managers do not have to be registered nurses. Many individuals with degrees in social work and human resources, as well as registered nurses, are serving in the capacity of case managers. Perhaps the ideal situation would be to function as a **health-care team,** with both a registered nurse and a social worker coordinating all aspects of the client's care.

A Wide Range of Skills

As case managers, nurses are responsible for developing clinical pathways and for directing and guiding the overall health care of a specific group of clients. Case management includes not only overseeing the clients' care while they are in the hospital but also following clients through their rehabilitation at home, long-term follow-up, health-care practices, and developmental stages.

The knowledge and thinking required by an effective case manager go far beyond what is currently required of new graduates. Nurses must be able to understand not only the immediate disease process but also the long-term outcomes and factors that influence the disease. Case managers must also practice health-focused nursing and primary levels of intervention. Decisions will need to be made about care from a broad **database** as well as an understanding of the client's abilities, knowledge level, and even financial status.

Nursing education will be severely challenged to provide experiences to prepare students for this role. Students must be allowed to experience the authority, accountability, and responsibility of guiding a client's health care over an extended period. It might be beneficial to combine the learning experiences mentioned earlier in establishing the therapeutic relationship with the managed-care experience.

The Consumer in Authority

A consumer-driven health-care system is at one and the same time the nurse's dream and nightmare. Many widely used nursing models or theories claim to be client centered, which translates into being consumer driven. Yet, when these models are put into practice, the care given is more provider driven than anything else.

Care as Requested

A client/consumer-driven health-care system means that the care given and the outcomes are both determined by the consumer. The nurse must be able to accept the authority of the group or community as a determinant of health care. The nurse's role becomes one of a partner in guiding, implementing, and overseeing ways to deliver requested health care for a given community.

Many nursing programs, particularly baccalaureate programs, include a course in community health and home health-care nursing. Often, a requirement of this course is to have the students perform a community survey in which they determine the needs of the community as they perceive them. Many of these courses have been modified so that the students learn the community members' perceptions of their own needs.

Paradigm shifting is never easy. Major paradigm shifts in thinking and acting are even more difficult. Nursing education is currently dealing with a huge paradigm shift. How educators are meeting these challenges will, to a large extent, shape the future of professional nursing.

AMERICAN NURSES ASSOCIATION POSITION PAPER ON EDUCATION FOR NURSES

A Historical Perspective

After evaluating the changes that occurred in the health-care system during the 1950s and studying the projected educational needs for nurses, the ANA published a paper in 1965 that took a stand on an issue that was, and still is, highly controversial. Although written more than 40 years ago, this document is still relevant to many of the issues in nursing education today.

For full appreciation of the significance of this paper, it must be examined from a historical perspective. The overall purpose of the ANA has always been to ensure high-quality nursing care to the public by fostering high standards of nursing practice. In addition, the ANA was concerned with furthering the professional and educational advancement of nurses as well as protecting their occupational welfare. To achieve these goals, the ANA took responsibility for establishing the scope of practice for nurses and for guaranteeing the competence of those who claim the title of nurse.

After World War II, there was an explosion of scientific and technological knowledge used in health care. The educational level of the population was also increasing, resulting in greater public demand for higher-quality health care. In re-evaluating the nature and scope of nursing practice and the type and level of quality of education needed to meet these new demands, the ANA reached the conclusions that are presented in its position paper.

Support for the Bachelor's Degree

Since 1965, the ANA has upheld the belief that baccalaureate education should be the basic level of preparation for professional nurses. Specifically, the ANA concluded that:

> The education for all those who are licensed to practice nursing should take place in institutions of higher education; minimum preparation for beginning professional nursing practice at the present time should be the baccalaureate degree education in nursing; minimum preparation for beginning technical nursing practice at the present time should be associate degree education; education for assistants in the health care service occupations should be short, intensive preservice programs in vocational education institutions rather than on the job training.[4]

Nursing education will need to prepare students for more advanced critical thinking by exposing them to real-life situations that require the use of creativity, intuition, analysis, and deductive and inductive reasoning.

There were several assumptions on which the ANA based this position paper:

- Nursing is a helping profession and, as such, provides services that contribute to people's health and well-being.
- Nursing is of vital significance to the individual receiving services; it meets needs that cannot be met by the client, the family, or other persons in the community.
- The demand for the services of nurses will continue to increase.
- The professional practitioner is responsible for the nature and quality of all nursing care that clients receive.
- The services of professional practitioners of nursing will continue to be supplemented and complemented by the services of nurse practitioners who will be licensed.

- Education for those in the health-care professions must increase in depth and breadth as scientific knowledge expands.
- The health care of the public, in the amount and to the extent needed and demanded, requires the services of large numbers of health occupation workers, in addition to those licensed as nurses, to function as assistants to nurses. These workers are presently designated nurses' aides, orderlies, assistants, and attendants.
- The professional association must concern itself with the nature of nursing practice, the methods for improving nursing practice, and standards for membership in the professional association.[4]

Specialization and Interdependence

The rationale for taking such a strong stand on the future of nursing education derived from recognition by the profession of its heritage, its immediate problems, emerging social issues and trends, the nature of nursing practice, and the extent to which nurses could realistically enact changes for continued professional progress. The ANA drew on Florence Nightingale's vision of nursing and nursing education, which emphasized the value of education for the development of the profession. It was important to Nightingale that schools of nursing be independent of hospitals and have a strong theoretical component on which to base clinical practice.

By recognizing the increasing complexity of society, the ANA realized that nursing was not only becoming more specialized but also moving toward greater interdependence with other groups in society. One of these key groups was the U.S. government. As the federal government began increasing aid for nursing education, educational facilities expanded, providing greater opportunities for professional advancement. Larger numbers of students with more varied backgrounds were recruited into the profession, requiring greater flexibility in nursing education programs to accommodate their needs.

More recently, consumer groups have added their voice to the call for higher-quality and better-educated nurses. Huge numbers of medication errors and mistakes that lead to injury and death of clients have even attracted the attention of the U.S. Congress.

Schools of nursing were, at the same time, hard-pressed to meet the attendant demands of science and technology that were changing the traditional role of nurses. In addition to expanding roles for nurses, greater consumer awareness and expectations were placing new demands on nurses' abilities.

Even in 1965, the ANA recognized that nurses were required to master a very large and extremely complex body of knowledge. In addition, nurses were being increasingly called on to make critical and independent decisions about client care.

Effects of the ANA Paper

The implications of the ANA paper were far reaching and highly controversial. This paper affected many different elements of society and the health-care industry.

A Changing Role for Hospitals

Hospitals recognized that they would no longer retain their traditional role of preparing nurses for practice. Even though pressure to move nursing education from hospital-based diploma schools to institutions of higher education had been building for some time, in the mid-1960s, 75 percent of the graduating nurses were from hospital-based diploma programs.[5]

Colleges Under Pressure

Colleges and universities were pushed to quickly develop undergraduate and graduate curricula for increasing numbers of nursing majors. The relatively few baccalaureate programs in existence at the time were generally small and found it difficult to expand rapidly. It also became evident that a clear distinction between technical and professional programs needed to be made.

The Debate Continues

To this day, the ANA remains firmly committed to its stand that all nursing education should be housed in institutions of higher learning. More than 40 years have elapsed since this statement was made, and the profession of nursing is still trying to reach a consensus on the issue of basic educational preparation for entry into practice.

Over the past few years, several states have been looking at the BSN in Ten proposal, which would require graduates from ADN programs to obtain their BSN degrees within 10 years after graduating from the ADN program. As with almost all other proposals aimed at upgrading the education of professional nursing, this proposal has been met with fierce and concentrated opposition from ADN programs. Because of the superiority of numbers of the ADN programs, and some misguided support from medical and hospital associations, it appears at this time that the proposal will die a quiet and largely unnoticed death.

An examination of the current entry into practice debate from an educational perspective reveals a number of similarities in the social and political pressures felt by nursing in 1965. Not only do these same challenges exist in today's health-care system but also many new challenges have developed because of fast-paced technology developments and social changes.

> " *A consumer-driven health-care system is at one and the same time the nurse's dream and nightmare.* "

Defining a Profession

A similar resolution defining entry into practice was proposed by the ANA in 1985, but it also met strong opposition and was never enacted. In 1996, the American Association of Colleges of Nursing (AACN) presented its own position paper emphasizing the belief that the baccalaureate degree should be the minimal requirement for entry into the nursing profession. The discussion remains ongoing with seemingly little hope for resolution. The most influential reasons these proposals have not been adopted are economic, not conceptual. Although some experts believe it is time to leave the old debate behind and work toward developing a better-educated profession in general, many others see the issue as important to the definition of nursing as a profession.

Continuing the discussion and efforts to bring about collaborative agreement on nursing education is a goal that the profession must work toward. Only after the issue of basic entry-level education for professional nursing is resolved, and when nurses, like all other professionals, obtain their knowledge from recognized schools of higher education, will nursing as a profession be able to resolve its other important problems. Advancement of clinical practice, preparation for advanced practice roles, and an increased body of nursing knowledge all depend on baccalaureate entry-level education for professional nurses.

DIPLOMA SCHOOLS

No Academic Degree
The Nightingale School of Nursing was a diploma school in the strict use of the term. When nurses graduated from this school they were given a certificate or diploma noting their graduation, but no academic degree. The first graduates from the Nightingale School soon began to establish their own schools of nursing based on the Nightingale model and adhered to her philosophy of nursing education. These were also diploma schools.

An Improvement in Care
After an initial period of uncertainty and trepidation, both physicians and hospital administrators began to recognize that when the education of nurses improved, so too did the overall quality of the care provided by their hospitals. They also understood that these types of schools that were closely associated with hospitals could provide a source of free, or inexpensive, labor in the form of nursing students.

Diploma schools sprang up throughout Europe so that, in time, each hospital had its own school of nursing. Many of Nightingale's principles and concerns about nursing education were abandoned during this period of growth.

Catching Up to Europe
In the United States, developments in nursing education, as with health care in general, lagged behind those in Europe. It was not until the mid-1870s that the first school of nursing was established in the United States. This was a diploma school attached to the New England Hospital for Women.[6]

As in Europe, the idea of diploma schools quickly caught on, and within 10 years almost every large hospital in the United States had its own diploma school of nursing. These schools had very little in common with the Nightingale School of Nursing. There was no uniformity in curriculum, length of program, or requirements. To guarantee adequate enrollment, candidates were again being recruited from the lowest levels of society.

Learning on the Job
A Source of Cheap Labor
In early hospital-based diploma schools of nursing, hospitals used the student nurses as a major source of free labor for their facilities. There was little or no classroom or theoretical study. The students learned exclusively by hands-on experience during their 12- to 14-hour, 7-day-a-week work shifts.

Most of the students were young, single women recruited just after they graduated from high school. They were confined to dormitories on the hospital property. The dormitories were monitored closely by a housemother who enforced the rigorous rules of behavior covering all aspects of the students' lives and dismissed students for even minor infractions of the rules. The early diploma schools of nursing were organized and administered on a model that was similar to the strictest of the religious orders.

Submission to Authority
The nurses who graduated from these schools were proficient in basic nursing skills and could assume positions in the hospital where they were trained or in home nursing, where they worked on a case-by-case basis without any additional orientation or education. Because of the 24-hour-a-day, 7-day-a-week socialization process administered by these schools, diploma graduate nurses tended to be very submissive to authority and willing to carry out any duty to please the physician, administrator, or head nurse. Before the advent of licensure examinations and standardization of practice, nurses from diploma schools were often limited to employment in their own training institutions or in home health-care settings.

A Move Toward Accreditation
Diploma schools of nursing remained relatively unchanged in the United States until 1949, when the National Nursing Accrediting Service, working under the guidance of the National League for Nursing Education, became the licensing body for all schools of nursing that voluntarily sought accreditation.

The first formal accreditation of nursing schools occurred in the early 1950s. In 1952, the National League for Nursing (NLN) assumed accrediting responsibilities for all schools of nursing.[7] Accreditation by the National League for Nursing Accrediting Commission (NLNAC) has always been and remains a voluntary undertaking.

Outcome Criteria

To be accredited by the NLN, schools of nursing had to meet specific **outcome criteria** and teach specific content in their curricula. Many of the diploma schools of nursing could not or would not comply with these criteria and eventually closed. Some of the requirements for the schools that did choose to comply with the NLN included:

• Implementing a 3-year course of study meeting the criteria established by the state board of nursing using only faculty with baccalaureate or higher degrees in nursing
• Developing a philosophy and demonstrating how that philosophy was implemented through learning objectives, course objectives, and outcome criteria
• Showing an adequate pass rate on the State Board or National Council Licensure Examination (NCLEX)

A Jump in Expense

One of the key factors that all state boards of nursing were concerned about was that the school be able to demonstrate that the students were not being used as unpaid hospital personnel while they were in their education and training programs. When students could no longer be used as free labor, diploma nursing schools went from being virtually free to the hospital to being very expensive.

Not only did the hospitals still have to pay for the room and board of the students, but they also now had to hire and pay additional staff because the students could no longer be included in the overall staff numbers. Even more diploma schools closed because of the financial burdens to the hospitals. The schools that stayed open began increasing their tuition rates to the point that they were as expensive as programs granting academic degrees.

> *Continuing the discussion and efforts to bring about collaborative agreement on nursing education is a goal that the profession must work toward.*

CONVERTING THE CURRICULUM

During the 1960s and 1970s, many diploma schools became associated with universities and converted their curricula into degree-granting programs. According to recent data published by the NLN, approximately 100 accredited diploma programs remain open in the United States. They are of universally high quality and meet all the standards necessary for NLN accreditation. The main emphasis remains on preparing nurses who are highly competent in technical nursing skills through extensive hands-on practice in the clinical setting, but elements of leadership, humanities, and general sciences are also included in the classroom setting.[8]

ASSOCIATE DEGREE NURSING

The **associate degree nursing (ADN) program** was developed by Mildred Montague as a short-term solution to the nursing shortage experienced after World War II.[9] Originally designed to prepare students for technical nursing practice, the 2-year ADN programs were offered through community colleges with an emphasis on developing the skills necessary to provide high-quality bedside care in less time than BSN programs.

Technical Orientation

A successful pilot program for ADNs was conducted by Montague at Teachers' College in Columbia University in New York City in 1952 to prepare technical nurses who could assist professional nurses. It demonstrated that community college–based programs could attract large numbers of students, prove cost effective, and produce skillful technical nurses in half the time required for BSN programs.[10]

Which Exam to Take?

Early on, there was some heated debate concerning licensure and titling for this group of nurses. The technical orientation of the curriculum was, and remains, very similar to that found in programs that prepare LPNs, but the location of the programs in the community college setting and the increased theoretical orientation seemed to elevate these programs to a higher educational plane. It was finally decided that the ADN graduates should take the registered nurse (RN) licensure examination rather than the LPN/LVN examination.

A Proven Track Record

The emphasis on technical skills of the ADN programs met a need in the health-care system of the 1960s and 1970s. By the early 1980s, there were more than 800 ADN programs across the United States; as of 2007, the number was close to 900, with more than 63,000 students attending.[11] Graduates from these programs soon exceeded the number of graduates from all the diploma, BSN, and LPN/LVN programs combined.

Although it is possible to complete the requirements for an ADN in 2 academic years, most programs take at least 3 years to complete for a new student who has no prior college credit.[11] ADN graduates have a proven track record for providing safe bedside care for clients from the first day they are hired. They function well as team members and, after a period of orientation, can assume responsibility for the care of clients who are more acutely ill.

> *In early hospital-based diploma schools of nursing, hospitals used the student nurses as a major source of free labor for their facilities. There was little or no classroom or theoretical study.*

BACCALAUREATE EDUCATION

A Slow Increase

The development of schools of nursing in the university and college setting was a gradual process that extended over several decades. Only a few collegiate nursing programs were established during the years when the diploma programs were expanding. Some of these early collegiate programs were a hybrid mixture of college-level classes and diploma school clinical experiences that still granted only a diploma rather than an academic degree.

Early attempts at college-level nursing programs sometimes took the form of "pre-nursing" courses over a 1- or 2-year period that prepared students to enter upper-division schools of nursing.

Generally acclaimed as the first university program to be completely conducted in the higher education setting, the University of Minnesota School of Nursing was opened in 1909. In 1923, the Yale School of Nursing began accepting students; it is considered the first autonomous college of nursing in the United States.

The number of university-based nursing programs gradually increased over the years, and by the beginning of World War II, there were 76 programs granting baccalaureate degrees in nursing. These programs tended to specialize in preparing nurses for public health nursing, teaching, administration, and supervisory positions in hospitals. Although all these programs included a clinical component, the emphasis was more on theoretical knowledge, development of critical thinking, decision-making skills, and leadership.

Universities in general enjoyed rapid growth immediately after World War II, and higher-education nursing programs expanded along with the universities. Many military nurses, prepared by the Cadet Nurse Corps during World War II, went back to school under the G. I. Bill to complete their baccalaureate degrees, thus providing the framework for current ADN to BSN programs.

Education for a Profession

During this rapid growth period, these **baccalaureate degree nursing programs** were plagued with problems similar to those found in the diploma programs during their own rapid expansion period. Primarily, the lack of uniformity in content, curriculum, and even length of programs was problematic. It was difficult to find qualified faculty because most of the nurses up to this time had received their education in diploma programs. No doctorate degrees existed in nursing, few nurses had master's degrees, and only a smattering of nurses had baccalaureate degrees.

During the late 1940s and early 1950s, awareness began to develop that there was a need to stratify nursing education programs into technical levels and professional levels. It became apparent that all health-care professionals should have, at minimum, a baccalaureate degree.[12]

The NLN began to develop strict criteria for the accreditation of baccalaureate nursing programs. These criteria included courses in general education, general sciences, humanities, and language as well as specific nursing courses. They required a certain number of hours to be spent in the clinical setting practicing nursing skills, a faculty prepared at the master's degree level, and the availability of laboratory and library facilities for the students. Faculty-to-student ratios were limited, particularly in the clinical setting, and outcome criteria were required for the students.[13]

Different Approaches

Although all university-level baccalaureate degrees in nursing have the same number of required credit hours and educational requirements, there are three avenues for attaining this degree.

The Professional Degree

The BSN degree fulfills the criteria of a professional degree. It meets the overall requirements for a college baccalaureate degree (120 to 124 credit hours, 65 hours of nursing major, and most of the general education requirements), but does not meet all the general education requirements for an academic bachelor of science (BS) degree. Although this degree is usually obtained in a traditional college setting, it can also be obtained through an **external degree** program in which the student has to meet the criteria for the BSN.

The Full Academic Degree

The second approach is found in programs that offer a bachelor of science degree with a major in nursing (BS Nursing). This degree is the full academic college degree and guarantees that the person holding it has met all of the general education, science, and major subject requirements. According to statistics published by the NLN for academic year 2007, there were more than 535 accredited programs offering baccalaureate degrees in nursing.

A third avenue that may be pursued is sometimes called the career ladder program (see the section, Ladder Programs, later in this chapter).

> *During the late 1940s and early 1950s, awareness began to develop that there was a need to stratify nursing education programs into technical levels and professional levels. It became apparent that all health-care professionals should have, at minimum, a baccalaureate degree.*

PRACTICAL/VOCATIONAL NURSING

The practical/vocational nurse, in one form or another, has been a part of the health-care system in the United States for well over 100 years. Although the earliest formal schools of practical/vocational nursing were started around 1890, informal training programs for this level of nursing probably existed well before that time—for example, in the Young Women's Christian Association (YWCA), particularly in New York City.

A Useful Trade

These programs took uneducated girls who had migrated from rural areas and farms to the cities in search of employment and taught them a useful trade with which they could support themselves. With no regulation or accreditation for the early practical/vocational nurse programs, there were wide variations in the quality, length, and focus of what was being taught. Generally, the students were taught to provide home care, similar to that given by private duty nurses, for clients ranging from newborns to elderly and invalid individuals.

The number of **practical/vocational nursing programs** gradually increased during the next 50 years. Graduates of these 3-month programs were beginning to find employment in hospitals and nursing homes as well as in areas of private duty. During the nurse shortage after World War I, many hospitals found that these relatively undereducated nurses, after receiving on-the-job training in the hospital, could function at a fairly high level of skill, and at a much reduced cost. The word got around, and soon the number of these unlicensed nurses grew.

Compulsory Licensure

By the late 1930s, the ANA saw the need to regulate the quality of the practical/vocational nursing programs to protect public safety. It was not until 1938 that the State of New York took seriously the ANA's recommendation for compulsory licensure for practical/vocational nurses and enacted the first law requiring such licensure.

In 1960, all practical/vocational nurses were required to pass a licensure examination before they could practice. These nurses are now referred to as licensed practical nurses (LPNs). In Texas and California, these nurses are called licensed vocational nurses (LVNs).

The Importance of Technique

Although education for LPNs and LVNs varies slightly from one state to another, there are some common characteristics. Most of the programs are from 9 to 12 months and are measured in clock hours rather than academic hours. They are often offered in hospitals, high schools, vocational schools, or trade schools, although some programs are conducted in community colleges or even in universities.

Orientation of the curricula in these programs is highly technical and emphasizes the learning of skills in the setting of a hospital or nursing home, with less emphasis on theoretical knowledge. Because they are **technicians,** it is much more important for practical/vocational nurses to learn *how* to do something than *why* it is being done.

Filling a Shortage

The stated scope of practice for the practical/vocational nurse involves providing care for clients in hospitals, nursing homes, or the home setting for those who have stable conditions. LPNs/LVNs are to be under the supervision of an RN or a licensed physician.

However, in the real world, LPNs/LVNs are often required to provide care well outside their scope of practice, leaving them vulnerable to lawsuits. They often function in leadership roles or provide care in acute settings with highly unstable clients. LPNs/LVNs are often hired when there are shortages of RNs to fill the gaps in client care.

Many associate degree RN programs have developed a ladder curriculum whereby an LPN/LVN can go back to school for a shorter period, often receiving credit for years of experience, complete the program in 1 year, and then take the RN licensure examination.

LADDER PROGRAMS

Upward Mobility

Career ladder, educational ladder, **articulation,** or educational mobility programs have become increasingly popular as a result of an interest in **upward mobility,** educational articulation, and **career mobility.** A ladder program allows nurses to upgrade their education and move from one educational level to another with relative ease by granting credit for previous course work and experience and without loss of credits from previous education.

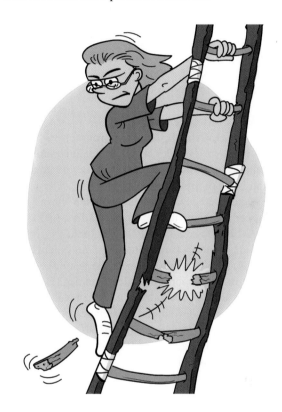

Each ladder program is developed according to the philosophy of the particular nursing school, may use any one of a number of curricular patterns, uses one of several means of **advanced placement** or credit granted for previous education, and must meet NLNAC accreditation standards.

Ladder programs take several different forms. Some ladder programs provide a **competency-based education** that allows the students to proceed at their own pace as long as they fulfill required educational outcomes. Ladder programs have become increasingly popular as colleges move toward Web-based courses and programs.

The Associate Ladder

The LPN/LVN-to-ADN ladder allows individuals who have been licensed as LPNs/LVNs to take a minimal number of courses in an associate degree program to obtain their ADN and then take the NCLEX-RN, CAT to become licensed as registered nurses. Programs vary widely as to how many credits they will accept from the LPN/LVN programs and how many courses the students take to complete the degree. Some of the requirements for number of hours are out of the control of the nursing programs because they have been established as general education requirements of the college or are state regent's requirements. These programs are highly compatible because of the similarity of curricula and the technical orientation of both types of programs.

The Baccalaureate Ladder

Some LPN/LVN-to-BSN ladder programs either allow licensed LPNs/LVNs to challenge a number of courses or grant them credit for nursing courses on the basis of previous experience and demonstrated competency. Students who enter these types of ladder programs usually spend more time in school than those in the LPN/LVN-to-ADN programs. In addition to meeting the requirements of the BSN, they also have to meet the general education requirements for a baccalaureate degree and complete 120 to 124 hours of college-level courses. One problem in developing these types of ladder programs is that many states' boards of regents do not recognize courses taken at the vocational-technical level as higher education courses and therefore will not transfer them into the college setting. One way around this requirement is for students to take challenge examinations in both general education courses and nursing courses. Once the students pass the test, they are granted college-level credit for the course. These examinations tend to be difficult and are really a type of outcome-based learning. However, they do not require the student to attend classes and are much cheaper than a regular college course.

Two Plus Two

Nursing education has seen a marked increase in the number of ADN-to-BSN and diploma-to-BSN ladder programs, sometimes called **two plus two (2 + 2) programs.** These programs admit individuals who are already licensed as registered nurses but who have either a diploma or an associate degree.

These programs may take several different forms. Upper-division baccalaureate programs work exclusively with RNs, have no generic students, and are designed exclusively to meet the educational needs of students who are already RNs. Many of these programs have adopted or are moving toward a totally online format: students take all of the classes on their home computers, with only minimal requirements for class attendance on campus. These types of classes work particularly well for students who work full-time and may have family responsibilities.

Other programs accept ADN or diploma graduates as students, in addition to generic students. These schools often have separate programs for ADNs or diploma RNs that allow them to take examinations to prove educational knowledge and nursing proficiency (**challenge examinations**) in specific classes, thus granting credit for their nursing experience. The RNs then take advanced-level nursing courses, such as Community Health/Home Health Care, Leadership, and Critical Care, which are not commonly found in diploma or ADN programs. Many of these programs also are online.

In either case, on completion of the degree requirements, these nurses are granted a baccalaureate degree. Some of these programs have an **open curriculum** that allows students to enter and leave the program freely. There are 418 such programs accredited by the NLNAC, and the number continues to grow.[11] The capacity to accept ADN graduates in to these completion programs is almost unlimited. Should the BSN in Ten proposal ever gain a toehold, there will be more than enough spaces for students coming from ADN programs.

Fast-Track Options

Some nursing programs have gotten creative in their attempt to educate nurses at the baccalaureate level. One approach is to place students who have a BS or BA degree in another major, such as biology or English, in fast-track programs that allow them to obtain their nursing degree in 1 or 2 years. In many ways, these programs are similar to the RN-to-BSN programs, but they also teach the basic nursing skills that ADN graduates already have.

The Master's Ladder
For the ADN

A growing trend in educational ladder programs is the ADN-to-MSN programs. Schools that offer this type of ladder must have an MSN program in place. The ADN students who enter these programs are given credit for prior classes and work experience and take both undergraduate- and graduate-level courses, receiving a BSN along the way to obtaining the MSN.

These programs vary a great deal from school to school and may require from three to five semesters of classes. Often they are offered on a part-time basis, with many evening and weekend classes or Web-based classes available to meet the needs of working students.

For the Nurse Practitioner

A less common type of educational ladder program is the nurse practitioner (NP)–to-MSN program. These programs admit nurse practitioners who graduated from programs that certified students but did not include enough credit hours for a master's degree. Again, the students are granted credit for past classes and work experience and often are allowed to challenge a certain number of core courses. Then they take the remaining required courses and are granted an MSN at graduation.

MASTER'S- AND DOCTORAL-LEVEL EDUCATION

The baccalaureate degree is considered a generalist degree that exposes a student to a wide range of subjects during the 4 years spent in college. The master's degree, on the other hand, is a specialist's degree.[14] Students who pursue a master's degree concentrate their study in one particular subject area and become expert in that given area.

> *Some early and current nurse leaders have stated that the master's degree in nursing should be the entry-level degree for the profession.*

Master's Degree Programs

Master's degree nursing programs have been in existence almost from the time baccalaureate-level nursing programs were started. Some early and current nurse leaders have stated that the master's degree in nursing should be the entry-level degree for the profession. The early master's degrees in nursing programs were designed for students who had baccalaureate degrees in other majors, such as biology, and wanted to become nurses. After completion of an additional 36 to 42 credit hours in nursing courses only, these students were awarded the MSN and could then take the licensure examination for registered nurses.

Experience Required

Today, most master's degrees in nursing programs are restricted to registered nurses who have the baccalaureate degree. Many of these programs require at least 1 year of clinical practice after the BSN and require an additional 36 to 46 college credit hours. Most students who enter master's degree programs attend classes on a part-time basis while they are working and may take up to 5 years to complete the requirements. Many universities have recognized this trend and have tailored their programs to meet the needs of these part-time students; universities now offer courses over the Internet, distance education in the evening and on weekends, or 1-day-a-week programs. There are 296 accredited master's degree programs in the United States.[11]

There are a number of available areas of study for those pursuing master's degrees in nursing. Some of the more popular areas include nursing administration, community health, psychiatric mental health, adult health, maternal–child health, gerontology, rehabilitation care, nursing education, and some more advanced areas of practice, such as anesthesiology, pediatric nurse practitioner (PNP), family nurse practitioner, geriatric nurse practitioner (GNP), and obstetric–gynecological nurse practitioner.[15] Many of these programs require the student to pass a comprehensive written or oral examination. Some courses require the student to write an extensive research thesis before graduation, although some programs are requiring a published journal manuscript in lieu of the thesis.

Professional and Academic Degrees

There are two basic types of master's degree in nursing. The master's of science in nursing (MSN) is the professional degree, and the master's of science with a major in nursing degree (MS Nursing) is the formal academic degree.[16] In practice, however, little differentiation is made between the two. Almost all master's programs accredited by the NLNAC require the applicant to have at least a 3.0 grade point average and to demonstrate academic proficiency by achieving a satisfactory score on the Graduate Record Examination (GRE) or the Miller's Analogy Test before admission. The GRE is also used to recommend remedial coursework needed to correct deficiencies before the master's program is undertaken.

What Do You Think?

Have you ever been to an advanced practice nurse for care? How would you rate the quality of that care? If you have not been to an advanced practice nurse, would you consider going to one for care? Why or why not?

Doctoral Programs

In the evolution of the various levels of education, the baccalaureate degree is a generalist's degree, the master's degree is a specialist's degree, and the academic doctoral degree is a generalist's degree, although at a much higher academic level than the baccalaureate degree. The major purpose of early doctoral degrees was to prepare the individual to conduct advanced research in a particular area of interest. Nurses holding these degrees conduct much of the research used in evidence-based practice (EBP). Currently, doctoral degrees for nursing practice are becoming popular and are considered specialists' degrees.

A Wide Range of Choices

Academic Doctorates

Currently there is a wide range of available doctoral degrees for nurses. The doctor of philosophy (PhD) degree is the most accepted academic degree and is designed to prepare individuals to conduct research. The doctor of education (EdD) degree is considered a professional degree, although in many programs there is little difference between the courses of study taken by the EdD and PhD candidates. In other programs, the PhD focuses primarily on research, whereas the EdD focuses more on administration in the educational setting. The classes and research credits differ somewhat between the two degrees.

Almost all PhD in Nursing programs have an additional focus on education because most PhD graduates will be teaching nursing in institutions of higher education. Nurses with PhDs learn about classroom teaching, curriculum development, and the evaluation process. Some programs require "nursing student teaching" for their candidates during their capstone courses to evaluate their teaching methodologies and techniques.

Professional Practice Doctorates

Since the 1970s, other doctoral programs for nurses have been developed to stress the clinical rather than the academic nature of nursing.[17] These include the doctor of nursing science (DNSc) and the doctor of science in nursing (DSN), which is a clinically oriented nursing degree. The doctor of nursing (DN or ND) degree is for the person with a BS or MS in a field other than nursing who wants to pursue nursing as a career. It is a generalist's degree at a basic level of education.

The Doctor of Nursing Practice degree (DNP) was first granted almost 20 years ago at Case Western University. However, at that time very few schools of nursing granted it, and there was a great deal of confusion about what the degree was and what nurses holding it could do. Very few nurses opted for the degree. The DNP is now being considered as the terminal degree for advanced practice nurses.

In recent years, there has been some discussion of making these degrees the basic entry-level degree into the profession of nursing. An additional degree for nurses who wish to pursue a career in higher education, the doctor of nursing education (DNEd) degree, is available.

Few Programs, Tough Requirements

Despite the wide range of doctoral degrees in nursing, relatively few programs across the United States offer these degrees. Many nurses who seek them may obtain them in fields such as higher education, psychology, college teaching, and adult education. Fewer than 2 percent of nurses hold doctoral degrees.

The requirements for all doctoral education degrees are similar, even though the specific degrees being sought may be different. The student must have attained a master's degree and must have achieved a satisfactory score on the GRE. Often candidates must go through an admission interview and preprogram examination before they can be formally admitted to the program. Doctoral programs are at least 60 college credit hours in length, require many statistics and research courses, and often have a residency requirement. Before the doctoral degree can be granted, the student must successfully complete both oral and written comprehensive examinations, as well as write a doctoral dissertation explaining the conducting of a major research project.

Many individuals now pursue doctoral degrees on a part-time basis while they are working full-time, whereas others attend classes full-time while working full-time, often completing the program in 3 to 4 years. Many programs have gone to a totally online format. Some programs require that the individual complete all the requirements within 10 years. Although this may seem like a long time, it is not unusual for the dissertation process itself to take 2 to 3 years.

Leaders in the Profession

Nurses with master's or doctoral degrees are regarded as leaders in the profession of nursing. Many of the larger hospitals in the United States require their unit managers and supervisors to have master's degrees and their directors of nursing or vice presidents of nursing to have doctorates. Of course, in baccalaureate programs, the minimal requirement for teaching is the master's degree, and the doctorate is preferred. Nurses with these advanced degrees provide direction and leadership for the profession through their publications, research, and theory development. As health-care delivery becomes more complicated, larger numbers of nurses with advanced degrees will be required.

EDUCATION FOR ADVANCED PRACTICE

> *In the evolution of the various levels of education, the baccalaureate degree is a generalist's degree, the master's degree is a specialist's degree, and the doctoral degree is a generalist's degree, although at a much higher academic level than the baccalaureate degree.*

"Advanced practice" is one of those often misused terms in nursing that add to the public's confusion about educational levels of those in the profession. The Advance Practice Registered Nurse (ARNP) certification has become the recognized credential for nurses receiving a master's degree in a specialized expanded practice role. It is also sometimes referred to as expanded role or expanded practice. Nurses who obtain certification are allowed to practice at a higher and more independent level depending on the nurse practice act of their individual state. Advanced practitioners diagnose illnesses, prescribe medications, conduct physical examinations, and refer clients to specialists for more intensive follow-up care. These nurses practice under their own licenses as independent practitioners but often work closely with a physician so that they can quickly refer clients who have medical problems that lie outside their scope of practice.

The Nurse Practitioner

The nurse practitioner levels of nursing are most widely accepted as advanced practice areas for nursing. These include the pediatric nurse practitioner (PNP), the neonatal nurse practitioner (NNP), the geriatric nurse practitioner (GNP), the obstetric–gynecological (OB-GYN) nurse practitioner, the family nurse practitioner (FNP), the rehabilitation nurse practitioner (RNP), the psychiatric nurse practitioner, and the nurse midwife.

The certified registered nurse anesthetist (CRNA) and nurse midwife are the oldest of the advanced practice specialties for nurses and are already well accepted in the medical community. Other advanced practice nurses experience varying levels of acceptance from physicians, although the public in general likes the care they receive from advanced practice nurses. All states now have granted some type of **prescriptive authority** to nurse practitioners.

In the past, nurses with baccalaureate degrees could attend highly concentrated courses of study for 1 to 2 years and increase their proficiency in a particular specialty area without obtaining an MSN. They could then take the certification examination and become certified as nurse practitioners. Currently, most nurse practitioner programs are offered in major universities, requiring students to complete the master's degree before allowing them to take the certification examination.[18]

The Clinical Nurse Specialist/Clinical Nurse Leader

One level of nursing that falls under the umbrella of advanced practice is the **nurse specialist,** or **clinical nurse specialist (CNS).** Although relatively few schools offer specific CNS curricula, these nurses are self-classified as CNSs after completing a master's degree, or some additional education, in a particular clinical area. However, in a few states, such as Ohio, the CNS designation requires a master's degree and a special licensing examination. CNSs are usually hired by hospitals and often function as in-service educators for the hospital. The clinical nurse leader (CNL) is an emerging role that advanced practice registered nurses (APRNs) can assume. The CNL is a generalist with a master's degree who can coordinate care for clients, use EBP in care, focus on quality improvement, and oversee risk management and client safety.[19]

The Scope of Advanced Practice

In 1988, an amendment to the New York Nurse Practice Act established a separate scope of practice and title protection for nurse practitioners (NPs). Subsequent to the NP amendment, there has been some confusion regarding which of the advanced nursing practice categories are included within the scope of practice, particularly clinical nurse specialists, nurse midwives, and certified nurse anesthetists. This confusion, especially in psychiatric mental health nursing and nurse anesthesia, is related to the legal interpretations of the NP amendment. The resultant debate about this issue has led to a clearer definition and understanding of the term *advanced practice registered nurse* (APRN).

The career opportunities for advanced practice nurses are numerous.[18] Many nurse practitioners work for county health departments, for rural clinics, and on Native American reservations; others work in hospitals, with physicians in private practice, and in rehabilitation centers. Some have even established their own independent clinics. APRNs often serve populations in areas where there is a lack of primary care physicians by providing primary health-care services. Although many of these areas are traditionally rural, today inner-city areas also often need this type of health care. With the passage of the Health Care Reform Act in 2010, the opportunity for APRNs will continue to grow. Health-care reform often requires that a client seeking entry into the health-care system be evaluated by a primary health-care practitioner before referral to a specialized practitioner. Although the family practice physician, or general practitioner, is the most common primary health-care provider to evaluate the client, the nurse practitioner can also function in this role.

DNP for the APRN?

Is the Master's Enough?

As the number of nursing schools granting the APRN increased and the number of APRNs grew, nursing leaders began to question whether all these nurse practitioners were prepared to meet the complexities of today's health-care system. These nursing leaders noticed that unlike dentists, physical therapists, or pharmacists, APRNs had no terminal degree. Because of the high level of skills and knowledge required for APRNs, many of whom can practice independently, they surmised that a clinical terminal degree focusing on practice expertise should be required for entry into the APRN level.[20]

Out of the many practice-oriented doctoral degrees discussed previously, the DNP seems best suited to meet the requirements of a terminal advanced practice doctoral degree. As a result, the AACN decided in 2004 that all advanced practice nursing master's degrees should transition to the DNP by the year 2015.[19] Currently practicing APRNs would not be affected except to be exempted into the new status. More than 50 other nursing organizations and societies have endorsed the proposal. However, questions linger.

Does It Make Sense?

Those who favor the transition to the DNP point out that practitioners need the highest levels of education to care for clients in today's complex and demanding health-care system. Requiring the DNP is the only way to guarantee high-quality and safe care. Credentialing all APRNs at the DNP level would provide better consistency in both the educational requirements and the titling of what is now a confusing array of programs and certifications. Those in favor also argue that current master's APRN programs have added so much practice and theoretical content in an attempt to keep current with the practice setting that they are almost at the doctoral level anyway.[21] Almost all professional practice specialty areas, except for nursing, now require a terminal degree. The DNP would seem the logical degree to demonstrate the high skill levels, knowledge, and expertise for nurses.

Those who do not support the DNP degree ask the questions: "How does the degree improve the practice of the APRN?" "Doesn't adding another degree only make it more confusing for the public?" Although no research has been conducted so far, it would be interesting to ask currently practicing APRNs if they believe they are practicing at the top levels of skills and knowledge and if an additional degree will make them "better." An additional degree does not necessarily make a higher-quality APRN. Then there is the question of cost.[22] Again, no research has been conducted to date about how much more it will cost to obtain a DNP than a master's degree. If a program converts an MSN to a DNP and only offers the DNP, the additional cost may be onerous. However, this is not known at this time.

The Long-Term Effect

The bigger objection to the DNP degree is its long-term effect on nursing education. The PhD has been the gold standard for nursing education since the beginning of college-level nursing baccalaureate degrees. Deans and chairpersons of nursing programs had to hold a PhD to earn accreditation from a national organization. Currently, at some schools, nurses holding the DNP degree are being appointed to dean and chairperson positions. Also, nurses with the DNP are now being hired as faculty with a terminal degree.[23] The intent is not to imply that any particular individual is unqualified for his or her job. However, because the DNP is advertised as a "practice" degree and not an educational degree, the DNP programs are not providing the content required for teaching or administering nursing programs. Most college and university administrators do not understand the difference between a PhD and a DNP. To them, a doctoral degree is a doctoral degree. They do recognize how difficult it is to find nurses with any type of post-master's degree, so finding a nurse with any kind of doctorate is like finding hidden treasure.

> *Most college and university administrators do not understand the difference between a PhD and a DNP. To them, a doctoral degree is a doctoral degree is a doctoral degree.*

The long-term impact on nursing education could be disastrous. In the short term, the negative effects are muted because all programs still have a mix of PhD and Master's in Nursing Education faculty along with DNP faculty. However, as time goes on and the current aging PhD population is replaced by DNP deans and faculty, the expertise and knowledge in areas such as curriculum development, evaluation, and teaching methodologies will be lost. Also, because much of the research currently used as the basis for EBP is conducted by PhD-prepared nurses, over time the profession will lose the ability to maintain its body of knowledge at a rate that matches the growth in technology and in medical and nursing knowledge.

The debate will go on; however, the change over to the DNP seems to be a certainty. It is extremely important for students who are thinking about obtaining advanced nursing degrees to consider the direction of their professional future. If they are truly interested in clinical practice as a lifelong career, the DNP is the degree to obtain. However, if they are even considering a career in education at some point in the future, the MSN in Nursing Education and the PhD are the way to go.[24]

Conclusion

In today's rapidly changing health-care environment, there is an ever-increasing need for health-care professionals who are educated to practice at the highest levels.[1] It is imperative that the schools that will be educating future nurses be responsive to the changes, challenges, and demands of an ever more sophisticated and technologically advanced health-care system. Nursing education is an important part of a much larger network of health-care systems, including the service and practice sector, government and regulatory agencies, and licensing and credentialing institutions. All of these interact with each other and together form what is called the health-care system.

The nursing profession has, over the years, developed a number of different types of education programs in an attempt to meet the demands of a growing health-care system. Some of the programs developed for specific needs that no longer exist should be examined for their usefulness and viability in today's advanced health-care atmosphere. Perhaps their resources could be rechanneled to programs that are more in tune with current needs. Students should carefully evaluate programs they might enter and decide which one best meets their care goals.

Meanwhile, nursing education continues to develop innovative approaches to help nurses meet the demands for more education, more technical

(continued)

Conclusion—cont'd

skills, and more leadership ability. The ladder programs are a good example. By recognizing the dynamic state of nursing education, and implementing changes that respond to or even anticipate changes in the health-care system, the nursing profession will continue as one of the pillars of the health-care system.

Educators in nursing have begun to recognize that it is impossible to teach nursing students everything they need to know in the short time allowed for formal education. The demands of the changing health-care system will make that goal even more difficult. However, it may not be necessary to teach nursing students everything. It is more important to teach these students the thinking, decision-making, and management skills that will allow them to adjust to an ever-changing and developing health-care system.

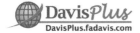

DavisPlus.fadavis.com

Critical Thinking Exercises

- Discuss why the current educational system for nurses leads to confusion over the role and scope of practice for nurses.
- The literature reports that there will be a nursing shortage well into the 21st century. What aspects of health-care reform are likely to produce changes in nursing education? Identify possible changes that may occur in nursing education because of the projected nursing shortage. Will these changes be beneficial or harmful to the profession of nursing?
- Are nurses holding the DNP degree better practitioners than those with an MSN? Defend your position.
- What should the minimum level of education be for the professional nurse—ADN, BSN, or MSN? Defend your position.

Issues Now

QSEN Competencies Guide Nursing Curriculum

The large numbers of medication and medical errors that occur in today's health-care system lead to the injury and death of as many as 90,000 clients per year. Driven by community and professional concerns, the Robert Wood Johnson Foundation undertook a three-phase project to improve the quality and safety of client care by focusing nursing education on student competency. The project, Quality and Safety Education for Nurses (QSEN), is built on five competencies developed initially by the Institute of Medicine (IOM).

Phase I began in 2005 with a $590,000 grant to the University of North Carolina at Chapel Hill School of Nursing. The goal of Phase I was to develop the theoretical foundations for QSEN, including student competencies; the knowledge, skills, and attitudes (KSAs) necessary to maintain a safe health-care system; and measurable outcomes for graduates of nursing programs. During Phase I, an additional competency (safety) was added to the five IOM competencies, bringing the total to six. These competencies are:

- Client-Centered Care
- Teamwork and Collaboration
- Evidence-Based Practice (EBP)
- Quality Improvement (QI)
- Safety
- Informatics

A thorough and extensive set of KSAs was developed for each competency for undergraduate students (www.qsen.org). In addition, Phase I established an electronic resources center, supported by the grant, that contains materials on client safety and quality initiatives.

Although Phase I was still ongoing, Phase II kicked off in 2007 with the goals of developing KSAs for graduate students and developing QSEN-based curricula in 15 selected schools. The 15 pilot schools are exploring the difficulties in implementing QSEN in their programs.

The Competency Outcomes Performance Assessment (COPA) model, developed in the early 1990s, has been used by medical schools and some schools of nursing to validate the skills and knowledge of their graduates. It is designed to promote competency for clinical practice at all levels. With a few modifications, the COPA model fits well with QSEN and can be used as the evaluation tool for graduates of these schools.

Phase III began in 2009 and is still ongoing. The goals of Phase III are:

- Developing nursing faculty knowledge and skills in teaching QSEN competencies
- Writing textbooks that include the six competencies
- Working with licensing, accreditation, and certification agencies to develop standards that reflect QSEN competencies
- Developing ongoing innovative methods to implement QSEN

Phase III will be in development for many years to come. Some of the pilot schools are beginning to publish information about their experiences implementing QESN as their curricular model. Overall, the conversion seems to be

Issues Now   continued

going smoothly and successfully. Nursing faculty resistance to change is an ever-present challenge.

One issue troubling some nursing leaders is that the QSEN competencies are based on a model developed by the IOM (i.e., a medical model). All agree on the need for quality and safety measures to reduce harm to clients, and QSEN certainly meets that need. However, for many years, the AACN's *Essentials of Baccalaureate Education for Professional Nursing Practice* has been the gold standard for outcomes for nursing programs. Is there a clearcut advantage in using the QSEN competencies over the *Essentials* as a curricular model?

Some nursing leaders believe that by conforming to QSEN-based curricula, they will transform the professional identity of nursing into something other than nursing. What about the competencies of caring, integrity, and client advocacy? What about research and scholarship? Where does prevention, a key nursing role since the time of Florence Nightingale, fit in? Those who support QSEN believe that if a nurse is providing high-quality and safe care, caring and integrity are already included. Others believe that a seventh competency, "Professional Person," should be added to include those aspects of nursing that make it unique and separate from the medical profession.

In fall 2010, a report by the ANA and the Constituent Member Associations (CMA) moved the discussion to a new level by outlining the key messages from the IOM Report on the Future of Nursing. This report is part of an ongoing project aimed at using evidence-based practice to advance the nursing profession so that nursing can keep pace with health-care reform activities. Although not entirely new, the four key messages from the report are:

- *Nurses should practice to the full extent of their education and training.* A fundamental element of this goal is to revise states' nurse practice acts by removing unnecessary scope-of-practice restrictions. Work initiated in the 11th Congress is continuing and will promote this issue in various health-care settings.
- *Nurses should achieve higher levels of education and training through an improved education system that promotes seamless academic progression.* Fundamental to this message are the goals of increasing to at least 80% the number of RNs with baccalaureate degrees by 2020 (up from the current 50%), doubling the number of nurses with doctorates by 2020, and having nurses commit to lifelong learning. Another goal is to increase the diversity of nurses to better meet the needs of an increasingly diverse U.S. population. Expanded residency programs, focused on easing the transition into practice, are fundamental to the progression of newly licensed nurses into successful professionals.
- *Nurses should be full partners with physicians and other health professionals in redesigning health care in the United States.* For a long time, nurses have needed expanded opportunities to demonstrate their leadership and management skills as key members of the health-care team. In collaboration with physicians and other team members, nurses need to be involved in redesigning the health care system through such activities as conducting research, improving practice environments, developing care systems, and improving quality of care.
- *Effective workforce planning and policy-making require better data collection and an improved information infrastructure.* Collaboration between national,

(continued)

Issues Now continued

state, and local initiatives in collecting and analyzing data can make the data more useful to all health-care providers.

• *Nursing education has long strived to be relevant and vibrant in a rapidly changing health-care system.* The shift in recent years to a consumer-driven health-care system, which demands an increased level of safety and high-quality care at all times, has led to the development of the QSEN competency model for nursing curricula. The success or failure of the QSEN model will be demonstrated as more and more nursing programs adopt it and as graduates of these programs enter the health-care system.

Competency/Outcome Comparison: IOM; QSEN; AACN Essentials

IOM Competencies	QSEN Competencies	AACN Essentials
Client-centered care	Client-centered care	Liberal education for baccalaureate generalist nursing practice
Interdisciplinary teamwork	Teamwork and collaboration	Basic organizational and systems leadership for high-quality care and client safety
EBP	EBP	Scholarship for EBP
QI	QI	Information management and application of client-care technology
Informatics	Safety	Health-care policy, finance and regulatory environments
	Informatics	Interprofessional communication and collaboration for improving health outcomes
		Clinical prevention and population health
		Professionalism and professional values
		Baccalaureate generalist nursing practice

AACN = American Association of Colleges of Nursing; EBP = evidence-based practice; IOM = Institute of Medicine; QI = quality improvement; QSEN = Quality and Safety Education for Nurses.

Sources: American Association of Colleges of Nursing: Essentials of baccalaureate education for professional nursing practice: Faculty tool kit, 2009. Retrieved August 2010 from http://www.AACN.nche.edu.

Armstrong GE, Spencer TS, Lenburg CB: Using quality and safety education for nurses to enhance competency outcome performance assessment: A synergistic approach that promotes patient safety and quality outcomes. Journal of Nursing Education 48(12):686–693, 2009.

Brown R, Feller L, Benedict L: Reframing nursing education: The Quality and Safety Education for Nurses Initiative. Teaching & Learning in Nursing 5(3):115–118, 2010.

Carlton G, Blegen MA: Medication-related errors: A literature review of incidence and antecedents. Annual Review of Nursing Research 24:19–38, 2006.

Cronenwett L, Sherwood G, Gelmon SB: Improving quality and safety education: The QSEN Learning Collaborative. Nursing Outlook 57(6):304–312, 2009.

Lenburg CB, Klein C, Abdur-Rahman V, Spencer T, Boyer S: The COPA Model: A comprehensive framework designed to promote quality care and competence for patient safety. Nursing Education Perspectives 30(5):312–317, 2009.

Nursing Workforce Centers: ANA and CMA activities reflected in the IOM recommendations, Retrieved October 2010 from http://www.nursingworkforcecenters.org.

Pohl JM, Savrin C, Fiandt K, Beauchesne M, Drayton-Brooks S, Scheibmeir M, Brackley M, Werner KE: Quality and safety in graduate nursing education: cross-mapping QSEN graduate competencies with NONPF's NP core and practice doctorate competencies. Nursing Outlook 57(6):349–354, 2009.

Sullivan DT: Quality and safety education for nurses: A national initiative funded by the Robert Wood Johnson Foundation. Creative Nursing 15(2):111, 2009. Retrieved August 2010 from http://www.qesn.org.

6

Critical Thinking

Joseph T. Catalano

Learning Objectives

After completing this chapter, the reader will be able to:

- Demonstrate logical, rational, and creative critical thinking.
- Describe the steps of the critical thinking process in resolving a client-care issue.
- Apply critical thinking to client care.
- List five characteristics of critical thinking.

A DECISION PROCESS

The Art of Thinking

One of the most important responsibilities that nurses have is to make correct and safe decisions in a variety of client-care situations. The decisions made by nurses affect the health status, recovery time, and even the survival or death of a client. For example, the critical care nurse must decide when to give certain medications on the basis of changes in the client's condition. The emergency department (ED) nurse must decide which clients to treat first by assessing the extent of their injuries. The hospital staff nurse must decide what prn medication to give for which set of symptoms. The home health nurse must decide when to call the physician about a change in a client's condition.

The process by which these decisions are made involves the use of critical thinking. Critical thinking is based on reason and reflection, knowledge, and instinct derived from experience. It has also been defined as "the art of thinking about thinking." It is both an attitude about and an approach to solving problems. Critical thinking helps nurses make decisions about problems for which there are no simple solutions. Often nurses have to make these decisions with less than complete information.

An Essential Element

Although critical thinking has always been used by nurses to some degree and is recognized as important in the provision of care, its status increased greatly when the National League for Nursing Accrediting Commission (NLNAC) designated critical thinking as one of its mandatory outcome objectives in 1992. It was removed as an outcome criterion in 1999 but remains an element that nursing schools must demonstrate as an essential part of the curriculum. Most of the questions on the National Council Licensure Examination (NCLEX) examination require graduates to use critical thinking in making decisions about client-care situations. If nursing students begin to develop critical thinking skills early in their education, those skills will help them throughout the program and prepare them for licensure and practice.

Schools of nursing have been challenged to demonstrate where and how they teach and measure critical thinking in the curriculum. It is fairly easy to claim, "Yes, we teach our students how to think critically," but much more difficult to accurately define what critical thinking is and then demonstrate that the graduates of the program have attained and can use the skill.

Can We Define it?

A definition is a short statement that identifies and distinguishes something from all other things so that it can be recognized. Generally, things that are easy to define have one or a few definitions. Things that are more difficult to define tend to have many definitions that may or may not overlap. Critical thinking falls into the latter category. At least 10 primary definitions for critical thinking have been developed over the years by various experts on the subject. Perhaps a better approach to recognizing and developing critical thinking is to look at the characteristics that seem common to most of the definitions.

CHARACTERISTICS OF CRITICAL THINKING

Critical Thinking Is Creative

Nurses who think creatively explore new ideas and alternative ways of solving client-care problems. Creative thinkers are able to bring together bits of knowledge or information that may initially seem unrelated and formulate them into a plan that leads to effective decision-making and solves the problem by finding connections between the thoughts and concepts. This process is similar to the linear approach used in the nursing process. All the situational variables must be considered, and decision-making becomes more complex as the number of variables increases.

Example of Creative Thinking

In a small hospital, a policy was instituted that required all post–cesarean delivery clients to be monitored in the recovery room just like all other postoperative clients. Because the operating room (OR) nurses were on call for the recovery room, they thought that they were being required to do more work with no additional staff. The circulating and scrub obstetric (OB) nurses could go home after the delivery. The OR nurses became very resentful of the extra call for the postdelivery clients and often called in sick the day after they were required to attend a post–cesarean delivery client. This practice left the OR short-staffed during the day and led to increased tension and frequent unfriendly confrontations between the OR and OB nurses.

The nurse managers of the OB and OR units resolved the problem by instituting a policy of "cross-training" with the OR and OB nurses. OB nurses were taught how to monitor the recovery of postoperative clients and were rotated through recovery for 1 week every 2 months to keep these skills current. The OR nurses were taught how to assist at cesarean deliveries and were rotated through the OB unit for 1 week every 2 months. This system kept the staffing levels constant and allowed the OB nurses to assist with the post–cesarean delivery clients. As often happens with these types of decisions, not everyone was happy with the change, but it did reduce the resentment levels between the two units and gave the nurses a better appreciation of the other nurses' responsibilities.

> *Creative thinkers are able to bring together bits of knowledge or information that may initially seem unrelated and formulate them into a plan that leads to effective decision-making and solves the problem by finding connections between the thoughts and concepts.*

What Do You Think?

Identify two situations that you have been involved with that required critical thinking. How did you resolve these situations? What elements of critical thinking did you use?

Critical Thinking Is Logical, Rational, and Reflective

Although the critical thinking process is often expanded beyond fundamental logical thinking, it must always be based on rationales and facts rather than emotions or egocentric impulses. Intuition can play a part in critical thinking when it is recognized as a rational thought process that brings together and processes a number of factors at the subconscious level rather than a simple "gut feeling."

If at all possible, critical thinkers must take the time to collect as much data as they can and examine them under the light of reason before making a decision or taking an action. Decisions must at times be made on a limited amount of information in situations in which there is a high degree of risk and ambiguity. In these situations, the nurse's past experiences resolving similar situations, as well as intuition, can help. However, in most cases, merely jumping to conclusions often produces poor decisions and negative results. Logical reasoning is often divided into deductive and inductive reasoning.

Example of Deductive Reasoning

Deductive logic or reasoning is a process whereby the individual proceeds from the general to the particular. The conclusions reached by deductive reasoning based on true arguments or premises are certain and true (i.e., valid):

Either John Smith or George Jones is to be given a dose of IV penicillin before surgery.
There was no order for IV penicillin for John Smith before surgery.
Therefore, George Jones is to be given IV penicillin before surgery.

The conclusion is certain. The rationale is that all of the information in the conclusion is found in the premises; therefore, the conclusion must logically follow and be true if the premises are true. If the argument is both certain and true; it is also valid.

Example of Inductive Reasoning

Inductive logic or reasoning involves proceeding from the particular to the general. The conclusions reached by inductive reasoning are probable or contingent. Inductive reasoning is more frequently used than deductive reasoning in health-care situations because the wide range of variables involved in client care almost always introduces a degree of uncertainty.

Mr. Jones has bacterial lobar pneumonia.
Antibiotics are usually used to treat this disease.
Therefore, Mr. Jones should probably be given an antibiotic.

The conclusion is valid. The rationale is that the conclusion is uncertain because the use of the word "usually" in the premise leaves room for alternative conclusions. For example, what if the cause of the lobar pneumonia was a viral infection? Then antibiotics would not be an appropriate treatment for the condition.

Errors in Reasoning

Keep in mind that all critical thinking, including both inductive and deductive reasoning, is open to fallacies. A fallacy is generally defined as an error in reasoning that leads to a conclusion that does not follow from its premises, or to a conclusion that is invalid because of false premises.[1] A conclusion may be certain because all the necessary information is in the premises; however, it can still be untrue, thereby rendering the whole argument invalid. As a fundamental principle, if any information in the premises is false, the conclusion will be false also.

For example, a nurse working in the ED has observed that all the clients she has seen with sexually transmitted diseases (STDs) also have had low moral values. A new client, Staci, is admitted for treatment of an STD; therefore, the nurse concludes that Staci must also have low moral values. The conclusion is certain because all the information is contained in the premises; however, it is false because the first statement is not true. It is possible for some clients to have an STD and also have high moral values.

The Non Sequitur

One of the most common types of fallacy seen in nursing is the non sequitur, a fallacy in which the conclusion does not follow from the arguments or premises, or in which a cause-and-effect relationship is seen but really does not exist. For example, a 28-year-old client is admitted with type 1 diabetes mellitus. He has been drinking five to six cans of nondiet cola a day since he was 16 years old. The nurse concludes that drinking large amounts of nondiet cola drinks causes type 1 diabetes.

Another common example of this type of fallacy is seen during staffing shortages. It is not unusual for a nursing supervisor to say to a staff nurse, "We need you to work this extra shift because everyone else called in. I know you take classes in the evening, but if you don't work you will be abandoning the clients. Therefore, if you decide not to work the extra shift, you might as well start looking for employment elsewhere."

How Fallacies Happen
People commit fallacies for various reasons. In some cases, individuals have such a strong ideological commitment to a religious, economic, or political belief that they refuse to listen to any ideas or opinions that contradict what they believe. Basically, their minds are closed to any alternative conclusions; thus, they stick to their own conclusions regardless of the reasoning process. Some individuals have difficulty acknowledging that they have made a mistake and refuse to see the lack of logic in their reasoning and conclusions. Still others must "win" at all costs and subvert the critical thinking process and logic by abuse, twisting the other person's words, and using personal attacks. Being able to recognize conclusions that are valid or invalid is an important part of critical thinking.

Critical Thinking Is Independent

Nurses who think critically are not easily influenced by others with strong opinions. They demonstrate their autonomy by thinking for themselves and not passively succumbing to peer pressure or the belief system of the majority.

Example of Independent Thinking

An 82-year-old woman was brought into the ED by her family with complaints of "difficulty urinating." During the initial assessment, the RN noted that the client had 2+ pitting edema of her ankles and feet, congested lung sounds, and shortness of breath. The ED physician ordered a urinary catheter to be inserted, urinalysis, and a consultation with a urologist for the urinary complaint. The RN pointed out the client's history of congestive heart failure (CHF) and current symptoms and also the fact that only 10 mL of urine was obtained when the catheter was inserted. The ED physician insisted that the problem was urinary and refused to discuss the client's condition any more.

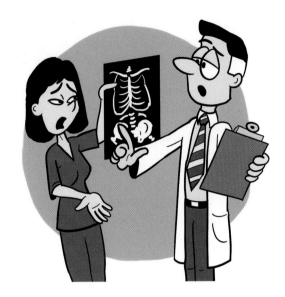

While waiting for the urinalysis results, the client became increasingly short of breath and restless. The RN called for a chest x-ray and measurement of arterial blood gases (ABGs). The chest x-ray showed that 75 percent of the client's lung fields were filled with fluid, and the ABGs showed respiratory acidosis with hypoxia. The nurse asked the physician to order furosemide for the client on the basis of these findings. The physician became angry, accused the nurse of practicing medicine, and refused to write the order. The nurse then called the client's attending physician, who decided to admit the client to the hospital and begin treatment with IV furosemide for the obvious congestive heart failure.

Critical Thinking Challenges Custom

A healthy, constructive questioning of long-used health-care practices prevents the nurse from mindlessly providing rote care. Improvement and advances in health-care practices occur only when nurses understand the rationale behind the practices, and then accept or reject them on evidence that they either do or do not work as intended.[2]

Example of Challenging Custom

A newly hired nurse was beginning her first shift on the obstetric unit when a 28-year-old client in her sixth month of pregnancy was admitted with abdominal cramps and vaginal bleeding. A spontaneous abortion was suspected. Another nurse who had worked on the OB unit for 10 years knew the client and her family. She told the newly hired nurse to call the client's sister (her number was on the chart) even though the client had not requested it. The newly hired nurse felt uncomfortable making the call and refused on the grounds that it was a violation of client **confidentiality.** The experienced nurse became angry at the refusal and berated the new nurse with the statement, "We've been notifying the families of our clients for years, and you're not going to change that practice."

The next day, the newly hired nurse had a conference with the OB unit nurse manager. The nurse manager decided that a series of in-service presentations on the right to privacy, and the code of ethics, and requirements of the Health Insurance Portability and Accountability Act (HIPAA), should be attended by all members of the unit.[3]

Critical Thinking Is Free of Bias and Prejudice

Biases are unjustified personal opinions. When a bias, as well as **stereotype,** is taken as fact, it becomes a prejudice. A belief is not necessarily true just because it has been in existence for a long period of time or because many people believe it. To use effective critical thinking, biases and stereotypes must be identified and eliminated.

> *People commit fallacies for various reasons. In some cases, individuals have such a strong ideological commitment to a religious, economic, or political belief that they refuse to listen to any ideas or opinions that contradict what they believe.*

Analyzing and viewing a situation from all points of view before arriving at a conclusion prevents the nurse from making one-sided decisions. It also helps identify bias or prejudice on the part of physicians, nurses, and even clients and the backlash effect that it may produce on other decision makers.

Recognition of bias does not always eliminate it, but it helps the decision maker compensate for it when making the final decision.

Example of Bias- and Prejudice-Free Thinking

A homosexual, HIV-positive client with full-blown symptoms of AIDS is admitted to a medical-surgical unit for care. The nurse assigned to care for the client has very strong religious beliefs about homosexuality. She believes that her obligation as a nurse requires her to care for this client despite his diagnosis and sexual preference, yet she also believes that caring for this client would tacitly condone his sexual preferences and lifestyle. She tries to place herself in the client's situation and recognizes that an ill client deserves high-quality care without consideration of his beliefs or background.

Critical Thinking Is Action Oriented

The goal of critical thinking in health care should always be the resolution of a problem or a method to improve client care. Critical thinking is used at all levels of the health-care system and is essential to the formulation and evaluation of policies and procedures, use of effective communication, and resolution of management and personnel conflicts.

Example of Action-Oriented Critical Thinking

A physician with a reputation for striking fear in the hearts of the nurses in the medical-surgical unit was in a particularly bad mood one day. After making his rounds, the physician loudly and publicly criticized the care that the nurses were giving to his clients and proceeded to announce numerous mistakes that the nurses had made over the past year. The unit manager took the physician aside and told him that if he was having problems with the nurses on the unit, he should follow correct channels to file complaints and not make a scene in the nurses' station where many of the clients could hear him.

The physician became even more irate, stormed out of the unit, and went directly to the office of the vice president of nursing services (VPNS). He told the VPNS that he was filing an official **complaint** against the unit manager for unprofessional behavior, disrespect for a physician, and failure to follow medical orders. The VPNS told him that she would investigate the complaint and take appropriate action.

After talking with all the nurses on the medical-surgical unit and nurses on other units, as well as a number of physicians, the VPNS discovered that the physician who filed the complaint was well known for his capricious and obnoxious behavior toward nurses. He was referred to the hospital medical board, reprimanded for his behavior toward the nurses, and required to drop the complaint about the manager of the medical-surgical unit. In addition, a special meeting was called for all the physicians practicing in the hospital to discuss the problem and to better understand what was involved regarding professional behavior.

CRITICAL THINKING SKILLS

Although there are different approaches to developing critical thinking, certain concepts are common to the skill. Some individuals seem to have an innate ability to master these concepts, whereas others have difficulty with them. As with most skills, practice and repetition increase efficiency and the ability to make safe decisions in complex nursing situations in which there are multiple variables that affect the client's health status.

> *To use effective critical thinking, biases and stereotypes must be identified and eliminated.*

Identify the Problem
The saying "It's hard to know when you have arrived if you don't know where you are going" applies particularly well to critical thinking. If the underlying problem has not been identified, it is almost impossible to develop a plan to solve it. One way to identify the underlying problem is to try to restate the issue as a declarative statement. For example, a public health nurse may identify that "STDs among teenagers in our society are increasing at a rapid rate."

Gather Pertinent Data
It sometimes happens that, in applying critical thinking to the resolution of a problem, there is only a small amount of information that relates to the situation. On the other hand, in our information-oriented society, there may be an overabundance of data. It becomes necessary for the nurse to sort through the data, use the data that relate to the problem, and reject the data that are extraneous and perhaps misleading.

What Do You Think?

What five values are most important to you? How do these influence the way you act? What happens when these values conflict?

In the example of STDs in teenagers, the Internet can provide copious data, including general population statistics, racial and ethnic breakdowns, STD incidence by region, the most common STDs, treatment regimens, and even projections for the future.

Rational analysis and consideration of the data may produce a reexamination and refocusing of the problem. For example, after examining the abundance of information about teenage STDs, the community health nurses may decide to focus their efforts on dealing with the problem in their community rather than the entire state.

Your Values
in Context
Contextual Awareness
The Influence of Belief
Developing a contextual awareness requires primarily the use of deductive reasoning.

Contextual awareness is a very broad concept that is not merely limited to values but includes everything that may affect the client, such as physical symptoms and environment. Everyone, including nurses, has feelings and beliefs about all issues. Some of these beliefs are personal; some are cultural; some are stated overtly, whereas others remain deeply rooted but hidden in the subconscious. In any case, these beliefs influence how situations are perceived and what decisions are made.

Values Clarification
To make solid decisions based on critical thinking, nurses must examine their own philosophies, beliefs, and value systems. **Values clarification** is an important element in critical thinking. At some point, preferably early in their careers, nurses should make a list of all the things they consider valuable (Box 6.1). It should also be recognized that values are not static and will be added or deleted or will change in priority with time.

Box 6.1

Personal Values

Listed below are a number of values that almost everyone has. Circle the ones that are important to you, including additional values as necessary. Then rank the values according to priority.

Family	Flexibility
Education	Trust
Career	Teamwork
Honesty	Dependability
Good health	Punctuality
Respect	Accountability
Leisure time	Self-determination
Nonjudgmental attitude	Independence
Cooperative work relationships	Veracity
Professional integrity	Justice
Competency	Commitment
Empathy	

In addition, nurses must examine their own philosophy of nursing and health care as it relates to that of the agency for which they are working. Then they need to compare how societal values relate to their personal philosophy and that of the agency. Do societal values reflect or contradict the philosophy? How do the standards of care, the nurse practice act of the state, facility **protocols,** and even the code of ethics affect the care being provided?

Challenging Assumptions and Rituals
Does the Old Approach Really Work?
Challenging assumptions and rituals of care requires use of inductive reasoning. The nurse needs to ask whether there are any assumptions about the care provided, what they are, how they affect care, and whether any of these assumptions can be challenged.

In much the same way, rituals about care should also be identified and challenged. What are

the rituals that are done routinely without much thought? Are they beneficial, or can they be changed or eliminated?

The community health nurse, for example, may have the philosophy that STDs among teenagers represent a dangerous and serious threat to the health of the community. On the other hand, the community may have an underlying philosophy that teenage STD is to be expected and is one of the rites of passage that must be experienced. Where such a major difference in philosophy exists, it would be extremely difficult for the nurse to implement any action that would resolve the problem.

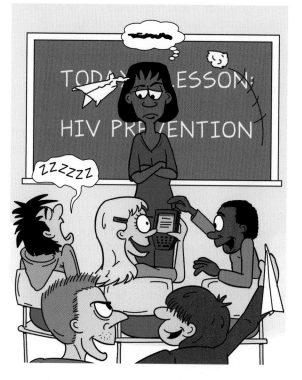

What Really Caused the Problem?
Some assumptions that could be challenged might revolve around the cause of the problem. An increase in STDs among teenagers may be caused by (1) a lack of sexual education in school, (2) a lack of morals in our society, or (3) an atmosphere of permissiveness and egocentrism that is projected in the media.

One health department philosophy about teenagers that may need to be challenged might be that all teenagers are rebellious, uncooperative, and promiscuous, when in reality, many teenagers work well with others, are highly productive, and have high moral standards.

Nurses also need to learn about and evaluate the value systems of those with whom they are working. Even though they may not agree with those values, it is important to recognize them and work with them when attempting to affect health. For example, when teaching a group of high-school students about STDs, it would be essential to know what their attitudes toward sex and health are. In all likelihood, these attitudes would be different from those of the nurse. An education program organized around only the nurse's belief and value system would be doomed to failure. Presenting the information from the students' viewpoint would help them better understand and perhaps be more willing to accept it.

Imagine and Explore Alternatives Creatively

Once the nurse has identified the problem and explored the assumptions and rituals, he or she needs to consider the possible alternatives to care delivery. However, the nurse does not need to do this alone.

> *A healthy, constructive questioning of long-used health-care practices prevents the nurse from mindlessly providing rote care.*

This information can be obtained from a variety of sources, such as written reports, surveys, and published articles. Information may also be obtained informally from others, such as in discussions with individuals who work in the field or have dealt with a similar problem before, or through feedback from the clients who are receiving the care. No matter what the source of information, it needs to be evaluated critically for accuracy, consistency, cause and effect, and biases.[4]

A nurse using critical thinking will often be able to identify more than one solution to a problem. For example, possible solutions to the teenage STD problem may include providing condoms for all high-school students, performing tubal ligations on sexually active girls, or establishing strict nighttime curfews.

Although all these solutions may be effective, the nurse would have to evaluate the cause-and-effect relationship, value, and consequences of each of these courses of action. A nurse who is a critical thinker would consider each one of these before implementing a course of action.

CRITICAL THINKING IN DECISION-MAKING

Although critical thinking is used in all aspects of decision-making, it is particularly important in the nursing process. It is important to remember that although the nursing process and critical thinking are interrelated and interdependent, they are not identical.

As a way of looking at the world, critical thinking allows the nurse to consider new ideas and then evaluate those ideas in light of accepted information as well as client and personal value systems. Nurses are constantly making decisions in both their professional and personal lives. By viewing critical thinking as a purposeful mental activity in which ideas are evaluated and decisions reached, nurses will be able to make ethical, creative, rational, and independent decisions related to client care.[5]

Critical thinking, when applied to the nursing process, makes it a powerful client problem-solving tool. Critical thinking expands the usual linear nursing process into a gestalt that allows the nurse to sort through the multiple variables that are often encountered in client care. Effective use of critical thinking within the nursing process is evident when the nurse successfully applies knowledge from other disciplines in the resolution of client problems, deals with stressful environments, and creatively resolves unique nursing care problems.

Conclusion

Nurses practicing in today's health-care system are required to master many skills. Critical thinking underlies many of these skills. By examining assumptions, beliefs, propositions, and meanings, nurses are able to make sound and valid decisions about client care. Critical thinking both underlies and expands the nursing process in the practical provision of nursing care. When students and nurses master critical thinking concepts and skills, they open their perspectives on client care. An important transformation occurs when students are taught how to think rather than what to think.

The profession of nursing is in an active state of change, continually developing new theories, redefining its practice, and adapting to changing public policy and social mandates. Nurses who use critical thinking in making nursing judgments tend to consider the client's human rights and be effective client advocates. These nurses will also be able to adapt the rules of the nursing process to meet a wide range of client needs.

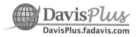
DavisPlus.fadavis.com

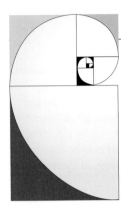

Issues in Practice

National Safe Staffing Bill

Try this out for deductive reasoning:

Research has shown that poor staffing leads to nurses working overtime and long shifts.

Research has also shown that overtime and long shifts lead to an increase in medication and other types of medical errors that cause injury and death to clients.

Therefore, poor staffing increases injury and death of clients.

Recent emphasis has been placed on educating nurses to be safe practitioners through efforts such as the Institute of Medicine (IOM) and Quality and Safe Education for Nurses (QSEN) competencies (see Chapter 5). Nursing schools are gradually incorporating these into their curricula and will without a doubt be educating nurses to practice more safely and with higher quality, which should reduce errors to some degree. However, the sad truth is that, even with the safest and most educated nurses in the world working in your unit, if it is not staffed at a safe level, the number of errors is going to increase.

Over the past decade, a number of states have enacted laws that deal with staffing ratios in hospitals. Some, such as California's law, actually mandate a certain number of nurses for a certain number of clients, depending on the units. Other states have less prescriptive laws. These efforts have proved somewhat effective. But if poor staffing is such a major problem, why hasn't there been a national bill to deal with it?

In June 2010, a bill was reintroduced in both the U.S. House of Representatives and the Senate to address the staffing issue. Called the Registered Nurse Safe Staffing Act of 2010 (S. 3491/H.R. 5527), it was initially introduced in the 2003–2004 session of Congress and reintroduced in the 2007–2008 session, but was quickly dismissed by the Republican majority. It is hoped that the bill will find a more favorable reception with a Democratic majority in the Senate, if not in the House. This bill does not mandate staffing levels but rather demands accountability by hospitals to maintain safe levels. The bill calls for hospitals to make information available to the public about their staffing plans for each unit in the facility. These staffing plans would take into account the number of clients and their level of illness, the education level of the nurses providing care, and the availability of support technologies. The decision about staffing levels would be made by a committee of 55% of nurses providing direct client care.

Other provisions include whistle-blower protection for nurses who report understaffing or refuse an assignment they believe to be dangerous because of understaffing. Other protections include the ability to follow through on such complaints and guarantees that nurses cannot be forced to work in units where

Issues in Practice   continued

they do not usually work. As with other bills that deal with nursing staffing issues, this one is likely to receive much opposition from the lobbyists for the American Medical Association and the Hospital Association.

What can you do? Get politically active! Write, call, or e-mail your senator or representative and tell him or her that you and all your nurse friends support this bill. Get the public and media involved. Bills such as this show that nurses are concerned for client safety and well-being.

Sources: Assadian O: Implications of staffing ratios and workload limitations on healthcare-associated infections and the quality of patient care. Critical Care Medicine 35(1):296–298, 2007.

Crouch BI, Caravati EM, Moltz E: Tenfold therapeutic dosing errors in young children reported to U.S. poison control centers. American Journal of Health-System Pharmacy 66(14):1292–1296, 2009.

Hoffmann B, Rohe J: Patient safety and error management: What causes adverse events and how can they be prevented? Deutsches Ärzteblatt International 107(6):92–99, 2010.

Mark BA, Belyea M: Nurse staffing and medication errors: Cross-sectional or longitudinal relationships? Research in Nursing & Health 32(1):18–30, 2009.

The Registered Nurse Safe Staffing Act (full text). Retrieved August 2010 from http://www .washingtonwatch.com.

Critical Thinking Exercises

Use the steps in the nursing process to provide a plan of care, including at least two nursing diagnoses, for the following client situation:

Mr. Y is 49 years old and has been complaining of chest pain starting in the center of his chest and radiating to his left arm and hand for 2 hours. He is having trouble breathing, is very pale, and has cool and moist skin. His pulse is 134 bpm and irregular, his blood pressure is 92/50 mm Hg, and his respiratory rate is 24 breaths per minute. He is very anxious and expresses concern about having to leave his job as an accountant because of these symptoms. He is diagnosed as having an acute anterior myocardial infarction and is admitted to the intensive care unit.

- What key assessment does the nurse need to identify as essential to this client's problem?
- What problems does this client have that a nurse can treat independently? Write nursing diagnoses for these problems.
- What can be accomplished in the nursing treatment of this client's problems (goals)?
- What type of activity can the nurse undertake to achieve the goals (intervention)?
- What does the nurse need to look for to see whether the interventions have worked (evaluation)?

2

Making the Transition to Professional

7

Ethics in Nursing

Joseph T. Catalano

Learning Objectives

After completing this chapter, the reader will be able to:

- Discuss and analyze the difference between law and ethics.
- Define the key terms used in ethics.
- Discuss the important ethical concepts.
- Distinguish between the two most commonly used systems of ethical decision-making.
- Apply the steps in the ethical decision-making process.

A LEARNED SKILL

Nurses who practice in today's health-care system soon realize that making ethical decisions is a common part of daily nursing care. However, experience shows that in the full curricula of many schools of nursing, the teaching of ethical principles and ethical decision-making gets less attention than the topics of nursing skills, core competencies, and electronic charting. As health-care technology continues to advance at a rapid pace, nurses will find it more and more difficult to make sound ethical decisions. Many nurses feel the need to be better prepared to understand and deal with the complex ethical problems that keep evolving as they attempt to provide care for their clients.[1]

Ethical decision-making is a skill that can be learned. The ability to make sensible ethical decisions is based on an understanding of underlying ethical principles, ethical theories or systems, a decision-making model, and the profession's code of ethics. This skill, like others, involves mastery of the theoretical material and practice of the skill itself. This chapter presents the basic information required to understand ethics, the code of ethics, and ethical decision-making. It also highlights some of the important bioethical issues that confront nurses in the current health-care system.

IMPORTANT DEFINITIONS

In Western cultures, the study of ethics is a specialized area of philosophy, the origins of which can be traced to ancient Greece. In fact, certain ethical principles articulated by Hippocrates still serve as the basis of many of the current debates. Like most specialized areas of study, ethics has its own language and uses terminology in precise ways. The following are some key terms that are encountered in studies of health-care ethics.

Values

Values are ideals or concepts that give meaning to the individual's life. Values are derived most commonly from societal norms, religion, and family orientation and serve as the framework for making decisions and taking action in daily life. People's values tend to change as their life situations change, as they grow older, and as they encounter situations that cause value conflicts. For example, before the 1950s, pregnancy outside of marriage was unacceptable, and unmarried women who were pregnant were shunned and generally separated from society. Today this situation is much more accepted, and it is not uncommon to see pregnant high-school students attending classes.

Values are usually not written down; however, at some time in their professional careers, it may be important for nurses to make lists of their values. This value clarification process requires that the nurse assess, evaluate, and then determine a set of personal values and prioritize them. This will help the nurse make decisions when confronted with situations in which the client's values differ from the nurse's own values.

Value conflicts that often occur in daily life can force an individual to select a higher-priority value over a lower-priority one. For example, a nurse who values both career and family may be forced to decide between going to work and staying home with a sick child.

> *Values are usually not written down; however, at some time in their professional careers, it may be important for nurses to make lists of their values.*

Morals

Morals are the fundamental standards of right and wrong that an individual learns and internalizes, usually in the early stages of childhood development. An individual's moral orientation is often based on religious beliefs, although societal influence plays an important part in this development. The word *moral* comes from the Latin word *mores*, which means customs or values.

Moral behavior is often manifested as behavior in accordance with a group's norms, customs, or traditions. A moral person is generally someone who responds to another person in need by providing care and who maintains a level of responsibility in all relationships.[1] In many situations in which moral convictions differ, it is difficult to find a rational basis for proving one side right over the other. For example, animal rights activists believe that killing animals for sport, their fur, or even food is morally wrong. Most hunters do not even think of the killing of animals as a moral issue at all.

What Do You Think?

What type of value conflicts have you experienced in the past week? How did you resolve them? Were you satisfied with the resolution, or did it make you feel uncomfortable?

Laws

Laws can generally be defined as rules of social conduct made by humans to protect society, and these laws are based on concerns about fairness and justice. The goals of laws are to preserve the species and promote peaceful and productive interactions between individuals and groups of individuals by preventing the actions of one citizen from infringing on the rights of another. Two important aspects of laws are that they are enforceable through some type of police force and that they should be applied equally to all persons.

Ethics
A System of Morals

Ethics are declarations of what is right or wrong and of what ought to be. Ethics are usually presented as systems of value behaviors and beliefs; they serve the purpose of governing conduct to ensure the protection of an individual's rights. Ethics exist on several levels, ranging from the individual or a small group to the society as a whole. The concept of ethics is closely associated with the concept of morals in the development and purposes of both. In one sense, ethics can be considered a system of morals for a particular group. There are usually no systems of enforcement for those who violate ethical principles.[2]

A **code of ethics** is a written list of a profession's values and standards of conduct. The code of ethics provides a framework for decision-making for the profession and should be oriented toward the daily decisions made by members of the profession.

A Dilemma

An **ethical dilemma** is a situation that requires an individual to make a choice between two equally unfavorable alternatives. The basic, elemental aspects of an ethical dilemma usually involve conflict of one individual's rights with those of another, conflict of one individual's obligations with the rights of another, or combined conflict of one group's obligations and rights with those of another group.

Principles in Conflict

By the very nature of an ethical dilemma, there can be no simple correct solution, and the final decision must often be defended against those who disagree with it.

> For example, a client went to surgery for a laparoscopic biopsy of an abdominal mass. After the laparoscope was inserted, the physician noted that the mass had metastasized to the liver, pancreas, and colon, and even before the results of the tissue biopsy returned from the laboratory, the physician diagnosed metastatic cancer with a poor prognosis. When the client was returned to his room, the physician told the nurses about the diagnosis but warned them that under no circumstances were they to tell the client about the cancer.
>
> When the client awoke, the first question that he asked the nurses was, "Do I have cancer?" This posed an ethical dilemma for the nurses. If they were to tell the client the truth, they would violate the principle of fidelity to the physician. If they lied to the client, they would violate the principle of veracity.

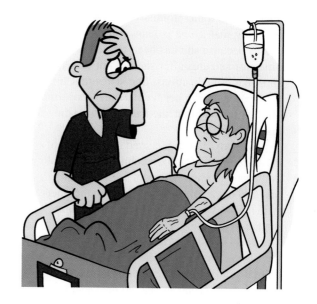

KEY CONCEPTS IN ETHICS

In addition to the terminology used in the study and practice of ethics, several important principles often underlie ethical dilemmas. These principles include autonomy, justice, fidelity, beneficence, nonmaleficence, veracity, standard of best interest, and obligations.

Autonomy

Autonomy is the right of self-determination, independence, and freedom. Autonomy refers to the client's right to make health-care decisions for himself or herself, even if the health-care provider does not agree with those decisions.

Autonomy, as with most rights, is not absolute, and under certain conditions, limitations can be imposed on it. Generally these limitations occur when one individual's autonomy interferes with another individual's rights, health, or well-being. For example, a client generally can use his or her right to autonomy by refusing any or all treatments. However, in the case of contagious diseases (e.g., tuberculosis) that affect society, the individual can be forced by the health-care and legal systems to take medications to cure the disease. The individual can also be forced into isolation to prevent the disease from spreading. Consider the following situation:

> June, who is the 28-year-old mother of two children, is brought into the emergency department

(ED) after a tonic-clonic–type seizure at a shopping mall. June is known to the ED nurses because she has been treated several times for seizures after she did not take her antiseizure medications. She states that the medications make her feel "dopey" and tired all the time and that she hates the way they make her feel.

Recently, June has started to drive one of her children and four other children to school in the neighborhood car pool 1 day a week. She also drives 62 miles one way on the interstate highway twice a week to visit her aging mother in a nursing home in a different city. The nurse who takes care of June this day in the ED knows that the state licensing laws require that an individual with uncontrolled seizures must report the fact to the Department of Motor Vehicles and is usually ineligible for a driver's license. When the nurse mentions that she is going to have to report the seizure, June begs her not to report it. She would have no means of taking her children to school or visiting her mother. She assures the nurse that she will take her medication no matter how it makes her feel.

> By the very nature of an ethical dilemma, there can be no simple correct solution, and the final decision must often be defended against those who disagree with it.

Justice

Justice is the obligation to be fair to all people. The concept is often expanded to what is called distributive justice, which states that individuals have the right to be treated equally regardless of race, gender, marital status, medical diagnosis, social standing, economic level, or religious belief. The principle of justice underlies the first statement in the American Nurses Association (ANA) Code of Ethics for Nurses:

The nurse provides services with respect for human dignity and the uniqueness of the client unrestricted by considerations of social or economic status, personal attributes, or the nature of health problems.[3]

Distributive justice sometimes includes ideas such as equal access to health care for all. As with other rights, limits can be placed on justice when it interferes with the rights of others.

For example, a middle-aged homeless man who was diagnosed with type 1, insulin-dependent diabetes mellitus demanded that Medicaid pay for a pancreas transplantation. His health record showed that he refused to follow the prescribed diabetic regimen, drank large quantities of wine, and rarely took his insulin. The transplantation would cost $108,000, which is the total cost of immunizing all the children in a state for 1 year.

Fidelity

Fidelity is the obligation of an individual to be faithful to commitments made to himself or herself and to others. In health care, fidelity includes the professional's faithfulness or loyalty to agreements and responsibilities accepted as part of the practice of the profession. Fidelity is the main support for the concept of accountability, although conflicts in fidelity might arise from obligations owed to different individuals or groups.

For example, a nurse who is just finishing a very busy and tiring 12-hour shift may experience a conflict of fidelity when she is asked by a supervisor to work an additional shift because of the hospital's being short-staffed. The nurse has to weigh her fidelity to herself against fidelity to the employing institution and against fidelity to the profession and clients to do the best job possible, particularly if she feels that her fatigue would interfere with the performance of those obligations.

Beneficence

Beneficence, one of the oldest requirements for health-care providers, views the primary goal of health care as doing good for clients under their care. In general, the term *good* includes more than providing technically competent care for clients. Good care requires that the health-care provider take a holistic approach to the client, including the client's beliefs, feelings, and wishes as well as those of the client's family and significant others. The difficulty in implementing the principle of beneficence is in determining what exactly is good for another and who can best make the decision about this good.

> *Fidelity is the main support for the concept of accountability, although conflicts in fidelity might arise from obligations owed to different individuals or groups.*

Consider the case of the man involved in an automobile accident who ran into a metal fence pole. The pole passed through his abdomen. Even after 6 hours of surgery, the surgeon was unable to repair all the damage. The man was not expected to live for more than 12 hours. When the man came back from surgery, he had a nasogastric tube inserted, so the physician ordered that the client should have nothing by mouth (NPO) to prevent depletion of electrolytes.

Although the man was somewhat confused when he awoke postoperatively, he begged the nurse for a drink of water. He had a fever of 105.7°F. The nurse believed the physician's orders to be absolute; thus she repeatedly refused the client water. He began to yell loudly that he needed a drink of water, but the nurse still refused his requests. At one point, the nurse caught the man attempting to drink water from the ice packs that were being used to lower his fever. This continued for the full 8-hour shift until the man died.

Nonmaleficence

Nonmaleficence is the requirement that health-care providers do no harm to their clients, either intentionally or unintentionally. In a sense, it is the opposite side of the concept of beneficence, and it is difficult to speak of one term without referring to the other. In current health-care practice, the principle of nonmaleficence is often violated in the short term to produce a greater good in the long-term treatment of the client. For example, a client may undergo painful and debilitating surgery to remove a cancerous growth to prolong his life.[4]

By extension, the principle of nonmaleficence also requires that health-care providers protect from harm those who cannot protect themselves. This protection from harm is particularly evident in groups such as children, the mentally incompetent, the unconscious, and those who are too weak or debilitated to protect themselves. In fact, very strict regulations have developed around situations involving child abuse and the health-care provider's obligation to report suspected child abuse. (This issue is discussed in more detail in Chapter 8.)

Veracity
A Right to Know

Veracity is the principle of truthfulness. It requires the health-care provider to tell the truth and not to deceive or mislead clients intentionally. As with other rights and obligations, limitations to this principle exist. The primary limitation occurs when telling the client the truth would seriously harm (principle of nonmaleficence) the client's ability to recover or would produce greater illness.

Health-care providers often feel uncomfortable giving a client bad news, and they tend to avoid answering these questions truthfully. An uncomfortable feeling is not a good enough reason to avoid telling clients the truth about their diagnosis, treatments, or prognosis. Clients have a right to know this information.

One common situation in which veracity is violated is in the use of placebo medications. At some point during their careers, most health-care providers will observe the placebo effect among some clients.

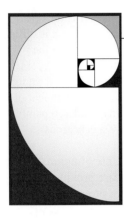

Issues in Practice

A Question of Distributive Justice

Jessica B was diagnosed with acute lymphocytic leukemia at age 4. She is now 7 years old and has been treated with chemotherapy for the past 3 years with varying degrees of success. She is currently in a state of relapse, and a bone marrow transplantation seems to be the only treatment that might improve her condition and save her life. Her father is a day laborer who has no health insurance, so Jessica's health care is being paid for mainly by the Medicaid system of her small state in the Southwest.

The current cost of a bone marrow transplantation at the state's central teaching hospital is $1.5 million, representing about half of the state's entire annual Medicaid budget. Although bone marrow transplantations are an accepted treatment for leukemia, this therapy offers only a slim chance for a total cure of the disease. The procedure is risky, and there is a chance that it may cause death. The procedure will involve several months of post-transplantation treatment and recovery in an intensive care unit far away from the family's home and will require the child to take costly antirejection medications for many years.

The family understands the risks and benefits. They ask the nurse caring for Jessica what they should do. How should the nurse respond? Does the nurse have any obligations toward the Medicaid system as a whole?

Sometimes, when a client is given a gel capsule filled with sugar powder and it seems to relieve the pain, the placebo has the same effect as a narcotic, but without the side effects or potential for addiction. Of course, if the client was told that it was just a sugar pill (veracity), it would not have the same effect. How should nurses feel about this practice?

Costly Errors

Another issue that has come into the public eye recently is medical errors. Some studies indicate that the incidence of medical errors in the current health-care system is extremely high and accounts for as many as 44,000 deaths per year and almost 90,000 injuries. Nurses are often involved in these incidents. What is the nurse's ethical obligation to reveal this information? Some believe that if there is no injury to clients, the error need not be revealed.

Consider the following case study from the viewpoint of veracity:

Tisha S, a senior nursing student, was acting as the team leader during her final clinical experience. Jamie D, a close friend of Tisha's, was one of three junior nursing students on Tisha's team that day. Because of some personal problems, Jamie had been late and unprepared for several clinical experiences. She was informed by her instructor that she might fail unless she showed marked improvement during clinical training.

Claire B, a 64-year-old woman with diabetes and possible renal failure, was one of Jamie's clients. Mrs. B was having a 24-hour urine test to help determine her renal function. After the test was completed later that afternoon, she was to be discharged and treated through the renal clinic. Jamie understood the principles of the 24-hour urine test and realized that all the urine for the full 24 hours needed to be saved, but she became busy caring for another client and accidentally threw away the last specimen before the test ended. She took the specimen container to the laboratory anyway.

At the end of the shift, when Jamie was giving her report to Tisha, she confided that she had thrown away the last urine specimen but begged Tisha not to tell the instructor. This mistake would mean that the test would have to be started over again, and Mrs. B would have to spend an extra day in the hospital. Out of friendship, Tisha agreed not to tell the instructor, rationalizing that they had collected almost all the urine

and she was going to be treated for renal failure anyway. When the instructor asked Tisha for her final report for the day, she specifically asked if there had been any problems with the 24-hour urine test. What would be the consequences of telling the truth and of not telling the truth?

Standard of Best Interest
The Client's Wishes

Standard of best interest describes a type of decision made about a client's health care when the client is unable to make the informed decision regarding his or her own care. The standard of best interest is on the basis of what health-care providers and the family decides is best for that individual. It is very important to consider the individual client's expressed wishes, either formally in a written declaration (e.g., a living will) or informally in conversation with family members.

A Designated Person

Individuals can also legally designate a specific person to make health-care decisions for them in case they become unable to make decisions for themselves. The designated person then has what is called durable power of attorney for health care (DPOAHC). The Omnibus Budget Reconciliation Act (OBRA) of 1990 made it mandatory for all health-care facilities, such as hospitals, nursing homes, and home health-care agencies, to provide information to clients about the living will and DPOAHC.

The standard of best interest should be based on the principle of beneficence. Unfortunately, when clients are unable to make decisions for themselves and no DPOAHC has been designated, the resolution of the dilemma can be a unilateral decision made by health-care providers. Health-care providers' making a unilateral decision that disregards the client's wishes implies that the providers alone know what is best for the client; this is called paternalism.

Obligations

Obligations are demands made on an individual, a profession, a society, or a government to fulfill and honor the rights of others. Obligations are often divided into two categories.

Legal Obligations

Legal obligations are those that have become formal statements of law and are enforceable under the law. For instance, a nurse has a legal obligation to provide safe and adequate care for clients assigned to him or her

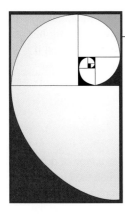

Issues in Practice

The nurse is caring for a critically ill client in the surgical intensive care unit (ICU) after radical neck surgery. The client is connected to a ventilator and is on a sedation protocol with continuous IV infusion of midazolam (Versed), a powerful sedative that requires constant monitoring and titration to maintain the required level of sedation. During the night shift, the nurse discovers that the medication bag is almost empty, and the pharmacy, which is closed, did not send up another bag. She looks the medication up in a drug guide and proceeds to mix the drip herself. The night charge nurse is busy supervising a cardiac arrest situation out of the ICU and is unavailable to double-check how the medication was mixed.

Inadvertently, the nurse mixes a double-strength dose of the medication. Thirty minutes after she hangs the new drip, the client's blood pressure is 44/20 mm Hg. The client requires a saline bolus and a dopamine drip to stabilize the blood pressure. The family is notified that the client has "taken a turn for the worse" and that they should come to the hospital immediately. In backtracking for the cause of the hypotension, the nurse realizes that she has mixed the sedative double-strength and reduces the rate by half.

When the family arrives, the client's blood pressure has started to return to normal. They ask the nurse what happened and why their mother was on the new IV medication. Should the family be told about the error? Who should tell them? The nurse? The physician? What approach should be used?

Source: Gallagher TH: Disclosing harmful medical errors to patients. New England Journal of Medicine 356(26):2713–2719, 2007.

Moral Obligations.

Moral obligations are those based on moral or ethical principles that are not enforceable under the law. In most states, no legal obligation exists for a nurse on a vacation trip to stop and help an automobile accident victim.

Rights

Rights are generally defined as something owed to an individual according to just claims, legal guarantees, or moral and ethical principles. Although the term "right" is frequently used in both the legal and ethical systems, its meaning is often blurred in daily use. Individuals sometimes mistakenly claim things as rights that are really privileges, concessions, or freedoms. Several classification systems exist in which different types of rights are delineated. The following three types of rights include the range of definitions.

Welfare Rights

Welfare rights (also called **legal rights**) are based on a legal entitlement to some good or benefit. These rights are guaranteed by laws (e.g., the Bill of Rights of the U.S. Constitution), and violation of such rights can be punished under the legal system. For example, citizens of the United States have a right to equal access to housing regardless of race, sexual preference, or religion.

Ethical Rights

Ethical rights (also called **moral rights**) are based on a moral or ethical principle. Ethical rights usually do not need to have the power of law to be enforced. Ethical rights are, in reality, often privileges allotted to certain individuals or groups of individuals. Over time, popular acceptance of ethical rights can give them the force of a legal right.

An example of an ethical right in the United States is the belief in universal access to health care. In the United States, it is really a long-standing privilege, whereas in many other industrialized countries, such as Canada, Germany, Japan, and England, universal health care is a legal right.

> *Health-care providers' making a unilateral decision that disregards the client's wishes implies that the providers alone know what is best for the client; this is called paternalism.*

Option Rights

Option rights are rights that are based on a fundamental belief in the dignity and freedom of humans. These are **basic human rights** that are particularly evident in free and democratic countries, such as the United States, and much less evident in totalitarian and restrictive societies, such as Iran. Option rights give individuals freedom of choice and the right to live their lives as they choose, but within a given set of prescribed boundaries. For example, people may wear whatever clothes they choose, as long as they wear some type of clothing.

ETHICS COMMITTEES

Physicians, nurses, and other staff members often encounter ethical conflicts they are unable to resolve on their own. In these cases, the interdisciplinary ethics committee can help the health-care provider resolve the dilemma. An increasing number of health-care facilities, particularly hospitals, have instituted ethics committees that make their consultation services available to health-care providers.

The people who belong to the ethics committee vary somewhat from one institution to another, but almost all include a physician, a member of administration, an RN, a clergy person, a philosopher with a background in ethics, a lawyer, and a person from the community. Members of ethics committees should not have any personal agenda that they are promoting and should be able to make decisions without prejudice on the basis of the situation and ethical principles.

Depending on the institution, the scope of the ethics committee's duties can range widely, from very limited activity with infrequent meetings on an ad hoc basis to active promotion of ethical thinking and decision-making through educational programs. Other common functions of ethics committees include evaluating institutional policies in the light of ethical considerations, making recommendations about complex ethical issues, and providing education programs for medical and nursing schools as well as the community. It is extremely important that nurses participate in these committees and that the ethical concerns of the nurses are recognized and addressed.

Case Study
When to Tell

A 48-year-old woman was scheduled for a below-the-knee amputation due to complications from diabetes. She was admitted to the preoperative area, signed a number of surgical permits, and was given her preoperative sedative medication. Because clients undergoing this type of surgery usually lose a significant amount of blood, several units of blood had been typed and cross-matched and placed on standby for her. After she was moved to the operating room and anesthetized, the nurse anesthetist rapidly administered the first unit of blood in preparation for the anticipated blood loss during surgery.

The circulating nurse was checking the paper work before the beginning of the operation and noticed that there was no consent signed for the administration of blood products. In examining the chart further, she noted that under the "Religion" section was listed "Jehovah's Witness." The Jehovah's Witness religion does not allow blood transfusions or transplantation of any tissue or organs. The circulating nurse told the nurse anesthetist about the client's religion, and his response was, "Holy cow—I can't believe this is happening!"

The family did not know about the blood transfusion, and obviously the client, who was under anesthesia, did not know she had received a unit of blood. The nurse anesthetist announced that it was not his fault because he was never told about the client's religion and was not going to tell the family or client about the mistake. The circulating nurse felt that because she did not administer the blood, she should not be the one to inform the family. The unit manager was called in, and the consensus was that she should be the one to reveal the information because she was ultimately responsible for what occurred in the surgical unit. Her feeling was that because no physical harm was

done to the client, the whole incident should just be kept quiet.

QUESTIONS

1. Using the ethical decision-making model listed, work through the decision-making process for this ethical dilemma.

2. What are the key ethical principles involved in this dilemma?

3. What are the possible solutions to the dilemma and their consequences?

4. How would you resolve the dilemma? How would you defend your decision?

ETHICAL SYSTEMS

An ethical situation exists every time a nurse interacts with a client in a health-care setting. Nurses continually make ethical decisions in their daily practice, whether or not they recognize it. These are called normative decisions.

Normative Ethics.
Normative ethics deal with questions and dilemmas that require a choice of actions when there is a conflict of rights or obligations between the nurse and the client, the nurse and the client's family, or the nurse and the physician. In resolving these ethical questions, nurses often use just one ethical system, or they may use a combination of several ethical systems.

The two systems that are most directly concerned with ethical decision-making in the health-care professions are utilitarianism and deontology. Both apply to bioethical issues: the ethics of life (or, in some cases, death).

Bioethics. **Bioethics** and **bioethical issues** are terms that are in common use. These terms have become synonymous with health-care ethics and encompass not only questions concerning life and death but also questions of quality of life, life-sustaining and life-altering technologies, and biological science in general. It is in the context of bioethics that the following discussion of these two systems of ethics is undertaken.

Utilitarianism
Ethical Precepts

Utilitarianism (also called **teleology,** consequentialism, or situation ethics) is referred to as the ethical system of utility. As a system of normative ethics, utilitarianism defines good as happiness or pleasure. It is associated with two underlying principles: "the greatest good for the greatest number" and "the end justifies the means." Because of these two principles, utilitarianism is sometimes subdivided into rule utilitarianism and act utilitarianism.

Rule Utilitarianism

According to rule utilitarianism, the individual draws on past experiences to formulate internal rules that are useful in determining the greatest good. With act utilitarianism, the particular situation in which a nurse finds himself or herself determines the rightness or wrongness of a particular act. In practice, the true follower of utilitarianism does not believe in the validity of any system of rules because the rules can change depending on the circumstances surrounding whatever decision needs to be made.

Act Utilitarianism

Situation ethics is probably the most publicized form of act utilitarianism. Joseph Fletcher, one of the best-known proponents of act utilitarianism, outlines a method of ethical thinking in which the situation itself determines whether the act is morally right or wrong. Fletcher views acts as good to the extent that they promote happiness and bad to the degree that they promote unhappiness. Happiness is defined as the happiness of the greatest number of people, yet the happiness of each person is to have equal weight.

Abortion, for example, is considered ethical in this system in a situation in which an unwed mother on welfare with four other children becomes pregnant with her fifth child. The greatest good and the greatest amount of happiness are produced by aborting this unwanted child.

Because utilitarianism is based on the concept that moral rules should not be arbitrary but should rather serve a purpose, ethical decisions derived from a utilitarian framework weigh the effect of alternative actions that influence the overall welfare of present and future populations. As such, this system is oriented toward the good of the population in general and toward the individual in the sense that the individual participates in that population.

Advantages

The major advantage of the utilitarian system of ethical decision-making is that many individuals find it easy to use in most situations. Utilitarianism is built around an individual's needs for happiness in which the individual has an immediate and vested interest. Another advantage is that utilitarianism fits well into a society that otherwise shuns rules and regulations.

A follower of utilitarianism can justify many decisions based on the happiness principle. Also, its utility orientation fits well into Western society's belief in the work ethic and a behavioristic approach to education, philosophy, and life.

> *Over time, popular acceptance of ethical rights can give them the force of a legal right. An example of an ethical right in the United States is the belief in universal access to health care. In the United States, it is really a longstanding privilege. . . .*

Telling a Sad Truth?

The follower of utilitarianism will support a general prohibition against lying and deceiving because ultimately the results of telling the truth will lead to greater happiness than the results of lying. Yet truth telling is not an absolute requirement to the follower of utilitarianism. If telling the truth will produce widespread unhappiness for a great number of people and future generations, it would be ethically better to tell a lie that will yield more happiness than to tell a truth that will lead to greater unhappiness.

Although such behavior might appear to be unethical at first glance, the strict follower of act utilitarianism would have little difficulty in arriving at this decision as a logical conclusion of utilitarian ethical thinking.

Disadvantages
Who Decides?

Some serious limitations exist in using utilitarianism as a system of health-care ethics or bioethics. An immediate question is whether happiness refers to the average happiness of all or the total happiness of a few. Because individual happiness is also important, one must consider how to make decisions when the individual's happiness is in conflict with that of the larger group.

More fundamental is the question of what constitutes happiness. Similarly, what constitutes the greatest good for the greatest number? Who determines what is good in the first place? Is it society in general, the government, governmental policy, or the individual? In health-care delivery and the formulation of health-care policy, the general guiding principle often seems to be the greatest good for the greatest number. Yet where do minority groups fit into this system?

Also, the tenet that the ends justify the means has been consistently rejected as a rationale for justifying actions. It is generally unacceptable to allow any type of action as long as the final goal or purpose is good. The Nazis in the 1930s and 1940s used this aphorism to justify many actions that may be viewed by others to be considerably less than good.

What Is Good?

The other difficulty in determining what is good lies in the attempt to quantify such concepts as good, harm, benefits, and greatest. This problem becomes especially acute in regard to health-care issues that involve individuals' lives. For example, an elderly family member has been sick for a long time, and that course of illness has placed great financial hardship on the family. It would be ethical under utilitarianism to allow this client to die or even to euthanize her to relieve the financial stress created by her illness.

Utilitarianism as an ethical system in the health-care decision-making process requires use of an additional principle of distributive justice as an ultimate guiding point. Unfortunately, whenever an unchanging principle is combined with this system, it negates the basic concept of pure utilitarianism.

Pure utilitarianism, although easy to use as a decision-making system, does not work well as an ethical system for decision-making in health care because of its arbitrary, self-centered nature. In the everyday delivery of health care, utilitarianism is often combined with other types of ethical decision-making in the resolution of ethical dilemmas.[5]

> *Another advantage is that utilitarianism fits well into a society that otherwise shuns rules and regulations. A follower of utilitarianism can justify many decisions based on the happiness principle.*

Deontology
Ethical Precepts

Deontology is a system of ethical decision-making based on moral rules and unchanging principles. This system is also termed the formalistic system, the principle system of ethics, or duty-based ethics. A follower of a pure form of the deontological system of ethical decision-making believes in the ethical absoluteness of principles regardless of the consequences of the decision.

The Categorical Imperative. Strict adherence to an ethical theory, in which the moral rightness or wrongness of human actions is considered separately from the consequences, is based on a fundamental principle called the categorical imperative. It is not the results of the act that make it right or wrong, but the principles by reason of which the act is carried out. These fundamental principles are ultimately unchanging and absolute and are derived from the universal values that underlie all major religions. Focusing on a concern for right and wrong in the moral sense is the basic premise of the system. Its goal is the survival of the species and social cooperation.

Unchanging Standards

Rule deontology is based on the belief that standards exist for the ethical choices and judgments made by individuals. These standards are fixed and do not change when the situation changes. Although the number of standards or rules is potentially unlimited, in reality—and particularly in dealing with bioethical issues—many of these principles can be grouped together into a few general principles.

These principles can also be arranged into a type of hierarchy of rules and include such maxims as the following: People should always be treated as ends and never as means; human life has value; one is always to tell the truth; above all in health care, do no harm; humans have a right to self-determination; and all people are of equal value. These principles echo such fundamental documents as the Bill of Rights and the American Hospital Association's Patient's Bill of Rights.

Advantages

The deontological system is useful in making ethical decisions in health care because it holds that an ethical judgment based on principles will be the same in a variety of given similar situations regardless of the time, location, or particular individuals involved. In addition, deontological terminology and concepts are similar to the terms and concepts used by the legal system.

The legal system emphasizes rights, duties, principles, and rules. Significant differences, however, exist between the two. Legal rights and duties are enforceable under the law, whereas ethical rights and duties are usually not. In general, ethical systems are much wider and more inclusive than the system of laws that they underlie. It is difficult to have an ethical perspective on law without having it lead to an interest in making laws that govern health care and nursing practice.

Disadvantages

The deontological system of ethical decision-making is not free from imperfection. Some of the more troubling questions include the following: What do you do when the basic guiding principles conflict with each other? What is the source of the principles? Is there ever a situation in which an exception to the rule will apply?

Although various approaches have been proposed to circumvent these limitations, it may be difficult for nurses to resolve situations in which duties and obligations conflict, particularly when the consequences of following a rule end in harm or hurt being done to a client. In reality, there are probably few pure followers of deontology because most people will consider the consequences of their actions in the decision-making process.

APPLICATION OF ETHICAL THEORIES

Ethical theories do not provide recipes for resolution of ethical dilemmas. Instead, they provide a framework for decision-making that the nurse can apply to a particular ethical situation.

A Framework for Decisions

At times, ethical theories may seem too abstract or general to be of much use to specific ethical situations. Without them, however, ethical decisions may often be made without reasoning or forethought and may be based on emotions. Most nurses in attempting to make ethical decisions combine the two theories presented here.

What Do You Think?

Identify a situation in which you were faced with an ethical dilemma. Which system of ethical decision-making did you use? Why did you select that system?

Nursing Code of Ethics

A code of ethics is generally defined as the ethical principles that govern a particular profession. Codes of ethics are presented as general statements and thus do not give specific answers to every possible ethical dilemma that might arise. These codes do, however, offer guidance to the individual practitioner in making decisions.

> *Ethical theories do not provide recipes for resolution of ethical dilemmas. Instead, they provide a framework for decision-making that the nurse can apply to a particular ethical situation.*

A Periodic Review

Ideally, codes of ethics should be reviewed periodically to reflect necessary changes in the profession and society as a whole. Although codes of ethics are not judicially enforceable as laws, consistent violations of the code of ethics by a professional in any field may indicate an unwillingness to act in a professional manner and will often result in disciplinary actions ranging from reprimands and fines to suspension of licensure.

Although they are similar, there are several different codes of ethics that nurses may adopt. In the United States, the ANA Code of Ethics is the generally accepted code. After several years of work, the ANA revised the Code of Ethics in 2001 to be more reflective of the health-care challenges in the new century (Box 7.1). There is also a Canadian Nurses Association Code of Ethics.

Box 7.1

The American Nurses Association Code of Ethics

1. The nurse in all professional relationships practices with compassion and respect for the inherent dignity, worth, and uniqueness of every individual, unrestricted by considerations of social or economic status, personal attributes or the nature of health problems.
2. The nurse's primary commitment is to the patient, whether an individual, family, group, or community.
3. The nurse promotes, advocates for, and strives to protect the health, safety, and rights of the patient.
4. The nurse is responsible and accountable for individual nursing practice and determines the appropriate delegation of tasks consistent with the nurse's obligation to provide optimum patient care.
5. The nurse owes the same duties to self as to others including the responsibility to preserve integrity and safety, to maintain competence, and to continue personal and professional growth.
6. The nurse participates in establishing, maintaining, and improving health-care environments and conditions of employment conducive to the provision of quality health care and consistent with the values of the profession through individual and collective action.
7. The nurse participates in the advancement of the profession through contributions to practice, education, administration, and knowledge development.
8. The nurse collaborates with other health professionals and the public in promoting community, national, and international efforts to meet health needs.
9. The profession of nursing, as represented by associations and their members, is responsible for articulating nursing values, for maintaining the integrity of the profession and its practice, and for shaping social policy.

Source: Code for Nurses With Interpretive Statements. Washington DC, American Nurses Publishing, American Nurses Foundation/American Nurses Association, 2001, p 1, with permission.

Clearly Stated Principles

The ANA Code of Ethics has been acknowledged by other health-care professions as one of the most complete. It is sometimes used as the benchmark against which other codes of ethics are measured. Yet a careful reading of this code of ethics reveals only a set of clearly stated principles that the nurse must apply to actual clinical situations.

For example, the nurse involved in resuscitation will find no specific mention of **no-code orders** in the ANA Code of Ethics. Rather, the nurse must be able to apply general statements to the particular situation. For example:

The nurse . . . practices with compassion and respect for the inherent dignity, worth, and uniqueness of every individual, unrestricted by considerations of social or economic status, personal attributes or the nature of health-care problems.

The nurse is responsible and accountable for individual nursing practice and determines the appropriate delegation of tasks consistent

with the nurse's obligation to provide optimum patient care.

The ANA Code Revised

The revised Code of Ethics restates and reinforces the basic values and commitments that have been and remain essential to the profession of nursing (see Box 7.1). Traditional ethical principles such as veracity, justice, beneficence, and autonomy are re-emphasized. The nurse is still expected to practice with cooperation, wisdom, compassion, honesty, courage, and respect for the client's privacy. However, the revised code, in response to current health-care practices, defines new boundaries of duty and loyalty. Ethical challenges, such as cost containment, delegation, and information technology, require nurses to look at health care from new perspectives.

The revised code supports nurses in their attempts to upgrade their employment conditions and environment through measures such as collective bargaining. The revised code addresses and supports nurses who are involved in whistle-blowing when dealing with health-care team members who may be chemically impaired or otherwise incompetent in practice. It also supports nurses in their right to refuse to practice in treatments that violate their beliefs.

The revised code also expands nursing duties beyond individual nurse–client interactions. It recognizes that professional nurses now work in multiple practice areas; therefore, they are responsible for developing and using their knowledge in these expanded areas through research and collaborative practice. The 2001 Code for Nurses is an important document that nurses need to be familiar with, both to help ensure ethical practice and to shape an improved future for the profession of nursing.

THE DECISION-MAKING PROCESS

Nurses, by definition, are problem solvers, and one of the important tools that nurses use is the nursing process. The nursing process is a systematic step-by-step approach to resolving problems that deal with a client's health and well-being.

Although nurses deal with problems related to the physical or psychological needs of clients, many feel inadequate when dealing with ethical problems associated with client care. Nurses in any health-care setting can, however, develop the decision-making skills necessary to make sound

ethical decisions if they learn and practice using an ethical decision-making process.

Modeling the Nursing Process

An ethical decision-making process provides a method for nurses to answer key questions about ethical dilemmas and to organize their thinking in a more logical and sequential manner. Although there are several ethical decision-making models, the problem-solving method presented here is based on the nursing process. It should be a relatively easy transition from the nursing process used in resolving a client's physical problems to the ethical decision-making process for the resolution of problems with ethical ramifications.

The chief goal of the ethical decision-making process is to determine right and wrong in situations in which clear demarcations are not readily apparent. This process presupposes that the nurse making the decision knows that a system of ethics exists, knows the content of that ethical system, and knows that the system applies to similar ethical decision-making problems despite multiple variables. In addition to identifying their own values, nurses need an understanding of the possible ethical systems that may be used in making decisions about ethical dilemmas.

The following ethical decision-making process is presented as a tool for resolving ethical dilemmas (Fig. 7.1).

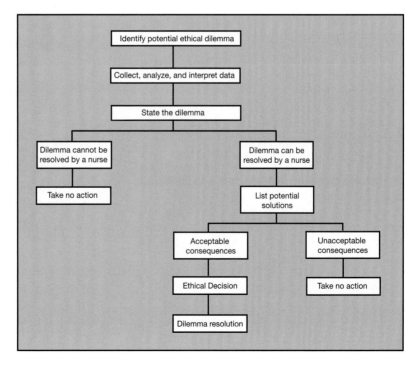

Figure 7.1 Ethical decision-making algorithm. (Adapted with permission from Catalano JT: Ethical decision making in the critical care patient. Critical Care Nursing Clinics of North America 9(1):45–52, 1997.)

Step 1: Collect, Analyze, and Interpret the Data

Obtain as much information as possible concerning the particular ethical dilemma. Unfortunately, such information is sometimes very limited. Among the important issues are the client's wishes, the client's family's wishes, the extent of the physical or emotional problems causing the dilemma, the physician's beliefs about health care, and the nurse's own orientation to issues concerning life and death.

What Do You Think?

identify a health-care–related ethical situation that is currently in the news. What are the key elements of the dilemma? Discuss how to resolve it with your classmates.

Many nurses, for example, face the question of whether or not to initiate resuscitation efforts when a terminally ill client is admitted to the hospital. Physicians often leave instructions for the nursing staff indicating that the nurses should not resuscitate the client but should, instead, merely go through the motions to make the family feel better, which is sometimes referred to as a **slow-code order.** The nurse's dilemma is whether to make a serious attempt to revive the client or to let the client die quietly.

Important information that will help the nurse make the decision might include:

• The mental competency of the client to make a no-resuscitation decision
• The client's desires
• The family's feelings
• Whether the physician previously sought input from the client and the family
• Whether there is a living will or DPOAHC

Many institutions have policies concerning no-resuscitation orders, and it is wise to consider these during data collection. After collecting information, the nurse needs to bring the pieces of information together in a manner that will give the clearest and sharpest focus to the dilemma.

Step 2: State the Dilemma

After collecting and analyzing as much information as is available, the nurse needs to state the dilemma as clearly as possible. In this step, it is important to identify whether the problem is one that directly involves the nurse or is one that can be resolved only by the client, the client's family, the physician, or the DPOAHC.

Recognizing the key aspects of the dilemma helps focus attention on the important ethical principles. Most of the time, the dilemma can be reduced to a few statements that encompass the key ethical issues. Such ethical issues often involve a question of conflicting rights, obligations, or basic ethical principles.

In the case of a no-resuscitation order, the statement of the dilemma might be "the client's right to death with dignity versus the nurse's obligation to preserve life and do no harm." In general, the principle that the competent client's wishes must be followed is unequivocal. If the client has become unresponsive before expressing his or her wishes, the family members' input must be given serious consideration. Additional questions can arise if the family's wishes conflict with those of the client.

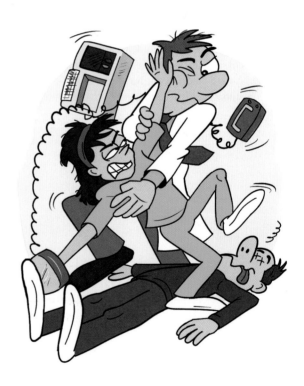

Step 3: Consider the Choices of Action

After stating the dilemma as clearly as possible, the next step is to attempt to list, without consideration of their consequences, all possible courses of action that can be taken to resolve the dilemma. This brainstorming activity, in which all possible courses of action are considered, may require input from outside sources such as colleagues, supervisors, or even experts in the ethical field. The consequences of the different actions are considered later in this chapter.

Some possible courses of action for the nurse in the resuscitation scenario might include the following:

- Resuscitating the client to the nurse's fullest capabilities despite what the physician has requested
- Not resuscitating the client at all
- Only going through the motions without any real attempt to revive the client
- Seeking another assignment to avoid dealing with the situation
- Reporting the problem to a supervisor
- Attempting to clarify the question with the client
- Attempting to clarify the question with the family
- Confronting the physician about the question
- Consulting the institution's ethics committee

Recognizing the key aspects of the dilemma helps focus attention on the important ethical principles. Most of the time, the dilemma can be reduced to a few statements that encompass the key ethical issues.

For nurses who are unsure about which issues can be referred to the ethics committee, the facility's policy and procedure manual can give direction.

Step 4: Analyze the Advantages and Disadvantages of Each Course of Action

Some of the courses of action developed during the previous step are more realistic than others. The identification of these actions becomes readily evident during this step in the decision-making process, when the advantages and the disadvantages of each action are considered in detail. Along with each option, the consequences of taking each course of action must be thoroughly evaluated.

Consider whether initiating a discussion might anger the physician or cause distrust of the nurse involved. Both these responses may reinforce the attitude of submission to the physician, and either could create difficulty in continuing to practice nursing at that institution. The same result may occur if the nurse successfully resuscitates a client despite orders to the contrary. Failure to resuscitate the client has the potential to produce a lawsuit unless a clear order for no resuscitation has been given. Presenting the situation to a supervisor may, if the supervisor supports the physician, cause the nurse to be considered a troublemaker and thus have a negative effect on future evaluations. The same process could be applied to the other courses of action.

When considering the advantages and disadvantages, the nurse should be able to narrow the realistic choices of action. Other relevant issues need to be examined when weighing the choices of action. A major factor would be choosing the appropriate code of ethics. The ANA Code of Ethics should be part of many client-care decisions affected by ethical dilemmas.

Step 5: Make the Decision and Act on it

The most difficult part of the process is actually making the decision, following through with action, and then living with the consequences. Decisions are often made with no follow-through because nurses are fearful of the consequences of their decisions. By their nature, ethical dilemmas produce differences of opinion, and not everyone will be pleased with the decision.

In the attempt to solve any ethical dilemma, there will always be a question of the correct course of action. The client's wishes almost always supersede independent decisions on the part of health-care professionals. A collaborative decision made by the client, physician, nurses, and family about resuscitation is the ideal situation and tends to produce fewer complications in the long-term resolution of such questions.

Conclusion

Ethical dilemmas, by definition, are difficult to resolve. Rarely will a nurse find ethical dilemmas covered in policy, procedure, and protocol manuals, but nurses can develop the skills necessary to make appropriate ethical decisions. The key to developing these skills is the recognition and frequent use of an ethical decision-making model and application of the appropriate ethical theories to the dilemma. As an orderly approach in solving the often disorderly aspects of ethical questions encountered in nursing practice, the decision-making model presented in this chapter can be applied to almost every type of ethical dilemma. Although each situation is different, ethical decision-making based on ethical theory can provide a potent tool for resolving dilemmas found in client-care situations.

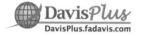
DavisPlus.fadavis.com

Critical Thinking Exercises

1. Ask the facility where you work or have clinical rotations what code of ethics they use. How does that differ from the ANA Code?

2. Ask your faculty what code of ethics is used for your evaluation.

3. Compare and contrast ethics with laws by delineating the purposes, scopes, and methods of enforcement of each.

4. Distinguish between the two types of obligations.

5. Compare the three categories of rights.

6. Analyze the following ethical dilemma case study using the ethical decision-making process:

- What are the important data in relation to this situation?
- State the ethical dilemma in a clear, simple statement.
- What are the choices of action and how do they relate to specific ethical principles?
- What are the consequences of these actions?
- What decision can be made?

Bill L, a veteran ED nurse, called the resident physician about a client just admitted to the ED after a fall from a ladder. The client, a 52-year-old man, had been fixing his roof when the accident occurred. He had suffered a minor head injury, a twisted ankle, and a badly bruised arm. He also had a long history of asthma and heavy smoking. Not long after his admission to the ED, the client became cyanotic, dyspneic, and semiconscious. By the time the resident physician arrived, the nurse had prepared the client for endotracheal intubation and had already notified the personnel in the medical intensive care unit (MICU) that they would be receiving this client.

After a hasty evaluation of the client, the resident decided to perform an emergency tracheostomy before transporting the client to the MICU. While performing the tracheostomy, the physician severed a major blood vessel, and the client hemorrhaged profusely. After several tense minutes, the endotracheal tube was inserted, and the client was quickly transported to the MICU. The client remained cyanotic and had great difficulty breathing. Shortly after he left the ED, the nurse realized that the oxygen tank that the client had been connected to was empty. The client never regained consciousness and died 3 days after admission. His death was due to respiratory failure and not to the injuries sustained in the fall.

When the client's wife came to the unit to collect the deceased's belongings, the nurse was torn between telling her about the mistakes that were made in the treatment of her husband and remaining silent. What are the key ethical principles involved in this situation? Are there any statements in the ANA Code of Ethics that may help resolve this dilemma? What would be the consequences of informing the client's wife of the truth? What are the consequences of not informing her?

8

Bioethical Issues

Joseph T. Catalano
Sarah T. Catalano

Learning Objectives

After completing this chapter, the reader will be able to:

- Discuss the key ethical principles involved in:
  Abortion
  Genetic research
  Fetal tissue research
  Organ transplantation
  Use of scarce resources
  Assisted suicide
  Acquired immunodeficiency syndrome (AIDS)
  Children's issues
- Discuss the nurse's role in these ethical dilemmas.
- Analyze and make a thoughtful ethical decision in a complex situation.

THE CLIENT'S WELL-BEING

In the recent history of nursing, numerous biomedical and ethical dilemmas have arisen. Historically, nurses have been concerned with moral responsibility and ethical decision-making. The nursing code of ethics and its frequent revisions demonstrate the profession's concern with providing ethical health care.

The earliest codes of ethics made obedience to the physician the nurse's primary responsibility. The present code of ethics recognizes that the primary responsibility of the nurse is the client's well-being. This change in emphasis reflects the profession's increased self-awareness, independence, and growing accountability for its actions. Unfortunately, this new attitude has also heralded an era of increased tension, self-doubt, and ethical confusion. By examining the issues and identifying the key moral and ethical conflicts, nurses will be able to accept their moral responsibilities and make good ethical decisions.

In the course of their careers, nurses are likely to encounter any number of ethical dilemmas. Although a complete analysis of every issue is beyond the scope of this book, some of the more common situations and their important ethical features are presented as examples of ways to analyze such dilemmas and to make informed decisions. The resolution of ethical dilemmas is never an easy task, and it is likely that someone may disagree with the decision.

ABORTION

A Polarizing Issue

Few issues evoke as strong an emotional reaction as abortion. Because of its religious, ethical, social, and legal implications, the abortion issue touches everyone in one way or another. There seems to be very little middle ground. People are either strongly in favor of abortion or oppose it completely. Even in presidential elections, abortion has become a central issue, and the outcomes of some elections may very well be decided by the candidates' positions on the law that supports the practice.

What Do You Think?

Do you support or reject elective abortion? On what ethical principles do you base your belief? What advice would you give to a pregnant teenager who wanted to have an abortion?

A Matter of Convenience?

Elective abortion is the voluntary termination of a pregnancy before 24 weeks of gestation. An elective abortion may be either therapeutic or self-selected. Late-term abortion is the termination of a pregnancy after 24 weeks of gestation up to the day of delivery. Strictly speaking, a therapeutic abortion would be one performed in consultation with and on the recommendation of a physician or psychiatrist, based on the conclusion that the mother's health or psychological state would be damaged without the abortion.

Self-selected, or elective, abortions are those performed solely on the mother's own decision, without consultation with a physician or psychiatrist, usually for economic or convenience reasons. In the case of *Roe v. Wade* in 1973, the Supreme Court changed the legal status of elective abortion in the United States, but the ethical basis and moral status of this decision remain controversial.

A careful reading of the court's decision in *Roe v. Wade* reveals that the justices made no decision about the ethics or morality of elective abortion. Rather, the court said that, according to the U.S. Constitution, all people have a right to determine what they can do with their bodies (i.e., the right to self-determination) and that such a right includes termination of a pregnancy.

A Conflict of Rights?

The fundamental issues at the heart of the abortion debate center on the question of when life begins and the right of freedom of choice. Those who argue against abortion believe that life begins at the moment of conception and therefore hold that abortion is an act of killing. Proponents of abortion argue that the fetus is not really human until it reaches the point of development when it can live outside the mother's body (i.e., the age of viability, about 20 weeks). From a deontological standpoint, abortion represents a basic conflict of rights.

On one hand, a woman's rights to privacy, self-determination, and freedom of choice are at issue. In the United States, these rights are fiercely held and are considered to be issues of public policy and **constitutional law.** Indeed, these rights form the basis of the *Roe v. Wade* decision.

The conflicting right from the antiabortion side of the dilemma is the fetus's right to life. In most Western civilizations, particularly those that are based on Judeo-Christian beliefs, the casual and intentional taking of a human life is strongly prohibited. Life is the most basic good because without it there can be no other rights. In general, the right to life is considered to be the most profound of the rights and is absolute in most situations.

When one is attempting to resolve the ethics and morality of abortion, these two conflicting rights need to be weighed against each other. Nurses are often placed in situations in which they must help clients make decisions about abortion. Just as frequently, they are asked to participate in the procedure itself.

Where Your Values Fit in

In practice, ethical issues are always affected by the health-care provider's moral values. In the dilemma over abortion, nurses must analyze their own values and perceptions of their roles to make the best decisions. As a client **advocate,** should a nurse be for or against abortion? How can a nurse avoid influencing the woman's decision about abortion? Can a nurse ethically and legally refuse to assist at abortions? Should the client's reason for wanting an abortion or her stage of pregnancy (i.e., first or second trimester, or later, requiring a partial-birth procedure) have any influence on the nurse's decision?

These questions are not easily answered, but understanding the underlying principles involved in the issue may help defuse some of the emotional impact that often surrounds this topic. As in all complicated ethical dilemmas, the nurse needs to remember that the client must receive competent, high-quality care regardless of the nurse's own personal values or moral beliefs.

GENETICS AND GENETIC RESEARCH

The ability to alter genetic material to produce organisms that differ greatly from their original form is now a reality. Scientific and popular literature is filled with reports of new ways to identify and change the genetic material of all types of living creatures.

The Future is Now

Currently, genetically altered bacteria (e.g., *Escherichia coli*) are used to produce various medications, including a purer form of insulin. Genetically altered corn is now growing in very hot, dry places and is resistant to most insects. Abnormal genes that indicate individuals who are at risk for various types of cancer, Alzheimer's disease, Parkinson's disease, and Down syndrome have been identified. Recently, "artificial" bacteria have been produced in the lab by chemically generating DNA segments and then assembling them into larger structures. The process is called *homologous recombination* and has been used experimentally for several years to repair damaged chromosomes in yeast. Scientists view this process as the first step to understanding how life developed on earth and eventually as a way to create designer bacteria that can produce everything from medicines to biofuels. Detractors fear the development of bioweapons that will not be able to be controlled.

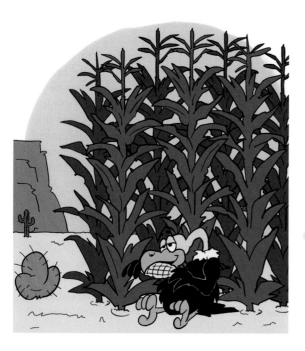

In the 20th century, society became so accustomed to the idea that science should be allowed to do whatever it is capable of doing that very few questions were asked about the ethics of genetic engineering and research. As with most scientific research and techniques, the techniques of genetic engineering are ethically neutral. Procedures such as refining recombinant DNA, gene therapy, altering germ cells, and cloning other cells are neither good nor bad in themselves. The potential for misuse of these procedures is so great, however, that it may permanently alter or even destroy the human species.

Ethics of Genetic Research

Several ethical issues need to be considered when genetic engineering and research are being conducted, including those involving the safety of genetic research, the legality and morality of genetic screening, and the proper use of genetic information. In 2008, the Genetic Information Nondiscrimination Act (GINA) was passed to help guide healthcare workers in the use of genetic information and the protections for clients under the law. However, the law has several major limitations and does not protect all clients in all situations.[1] Other laws regulating genetic research have been proposed to prevent the production of a supervirus or superbacterium that could exterminate the entire human population.

Mandatory Screening

With current technology, it is possible to detect genetic patterns in newborn infants that are linked to breast and colon cancer, heart disease, Huntington's disease, and Parkinson's disease. The advantage to insurance companies, which could screen individuals as early as infancy for costly and potentially lethal diseases later in life, is obvious: these individuals could be excluded from health and life insurance coverage, thus saving the insurance companies a great deal of money.

What Do You Think?

Do you support genetic research? What restrictions, if any, would you place on this type of research? Are these restrictions plausible or enforceable?

Although this practice would most likely be unethical, the concept of mandatory genetic screening is not unrealistic. Because it requires just one blood sample from a person at some point during that person's life, it is possible that this type of screening could even be done without the individual's knowledge or consent.

Informed Consent

Informed consent is permission granted by a person with full knowledge of the risks and benefits of what is being done. The basic question is: Do parents violate the right of informed consent if they give permission to have gene testing performed on their newborn and have the results released to an insurance company? Do insurance companies violate informed consent if they somehow obtain the information without the knowledge of the client? (Informed consent is discussed in detail in Chapter 9.)

Confidentiality

Similarly, confidentiality is at great risk for being violated by genetic screening. The confidentiality, trust, and fidelity that exist between the health-care provider and the client have been the basis of the therapeutic relationship. In some cases, individuals may be denied employment because of the results of genetic testing. In this time of the information superhighway and vast computerized databases, very little of a client's health history remains confidential.[2] Recently, various state and federal law enforcement agencies have compiled DNA databases for identifying criminals. It is only a short step from using genetic samples for disease screening to placing DNA samples in a national database.

Emotional Impact

An important ethical implication for nurses is the emotional impact that genetic information may have on the client. Knowledge of the possible long-term outcome of one's health, particularly if that knowledge is negative, may cause a client **anxiety,** or the person may become depressed or suicidal. Nurses must further hone their teaching and counseling skills to assist clients in dealing with the implications of this type of information.

Obstetric nurses have been involved with genetic screening procedures for years. Some of the most important information obtained from amniocentesis deals with the genetic composition of the fetus. It is important that the mother understand the procedure and the type of information it may yield and that she give informed consent for this procedure.

Self-Determination

Nurses have a strict ethical obligation to refuse to participate in mandatory, involuntary screening programs, as well as a strict prohibition about revealing genetic test results to unauthorized individuals. Forcing testing on clients who are strongly opposed to finding out information about their genetic status is clearly a breach of those clients' right to self-determination.

> *In practice, ethical issues are always affected by the health-care provider's moral values. In the dilemma over abortion, nurses must analyze their own values and perceptions of their roles to make the best decisions.*

However, much as the current practice of routine screening for diseases such as tuberculosis, hepatitis, and blood lead levels promotes the general health of the population, so does the screening for genetic diseases. Clients who are strongly opposed to such genetic screening must be allowed the option to refuse it to maintain their right to self-determination.

Promise or Threat?

Now that the human genome has been decoded, a whole new world of possibilities—both positive and negative—has been opened for health-care providers. The impact of the Human Genome Project, cloning research, and other related genetic procedures is on par with the discovery of bacteria and antibiotics. The potential now exists for the cure of almost all known diseases, ranging from viral infections to cancer to the regeneration of spinal cord nerves.

On the other side of the issue, there is the potential for the development of superviruses that could wipe out the population of the earth. Nurses need to watch each development very closely and call their legal representatives when they believe science is moving into dangerous areas.[3]

USE OF FETAL TISSUE

Fetal tissue research has been conducted since at least the early 1990s. Traditional fetal tissue research has been generally limited to taking living cells from an aborted fetus and transplanting them into people who have chronic or severe diseases. The procedure has been found to be helpful to a limited extent in the treatment of Alzheimer's disease, Parkinson's disease, and spinal cord regeneration after traumatic injuries.

Growing Tissue on Demand
Artificial Conception
From 1997 to 2000, the Human Genome Project added a new twist to this research. Rather than using tissue from aborted fetuses, scientists are now growing their own fetal tissue in the laboratory through **artificial insemination** and in vitro fertilization procedures. These test-tube fetuses are then dissected. Various fetal tissues are used for genetic and other types of research. The legal system became aware of the potential abuses of these procedures and has passed legislation to control their use, including limiting the age of in vitro fetuses to 6 weeks. After 6 weeks, such fetuses will have to be destroyed.

Stem Cell Research
Stem cell research is a closely related issue. Stem cells are the very early cells present in the developing fetus that have not yet begun to differentiate; that is, all the cells are identical and contain all the genetic material needed to reproduce an identical individual. Stem cells can be separated and then placed in an environment where they will form more stem cells; or the genetic material from the stem cell can be removed and replaced; or the genetic material can be removed, manipulated, and then replaced. Recent federal administrative acts have lifted many of the restrictions put in place by the Bush administration. However, the types of research that can be conducted are still tightly restricted. There are no restrictions on privately funded stem cell research.[4]

For a number of years, research in stem cell technology has demonstrated that umbilical cord blood contains significant levels of stem cells. Because the placenta and umbilical cord are discarded after a baby is born, this source of stem cells would seem to lack the ethical implications of in vitro fertilization and embryonic research, which require the destruction of embryos. However, several ethical questions to consider are: Who owns the placenta and umbilical cord after the baby is born? Does the mother own it? Should she receive payment for it? Is it the baby's? Or is it just considered medical waste, like a tumor that has been removed?

Like stem cells, fetal tissue is highly desirable for research and transplantation because it lacks some of the genetic material that makes more mature tissues and organs more likely to cause rejection in the host. These fetal tissues are also in a rapid growth mode and naturally develop more quickly than do tissues from other sources. Scientists involved in this research see fetal tissue as one of the most important means of curing diseases.

Adult stem cell research has yielded a new source of stem cells without the ethical issues that swirl around fetal stem cells. However, initial research results indicate that adult stem cells are useful in only a few disease processes.

The Source of the Material
Even a superficial consideration of these procedures necessarily raises many important ethical issues. The source of the research material is basic to the ethics of this type of research. In the past, much of the material came from elective abortions.

Potential for Abuse
Because of the immaturity and lack of differentiation of cells during the first trimester of pregnancy, the best fetal tissue comes from fetuses aborted during the second trimester. Most scientists agree that second-trimester fetuses have well-developed nervous, cardiovascular, gastrointestinal, and renal systems and are capable of feeling pain. Even though fetal tissue research has not led to an increase in abortions, the potential for abuse is tremendous.

Paying for Fetuses?
It is also not definite whether the fetal tissue research scientists are paying others for these aborted fetuses. If payment is being made for aborted fetuses, it would seem to violate both the laws that prevent payment for organs used in transplantation and the moral respect for humanity. Questions also arise concerning who is giving permission for the use of fetuses in transplantation procedures. Does anyone really own them?

In Vitro Fertilization

Another important ethical issue concerns the use of in vitro fertilization as a source for fetal tissue. Many religious groups question the morality of the procedure itself. Even if in vitro fertilization is considered ethical for procedures such as surrogate motherhood, is it ethical to create fetuses that are going to be used only for research and transplantation? From whom are the ova and sperm coming? Have the people from whom these have been obtained given permission for such use of their tissues? What about the rights of a fetus that was created in a test tube without ever having a hope of a normal life?

The Nurse's Role

The 1988 directive, which was extended indefinitely in 1990 to prevent the Department of Health and Human Services from using federal money for fetal tissue research, was amended in 2001 to allow this type of research on a very limited basis with federal funding. This regulation was reinforced by the Obama administration in 2009. Local biomedical ethical panels can make decisions about this type of research. Many of these panels, which consist mainly of research scientists, have ruled in favor of continuing research.

Nurses may have an important role to play in issues involving fetal tissue research. Although they will not likely be involved directly in research, nurses are often employed in facilities where elective abortions are performed. Nurses employed in such places must become aware of the issues involved in abortion. They also should know where the aborted fetuses are taken and how they are disposed of. Nurses should remain informed about developing procedures and techniques regarding fetal tissue research; they should support legal and ethical efforts to control its abuses.

ORGAN TRANSPLANTATION

Despite widespread public and medical acceptance of organ transplantation as a highly beneficial procedure, ethical questions still remain. Whenever a human organ is transplanted, many people are involved, including the donor, the donor's family, medical and nursing personnel, and the recipient and his or her family. Transplantation is the only health-care field in which actions taken by a group of medical professionals in one part of the country affect their counterparts in another part of the country.

Society as a whole is affected by organ transplantation, mainly because of the high cost of the procedures, which usually are covered by federal funding from taxes or reimbursement from private insurance, which in turn increases insurance premiums. Whether it occurs on a popular medically oriented television series or in a movie where organ donation is the primary focus, the general public is exposed to organ donation more frequently now than in decades past.[5] This popular exposure increases awareness of the need for organ donation and calls attention to people or groups of people who are affected by every aspect of donation and transplantation. Each one of these persons or groups has rights that may directly conflict with the rights of others.

The Good of the Donor

Currently, the three primary sources for organ and tissue donations are living related donors, living unrelated donors, and **deceased,** formerly called **cadaveric, donors.** Transplantation centers and organizations involved in obtaining organs and tissues have developed complex procedures to cope with the ethical and legal issues involved in transplantation. Despite these efforts, some ethical uncertainties still surround the issue of organ transplantation.

When the Donor is a Child

Living pediatric organ donors exemplify a particularly sensitive issue. For example, when one sibling donates a kidney to another sibling, the procedure poses some serious risk for both donor and recipient. Parents are required to give consent for medical procedures for their children. By legal definition, a child younger than 18 years of age cannot give informed consent to such a procedure. It can be argued, however, that ethically the donor child, as a participant, should have input in making such a decision. At what age should a child have a say in the decision? Can a child be forced, for example, to donate a kidney even if he or she refuses? (See the discussion of children's ethics later in this chapter.)

One situation that illustrates this dilemma is that of a teenage girl who developed leukemia. The only way to save her life was to find a bone marrow donor who matched her genetic type. When no donor could be found, the parents decided to have another baby in the hope that the bone marrow of the second child would match that of the first child. After the baby was born, it was found that the bone marrow did indeed match, and when the child was old enough to donate safely, the bone marrow was taken and transplanted into the older child.

When Does Death Occur?

Despite the best efforts of the medical and legal community to establish criteria for death, some ethical questions still linger about what constitutes death. Because organs for transplantation such as the heart, lungs, and liver should ideally come from a donor whose heart is still beating, some clinicians fear that there will be a tendency for physicians to declare a person dead before death actually occurs. Many people also mistakenly believe that if they indicate they would like to be organ donors, and become sick or injured and admitted to the hospital, physicians will not work as hard to "save their lives."

The most widely accepted criterion for determining death in deceased donors is death by neurological criteria, formerly called brain death. The definition of death by neurological criteria in conjunction with organ donation is very clear, and health-care professionals use proven procedures to test for and determine death by neurological criteria. Because death by neurological criteria is defined by the complete cessation of function of the brain stem, brain death can be declared even when an electroencephalogram (EEG) shows continued cortical brain activity. Some researchers and health-care professionals struggle with the perceived ramifications of this determination of death. Should some other criteria be examined in conjunction with the neurological criteria for death?

Since 2006, the use of organs from non-heart-beating donors, also known as Donation after Cardiac Death (DCD), has become more readily accepted by the transplantation community as a viable alternative to narrowing the donation gap. DCD organ donation has its own set of ethical and legal considerations as well. Typically, only kidneys are recovered and transplanted from a DCD donor. However, progressive transplantation

programs have been successfully transplanting DCD livers and lungs.

Selecting the Recipient

One of the most difficult ethical issues involved in organ transplantation is the selection of recipients. Because fewer organs are available than the numerous people who need them, the potential ethical dilemmas are great. To give some perspective of the disparity of need versus availability, as of April 30, 2010, more than 100,000 people were listed on the transplant waiting list, whereas 9100 transplantations were performed from January 2010 through April 2010.[6]

Legislating Donation

The Uniform Anatomical Gift Act, passed in 1968, made the donation of organs, eyes, and tissue for transplantation a legal transaction involving a prespecified recipient. Later legislation prohibited prespecification of recipients by creating a federal entity to regulate the transplantation industry and made the sale of human organs illegal. This legislation, the National Organ Transplant Act, created the United Network for Organ Sharing (UNOS) to regulate organ allocation and maintain the national organ transplant waiting list. UNOS created a database of all people waitlisted for an organ and lists potential recipients using a prioritized computerized algorithm designed to ensure each recipient will benefit the most from a transplant. Transplant professionals create match-run lists for organ allocation based on the database and algorithm when a donor organ becomes available.

Additionally, each organ has its own requirements for allocation, and a match-run list for transplantation is generated according to the individual allocation policies for each organ. Important criteria for ranking potential recipients include stage of disease process, length of time spent waiting, tissue and blood type compatibility, size matching, and geographic proximity to the donor. The UNOS allocation policy is designed to provide organs for clients who have the greatest need as well as the best

> *Whenever a human organ is transplanted, many people are involved, including the donor, the donor's family, medical and nursing personnel, and the recipient and his or her family.*

projected outcome for a successful transplantation. Despite widespread public beliefs, the amount of money a potential recipient has, or the amount of publicity generated by a recipient and his or her family, does not have any bearing on the way organs are allocated.

There are 34 states that have passed First-Person Consent (or Donor Designation) laws, which are strictly upheld by local organ recovery agencies.[7] The federal legislation is known as the Revised Uniform Anatomical Gift Act (UAGA) and was designed to ensure the donor's wishes are honored at the time of death. This piece of legislation has created myriad ethical and legal issues, but all transplantation organizations agree that not accepting the donation from a medically suitable donor is a violation of this law. Additionally, failure to honor client wishes, in this case the donor's, may result in a risk management issue for the hospital in question. Recent revisions of the UAGA have strengthened the letter of the law to make the donor's wishes override all opposition and have given permission for organ procurement professionals to proceed with donation in the face of disapproving family members, many of whom threaten litigation (Box 8.1). A position paper from the National Organization for Transplant Professionals states, "From an ethical perspective, not accepting the donor's gift is a violation of their autonomy and a disregard for their wishes to help those in need."[8]

Box 8.1
Organ Donation

Have you ever called your hospital's attorney at 1:00 in the morning? I have. I also called my organization's lawyers, our medical director, and my executive director. The reason for all these early morning wake-up calls was that I had a brain-dead client on a ventilator who had declared her wish to be an organ donor on her driver's license and her heartbroken family was having none of it. They accepted her wish to be an organ donor, but they wanted the process to happen in 5 minutes. Despite what you see on television, that *never* happens in the world of organ donation. After learning that the donation would take time and that they could not override her wish, they became extremely upset and began yelling at me in the conference room of the unit. They were hostile to the hospital staff, and some family members were eventually escorted out by hospital security. Security also escorted me to my car when my shift ended at 8:00 a.m. because of threats made against me by the client's family.

I knew that I was doing the right thing by upholding the client's wish, but there were many times during the hours of confrontation with the family that I felt like backing down and "pulling the plug" on the whole situation. However, with every phone call I made, the answer was always the same: "Go ahead. Move forward. Proceed with the donation."

About 4 hours before taking the donor to the operating room, I called the client's family to see if they would like to return to the hospital to see her one last time before we took her away. Her husband, two sons, and one daughter returned to her bedside and said their tearful good-byes. After the surgical team took her to the operating room, I was able to have a sensible and more compassionate conversation with the family. Her husband dissolved into tears when I told him we were able to place her liver and both her kidneys. She saved three lives that day. Of course, they also had a lot of questions about her Donor Designation and why we had to do what we did.

This family was finally able to come to terms with the process of organ donation, and the fact that their loved one touched the lives of three others has been a great comfort to them in their grief. When I last spoke with them, they were working with an after-care specialist to facilitate a meeting with one of the kidney recipients. All because their wife and mother had a heart—on her driver's license.

Source: Sarah T. Catalano, Procurement Coordinator, New Mexico, Organ Procurement Organization.

The Nurse's Responsibility

All states have passed laws requiring health-care workers to refer all potential organ donors to the local organization responsible for organ recovery. The most important function of nurses in the organ donation process is to recognize and refer potential donors to the local organ procurement organization. Referral rates of potential organ donors within hospitals are tracked and reported to agencies such as The Joint Commission and the Centers for Medicare and Medicaid Services. Many nurses, particularly nurses who work in emergency departments and critical care units, care for clients who may potentially become organ donors. Such nurses should note that the referral of a client to the organ procurement organization for evaluation should not be viewed in any way as "giving up on the client" or "putting a nail in the coffin" for that client.

Organ donation professionals do not become involved in care of the client until after death has been declared by a physician or other designated health-care professional. Additionally, nurses should not hesitate to make a referral because of the physical or medical condition of the client. A referral is simply a notification of a client who meets or may meet criteria for organ donation. It is up to organ recovery professionals to determine whether the client is medically suitable for donation and to facilitate the donation process.

> *The most important function nurses perform in the organ donation process is the recognition and referral of a potential organ donor to the local organ procurement organization.*

When Should I Refer?

Although the exact requirements for referral vary by geographical service area, in general, clients meeting the following criteria should always be referred to the local organ procurement organization for evaluation for organ donation:

- Severe neurological insult or injury (i.e., hemorrhagic stroke, ruptured aneurism, head trauma such as gunshot wounds or motor vehicle accidents, and anoxic brain injury resulting from significant cardiac downtime)
- Glasgow Coma Scale score of 4 or less
- Intubated (on a ventilator) with a heartbeat
- When brain death evaluation is scheduled
- Before terminal extubation of a client meeting any of the above criteria[9]

Operating room nurses may help in surgical procedures to recover organs from a deceased donor and prepare them for transport and eventual transplantation into a recipient's body. Other nurses provide the postoperative care for clients who have received a transplant. Home health-care nurses give the follow-up care to such clients at home.

Many organ recovery agencies also train nurses to maintain the potential for organ donation in their clients and to deal with family members of potential donors in a compassionate, professional manner.

Nurses working with potential recipients should be sensitive to the potential for manipulation. Most people waiting for transplants are desperately ill or near death. They and their families can be easily manipulated or they themselves can become manipulative.

Obtain Permission Gently

On the other side, the families of potential organ donors are usually distraught about the sudden and traumatic loss of a loved one. They too are vulnerable to psychological manipulation. The emotionally fragile state of a trauma victim's family members predisposes them to feelings of guilt and grief. Health-care providers should avoid appealing to these emotions or becoming coercive when obtaining permission for organ donation. They are always welcome to participate in any discussion about donation with a potential donor's family. However, discussing organ, tissue, and eye donation and obtaining consent for these activities is generally best left to professionals who work exclusively for organ procurement organizations. They are specially trained, have time to spend with the families, and can make the organ donation process a positive experience for both the donor's family and the health-care professionals involved.

Nurses should avoid making statements or giving nonverbal indications of their approval or disapproval of potential recipients. Generally, neither the donor nor the family plays any part in selecting a recipient, and the identity of the recipient is carefully guarded by organ recovery professionals.

At times, organ recovery professionals can facilitate a process called Directed Donation, whereby a donor's family can indicate a particular recipient. Whether this process is successful depends on several factors, including geographical proximity, tissue and blood type compatibility, and whether the potential recipient is listed and has completed all the prerequisite tests to receive the organ. In cases in which Directed Donation is desired but not possible, the donated organs will be allocated according to UNOS policy.[9]

Tissue and Eye Donation

Although organ donation is done within a clinical setting, tissue and eye donation can take place in such venues as hospital morgues, funeral homes, and specialized recovery suites anywhere from 12 to 24 hours after cardiac death has occurred. Many families are approached regarding tissue and eye donation after they have left the hospital, if a death has occurred in a hospital, or on the arrival of the decedent's body at the funeral home. Recovery of donated tissue and corneas takes place in a sterile setting, and recovered tissues are often shipped to processors for storage and later dispersal.

Tissue and eye donation differs from organ donation in several respects. First, donated human tissue is regulated by the Food and Drug Administration as a medical implant or device and is subject to stringent quality control guidelines. Donated tissue undergoes rigorous testing before implantation to ensure the safety of the recipients. Tissue recovered from one cadaver can potentially be implanted in up to 2500 recipients, so testing for biohazards and infectious disease is of the utmost priority in tissue recovery and dispersal.

Second, recovered tissue typically does not have a predetermined recipient waiting on the other end for a transplant. Donated tissue, particularly bone, can be processed and stored for up to 10 years after recovery. Two exceptions to this rule are donated corneas, which can be transplanted up to 12 hours after recovery, and heart valves, particularly those recovered from children. Heart valves from pediatric donors go to pediatric recipients because heart valves must be implanted in a recipient heart of similar size.

Have a Heart

Since 2006, the world of organ donation has been quietly undergoing changes in functionality and technology. A movement solely focused on increasing the number of organ, tissue, and eye donors has gained significant momentum. As of 2009, 36 states and the District of Columbia have enacted Donor Designation laws and implemented some form of computerized database to maintain a statewide donor registry. In most cases, these databases are tied to the state's Department of Motor Vehicles (DMV), and the person's Donor Designation is indicated by a small red or pink heart or dot on the driver's license. In these states, Donor Designation is considered legally binding and includes consent for tissue and eye donation.

The DMV can enroll donors through driver's license applications, as well as ID cards and renewals. In states with mature systems, the DMV can export the donor enrollments to a registry database, and the database can accept online enrollments without DMV involvement. In all states with Donor Designation, transplant professionals can easily access the database to check for consent.

Although the creation of Donor Designation has succeeded in increasing the number of organ, tissue, and eye donors, legal and ethical considerations still arise—for example, what happens if a family objects strenuously to the donation? A grassroots movement against this particular aspect of Donor Designation focuses specifically on ensuring that families know the exact meaning of a heart on their relative's license.

USE OF SCARCE RESOURCES IN PROLONGING LIFE

In these days of huge federal budget deficits and attempts to control them by shrinking the healthcare budget, money for health care is becoming more difficult to obtain. It is recognized that most public money allocated for health care is spent during the last year of life for many elderly clients. Expensive procedures, therapies, technologies, and care are provided to terminally ill individuals to extend their lives by a few days or even a few hours. It is not unusual to spend as much as $5000 to $10,000 a day on a client receiving care in an intensive care unit.

Preserving Life at Any Cost

The traditional belief has been that life should be preserved at all costs and by any means available. Health-care providers feel uncomfortable when cost considerations are mentioned regarding treatments for terminally ill clients. Yet, in the context of current problems in society, such considerations are both economic and ethical realities. The necessity of conserving resources has forced society, through governmental action, to face this issue.

All proposed health-care plans, including the Patient Protection and Affordable Care Act and the Health Care and Education Reconciliation Act of 2010, take into consideration some type of cost-control measures related to restricting payment for client care. In addition, the **hospice care** movement and a growing number of physicians and other health-care professionals support **palliative** care for the terminally ill that provides pain relief and comfort measures but does not try to prolong the person's life.

In reality, the American health-care system has been rationing care to some degree for many years. People who are not covered by health insurance often do not seek health care. Groups such as the poor, who are covered by massive governmental programs, shy away from seeking health care because of the numerous restrictions placed on it. Individuals who are covered by insurance often have restrictions placed on them by the insurance companies.

The Ethics of Tube Feeding

The long-standing controversy over tube feedings periodically comes to public attention when the media become involved in cases such as those of Terri Schiavo, Karen Quinlan, and Nancy Cruzan. Tube feeding is a relatively simple procedure used in all areas of health care, from feeding premature infants in the neonatal intensive care unit to maintaining elderly postoperative clients under the supervision of home health-care staff. Additionally, it is a way of maintaining nutrition and hydration, two of the most basic needs of life. Nurses who work with terminally ill clients often believe that once a feeding tube has been inserted, it cannot be removed for any reason because that would constitute active euthanasia, or mercy killing.[10] But is that belief justified in all circumstances? Consider the following scenario:

Mrs. Ada Floral, 82 years old, had just suffered a massive stroke that rendered her unresponsive.

Her large family—consisting of her husband of many years, three sons, and two daughters—were very upset. Although she was breathing on her own, she had no voluntary movements and seemed to be completely paralyzed. Magnetic resonance imaging (MRI) showed a large area of bleeding around the midbrain and brain stem. Her pupils were constricted and unresponsive. The physician explained that the prognosis was extremely grave and that the likelihood of Mrs. Floral's survival was minimal.

However, the family members all agreed that "everything" should be done, so the physician reluctantly initiated aggressive medical therapy with intravenous (IV) glucocorticoids, osmotic diuretics, antihypertensives, and physical therapy. After a week, there was no change. The family wondered whether Mrs. Floral might be "starving to death" and asked the physician to have a feeding tube inserted and feedings started.

One month later, the still-unresponsive Mrs. Floral is being cared for at home by her family with the supervision of the local hospice and home health-care program. She is off all IV medications; however, she is receiving some medications, a commercially prepared feeding, and water through the feeding tube. Some of the family members are beginning to question whether they did the right thing by insisting that everything be done and wish to remove the feeding tube so that Mrs. Floral can die a peaceful and dignified death rather than just hanging on for months. Other family members feel that if they give permission for the tube's removal, they would be killing their mother and could not live with the guilt.

The hospice nurse in charge of the case has discussed the issue with the family. She too believes that once a feeding tube has been placed, it should not be removed, even if all the family agrees on its removal. She feels that it's not an issue a family can "just change their minds about." Although she is in frequent contact with Mrs. Floral's physician, she has not mentioned that the family is thinking about removing the feeding tube in fear that the physician might agree.

Is the hospice nurse correct in her belief about the removal of the feeding tube? When do tube feedings stop being beneficial to clients? Is there a right to death with dignity? What ethical rationales could be used for removal of the feeding tube in this case?

Should Care Be Restricted?

The use of public funds for health care is an ethical issue that revolves around the principle of distributive justice. In this context, distributive justice requires that all citizens have equal access to all types of health care, regardless of their income levels, race, gender, religious beliefs, or diagnosis. Many complex issues are involved in this dilemma.

These issues go far beyond the questions of who gets what type of care and where and how the care takes place. Although **universal health-care coverage** was not mandated for all Americans by the passage of the Health Care Reform Act, coverage has been expanded significantly. Is it fair that some individuals (taxpayers) pay for the health care of others? Should individuals who contribute to their own poor state of health by smoking, drinking, taking illicit drugs, or overeating be provided with the same type of care as those who do not put themselves at risk? Who is going to make the decisions about who gets expensive treatment such as organ transplantations, experimental medications, placement in intensive care units, or life-extending technologies?

The use of criteria such as age, potential for a high-quality life, and availability of resources for determining who receives life-extending technologies is gaining wider acceptance, but is this a valid ethical position? Nurses are often involved in situations in which terminally ill clients are brought to the hospital for end-of-life care. Nurses need to play an active role in helping formulate policies concerning the issues they face daily.

What Do You Think?

Do all U.S. citizens have a right to health care? How can that be achieved? Discuss your rationale for your position.

THE RIGHT TO DIE

The right-to-die issue is an extension of the right to self-determination issue discussed in Chapter 9. It also overlaps with the dilemma of **euthanasia** and assisted suicide. Health-care providers often become involved in the decision-making process when clients are irreversibly comatose, vegetative, or suffering from a terminal disease. The choices that the families of such clients often face are death or the extension of life using painful and expensive treatments.[11]

What is Extraordinary?

One of the difficulties in resolving right-to-die issues is understanding the terminology used. Often clients who have living wills state that they want no extraordinary treatments if they should become comatose or unable to make decisions involving health care. But what constitutes extraordinary treatments? A general definition of ordinary treatments includes any medications, procedures, surgeries, or technologies that offer the client some hope of benefit without causing excessive pain or suffering.

By this definition, extraordinary treatments (sometimes called *heroic measures*) are those treatments, medications, surgeries, and technologies that offer little hope for curing or improving the client's condition. Although these general definitions provide some guidelines for making decisions about ordinary and extraordinary treatments, discerning the nature of the specific modalities remains difficult.

Ventilation

For example, a ventilator is a machine that assists a client's breathing. In intensive care units (ICUs), it is a common mode of treatment for many types of clients, including postoperative clients, clients with cardiac and respiratory diseases, and victims of trauma. Does its widespread and frequent use make the ventilator an ordinary mode of treatment? Many would say yes, whereas others would say it is still extraordinary because of its invasive nature and complicated technology.

Cardiopulmonary Resuscitation

Another issue often included in the right-to-die debate is that of codes and "do-not-resuscitate" (DNR or no code) orders. Cardiopulmonary resuscitation (CPR) is widely taught to both health-care providers and the general public. It is often used to treat clients who have suffered heart attacks and gone into cardiac arrest as well as clients suffering from electrical shock, drowning, and traumatic injuries.

In the hospital setting, the nursing staff is obligated to perform CPR on all clients who do not have a specific DNR order. This leads to situations in which terminally ill clients may be subjected to CPR efforts several times before they die.

Advance Directives

As an issue of self-determination, it is essential that the client's wishes about health care be followed. All client communication to the nurse about desires for future care should be documented. If at all possible, the client should be encouraged to designate an individual to act as a moral surrogate—a designated decision maker—should the client become unable to make his or her own decisions. The expressed desires about future medical care are known as *advance directives*. They are the best means to guarantee that a client's wishes will be honored.

A Formal Document

Advance directives, in the form of a living will or durable power of attorney for health care, can and should specify which extraordinary procedures, surgeries, medications, or treatments can or cannot be used. These directives are often formal documents that need to be witnessed by two individuals who are not related to the client (Box 8.2).

As useful as advance directives are in helping the client decide on future care, clients often are unable to anticipate all the possible types of treatments used. For example, an elderly client with a long history of cardiovascular disease specified in his living will that he did not want CPR performed and did not want a ventilator. When his heart developed a potentially lethal dysrhythmia that rendered him unresponsive, his physician decided to use electrical cardioversion because this mode of treatment was not specifically forbidden by the client's living will. Strictly speaking, the physician did not violate the letter of the living will, but did he violate its spirit? Similarly, would the administration of a potent and potentially dangerous IV antidysrhythmic medication be in violation of the client's living will?

A Legal Requirement

Advance directives, which include living wills, are now a required part of the health care of all clients. The Omnibus Budget Reconciliation Act of 1990

Box 8.2

Checklist for Evaluating a Client's Living Will Document

1. Statement of intention: the document was written freely when the client was competent.
2. Statement of when the document goes into effect: usually when the client is no longer able to make decisions for himself or herself
3. Section specifying general health-care measures to be excluded from care
4. Open section for specific measures (ventilators, pacemakers, etc.) and any other specific instructions concerning care
5. Proxy statement (sometimes called *durable power of attorney*): optional, but a strong addition. Allows another person to make decisions in situations not anticipated in the living will. (Check your state law concerning details of proxy selection.)
6. Substitute proxy: optional. Specifies who can make decisions if first-choice proxy is not available
7. Legal statement that the proxy(s) may make decisions
8. Witness selection statement. Many states require that witnesses not be related or members of the health-care team.
9. Signature and date. Document must be signed and dated by the client. Some states have very specific regulations concerning how long the will is valid. It may range from a few months to 5 years.
10. Legal signatures of witnesses (required)
11. Notary seal, if required by state law. State laws differ on notary seal requirement. It is usually required if a proxy is selected.

requires that all hospitals, nursing-care facilities, home health-care agencies, and caregivers ask clients about advance directives and provide information concerning living wills and durable power of attorney (DPOA) to help clients make informed health-care decisions. However, the federal law mandates only the requirements and not the directives to implement the law. The actual implementation of the law is left to the individual states. Because of the vagueness of the law, a great deal of confusion exists, particularly with regard to living wills.

Nurses play an important role in ensuring that clients understand the implications of their choices pertaining to decisions that may prolong their lives during medical emergencies. Because of their "frontline" position as caregivers within the health-care system, nurses must understand this role, specifically as it pertains to living wills.

Ethical Difficulties of Living Wills
What Did the Client Know?

Although a living will seems a simple solution to a complex care situation, there are some ethical difficulties inherent in its use that nurses need to know about. Primary among these ethical difficulties is the question of the person's level of knowledge of potential and future health-care problems at the time the will was formulated. Because living wills are often formulated long before they are to be used, there may later be serious questions about how informed the person was about the disease states and treatment modalities that might later affect care. If there is any indication that the person did not understand the full implications of future therapies or potential medical problems, the validity of the living will is in question.

A Moral Conflict

A second ethical difficulty for nurses encompasses the principles of beneficence and nonmaleficence. The principle of beneficence states that a health-care professional's primary duty is to benefit or do good for the client. The principle of nonmaleficence states that health-care providers should protect the client from harm. It is sometimes difficult to determine whether the primary duty is to produce benefit or prevent harm.

Generally, most health-care providers think that the duty to avoid harming the client outweighs the concerns for providing benefit. When evaluated from the beneficence and nonmaleficence viewpoints, living wills seem to violate the principle of providing benefit to the client. This perception makes many health-care providers ethically uncomfortable. In some situations, the implementation of a living will might actually involve the termination of some modes of treatments already in use. Termination of treatments would seem to constitute harm to the client.

In either case, respecting a living will might often appear to health-care providers to be a violation of their duty to help clients and preserve life. Nurses, as well as other health-care providers, often experience a sense of frustration when they are not allowed to use all the skills they have learned to preserve life.

> *The expressed desires about future medical care are known as advance directives. They are the best means to guarantee that a client's wishes will be honored.*

Lack of Clarity

A third difficulty nurses and other health-care workers may have with living wills is their formulation and legal enforcement. In general, the language used in the standard living will document is broad and vague. Living wills are often not specific enough to include all the forms of treatments that are possible for the many types of illnesses that might render a person incompetent to make decisions. Health-care providers may have little direction as to the care they are to give if the circumstances at the time the living will was formulated are significantly different from the declared wishes of the client.

Furthermore, unless the particular state has enacted into law a special type of living will called a *natural death act*, the living will has no mechanism of legal enforcement. Also, when a client travels from one state to another, the legal effect of the living will may be in question. Does the nonresident state have an obligation to honor it?

In some states, a living will is considered only advisory, and the physician has the right to comply with the living will or treat the client as the physician deems most appropriate. There is no protection for nurses or other health-care practitioners

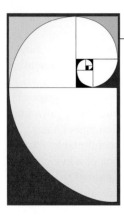

Issues in Practice

In the current health-care environment, nurses may encounter elderly clients who function independently at home and have not officially or legally been declared incompetent, but whose behavior might indicate that they are unable to make rational decisions about their care. Consider the following situation:

A 74-year-old client, Buster Mack, had been a long-haul truck driver for most of his life and was still driving his big rig into his 60s. He had been in relatively good health until 5 years earlier, when he was diagnosed with lung cancer. A lobectomy was performed at that time, and he was treated with follow-up radiation and chemotherapy, but the cancer had slowly metastasized to the bone. His current hospitalization was because of a syncopal episode witnessed by a neighbor in the front yard of Mr. Mack's home, where he lives by himself.

During the admission assessment, the nurse observed that Mr. Mack had trouble focusing on the questions, and often the answer was unrelated to the question or in the form of a long rambling account of something that happened many years ago. Although he knew he was in a hospital (he could not remember the name), he had no idea where it was or what the date was. His demeanor was cooperative and pleasant, and he laughed easily when the nurse joked with him. He could not remember whether he had any family left living, although the name and address of a son in a distant city were listed on the old records.

Mr. Mack signed all the admission papers and consent forms placed in front of him for a number of neurological tests. His physician was fearful that the cancer might have spread to his brain and wanted to do a magnetic resonance imaging (MRI) test, spinal tap, and brain scan. The MRI and brain scan showed a small tumor in an area of the brain where it could be removed rather easily. Mr. Mack's physician, in consultation with a neurosurgeon, felt that an immediate craniotomy with removal of the tumor was required. After explaining the procedure to Mr. Mack, the physicians placed the consent-to-operate form on his over-the-bed table and gave him a pen. He promptly signed and gave it back.

Later on that day during her shift assessment, the nurse checked on Mr. Mack. The neighbor who had found him unconscious was visiting at the time. When the nurse asked Mr. Mack whether he was ready for the surgery scheduled for the next morning, he had a blank look on his face. On further questioning, the nurse concluded that Mr. Mack had no idea about what was going to happen to him the next day. The neighbor, who helped Mr. Mack with his bills and other paperwork at home, stated: "He'll pretty much sign anything that you put in front of him." At this point the nurse felt that Mr. Mack was incapable of making an informed decision about the craniotomy.

The nurse called both the primary physician and the neurosurgeon about her observations. She was told bluntly that the consent had been signed and that they were going to operate on Mr. Mack the next day for his own good. If she wanted what was best for the client, she would just drop the issue.

Should the nurse just drop the issue? Is there anything she could do to resolve the problem? What ethical principles are involved with this situation?

against criminal or civil liability in the execution of living wills in states without a natural death act. Once a valid living will exists, it only becomes effective when the person who formulated it meets the qualifications for the natural death act. In most states, the individual must be diagnosed as having a terminal condition in which the continuation of treatment and life support would only prolong the client's dying process, but there is no clear consensus on the definition of *terminal condition.*

A Guide for the Care Provider

Despite all these difficulties, living wills are still a good way for a client to make health-care wishes known to providers. Documents that are specific about treatment modalities, are written in a "legal" format, and are signed by two or more witnesses tend to be treated with an increased level of respect by health-care providers (Fig. 8.1).

Nurses can help clients plan ahead for their care should they become unable to make decisions for themselves. Although the nurse should not make the decisions for the client, the nurse can provide important information about the various treatment modalities that the client is considering. The nurse also can help clients clarify their wishes and guide them through the process of formulating an advance directive.

EUTHANASIA AND ASSISTED SUICIDE

Although the term *euthanasia* simply means a "good" or peaceful death, it has taken on the connotation of some type of action that produces death. A distinction needs to be made between passive and active euthanasia. Passive euthanasia usually refers to the practice of allowing an individual to die without any extraordinary intervention. This umbrella definition includes practices such as DNR orders, living wills, and withdrawal of ventilators or other life support.

Active Euthanasia

Active euthanasia usually describes the practice of hastening an individual's death through some act or procedure. This practice is also sometimes referred to as *mercy killing* and takes many forms, ranging from use of large amounts of pain medication for terminal cancer clients to use of poison, a gun, or a knife to end a person's life.

The Case of Dr. Kevorkian

Assisted suicide—brought to public attention by Dr. Jack Kevorkian, a Michigan physician who publicly practiced it for many years—can be considered a type of active euthanasia or mercy killing. The central issue that Dr. Kevorkian demonstrated was whether it is ever ethically and legally permissible for health-care personnel to assist in taking a life. In most states, the practice is illegal. The legal definition of homicide—bringing about a person's death or assisting in doing so—seems to fit the act of assisted suicide. In the past, there has been a great deal of hesitation on the part of the legal system to prosecute persons who are involved in assisted suicide, and on the part of juries to convict physicians who participate in the activity.

A Killing on TV

In the fall of 1998, Dr. Kevorkian raised the legal and ethical stakes. On a nationally broadcast network news show, *60 Minutes,* he not only admitted to administering a lethal medication to a client without the client's assistance, but he also played a videotape that showed the whole episode.

The client, who had Lou Gehrig's disease (amyotrophic lateral sclerosis), had requested that Dr. Kevorkian help him end his life. The client had signed a **consent** form and release and was even given an extra 2 weeks to "think about it." The client waited for only 3 days before making his final request for the lethal medication.

Under Michigan law, Dr. Kevorkian could have been charged with **manslaughter** or even first-degree murder. Dr. Kevorkian admitted that his **motivation** for the act was to be tried under these laws as a test case for active euthanasia. He was arrested 2 weeks after the tape was broadcast, on a charge of first-degree murder. However, he believed that a jury would never convict him. The trial verdict was guilty of second-degree murder, and he served 10 years of a 25 years–to-life prison term. He was released on probation in 2007 and died on June 3, 2011. This verdict reinforced the belief of most health-care professionals that mercy killing or assisted suicide is always ethically wrong.

The unfortunate fallout from Dr. Kevorkian's conviction is that many physicians have become even more reluctant to write DNR orders or comply with clients' or families' wishes to allow clients to be removed from life support. Clearly they do not understand the distinctions between active and passive euthanasia.

INSTRUCTIONS	**PENNSYLVANIA DECLARATION**
PRINT YOUR NAME	I, _____, being of sound mind, willfully and voluntarily make this declaration to be followed if I become incompetent. This declaration reflects my firm and settled commitment to refuse life-sustaining treatment under the circumstances indicated below. I direct my attending physician to withhold or withdraw life-sustaining treatment that serves only to prolong the process of my dying, if I should be in a terminal condition or in a state of permanent unconsciousness. I direct that treatment be limited to measures to keep me comfortable and to relieve pain, including any pain that might occur by withholding or withdrawing life-sustaining treatment.
CHECK THE OPTIONS WHICH REFLECT YOUR WISHES	In addition, if I am in the condition described above, I feel especially strongly about the following forms of treatment: I ( ) do ( ) do not want cardiac resuscitation. I ( ) do ( ) do not want mechanical respiration. I ( ) do ( ) do not want tube feeding or any other artificial or invasive form of nutrition (food) or hydration (water). I ( ) do ( ) do not want blood or blood products. I ( ) do ( ) do not want any form of surgery or invasive diagnostic tests. I ( ) do ( ) do not want kidney dialysis. I ( ) do ( ) do not want antibiotics. I realize that if I do not specifically indicate my preference regarding any of the forms of treatment listed above, I may receive that form of treatment.
ADD PERSONAL INSTRUCTIONS (IF ANY)	Other instructions:
© 2000 **PARTNERSHIP FOR CARING, INC.**	

Figure 8.1 Sample advance directive. Because the laws on advance directives vary widely from state to state, there is no standard advance directive whose language conforms exactly with all states' laws. (Reprinted with permission of Partnership for Caring, formerly Choice in Dying, 200 Varick Street, New York. For more information visit http://www.partnershipforcaring.org.)

An Issue of Self-Determination
A Last Act of Control?

The fundamental ethical issue in these situations is the right to self-determination. In almost every other health-care situation, a client who is mentally competent can make decisions about what care to accept and what care to refuse. Yet, when it comes to the termination of life, this right becomes controversial.

Supporters of the practice of assisted suicide believe that the right to self-determination remains intact, even with regard to the decision to end one's life. It is the last act of a very sick individual to control his or her own fate. Many believe that medical personnel should be allowed to assist clients in this procedure, just as they are allowed to assist clients in other medical and nursing procedures.

APPOINTING A SURROGATE	**PENNSYLVANIA DECLARATION PAGE 2 OF 2**

Surrogate decisionmaking:

I ( ) do ( ) do not want to designate another person as my surogate to make medical treatment decisions for me if I should be incompetent and in a terminal condition or in a state of permanent unconsciousness.

PRINT THE NAME, ADDRESS AND PHONE NUMBER OF YOUR SURROGATE

Name: _____
Address : _____
Phone: _____

Name and address of substitute (if surrogate designated above is unable to serve):

PRINT THE NAME, ADDRESS AND PHONE NUMBER OF YOUR ALTERNATE SURROGATE

Name: _____
Address: _____
Phone: _____

PRINT THE DATE

I made this declaration on the_____ day of_____ .
                        (day)   (month, year)

SIGN THE DOCUMENT AND PRINT YOUR ADDRESS

Declarant's signature: _____
Declarant's address: _____

The declarant, or the person on behalf of and at the direction of the declarant, knowingly and voluntarily signed this writing by signature or mark in my presence.

WITNESSING PROCEDURE

YOUR TWO WITNESSES MUST SIGN AND PRINT THEIR ADDRESSES

Witness's signature: _____
Witness's address: _____

Witness's signature: _____
Witness's address:_____

© 2000 PARTNERSHIP FOR CARING, INC.

Courtesy of **Partnership for Caring, Inc.**   6/96
1620 Eye Street, NW. Suite 202, Washington, DC 20006 800-989-9455

Figure 8.1 cont'd

An Unacceptable Practice?

Those who oppose assisted suicide find these arguments unconvincing. Legally, ethically, and morally, suicide in U.S. society has never been an accepted practice. Health-care staff goes to great lengths to prevent suicidal clients from injuring themselves. In addition, individuals in the terminal stages of a disease, who are overwhelmed by pain and depressed by the thought of prolonged suffering, might not be able to think clearly enough to give informed consent for assisted suicide. Also, because the termination of life is final, it does not allow for spontaneous cures or for the development of new treatments or medications.

Nonmaleficence is the term that describes the obligation to do no harm to clients. Whether assisting in or causing the death of a client violates this principle is most likely to be an issue that will continue to be debated for some time. Several states have passed laws permitting assisted suicide, but these states have very strict guidelines. The American Nurses Association (ANA) and other nurses' organizations oppose assisted suicide as a policy and believe that nurses who participate in it are violating the code of ethics. For similar reasons, the ANA opposes nurses participating in executions of convicted criminals.

HUMAN IMMUNODEFICIENCY VIRUS AND ACQUIRED IMMUNODEFICIENCY SYNDROME

After several years of decrease, the number of human immunodeficiency virus (HIV) and acquired immunodeficiency syndrome (AIDS) cases has begun to rise again in the United States despite educational efforts on its prevention and spread. Several Asian countries are also seeing a recent dramatic increase in cases of HIV/AIDS. In some parts of Africa, it is estimated that as much as 60 percent of the population is infected with the virus.

An Emotional Issue

HIV and AIDS have evoked strong emotions both in the public and in the medical community. Nurses, who for years held strongly to the ethical principle that all clients regardless of race, gender, religion, age, or disease process should be cared for equally, are questioning their obligation to take care of clients who have AIDS.

The Right to Privacy

Several ethical issues underlie the HIV/AIDS controversy. One of the most important is the right to privacy. Although there is a general requirement to report infection with HIV/AIDS to the Centers for Disease Control and Prevention (CDC), many states have strict laws regarding the confidentiality of the diagnosis. Unauthorized revelation of the diagnosis of HIV/AIDS brings the possibility of a lawsuit against the health-care provider or institution. However, the right to privacy is not absolute. Diseases such as tuberculosis, gonorrhea, syphilis, and hepatitis, which are highly contagious and sometimes fatal, must be reported to public health officials.

> " *The central issue that Dr. Kevorkian demonstrated was whether it is ever ethically permissible for health-care personnel to assist in taking a life.* "

If the right to privacy can be violated when the public welfare is at stake, does HIV/AIDS represent this type of threat? Is it unjust to ask health-care providers to care for clients with this disease without knowing that the client has it? Is it just to violate a client's privacy when the disease carries with it a potential for social stigma and isolation? Does the client have a right to know that a health-care provider is infected with HIV/AIDS?

The Right to Care

Another important ethical issue is the right to care. Can a nurse refuse to care for a client with HIV/AIDS? Obviously, a fundamental right of a client is to receive care, and a fundamental obligation of a nurse is to provide care.

The Nurse's Own Interest

The first statement of the ANA Code of Ethics for Nurses is that a nurse must provide care unrestricted by any considerations. Most acute care facilities will make some exceptions for the treatment of clients with HIV/AIDS, for example, if the nurse is pregnant, is receiving chemotherapy, or has had other immunity problems. In most situations, however, the nurse is obligated to provide the best nursing care possible for all clients, including those with HIV/AIDS.

What Cost to Society?

What about the tremendous cost involved in treating individuals who have HIV/AIDS? The medical cost of treating a client with HIV/AIDS from the time of diagnosis to the time of death can run into millions of dollars. In the face of this crisis, governmental agencies, which bear the brunt of paying for HIV/AIDS treatment, will have to make some difficult decisions concerning this issue. With more than 2 million U.S. citizens already infected with this disease, the cost to American society is becoming astronomical.

Nurses have the obligation to care for all clients, including those with HIV/AIDS, but should physicians, hospitals, or governmental agencies also be held to this same precept? Should our society regard health care as a right or a privilege?

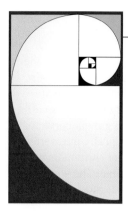

Issues in Practice

Nurses Legally Protected for Reporting Child Abuse

A newborn was admitted to the nursery with signs of drug withdrawal and tested positive for cocaine, although the mother denied using the drug before delivery. Hospital personnel are required by law to report suspected child abuse, and illegal drugs in the circulatory system of a newborn are one of the indicators for mandatory reporting. On the basis of this finding, the nurses in the newborn nursery filed a report with the local child protective services who investigated the case.

Child protective services removed the child from the home shortly after discharge from the hospital. The mother went to court a few days after the child was removed to plead her case before a family court judge. The judge upheld the decision to remove the child. The mother then became even more irate, still insisting she had not used cocaine, and filed a lawsuit against the hospital, the physicians, the nurses, and protective services. She cited that these entities were conspiring to keep her from exercising her constitutional rights.

Over the past decade, courts have been recognizing the integrity of the family and are beginning to make rulings that support it as a constitutional right. Because of this trend, the mother's lawyer felt that the case had merit and might result in a ruling in her favor with a large punitive settlement.

Looking at all the evidence, the higher court decided that there had been no attempt on the part of the hospital and staff to deprive the mother of her constitutional rights—the mother had been given the opportunity to plead in a lower court shortly after the child's removal from the home. The court upheld the nurses' requirement to report suspected child abuse and their immunity from civil lawsuits for caring out their obligations in good faith.

Source: Stewart v. Jackson County, 2009 WL 2922940 S.D. Miss., September 8, 2009.

ETHICS INVOLVING CHILDREN

Although children are universally acknowledged as the hope of the future, many children remain poorly fed, clothed, housed, and educated and are in dire need of all types of health care, even in affluent countries such as the United States. In the past few years, there has been a marked increase in the reporting of incidents of child neglect and abuse by parents.

The Power of Parents

Our society generally acknowledges the tremendous decision-making power that parents have on behalf of their children; however, there are limits to how parents may decide to act. These limits are sometimes obvious, as in cases of physical abuse and cruelty to children; however, they may also be less conspicuous, such as in cases of neglect or decisions about withholding medical care for religious reasons. Health-care professionals often find themselves trying to make decisions about the appropriateness of a parent's actions toward a child.

The legal and ethical factors surrounding the decisions that health-care providers must make about child health issues are complicated and sometimes contradictory, ranging from laws about reporting suspected abuse to obtaining permission for treatment. This section focuses on child abuse and the ethical issues that it creates for nurses and on the issues of informed consent as it pertains to children.

Issues involving children have always been an important consideration in our society. Whereas the political attention seems to focus on education, drug and alcohol abuse, and child health-care issues, ethical concerns in **pediatrics** are never forgotten and often serve as the unspoken basis for the more visible issues.

Child health ethical issues are numerous and diverse, ranging from mass screening for diseases to withholding permission for treatment.

> *Most acute care facilities will make some exceptions for the treatment of clients with AIDS, for example, if the nurse is pregnant, is receiving chemotherapy, or has had other immunity problems. In most situations, however, the nurse is obligated to provide the best nursing care possible for all clients, including those with AIDS.*

Child Abuse
Case Study

Emily, who is 8 months old, was brought to the hospital by her 17-year-old unemployed mother, who stated that the baby refused to eat at home and vomited a lot. Emily was very small for her age and was below the growth curve for weight. She was also neurologically introverted and showed little interest in her surroundings. She slept a great deal of the time. She was admitted to the hospital with a diagnosis of nonorganic failure to thrive.

During her stay in the hospital, Emily ate well and gained a significant amount of weight. Her neurological status also improved.

One nurse suspected that this was a case of neglect (a form of child abuse) and suggested to the physician that child protective services be notified to evaluate the case. The physician resisted because there was not enough evidence to make a definitive case and thought that it was unfair to the parents to make such a claim. The other nurses felt that by reporting the case they would lose the trust of the mother and cause her to avoid health care for Emily in the future. They also cited a case in which nurses and the hospital were sued when they reported a teenage mother for neglect; the accusation later proved to be false.

Emily was sent home after 3 weeks but was readmitted 1 month later with the same complaints of poor feeding. She had lost weight since her discharge from the hospital, and she was again neurologically withdrawn. The physician still refused to notify child protective services because of the lack of hard evidence. He thought that the available data did not warrant an investigation and possible removal of the child from the home. The nurse still believed that the mother should be reported on the basis of suspicions that could be substantiated legally.

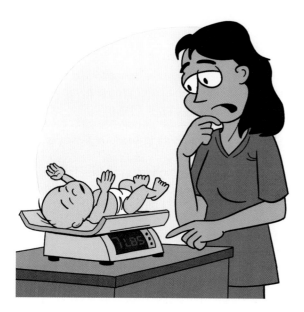

Ethics Regarding Child Abuse

There is a general legal requirement in most states that suspected child abuse must be reported by health-care providers as well as by anyone who suspects that child abuse has occurred. Abuse is more obvious when the child has physical injuries that do not fit the medical history or are atypical for the age group. However, in cases of neglect, the evidence may be very minimal or even nonexistent. Often nurses and physicians who specialize in the care of children rely on their experience in making decisions to report or not report suspected abuse.

A conflicting ethical principle sometimes forgotten in the reporting of suspected child abuse is the family's right to privacy and self-determination. It is an equally fundamental right that Emily's parents be allowed to live their lives according to their own values, free from intrusions.

Decisions about reporting suspected child abuse or neglect rest on the underlying ethical principles of beneficence and protection of the best interests of the child. It is always difficult to decide how far ranging these concerns for "best interest" should be. However, when the child is a client in the hospital, beneficence usually outweighs fidelity and veracity.

Physicians tend to focus on solving the immediate problem. Nurses have a more holistic viewpoint and tend to see children in relationship to their environments as well as the environments of the parents. Nurses also tend to think of themselves as saviors, protecting the unfortunate or disadvantaged from a malignant social system and often making value judgments about the lifestyles of others from their middle-class vantage point.

Resolving the Dilemma

How is the nurse going to resolve this dilemma? Should she report the case and go against the physician's decision? Should she just agree with the physician and defer to his greater experience and better judgment? Should she submit the problem to the hospital ethics committee? Are there any other possible options for action in this case?

It is likely that the physician was correct in his decision about this case, although his ethical reasoning may leave something to be desired. Legally, it is unlikely that there would be sufficient proof to remove the infant from the mother because home monitoring could achieve the same results. Therefore, how can the ethical obligations for the best interest of the child be met?

One very plausible solution is to monitor the child closely through frequent follow-up either at the physician's office or at the local health department. In addition, a follow-up and home evaluation could be arranged through a home health-care agency, which could also make available other community resources to help in Emily's care. If the infant continued to fail to gain weight, or if it was later determined that Emily's mother was indeed unable to care adequately for her, the case could then be referred to child protective services.

The role of the nurse who cares for the very young or abused child is one of client advocate. These children need help and protection, and at times, for their very survival, must be taken out of an abusive home setting. Nurses need to be aware of and use all the assets available in these situations, including the police, child protective services, welfare, and home health-care agencies.

Informed Consent and Children
Case Study

Peter, one of a pair of 7-year-old identical twins, developed severe bilateral glomerulonephritis after a streptococcal (strep) throat infection. The renal involvement was so severe

Determining the Greatest Good

Sherry is an RN who works for a rehabilitation center that deals mainly with developmentally delayed children. For several years, Sherry has been following the case of Margie N, who is now 8 years old and has Down syndrome and moderate retardation. Margie has made steady, if slow, progress in achieving basic motor and cognitive skills but still requires close supervision of all activities and care for all basic hygiene needs. Margie is still not advanced enough to participate in group activities at the center's day clinic.

Mrs. N, Margie's mother, a 42-year-old widow, has been providing a high level of care for Margie at home as well as meeting the child's demands for love and attention. Recently, Mrs. N has been diagnosed with systemic lupus erythematosus (SLE), which has displayed as its primary symptoms severe joint pain and stiffness. During the past several months, Mrs. N has been finding it increasingly difficult to care for Margie because of the progressive nature of the SLE.

Mrs. N is trying to make a decision about long-term care for Margie. She trusts Sherry's judgment completely and often relies on the information and teaching given by the nurse to make changes in Margie's care. Sherry is uncertain about what advice she should give. She recognizes that the high level of care and comfort provided by Mrs. N has been an essential part in the advances Margie has made up to this point, but she also recognizes that Mrs. N may soon reach a point at which that care can no longer be provided. It seems that to do what is good for Mrs. N (i.e., placing Margie in an institution) would be harmful to Margie, whereas doing what is good for Margie (i.e., leaving her at home) would be harmful to Mrs. N. What is the best course of action in this situation? Are there any alternative solutions to this dilemma?

that it did not respond to any medical treatment, and both of his kidneys had to be removed. Paul, Peter's identical twin, was evaluated for kidney donation and, as expected, matched on all six antigens as well as blood type and size. Paul seemed to understand what had happened to his brother and agreed to donate one of his kidneys to keep his brother alive.

However, the children's parents were having some trouble agreeing on whether Paul should donate a kidney to Peter. The twins' mother felt that the donation and transplantation should be permitted because it would indeed help keep Peter alive and would also make Paul feel that he was an important part of the process. She argued that if Peter ever did die, Paul would be overcome with guilt knowing that he could have saved his brother but did not.

The twins' father was not as certain about the transplantation procedure. He thought that Paul was too young to make a truly free decision of that type and that he did not really understand the serious nature of a kidney removal operation. He thought that Paul, because he was so young,

might have been unduly influenced by subtle yet powerful pressures from his family. No one had directly told Paul that he *must* donate one of his kidneys, yet the fact that his brother's survival might well depend on his decision could have had a major effect on his willingness to donate. Because Peter was being maintained on dialysis and seemed to be doing fairly well, the twins' father thought that he should be put on the transplant list to see whether a suitable nonrelated donor could be found.

The nurses on the unit where Peter was being cared for were equally divided about whether the transplantation should be performed. At various times during Peter's lengthy stay in the hospital, they had all been asked by the parents, usually one parent at a time, whether or not they should go ahead with the transplantation.

Case-Study Analysis

The question as related to the case study is, "Does a 7-year-old child have sufficient rational decision-making ability to decide to donate a kidney to his brother?" If, after careful assessment of the child, the answer is "yes," then under the rights-in-trust doctrine, the right to self-determination can be turned over to the child, and he can make his own decision. If the answer is "no," the child should not be permitted to donate the kidney.

Other ethical principles can be brought to bear on this decision. From a utilitarian viewpoint, the child should be allowed to donate the kidney because it would provide the greatest good or happiness for the greatest number of people. Similarly, love-based ethics, or the Golden Rule system of ethical decision-making, would also support the donation on the grounds that Paul identifies closely with his brother and appears to understand the issues involved in donation. However, from an egoistic or beneficent viewpoint, because the transplantation has little benefit for the donor and will surely cause pain and place him at risk for postoperative complications, the operation should not be permitted.

As with many ethical dilemmas, there is no perfect answer to this situation. The best that can be done is to ensure that the parents and children have as much necessary information as possible and to support their decisions.

By recognizing the rights of children as individuals, we also recognize their importance to society. However, parents and health-care professionals also have the duty to nurture, support, and guide children as they grow into adolescence and adulthood. Nurses who work with children are challenged to support their independence by encouraging them to be responsible for and participate in their own health care.

Ethical Principles Regarding Child Health Care

One important difference between adults and children that always needs to be included in ethical decisions about child health issues is that children are dependents. As dependents, they generally are not attributed the right to self-determination that is fundamental to adult decision making.

A Three-Way Relationship

Whenever there is an ethical dilemma involving child health-care issues, a three-way relationship develops involving the child, the health-care professional, and the parents. Generally, the parents have the primary role in deciding health-care issues for their underage, dependent children on the basis of what they consider to be in the child's best interests.

Current routine child health practices reinforce this principle. Young children are given immunizations and medications, have blood drawn for tests, and even have operations such as tonsillectomies or myringotomies, all without anyone asking for their permission. This exemption to the principle of self-determination in children is based on the belief that young children do not yet have the capacity to make fully rational decisions. Yet the final expectation for children is that at some point in their lives they develop the capacity to make informed, correct decisions. The primary questions then become, "When do they develop this capacity for rational decision-making?" and "How should they be treated until they develop this capacity?"

What Do You Think?

If you were the nurse, what would you suggest to the twins' parents? What ethical issues would be involved in your suggestions?

Safeguarding the Child's Rights

The legal system has fixed the age for rational decision-making at age 18 years. Children who are younger than 18 years of age, with a few exceptions, require the permission of the parent for any and all medical procedures. Children older than 18 years of age can make their own decisions about health care.

The difficulty with fixing an age is that it is arbitrary and does not reflect the reality of the individual child's development. From experience it can be observed that many children who are 9 or 10 years old exhibit rather advanced and adult-like decision-making skills, whereas other "children" who may be 18 or 19 years of age display a marked lack of this ability.

The more serious question, however, is, "How should underage children be treated?" One solution is to deny, because of their age, that they have rights and then treat them as being incompetent by bringing to bear paternalistic, best-interest interventions. Another approach is to say that children do have the same rights as adults except that these rights are temporarily suspended until the child is sufficiently mature to exercise them. This is called *rights-in-trust*, and the rights are turned over to the child at the appropriate time. The question then becomes, "When is the appropriate time?"

One approach is to turn over all the rights to the child at the same time, for example, when he or she reaches 18 years of age. Another approach is to gradually release individual rights as the child grows older and is prepared to exercise them. In either case, appropriate adults, including nurses, have the role of safeguarding the child's rights and act as guardians, protectors, and advocates of the children under their care.

Conclusion

Ethical issues are a factor in the daily practice of all nurses. Any time a nurse comes in contact with a client, a potential ethical situation exists. In today's world, with rapidly advancing technology and unusual health-care situations, ethical dilemmas are proliferating. Nurses can be prepared to deal with most of these dilemmas if they keep current with the issues and are able to follow a systematic process for

making ethical decisions. At some point, difficult decisions must be made, and we should not avoid making them. One of the worst elements of ethical decision making is that it is very unlikely that everyone involved in the dilemma will be happy with the decision. However, if the decision is made after the situation has been analyzed and if it is on the basis of sound ethical principles, it can usually be defended.

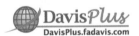

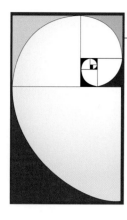

Issues in Practice

Case Study in Ethics

Analyze the following case study using the ethical decision-making process:

Sally Jones, RN, a public health nurse for a rural health department, was preparing to visit Mr. Weems, a 58-year-old client who was recently diagnosed with chronic bronchitis and emphysema. Mr. Weems was unemployed as a result of a farming accident and had been previously diagnosed with hypertension and extreme obesity. Ms. Jones was making this visit to see why Mr. Weems had missed his last appointment at the clinic and whether he was taking his prescribed antibiotics and antihypertensive medications.

As Ms. Jones pulled up in the driveway of his house, she noticed Mr. Weems sitting on the front porch smoking a cigarette. She felt a surge of anger, which she quickly suppressed, as she wondered why she spent so much of her limited time teaching him about the health consequences of smoking.

During the visit, Ms. Jones determined that Mr. Weems had stopped taking both his antihypertensive and antibiotic medications and rarely took his expectorants and bronchodilators. He coughed continuously, had a blood pressure of 196/122 mm Hg, and had severely congested lung sounds. Mr. Weems listened politely as Ms. Jones explained again about the need to stop smoking and the importance of taking his medications as prescribed. She also scheduled another appointment at the clinic in 1 week for follow-up.

As she drove away to her next visit, Ms. Jones wondered about the ethical responsibilities of nurses who must provide care for clients who do not seem to care about their own health. Mr. Weems took little responsibility for his health, refused to even try to stop smoking or lose weight, and did not take his medications. She wondered whether there was a limit to the amount of nursing care a noncompliant client should expect from a community health agency. She reflected that the time spent with Mr. Weems would have been spent much more productively screening children at a local grade school or working with mothers of newborn infants.

Critical Thinking Exercises

- What data are important in relation to this situation?
- State the ethical dilemma in a clear, simple statement.
- What are the choices of action and how do they relate to specific ethical principles?
- What are the consequences of these actions?
- What decisions can be made?

9

Nursing Law and Liability

Mary Evans
Tonia Aiken

Learning Objectives

After completing this chapter, the reader will be able to:

- Distinguish between statutory law and common law.
- Differentiate civil law from criminal law.
- Explain the legal principles involved in:
  Unintentional torts
  Intentional torts
  Quasi-intentional torts
  Informed consent
  Do-not-resuscitate (DNR) orders
- Describe the trial process.
- List methods to prevent litigation.
- Identify the elements in delegation.

THE LEGAL SYSTEM

For many nurses, the mere mention of the word *lawsuit* provokes a high level of anxiety. At first glance, the legal system often seems to be a large and confusing entity whose intricacies are designed to entrap the uninitiated. Many nurses feel that even a minor error in client care will lead to huge settlements against them and loss of their nursing license. In reality, even though the number of lawsuits against nurses has been increasing since the early 1990s, the number of nurses who are actually sued in court remains relatively small. However, many cases are settled out of court, often before any official legal action has been taken.

It is important to remember that the legal system is just one element of the health-care system. Laws are rules to help protect people and to keep society functioning. The ultimate goal of all laws is to promote peaceful and productive interactions among the people of that society.

An understanding of basic legal principles will augment the quality of care that the nurse delivers. In our litigious society, it is important to comprehend how the law affects the profession of nursing and the individual nurse's daily practice.

SOURCES OF LAW

There are two major sources of laws in the United States: statutory law and common law (Box 9.1). Most laws that govern nursing are state-level statutory laws because licensure is a function of the state's authority.

Statutory Law

Statutory law consists of laws written and enacted by the U.S. Congress, the state legislatures, and other governmental entities such as cities, counties, and townships. Legislated laws enacted by the

Box 9.1
Division and Types of Law

Statutory Law and Common Law
I. Criminal Law
   A. Misdemeanor
   B. Felony
II. Civil Law
   A. Tort Law
      1. Unintentional tort
      2. Intentional tort
      3. Quasi-intentional tort
   B. Contract Law
   C. Treaty Law
   D. Tax Law
   E. Other

U.S. Congress are called federal **statutes.** State-drafted laws are called state statutes. Individual cities and municipalities have legislative bodies that draft **ordinances,** codes, and regulations at their respective levels.

The laws that govern the profession of nursing are statutory laws. Most of these laws are written at the state level because licensure is a responsibility of the individual states. These laws include the nurse practice act, which establishes the state board of nursing, the scope of practice for nurses, individual licensure procedures, punitive actions for violation of the practice act, and the schedule of fees for nurse licensure in the state.

Common Law

Common law is different from statutory law in that it has evolved from the decisions of previous legal cases that form a **precedent.** These laws represent the accumulated results of the judgments and decrees that have been handed down by courts of the United States and Great Britain through the years.

Common law often extends beyond the scope of statutory law. For example, no statutes require a person who is negligent and causes injury to another to compensate that person for the injury. However, court decisions that have addressed the same legal issues, such as negligence, over and over have repeatedly ruled that the injured person should receive compensation. The way in which each case is resolved creates a precedent, or pattern, for dealing with the same legal issue in the future. The common laws involving negligence or malpractice are the laws most frequently encountered by the nurse.

Common law or case law is law that has developed over a long period. The principle of *stare decisis* requires a judge to make decisions similar to those that have been handed down in previous cases if the facts of the cases are identical. Common law decisions are published in bound legal reports. Generally speaking, common law deals with matters outside the scope of laws enacted by the legislature.

DIVISIONS OF LAW

In the U.S. legal system, there are many divisions in the law. A major example of such a division is the difference between criminal law and civil law, either of which may be statutory or common in origin.

Criminal Law
A System of Protection

Criminal laws are concerned with providing protection for all members of society. When someone is accused of violating a criminal law, the government at the county, city, state, or federal level imposes punishments appropriate to the type of **crime.** Criminal law involves a wide range of **malfeasance,** from minor traffic violations to murder.

Although most criminal law is created and regulated by the government through the enactment of statutes, a small portion falls under the common law. Statutes are developed and enacted by the legislature (state or federal) and approved by the executive branch, such as a governor or the president. Criminal law is further classified into two types of offenses: (1) **misdemeanors,** which are minor criminal offenses, and (2) **felonies,** which are major criminal offenses.

In the criminal law system, an individual accused of a crime is called the **defendant.** The prosecuting attorney represents the people of the city, county, state, or federal jurisdiction who are accusing the individual of a crime. A **criminal action** is rendered when the person charged with the crime is brought to trial and convicted. Penalties or sanctions are imposed on the violators of criminal law and are based on the scope of the crime. They can involve a range of punishment from community service work and fines to imprisonment and death.

Do you know anyone who has filed a malpractice suit or a health-care provider who was the defendant in a malpractice suit? What was the situation that caused the case? How was it resolved? If you have never been involved with a malpractice suit or do not know anyone who has, how would you feel if a lawsuit were to be brought against you?

The Nurse's Involvement

Nurses can become involved with the criminal system in their nursing practice in several ways. The most common violation by nurses of the criminal law is through failure to renew nursing licenses. In this situation, the nurse is in effect practicing nursing without a license, which is a crime in all states.

> *The most common violation by nurses of the criminal law is through failure to renew nursing licenses. In this situation, the nurse is in effect practicing nursing without a license, which is a crime in all states.*

Nurses also become involved with the illegal diversion of drugs, particularly narcotics, from the hospital. This is a more serious crime, which may lead to imprisonment. Recent cases involving intentional or unintentional deaths of clients and assisted suicide cases have also led to criminal action against nurses.

Civil Law

Nurses are much more likely to become involved in civil lawsuits than in criminal violations. **Civil laws** generally deal with the violation of one individual's rights by another individual. The court provides the forum that enables these individuals to have their disputes resolved by an independent third party, such as a judge or a jury of the defendant's peers.

The individual who brings the dispute to the court is called the **plaintiff.** The formal written document that describes the dispute and the resolution sought is called the complaint. The individual against whom the complaint is filed is the defendant, who, in conjunction with his or her attorney, prepares the **answer** to the complaint. In civil cases, the **burden of proof** rests with the plaintiff.

Civil law has many branches, including contract law, treaty law, tax law, and tort law. It is under the tort law that most nurses become involved with the legal system.

Tort Law

A **tort** is generally defined as a wrongful act committed against a person or his or her property independently of a contract. A person who commits a tort is called the **tort-feasor** and is **liable** for **damages** to those who are affected by the person's actions. The word *tort,* derived from the Latin *tortus* (twisted), is a French word for injury or wrong. Torts can involve several different types of actions, including a direct violation of a person's legal rights or a violation of a standard of care that causes injury to a person. Torts are classified as unintentional, intentional, or quasi-intentional.

Unintentional Torts
Negligence

Negligence is the primary form of **unintentional tort.** **Negligence** is generally defined as the **omission** of an act that a reasonable and prudent person would perform in a similar situation or the commission of something a reasonable person would not do in that situation. **Nonfeasance** is a type of negligence that occurs when a person fails to perform a legally required duty.[1]

Malpractice

Malpractice is a type of negligence for which professionals can be sued (professional negligence). Because of their professional status, nurses are held to a higher standard of conduct than the ordinary layperson. The standard for nurses is what a reasonable and prudent nurse would do in the same situation: Registered nurses must use the skill, knowledge, and judgment they have learned through their education and experience.[2]

    For instance, it is reasonable and prudent that the nurse put the side rails up on the bed of a client who has just received an injection of a narcotic pain medication because the drug causes drowsiness and sometimes confusion. If the nurse gave an injection of a narcotic medication but forgot to put the side rails up, and the client fell out of bed and fractured a hip, the nurse could be sued for the negligent act of forgetting to put the side rail up.

    Four elements are required for a person to make a claim of negligence:

1. A duty was owed to the client (professional relationship).
2. The professional violated the **duty** and failed to conform to the standard of care (breach of duty).
3. The failure to act by the professional was the **proximate cause** of the resulting injuries (causality).

4. Actual injuries resulted from the breach of duty (damages).

    If any of these elements are missing from the case, the client will probably not be able to win the lawsuit (Box 9.2).

Case Study
Consider the following situation:

Mr. Fagin, a 78-year-old client, was admitted from a nursing home for the treatment of a fractured tibia after he fell out of bed. After the fracture was reduced, a fiberglass cast was applied, and Mr. Fagin was sent to the orthopedic unit for follow-up care. While making her 0400 rounds, the night charge nurse, a registered nurse (RN), discovered that Mr. Fagin's foot on the casted leg was cold to touch, looked bluish-purple, and was swollen approximately

Box 9.2

Malpractice Considerations

Nursing malpractice is based on the legal premise that a nurse can be held legally responsible for the personal injury of another individual if it can be proved that the injury was the result of negligence.[2] Nursing malpractice is based on four elements: (1) duty, (2) breach of duty, (3) causation (the "but for" test), and (4) damage or injury.

    Inappropriate work assignment and inadequate supervision are a breach of duty and could be the basis for finding a nurse's actions to be negligent. Failure or breach of duty to delegate is established by proving that a reasonably prudent nurse would not have made a particular assignment or delegated a certain responsibility or that supervision was inadequate under the circumstances.

    The act of improper delegation of tasks or inadequate supervision must be evaluated in light of the "but for" test related to the injury. If the person who performed the injurious act had not been assigned or delegated to perform the task, or had been adequately supervised, the injury could have been avoided. Consequently, the nurse is not being held liable for the negligent act of her subordinate, *but for the lack of competence in performing the independent duties of delegation and supervision.*

Off-Site Consideration
Registered nurses who practice in public health, community, or home-care settings must rely frequently on written or telephone communication when delegating patient care duties to assistive personnel. The nurse who must supervise from off site has a particular duty to assess the knowledge, skills, and judgment of the assistive personnel before assignments are made. Regular supervisory visits and impeccable documentation will help the registered nurse ensure that care provided by assistive personnel is adequate.

Source: Aiken TD: Legal, Ethical, and Political Issues in Nursing. Philadelphia, FA Davis, 1994, pp 66–69.

1½ times normal size. The nurse noted these findings in the client's chart and relayed the information to the day-shift nurses during the 0630 shift report.

The charge nurse on the day shift promptly called and relayed the findings to Mr. Fagin's physician. The physician, however, did not seem to be concerned and only told the nurse to "Keep a close eye on him, and don't bother me again unless it is an absolute emergency." A short time later, Mr. Fagin became agitated, complained of severe pain in the affected foot, and eventually began yelling uncontrollably. The charge nurse called the emergency department (ED) physician to come to check on the client. The ED physician immediately removed the cast and noted an extensive circulatory impairment that would not respond to treatment. A few days later, Mr. Fagin's leg was amputated. His family filed a malpractice lawsuit against the hospital, the physician, and both the night and day charge nurses.

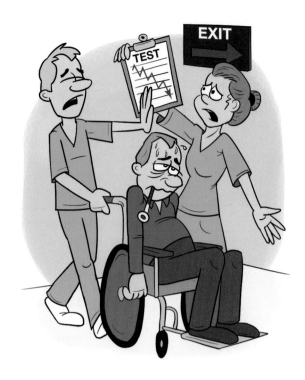

Are all the elements present in this case for a bona fide lawsuit? What could have been done to prevent this situation from happening? How should nurses deal with reluctant or hostile physicians?

Professional Misconduct

Malpractice is more serious than mere negligence because it indicates professional misconduct or unreasonable lack of skill in performing professional duties. Malpractice suggests the existence of a professional standard of care and a deviation from that standard of care. A professional **expert witness** is often asked to testify in a malpractice case to help establish the standard of care to which the professional should be held accountable.

A 1988 case in South Dakota presents an example of nursing malpractice. The nurse failed to question the physician's order to discharge a client when she discovered that the client had a fever. In this case, a supervisory nurse provided expert testimony and reported to the judge that the general standard of care for nurses is to report a significant change in a client's condition, such as an elevated temperature. It is the nurse's responsibility to question the physician's order as to appropriateness of discharge.

The records on this case indicated that the client's elevated temperature was charted after the physician had completed his rounds. The nurse did not notify the physician of the client's fever, and the client was subsequently discharged. The client was readmitted a short time after discharge and died in the hospital. The nurse was found negligent. The court held that negligence can be determined by failure to act as well as by the commission of an act.

Many other types of actions by nurses can produce malpractice lawsuits. Some of the more common actions include:

- Leaving foreign objects inside a client during surgery
- Failing to follow a hospital standard or protocol
- Not using equipment in accordance with the manufacturer's recommendations
- Failing to listen to and respond to a client's complaints
- Not properly documenting phone conversations and orders from physicians
- Failing to question physician orders when indicated (e.g., too large medication dosages, inappropriate diets)
- Failing to clarify poorly written or illegible physician orders

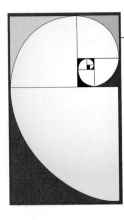

Issues in Practice

Nurse Malpractice in Client Fall

At a hospital in Washington State, a client with a recent leg amputation was still partially sedated after surgery. The nurse assigned to his care was called away from the room and failed to raise the bed rails. The client attempted to get out of bed, fell, and was injured.

The client sued the hospital for negligence. Using the hospital's own policies and procedures manual, the client's lawyer pointed out the requirement that satisfactory precautions be taken to restrain disabled or sedated clients.

The nurse's lawyer based the defense on the argument that the nurse was following the physician's standing orders to allow the client to ambulate postoperatively to hasten recovery and prevent complications.

The court agreed with the client and concluded that the nurse had an obligation, based on the hospital's policy and procedures, to assess the client's physical and mental condition. Nurses have an obligation not to leave clients unattended in an unsafe bed configuration.

All lawsuits alleging health-care provider negligence require expert witness testimony. Without expert witness testimony, courts will almost always dismiss a negligence case decided by a lay jury, even when it is as obvious as a fall from bed. In this case, the expert testimony not only supported the lawyer's contention that the hospital's policy and procedures upheld the suit but also emphasized the point that clients recently returned from surgery are disoriented from anesthesia and should never be left alone unless the bed rails are raised to their full upright position.

When the case was appealed, the court of appeals wrote the following ruling:

"A lawsuit against a hospital for negligence does not necessarily have to involve medical malpractice committed by a physician. A hospital's nurses have their own independent legal duties in assessing and caring for their patients.

"A hospital is not relieved of its own legal liability for negligence just because the hospital's staff nurses followed the physician's orders. That is, a hospital's nursing staff cannot necessarily rely on a physician's standing orders for a patient to be up and out of bed and leave the bed rails down.

"A patient freshly out of surgery who is taking pain and sedative medications must be evaluated continually by the staff. The patient's present physical and mental state is all that matters. The nurses may have to disregard the physician's standing orders and instead follow the hospital's policies and procedures for a restraint in the form of raised bed rails when necessary to insure the patient's safety."

Source: Greenberg v. Empire Health Services Inc., 2006 WL 1075574 Wash. App., April 25, 2006. Court of Appeals of Washington, April 25, 2006.

- Failing to assess and observe a client as directed
- Failing to obtain a proper informed consent
- Failing to report a change in a client's condition, such as vital signs, circulatory status, and level of consciousness
- Failing to report another health-care provider's **incompetency** or negligence
- Failing to take actions to provide for a client's safety, such as not cleaning up a liquid spill on the floor that causes a client to fall
- Failing to provide a client with sufficient and appropriate education before discharge[3]

If the Nurse is Liable

If a nurse is found guilty of malpractice, several types of action may be taken. The nurse may be required to provide monetary compensation to the client for general damages that were a direct result of the injury, including pain, suffering, disability, and disfigurement. In addition, the nurse is often required to pay for special damages that resulted from the injury, such as all involved medical expenses, **out-of-pocket expenses,** and wages lost by the client while he or she was in the hospital.

Optional damages, including those for emotional distress, mental suffering, and counseling expenses that were an outgrowth of the initial injury, may be added to the total settlement. If the client is able to prove that the nurse acted with conscious disregard for the client's safety or acted in a malicious, willful, or wanton manner that produced injury, an additional assessment of punitive or exemplary damages may be added to the award.

Intentional Torts

An **intentional tort** is generally defined as a willful act that violates another person's rights or property. Intentional torts can be distinguished from malpractice and acts of negligence by the following three requirements: (1) the nurse must intend to bring about the consequences of the act, (2) the nurse's act must be intended to interfere with the client or the client's property, and (3) the act must be a substantial factor in bringing about the injury or consequences.

> *Because of their professional status, nurses are held to a higher standard of conduct than the ordinary layperson.*

The most frequently encountered intentional torts are assault, battery, false imprisonment, abandonment, and intentional infliction of emotional distress. With intentional torts, the injured person does not have to prove that an injury has occurred, nor is the opinion of an expert witness required for adjudication. Punitive damages are more likely to be assessed against the nurse in intentional tort cases, and some intentional torts may fall under the criminal law if there is gross violation of the standards of care.

Assault and Battery

Assault is the unjustifiable attempt to touch another person or the threat of doing so. **Battery** is actual harmful or unwarranted contact with another person without his or her consent. Battery is the most common intentional tort seen in the practice of nursing.

For a nurse to commit assault and battery, there must be an absence of consent on the part of the client. Before any procedure can be performed on a competent, alert, and normally oriented client, the client must agree or consent to the procedure being done. Negligence does not have to be proved for a person to be successful in a claim for assault and battery.

A common example of an assault and battery occurs when a nurse physically restrains a client against the client's will and administers an injection against the client's wishes.

False Imprisonment

False imprisonment occurs when a competent client is confined or restrained with intent to prevent him or her from leaving the hospital. The use of restraints alone does not constitute false imprisonment when they are used to maintain the safety of a confused, disoriented, or otherwise incompetent client. In general, mentally impaired clients can be detained against their will only if they are at risk for injuring themselves or others. The use of threats or medications that interfere with the client's ability to leave the facility can also be considered false imprisonment.

Intentional Infliction of Emotional Distress

Intentional infliction of emotional distress is another common intentional tort encountered by the nurse. To prove this intentional tort, the following three elements are necessary: (1) the conduct exceeds what is usually accepted by society, (2) the health-care provider's conduct is intended to cause mental distress, and (3) the conduct actually does produce mental distress (causation). Any nurse who is charged with assault, battery, or false imprisonment is also at risk for being charged with infliction of emotional distress.

A 1975 case is an example of infliction of emotional distress. In *Johnson v. Women's Hospital,* a mother wished to view the body of her baby, who had died during birth. After she made the request, she was handed the baby's body floating in a gallon jar of formaldehyde.[1] The Johnson case demonstrates a clear lack of respect shown to the mother. If the mother in this delicate situation had been treated with dignity and respect, the situation would have been avoided.

Client Abandonment

Because of the ongoing nursing shortage, **abandonment** of clients has become an important legal and ethical issue for health-care providers. Abandonment occurs when there is a unilateral severance of the professional relationship with the client without adequate notice and while the requirement for care still exists. The nurse-client relationship continues until it is terminated by mutual consent of both parties.

From an ethical standpoint, the issue of abandonment falls under the umbrella of beneficence. From the legal view, client abandonment can be considered an intentional tort, breach of contract, or in some cases in which injury occurs, malpractice. The key phrase to keep in mind when discussing client abandonment is "without adequate notice." If the client knows that the nurse's shift is scheduled to end at 7:00 p.m., the client and the hospital both have adequate notice.

It is not uncommon for nurses in today's health-care system to be approached by nursing supervisors with the statement, "Everyone else called in, so you will have to work a double shift or you could be charged with client abandonment." In this case, the abandonment becomes the hospital's responsibility, not the nurse's. Nurses sometimes feel uncomfortable about going on strike because it seems to imply client abandonment; however, if there is adequate notice about the strike and if the facility has had time to make arrangements for care or discharge of clients, there is no client abandonment. The growing practice of emergency client diversion, occurring when facilities can no longer safely care for emergency clients because of lack of space or staffing, can potentially fall under the legal definitions of abandonment.

Quasi-Intentional Torts

A **quasi-intentional tort** is a mixture of unintentional and intentional torts. It is defined as a voluntary act that directly causes injury or distress without intent to injure or to cause distress. A quasi-intentional tort does have the elements of volition and causation without the element of intent. Quasi-intentional torts usually involve situations of communication and often violate a person's reputation, personal privacy, or civil rights (Box 9.3).

Defamation of Character

Defamation of character, which is the most common of the quasi-intentional torts, is harmful to a person's reputation. Defamation injures a person's

---

Box 9.3
Registered Nurse Licensure

The legislature of each state enacts laws that govern the practice of nursing. The purpose of licensing law is to ensure that the public is protected from unqualified practitioners by developing and enforcing regulations that define who may practice in the profession, the scope of that practice, and the level of education for the profession.

A fundamental premise of nursing practice is that a professional nurse is personally responsible for all acts or omissions undertaken within the scope of practice. The American Nurses Association defines delegation as "the transfer of responsibility for the performance of an activity from one person to another while retaining accountability for the outcome."[1] Additionally, the nurse is responsible for the adequate supervision of a task delegated to a subordinate. If the nurse fails to delegate appropriately or supervise adequately, any injuries resulting from the acts of the subordinate may result in licensure ramifications. The state licensing board may take disciplinary actions.

reputation by diminishing the esteem, respect, good will, or confidence that others have for the person. It can be especially damaging when false statements are made about a criminal act or an immoral act or when there are false allegations about a client's having a contagious disease. In *Schessler v. Keck* (1954), a nurse was found liable for defamation of character when she told a friend that a caterer for whom she was caring was being treated for syphilis. Even though the statement was false, when the information became public, it destroyed his catering business.[1]

Defamation includes **slander,** which is spoken communication in which one person discusses another in terms that harm that person's reputation. **Libel** is a written communication in which a person makes statements or uses language that harms another person's reputation. To win a defamation lawsuit against the nurse, the client must prove that the nurse acted maliciously, abused the principle of **privileged communication,** and wrote or spoke a lie.

Medical record documentation is a primary source of defamation of character. Through the years, the client's chart has been the basis of many defamation lawsuits. Discussion about a client in the elevators, cafeteria, and other public areas can also lead to lawsuits for defamation if negative comments are overheard.

Invasion of Privacy

Invasion of privacy is a violation of a person's right to protection against unreasonable and unwarranted interference with one's personal life. To prove that invasion of privacy has occurred, the client must show that (1) the nurse intruded on the client's seclusion and privacy, (2) the intrusion is objectionable to a reasonable and prudent person, (3) the act committed intrudes on private or published facts or pictures of a private nature, and (4) public disclosure of private information was made.[3] Examples of invasion of privacy include using the client's name or picture for the sole advantage of the health-care provider, intruding into the client's private affairs without permission, giving out private client information over the telephone, and publishing information that misrepresents the client's condition. Because of the Health Insurance Portability and Accountability Act (HIPAA) of 1996, health-care providers have become more aware than ever of the issue of confidentiality in the health-care setting.

Breach of Confidentiality

Privileged Communication

Confidentiality of information concerning the client must be honored. A breach of confidentiality results when a client's trust and confidence are violated by public revelation of confidential or privileged communications without the client's consent. Privileged communication is protected by law and exists in certain well-defined professional relationships, for example, physician–client, psychiatrist–client, priest–penitent, and lawyer–client.

Privileged communication ensures that the professional who obtains any information from the client cannot be forced to reveal that information, even in a court of law under oath. Nurses do not have privileged communication with clients. However, they can be bound, by extension, under the seal of privileged communication if they are in a room with a physician when the client reveals personal information.

Most breach of confidentiality cases involve a physician's revelation of privileged communications shared by a client. Nurses who overhear privileged communication or information, however, are held to the same standards as a physician with regard to that information.

Privileged client information can only be disclosed if it is authorized by the client. In accord with the HIPAA regulations, all health-care facilities must have specific guidelines dealing with client information disclosure. Disclosure of information to family members violates HIPAA regulations unless the client is under 18 years of age or gives permission for the disclosure. For instance, a client may not wish to disclose to a family member a specific diagnosis, such as cancer. If this is the case, the nurse should honor this request; otherwise, it is considered a violation of HIPAA regulations.

Electronic Pitfalls

Use of computerized documentation and telemedicine has led to several lawsuits based on breach of confidentiality and malpractice. (See Chapter 19 for examples.) The HIPAA regulations are the government's attempts to force the legal system to keep pace with the use of computers and electronic record-keeping. Cases exist in which medical records have been lost because of computer failure.

Other issues, such as correction of errors in **charting,** are complicated by use of computers. On paper charts, health-care providers had to draw a line through the erroneous entry, initial the entry, and date it. Many new computerized charting systems have attempted to address the "delete button" issue by including programs that track any changes made in the charting and indicate both the date and time of the change.

FACING A LAWSUIT

Because of the rapid proliferation of lawsuits since the 1990s, there is now a higher probability that a nurse, at some time in her or his career, will be involved either as a witness or as a party to a nursing malpractice action. Knowledge of the litigation process increases nurses' understanding of the way in which their conduct is evaluated before the courts.

The Statute of Limitations
A malpractice suit against a nurse for negligence must be filed within a specified time. This period, called the **statute of limitations,** generally begins at the time of the injury or when the injury is discovered and lasts until some specified future time. In most states, the limitation period lasts from 1 to 6 years, with the most common duration being 2 years. However, in cases involving children, the statute of limitations extends until the person reaches 21 years of age. If the client fails to file the suit within the prescribed time, the lawsuit will be barred.

> *Because of the rapid proliferation of lawsuits since the 1990s, there is now a higher probability that a nurse, at some time in his or her career, will be involved either as a witness or as a party to a nursing malpractice action.*

The Complaint
Filing the suit (also called the complaint) with the court begins the litigation process. The written complaint describes the incident that initiated the claim of negligence against the nurse. Specific allegations, including the amount of money sought for damages, are also stated in the **legal complaint.** The plaintiff, who is usually a client or a family member of a client, is the alleged injured party, and the defendant (i.e., the nurse, physician, or hospital) is the person or entity being sued. The first notice of a lawsuit occurs when the defendant (nurse) is officially notified or served with the complaint. All defendants are accorded the right of **due process** under constitutional law.

The Answer
The defendant must respond to the allegations stated in the complaint within a specific time frame. This written response by the defendant is called the answer. If the nurse had liability insurance in force at the time of the negligent act, the insurer will assign a lawyer to represent the defendant nurse. In the answer, the nurse can outline specific defenses to the claims against him or her.

The Discovery
After the complaint and answer are filed with the court, the discovery phase of the litigation begins. The purpose of discovery is to uncover all information relevant to the malpractice suit and the incident in question. The nurse may be required to answer a series of questions that relate to the nurse's educational background and emotional state, the incident that led to the lawsuit, and any other information the plaintiff's lawyer deems important. These written questions are called **interrogatories**.

In addition, the plaintiff's lawyer may seek requests for production of documents. These are documents related to the lawsuit, including the plaintiff's medical records, **incident reports,** card file, the institution's policy and procedure manual concerning the specific situation, and the nurse's job description. The plaintiff is also required to disclose information as part of the discovery process that includes the plaintiff's past medical history.

The Deposition
The next step in the process is the taking of a deposition from each party to the lawsuit, as well as any potential witnesses, to assist the lawyers in the trial preparation. A **deposition** is a formal legal process that involves the taking of testimony under oath and is recorded by a court reporter. These are usually wide ranging in scope and often include information not allowed in a trial, such as **hearsay** testimony. In some cases, videotaped depositions may be used. Nurses can prepare for a deposition by keeping some key points in mind (Box 9.4).

Box 9.4
Giving a Deposition

1. Do not volunteer information.
2. Be familiar with the client's medical record and nurse's notes.
3. Remain calm throughout the process and do not be intimidated by the lawyers.
4. Clarify all questions before answering; ask the lawyer to explain the questions if you do not understand.
5. Do not make assumptions about the questions.
6. Do not exaggerate answers.
7. Wait at least 5 seconds after a question is asked before answering it to allow objections from other lawyers.
8. Tell the truth.
9. Do not speculate about answers.
10. Speak slowly and clearly, using professional language as much as possible.
11. Look the questioning lawyer in the eye as much as possible.
12. If unable to remember an answer, simply state "I don't remember" or "I don't know."
13. Think before answering any question.
14. Bring a resume or curriculum vitae to the deposition in case it is requested.
15. Request a break if you are tired or confused.
16. Avoid becoming angry with the lawyers or using sarcastic language.
17. Avoid using absolutes in the answers.
18. If a question is asked more than once, ask the court recorder to read the answer given previously.
19. Be sure to read over the deposition just before the trial.

Source: Wagner KC, Hunter-Adkins D, Clifford R: Questions & answers. Effective preparation of the expert witness for deposition. Journal of Legal Nurse Consulting 19(4):26–29, 34, 2009.

The deposition **testimony** is reduced to a written document called an **affidavit** for use at trial. If a witness during the trial changes testimony from that given at the deposition, the deposition can be used to contradict the testimony. This process is called *impeaching the witness*. Impeaching a witness on a specific issue can create doubt about that witness's credibility and can thus weaken other areas in the witness's testimony. In some situations, witnesses can later be charged with **perjury** if it is proved that they gave false testimony under oath.

The Trial

The **trial** often takes place years after the complaint was filed. Once **jurisdiction** is determined, the *voir dire* process, more commonly called *jury selection*, begins. After jury selection, each attorney presents opening statements. The plaintiff's side is presented first. Witnesses may be served with **subpoenas** that require them to appear and provide testimony.

Each witness or party is subject to direct examination, cross-examination, and redirect examination. Direct examination involves open-ended questions by the attorney. Cross-examination is performed by the opposing lawyer, and questions are asked in such a way as to elicit short, specific responses. The redirect examination consists of follow-up questions to address issues that were raised during the cross-examination.

After both parties have presented their case, the lawyers deliver their closing arguments. The case then goes to a jury or a judge for deliberation. If the facts are not in dispute, the judge may render a **summary judgment.** The decision or ruling made about the case can be appealed if either party is not satisfied. The party appealing the decision is called the **appellant.**

POSSIBLE DEFENSES TO A MALPRACTICE SUIT

Contributory Negligence

Damages awarded vary from one state to another and also with the types of injuries sustained. In a state with contributory negligence laws, clients are not allowed to receive money for injuries if they contributed to those injuries in any manner. For example, a nurse forgot to raise the bed rail after administering an injection of a narcotic pain medication to a postoperative client but instructed the client to turn on the call light if he wanted to get out of bed. The client fell while attempting to go to the bathroom; because he did not use the call light, he contributed to his own injuries and thus could not receive compensation.

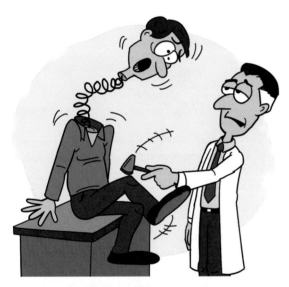

"I SUPPOSE THIS MEANS ANOTHER MALPRACTICE SUIT."

Comparative Negligence

In a state with comparative negligence laws, the awards are based on the determination of the percentage of fault by both parties. For example, in the aforementioned case, if $100,000 was awarded by the jury, it may be determined that the nurse was 75 percent at fault and the client was 25 percent at fault. In that case, the client would receive $75,000. In general, if the client is 50 percent or more at fault, no award will be made. As can be seen, determination of these types of awards is highly subjective, and an **appeal** about the decision is often made to a higher court.

Case Study

Consider the following case:

Ms. Gouge, a 44-year-old client who weighed 307 lb, was admitted to a large university medical center ED with complaints of chest pain and disorientation and a blood pressure of 208/154 mm Hg. She also displayed aphasia, hemiplegia, and loss of sensation and movement on her right side.

After a magnetic resonance imaging (MRI) scan of the head, it was discovered that she had an inoperable cerebral aneurysm. In addition to appropriate medical treatment for blood pressure and circulation, her family physician told her that she had to lose a significant amount of weight. The nurse in the physician's office instituted a weight loss teaching plan for Ms. Gouge, planned out a calorie-restricted low-fat diet, and gave her a large amount of information about healthy diet and a DVD of low-impact aerobic exercises. At a follow-up visit 1 month later, Ms. Gouge weighed 315 lb.

Six months later, Ms. Gouge's aneurysm ruptured, leaving her in a vegetative state. Ms. Gouge's family filed a lawsuit against the physician and his office nurse, claiming that they had failed to institute proper and appropriate preventive measures and that they had failed to inform the client of the seriousness of her condition.

Did the nurse's decisions or actions contribute to the filing of this suit? Is there any contributory negligence? What is the nurse's role in defending against this suit? What might the nurse have done to prevent the suit in the first place?

Assumption of Risk

When the client signs the informed consent form for a particular treatment, procedure, or surgery, it is implied that he or she is aware of the possible complications of that treatment, procedure, or surgery. Under the assumption-of-risk defense, if one of those listed or named complications occurs, the client has no grounds to sue the health-care provider. For example, a common complication from hip replacement surgery is some loss of mobility and range of motion of the affected leg. Even if a client, after having a hip replaced, is able to walk only using a walker, he or she still does not have any grounds for a lawsuit.

Good Samaritan Act

Health-care providers are sometimes hesitant to provide care at the scene of accidents, in emergency situations, or during disasters because they fear lawsuits. The **Good Samaritan Act** is designed specifically to protect health-care providers in these situations. A health-care professional who provides care in an emergency situation cannot be sued for injuries that may be sustained by the client if that care was given according to established guidelines and was within the scope of the professional's education.

For example, a nurse who finds a person in cardiac arrest administers cardiopulmonary resuscitation (CPR) to revive the person. In the process, she fractures several of the client's ribs. The client would not be able to sue the nurse for the fractured ribs if the CPR was administered according to established standards.

Good Samaritan laws do, however, have some limitations. They do not cover nurses for grossly negligent acts in the provision of care or for acts outside the nurse's level of education. For example, in the case of a person choking on a piece of meat, the nurse initially attempts the Heimlich maneuver but without success. As the person loses consciousness, the nurse decides to perform a tracheostomy. The client survives, but can sue the nurse for injuries from the tracheostomy because this is not a normal part of a nurse's education.

Unavoidable Accident

Sometimes accidents happen without any contributing causes from the nurse, hospital, or physician. For example, a client is walking in the hall and trips over her own bathrobe. She breaks an ankle. There were no puddles on the floor or obstacles in the hall, and the client was alert and oriented. Because no one is at fault, there are no grounds for a lawsuit.

Defense of the Fact

Defense of the fact is based on the claim that the actions of the nurse followed the standards of care, or that even if the actions were in violation of the standard of care, the actions themselves were not the direct cause of the injury.[4] For example, a nurse wraps a dressing too tightly on a client's foot after surgery. Later, the client loses his eyesight and blames the loss of vision on the nurse's improper dressing of his foot.

Going through the litigation process can produce high levels of anxiety. Placing every aspect of the nurse's conduct under scrutiny in a trial is very stressful. All aspects of the alleged negligent act will be examined and re-examined. Often events that happened years before can be brought in to establish a "pattern of behavior." Every word of the nurse's notes and the medical record will be closely analyzed and questioned. Nurses can survive the litigation process with the help of good attorneys and by being honest and demonstrating that they were acting in the best interests of the client. From this viewpoint, it is easy to see the importance of carrying nursing liability insurance.

> *Health-care providers are sometimes hesitant to provide care at the scene of accidents, in emergency situations, or during disasters because they fear lawsuits. The Good Samaritan Act is designed specifically to protect health-care providers in these situations.*

ALTERNATIVE DISPUTE FORUMS

Although most lawsuits against nurses are settled through the court system, there are other methods of settling them. Because of the large number of cases and the resultant overload of the judicial system, other methods of resolving disputes have become increasingly popular. These alternative forums of dispute resolution are being used for many types of conflict and are seen more frequently in the areas of torts, contracts, employment, and family law. Mediation and arbitration are the most commonly used alternatives to trial.

Mediation

Mediation is a process that allows each party to present his or her case before a mediator, who is an independent third party trained in dispute resolution. The mediator listens to each side individually. This one-sided session is called a caucus. The mediator's role is to find common ground between the parties and encourage resolution of the disputed matters by compromise and negotiation. The mediator aids the parties in arriving at a mutually acceptable outcome.

The mediator does not act as a decision maker, but rather encourages the parties to come to a "meeting of the minds."

Arbitration

Arbitration, in contrast, allows a neutral third party to hear both parties' positions and then make a decision or ruling on the basis of the facts and evidence presented. Arbitration, by agreement or by statutory definition, can be binding or nonbinding. **Arbitrators** or mediators can be, and frequently are, retired judges who work on an hourly-fee basis or practicing attorneys. In the family law area, they are frequently social workers or specially trained mediators. Negligence and malpractice issues are frequently resolved through arbitration and mediation.

COMMON ISSUES IN HEALTH-CARE LITIGATION

Informed Consent

Informed consent is both a legal and an ethical issue. Informed consent is the voluntary permission by a client or by the client's designated proxy to carry out a procedure on the client. Clients' claims that they did not grant informed consent before a surgery or invasive procedure can and do form the basis of a small percentage of lawsuits.

Although these lawsuits are most often directed against physicians and hospitals, nurses can become involved when they provide the information but are not performing the procedure. The person who is performing the procedure has the responsibility to obtain the informed consent. However, some physicians have gotten into the habit of giving nurses the consent forms and saying, "Get the client to sign this." Informed consent can only be given by a client after the client receives sufficient information on:

- Treatment proposed
- Material risk involved (potential complications)
- Acceptable alternative treatments
- Outcome hoped for
- Consequences of not having treatment

> *Nurses can reinforce the physician teaching and even supplement the information but should not be the primary or only source of information for the informed consent. It is often difficult to draw a clear distinction between where the physician's responsibility ends and that of the nurse begins.*

The physician should provide most of this information. Nurses can reinforce the physician teaching and even supplement the information but should not be the primary or only source of information for the informed consent. It is often difficult to draw a clear distinction between where the physician's responsibility ends and that of the nurse begins.

What Do You Think?

Have you ever had a surgical procedure where you signed an informed consent form? Did it meet all five criteria listed? Which ones were missing?

Exceptions to Informed Consent

There are two exceptions to informed consent:

1. Emergency situations in which the client is unconscious, incompetent, or otherwise unable to give consent.
2. Situations in which the health-care provider feels that it may be medically contraindicated to disclose the risk and hazards because it may result in illness, severe emotional distress, serious psychological damage, or failure on the part of the client to receive lifesaving treatment

Patient Self-Determination Act

The Patient Self-Determination Act of 1990, sponsored by Senator John Danforth, is a federal law that requires that all federally funded institutions inform clients of their right to prepare advance directives. The advance directives are meant to encourage people to discuss and document their wishes concerning the type of treatment and care that they want (i.e., life-sustaining treatment) in advance so that it will ease the burden on their families and providers when it comes time to make such a decision.

There are two types of advance directives: the living will and the medical durable power of attorney (Box 9.5). The **living will** is a document stating what health care a client will accept or refuse after the client is no longer competent or able to make that decision.

B o x   9 . 5
Common Questions About Advance Directives

Q. Which is better—a living will or a medical durable power of attorney for health care or health-care proxy?

A. The documents are different and allow the nurse to do two different things. The living will states what health-care procedures a client will accept or refuse after the client is no longer competent or able to make that decision. The medical durable power of attorney or health-care proxy allows a client to designate another person to make health-care choices for him or her.

Q. If I change my mind and have a living will, can I cancel the living will or durable medical power of attorney?

A. Yes, each state has ways that your advance directives can be cancelled or negated. Most states require an oral or written statement, destruction of the document itself, or notification to certain individuals, such as the physician. Again, each state's statute should be checked for the specific details required.

Q. If I have a living will in one state, is it good in all states?

A. It may or may not be, depending on that state's requirements for the living will. It is important that you have your living will checked by an attorney to determine whether or not it may be effective in the states in which you are traveling or working.

Q. If I have a living will and have a medical durable power of attorney, who should get copies?

A. Copies should be given to your next of kin, your physician, and your attorney so that more than one person has a copy and knows what your intentions are. Some states will allow you to register your living will with certain state agencies such as the Secretary of State. There are also national groups that will allow you to register your living will with them so that there is access to it.

The medical durable power of attorney, or health-care proxy, designates another person to make health-care decisions for a person if the client becomes incompetent or unable to make such decisions.

Each state outlines its own requirements for executing and revoking the medical durable power of attorney and living wills.

Incompetent Client's Right to Self-Determination

The courts are protective of incompetent clients and require high standards of proof before allowing a physician to terminate any life-sustaining treatment for that client.

Nancy Cruzan was 30 years old and in a persistent vegetative state. She had a gastrostomy feeding and hydration tube inserted to assist with feedings, which her husband consented to. Her parents, however, petitioned the court for removal of the tube. In the Cruzan case, the court held that the state had the right to err on the side of life. The U.S. Supreme Court recognized that a living will would have been sufficient evidence of Cruzan's wishes to sustain or to remove her feeding tube.

The issue before the U.S. Supreme Court was whether the state of Missouri could use its own standard of clear and convincing proof for removal of the tube or whether there was a 14th Amendment due process guarantee of a "right to die" that would override the state statute. It was decided that the constitutional right would not be extended and the state procedural requirement would be allowed, at which time the burden of proof was put on Cruzan's family to show that she would not have wanted to continue living in this manner.

Many aspects of the Terri Schiavo case in Florida parallel the Cruzan case. In the Schiavo case, after the feeding tube was removed by order of a Florida judge, the U.S. Congress became involved and passed a bill, signed by President George W. Bush, that required the case be heard by the U.S. Supreme Court. The goal was to have the tube reinserted until the high court could rule on the case. It is interesting to note that not much progress has been made in developing legal solutions for this type of case during the 20-plus years since the Cruzan case.

The Nurse's Role in Advance Directives

Because laws vary from state to state, it is important that nurses know the laws of the state in which they practice that pertain to advance directives, clients' rights, and the policies and procedures of the institution in which they work. Nurses must inform clients of their right to formulate advance directives and must realize that not all clients can make such decisions.

It is important for the nurse to establish trust and rapport with a client and the client's family so that the nurse can assist them in making decisions that are in the client's best interests. Nurses must also teach about advance directives and document all critical decisions, discussions with the client and client's family about such decisions, and the basis for the decision-making process. Also, it is essential to prevent discrimination against clients and their families based on their decisions regarding their advance directives.

It is important that nurses determine whether or not clients have been coerced into making advance directive decisions against their will. Nurses need to become involved in ethics committees at hospitals or nursing specialty groups at local, state, or national levels to help clients make decisions about advance directives.

> *Because laws vary from state to state, it is important that nurses know the laws of the state in which they practice that pertain to advance directives, clients' rights, and the policies and procedures of the institution in which they work.*

Do-Not-Resuscitate Orders

Protection for the Nurse

Although a DNR instruction may be included in an advance directive, DNR orders are legally separate from advance directives. For the health-care professional to be legally protected, there should be a written order for a "no code" or a DNR order in the client's chart.

Each hospital should have a policy and procedure that outlines what is required with regard to a client's condition for a DNR order. The DNR order should be reviewed, evaluated, and reordered. Different facilities have established different time periods for these reviews. Nurses must also know whether there is any law that regulates who should authorize a DNR order for an incompetent client who is no longer able to make this decision. Hospitals often have policies and procedures describing what must be done and which clients fit the requirements for a

DNR order. The American Nurses Association (ANA) has published a position statement on nursing care and DNR decisions.

Nurses face many legal dilemmas when dealing with confusing or conflicting DNR orders. For example, it may be difficult to interpret a DNR order when it has been restricted, for instance, "do not resuscitate except for medications and defibrillation" or "no CPR or intubation." Often a lack of proper documentation in the medical records indicating how the DNR decision was reached can be a crucial issue if a medical malpractice case is involved and it is disputed whether or not the client or family actually gave consent for the order.

Many facilities have developed DNR decision sheets. A DNR sheet may record information about DNR discussions or be dated and signed by the client and those family members who took part in the discussion. It then becomes a permanent part of the medical record.

Protection for the Client

It is very important that nurses not stigmatize clients by the use of indicators for DNR orders, such as dots on the wristband or over the bed. Health-care providers' attitudes often change because they feel that the client is "going to die anyway." This abandonment can jeopardize the care of a client designated with a DNR order. However, it is also important for the nurses and staff to know whether an order is to be honored and what the policies and procedures are with regard to transfer clients and DNR orders that accompany the incoming client.

Information about the DNR status of a client should be obtained during shift reports. If there has not been a periodic review, is the order still in effect? If a client is transferred from one facility to another and has a DNR order that is time limited and has not been reordered, what should a nurse do?

Standards of Care

A Measure of Action

Standards of care are the yardstick that the legal system uses to measure the actions of a nurse involved in a malpractice suit. The underlying principle used to establish standards of care is based on the actions that would probably be taken by a reasonable person (nurse) in the same or similar circumstances.

The standard usually includes both objective factors (e.g., the actions to be performed) and subjective factors, including the nurse's emotional and mental state. Specifically, a nurse is judged against the standards that are established within the profession and specialty area of practice. The ANA and specialty groups within the nursing profession, such as the American Association of Critical-Care Nurses (AACN), publish standards of care that are updated continually as health-care technology and practices change.

External Standards

Both external and internal standards govern the conduct of nurses. External standards include nursing standards developed by the ANA, the state nurse practice act of each jurisdiction, criteria from accrediting agencies such as The Joint Commission, guidelines developed by various nursing specialty practice groups, and federal agency regulations. Nurses are encountering an increasing number of incidents in which conflicts occur between institutional and professional standards, for example, in staffing ratios. These conflicts are difficult to resolve and may require deliberation and decisions from institutional committees. As a general rule, when a conflict exists, it is safer legally to follow professional standards.

Internal Standards

Internal standards include nursing standards defined in specific hospital policy and procedure manuals that relate to the nurse in the particular institution. The nurse's job description and employment contract are examples of internal nursing standards that define the duty of the nurse.

Criteria for Good Care

The rationale for advancing standards of care for the nurse is to ensure proper, consistent, and high-quality nursing care to all members of society. When nurses violate their duty of care to the client as established by the profession's standards of care, they leave themselves open to charges of negligence and malpractice. Until recently, nurses were held to the standards of the local community. National criteria have now replaced most **locality rule standards of care.** Individual nurses are held accountable not only to acceptable standards within the local community but also to national standards.

Although standards of care may appear to be specific, they are merely guidelines for nursing practice. Because every client's situation is different, the appropriate standard of care may be difficult to identify in a specific case. More than one course of nursing action may be considered appropriate under a proper standard of care. The final decision must be guided by the nurse's judgment and understanding of the client's needs.

The Nurse Practice Act

The nurse practice act defines nursing practice and establishes standards for nurses in each state. It is the most definitive legal statute or legislative act regulating nursing practice. Although nurse practice acts vary in scope from one state to another, they tend to have similar wording based loosely on the ANA model published in 1988. The nurse practice act provides a framework for the court on which to base decisions when determining whether a nurse has breached a standard of care.

> *Nurses are encountering an increasing number of incidents in which conflicts occur between institutional and professional standards, for example, in staffing ratios.*

Most state nurse practice acts define scope of practice, establish requirements for licensure and entry into practice, and create and empower a board of nursing to oversee the practice of nurses. In addition, nurse practice acts identify grounds for disciplinary actions such as suspension and revocation of a nursing license.[4]

The judicial interpretation of the nurse practice act and its relationship to a specific case provide guidance for decisions about future cases. Many state legislatures have responded to the expanded role of the nurse by broadening the scope of their nurse practice acts. For example, the addition of the term *nursing diagnosis* to many states' nurse practice acts reflects the legislature's recognition of the expansion of the nurse's role.

In addition, occupational roles such as nurse practitioner, **nurse clinician,** and clinical nurse specialist are beginning to be included in nurse practice acts. It is important to remember that as the nurse's role expands, so does the legal accountability of the role.

PREVENTING LAWSUITS

What can the nurse do to avoid having to go through the stressful, sometimes financially and professionally devastating, process of litigation? The following guidelines provide some ways to avoid a lawsuit.

Effective Communication
Situation–Background–Assessment–Recommendation (SBAR)

After many years of collecting data and analyzing sentinel and critical events, The Joint Commission concluded that miscommunication among health-care workers is the leading cause of health-care–related errors leading to injury, death, and lawsuits. The Commission called for a communication strategy that would be concrete, would provide a framework for communication between caregivers, and would be easy for all health-care workers to remember. It would need to work in all situations, from end-of-shift reports to exchanges in high-pressure critical care areas, when a nurse's immediate response and actions could make the difference between life and death. Care expectations could be communicated in a focused, simple way that allowed all team members to understand and respond quickly. The overall goal would be to develop a "culture of client safety" that would permeate any organization.[5]

The SBAR system (Situation–Background–Assessment–Recommendation, pronounced "S-Bar") was initially developed by the U.S. Navy to improve communications on the nuclear submarine fleet. Refined and adopted by Kaiser Permanente of Colorado in the late 1990s, SBAR is being incorporated into health-care facilities and is working its way into the nursing education system. SBAR has been proved useful when a client's status changes unexpectedly. A review of client charts in these emergency situations shows how confused the communication between the physician and the nurse can be. Fatigue, lack of experience, or reduced nursing education often leads to the omission of key information. In this type of situation, SBAR forms an outline for the communication of critical information.[6]

Each of the letters in SBAR stands for a step in the process:

S = Situation: Asks the question, "What is going on?" Information to provide or look for:
- Identify yourself, the hospital unit or health-care location, and the room number
- Identify the client by name, age, gender, and date of birth
- Describe the problem the client has that triggered the SBAR communication

B = Background: Provides key information that will help determine what actions to take:
- Give a short summary of the client's relevant past medical history
- Provide the client's diagnosis
- Describe the client's current mental status, current vital signs, complaints, pain level, oxygen saturation, and physical assessment findings.

A = Assessment: Allows the nurse to analyze the situation and isolate the specific problem:
- Note what vital signs are outside of parameters
- Give the nurse's clinical impressions of the client and additional concerns
- Rank the severity of the client's condition
- Identify specific client needs to resolve the situation

R = Recommendation: Identifies what actions will resolve the situation:
- Identify what needs to be done to resolve the client's problem
- Note how urgent the problem is and when action needs to be taken
- Suggest what action is to be taken
- State the desired client response

> *The medical record is the single most frequently used piece of objective evidence in a malpractice suit. In preparation for the trial, the lawyers attempt to reconstruct the events surrounding the incident in a minute-by-minute time line.*

Here is an example of how an SBAR communication could be used:

Situation: Hello, Dr. Nife, this is Crystal Beshear, RN, in the step-down unit, calling about Mr. Jenkins, who had the femoral bypass graft done yesterday. He was undergoing cardiac monitoring according to protocol, and within the last 15 minutes went from a sinus rhythm to an atrial fibrillation of 165 beats per minute.

Background: As you know, Mr. Jenkins, 68 years old, has a history of cardiac disease, including a myocardial infarction in 2005. He has type 1 diabetes and has had several deep vein thromboses over the past 3 years. Currently his vital signs are: blood pressure, 98/54; pulse, 165; respirations, 26; O_2 saturation, 89%; and urine output, 82 mL per hour. He has an intravenous (IV) infusion of D5 half-normal saline running at 125 mL per hour. He is complaining of some slight chest pressure. His incision site is clean and dry, and he has +2 pedal pulses in both feet.

Assessment: His blood pressure normally runs 136/76, pulse 90, respiration 18, and O_2 saturation 96%. This is the first time he has complained of chest pressure but ranks it as only a 2 on a 1-to-10 scale. The vital sign changes all occurred shortly after the change in his cardiac rhythm. His neurological status is unchanged, and the femoral graft has not been affected by the cardiovascular changes. He has been taking sips by mouth and tolerating it well.

Recommendations: It appears that restoring Mr. Jenkins to normal sinus rhythm is the highest priority. What would you think about restarting him on Lanoxin, 0.25 mg, which was discontinued preoperatively? We could give it either by IV or by mouth because he is tolerating water.

In general, nurses feel uncomfortable making medical recommendations to physicians. Also, some physicians do not handle recommendations from nurses very well. However, recommendations are part of the SBAR process, and the physician can always just say "No." Disguising the recommen-

> *Being direct, solving problems with the client, and helping the client become involved in his or her care are helpful in diffusing this negative behavior.*

dations in the form of a question softens the impact and meets with more success.[7]

Medical Record

Charting in the medical record is the best way to display the care provided and the communication between health-care workers. It is the single most frequently used piece of objective evidence in a malpractice suit. In preparation for the trial, the lawyers attempt to reconstruct the events surrounding the incident in a minute-by-minute time line. The client's **chart** is the most important source for this time line. Maintaining an accurate and complete medical record is an absolute requirement (Box 9.6).

In nursing and medical negligence claims, lawyers are beginning to ask whether the hospital has adopted the use of SBAR. They examine the materials used to educate the staff and any policies or procedures concerning the use of SBAR. They note any mention of SBAR communication in the medical record and see whether it is recorded properly.[8] Even if the facility has not adopted SBAR as a hospital-wide communication technique, nurses who know how can use it to help protect themselves in subsequent legal actions.

The old adage, "If it isn't written, it didn't happen" remains true in most situations; however, recent court trials have recognized some exceptions. Some judges and juries have begun to recognize that charting by exception is a valid form of health-care record-keeping. Charting by exception, very closely related to problem-oriented charting, was developed initially to save time for busy nurses and money for the facility by reducing the volume of documents created and stored. In institutions in which charting by exception is used, the nurse charts only those elements of client care that are abnormal or unusual or that constitute a health-care problem. If the client is stable and recovering as expected, there may be very little written in the chart about his or her physical or mental assessments.

Trying to recall specific events from 2 to 6 years ago without the benefit of written notes is almost impossible. In general, the client record should *not* contain personal opinion, should be legible, should be in chronological order, and should be

Box 9.6

Some Documentation Guidelines

Medications
- Always chart the time, route, dose, and response.
- Always chart prn medications and the client response.
- Always chart when a medication was not given, the reason (client in x-ray, physical therapy, etc.; do not chart that the medication was not on the floor), and the nursing intervention.
- Chart all medication refusals and report them to the appropriate source.

Physician Communication
- Document each time a call is made to a physician even if he or she is not reached. Include the exact time of the call. If the physician is reached, document the details of the message and the physician response.
- Read verbal orders back to the physician and confirm the client's identity as written on the chart. Chart only verbal orders that you have heard from the source, not those told to you by another nurse or unit personnel.

Formal Issues in Charting
- Before writing on the chart, check to be sure you have the correct client record.
- Check to make sure each page has the client's name and the current date stamped in the appropriate area.
- If you forgot to make an entry, chart "late entry" and place the date and time at the entry.
- Correct all charting mistakes according to the policy and procedures of your institution.
- Chart in an organized fashion following the nursing process.
- Write legibly and concisely and avoid subjective statements.
- Write specific and accurate descriptions.
- When charting a symptom or situation, chart the interventions taken and the client response.
- Document your own observations and not those that were told to you by another party.
- Chart frequently to demonstrate ongoing care and chart routine activities.
- Chart client and family teaching and the response.

Source: Tappen RM, et al: Essentials of Nursing Leadership and Management, 2nd ed. Philadelphia, FA Davis, 2001, p 169, with permission.

written and signed by the nurse. Although opinions have a relatively low value in legal proceedings, the documentation should indicate the nursing judgments made. An entry should never be obliterated or destroyed. If a nurse questions a physician's order, a record must be made that the physician was contacted and the order clarified.

Rapport with Clients
Establishing a rapport with the client through honest, open communication goes a long way in avoiding lawsuits. Treating clients and their families with respect and letting them know that the nurse really cares about them may well prevent a lawsuit. Many people are willing to forgive a nurse's error if they have good rapport and a trusting relationship with a nurse who they believe is interested in their well-being.

Current Nursing Skills
Keeping one's nursing knowledge and skills current is vital to preventing errors that may lead to lawsuits. It is better to refuse to perform an unfamiliar procedure than to attempt it without the necessary knowledge and skills. Taking advantage of in-service training, workshops, and continuing nursing education classes is an important part of maintaining the nurse's skill level. Nurses must practice within their level of competence and scope of practice.

Knowledge of the Client

Recognizing the client who is lawsuit prone can help reduce the risk for litigation. Some common characteristics of this type of client include constant dissatisfaction with the care given, constant complaints about all aspects of care, and negative comments about other nurses. This client often complains about the poor care given by nurses on the previous shift and may also have a history of lawsuits against nurses.

Being direct, solving problems with the client, and helping the client become involved in his or her care are helpful in diffusing this negative behavior. Also, even more careful documentation of the care provided and the client's responses to the care can be helpful if a lawsuit is filed later.

What Do You Think?

Think about being involved in a legal or courtroom activity as a defendant, complainant, witness, or juror. What would your role be in each situation?

LIABILITY INSURANCE

Maintenance of proper liability insurance is a necessity. Nurses who do not carry liability insurance place themselves at high risk. The nurse's personal assets, as well as wages, may be subject to a judgment awarded in a malpractice action. Even if the client does not win at the trial, the litigation process, including hiring a lawyer and paying the costs of experts, can be financially devastating.

A professional liability insurance policy is a contract with an insurer who promises to assume the costs paid to the injured party in exchange for payment of a premium (Box 9.7). There are two types of malpractice policies: claims made and occurrence. **Claims-made policies** protect only against claims made during the time the policy is in effect. **Occurrence policies** protect against all claims that occur during the policy period, regardless of when the claim is made. Generally, the

> *The nursing profession is responsible for monitoring and enforcing its own standards through the state licensing board.*

occurrence type of liability insurance offers more protection. Claims-made policy coverage can be broadened by purchasing a tail, a separate policy that extends the time of coverage.

Some hospitals have liability insurance policies for the nurse as a part of the nurse's employment package with the institution. This hospital policy may be limited to claims arising from the nurse's employment and might not apply in a situation in which a nurse renders care outside the institution, for instance, at an automobile crash site. It is preferable to have liability insurance coverage that includes all situations in which the nurse may be involved.

Individual indemnity insurance coverage independent of the facility's policy is recommended for all nurses. With passage of the **Federal Tort Claims Act** and similar state laws, nurses who were formerly protected from lawsuits by working at federal or state health-care facilities can now be sued for malpractice like nurses at any other facility.

REVOCATION OF LICENSE

Self-Enforced Standards

One of the most severe punishments that a nurse can experience is revocation of the license to practice nursing. The nursing profession is responsible for monitoring and enforcing its own standards through the state licensing board. These actions may or may not be related to tort law, contract law, or criminal charges. Each state's licensing board is charged with the responsibility to oversee the professional nurse's competence.

The state's nursing board receives its authority to grant and revoke licenses from specific statutory laws. The underlying rationale for establishment of a licensing board is to protect the public from uneducated, unsafe, or unethical practitioners. If nurses fail to adhere to the standards of safe practice and exhibit unprofessional behavior, they can be disciplined by the state nursing licensing board. One of the remedies that these boards can use is suspension or revocation of a nurse's license.

Box 9.7

What to Look for in an Insurance Policy

The following factors should be reviewed to determine what is the best policy for your type of nursing practice:

1. Type of insurance policy (claims-made or occurrence basis)
2. Insuring agreement. The insurance company's promise to pay in exchange for premiums is called the insuring agreement. The insurance company agrees to pay a money award to a plaintiff who is injured by an act of omission or commission by a health-care provider who is insured by the company.
3. Types of injuries covered. The language must be scrutinized to determine whether it is broad or limiting. Some companies will agree to pay only if the insured nurse is sued for damages, which means the nurse must be sued for a money amount or award. If the nurse is sued for a specific performance lawsuit or an injunctive relief action, which means that the nurse will either have to perform something or discontinue doing something, that particular insurance policy may not be adequate. Also, most insurance policies do not cover the nurse for disciplinary actions.
4. Exclusions. Items that are not covered by a policy are called exclusions. It is important to review the exclusions. Some of the more common exclusions include sexual abuse of a client, injury caused while under the influence of drugs or alcohol, criminal activity, and punitive damages. Punitive damages are used to punish the defendant for egregious acts or omissions.

Who Is Covered Under the Policy

The purchaser is the named insured and can be an individual, institution, or group. Others who may be covered by the policy are nurses, employees, agents, and volunteers, among others.

Limitations and Deductions

In exchange for payment of the premium, the insurance company agrees to pay up to a certain amount on behalf of the insured. This amount is called the limit of liability. It is usually expressed in two ways: the amount that can be paid per incident (per occurrence) and the amount that will be paid for the entire policy year. For example, if you have a policy that states $1,000,000/$3,000,000, it means that the company will pay up to $1 million per incident and a total of $3 million per policy year. The insurance industry relies on the A. M. Best Company to evaluate both the financial size and relative strengths of insurance companies. An A. M. Best rating of A or better should be a prerequisite for purchase of any policy.

The Right to Select Counsel

Some insurance companies allow nurses to select their own attorneys to represent them in a medical negligence claim. Others retain attorneys or law firms, and the nurse does not have the opportunity to make that selection.

The Right to Consent to Settlement

Some policies allow the nurse to decide whether a case should be settled or go to trial, whereas others do not.

The Disciplinary Hearing

A disciplinary hearing is held to review the charges of the nurse's unprofessional conduct. This hearing is less formal than the trial process, and the nurse is allowed to present evidence and be represented by legal counsel at the hearing. Due process requires that the nurse be notified in advance of the specific charges being made. The question of what constitutes unprofessional conduct is an issue frequently dealt with at the disciplinary hearing. Each respective state's nurse practice act provides guidance with regard to the specifics of unprofessional conduct.

Unprofessional conduct can be reported by a nursing peer, a supervisor, a client, or a client's family. Many cases are dismissed before the hearing takes place if the board finds there is no support for the allegation being made against the nurse. If a hearing is necessary, it is in the best interest of the nurse to seek legal counsel because of the potential risk of license revocation.

License revocation is a serious consequence for the nurse because it removes the nurse's right to practice. Drug abuse, administering medication without a prescription, practicing without a valid license, and any singular act of unprofessional or unethical conduct can constitute grounds for losing a nursing license.

Conclusion

The legal system and its effects on the practice of nursing are ever-present realities in today's health-care system. Nurses need to be aware of the implications of their actions but should not be so overwhelmed by fear that it reduces their ability to care for the client. The more advanced and specialized the nurse's practice becomes, the higher the standards to which the nurse is held. Nurses will be challenged throughout their careers to apply legal principles in the daily practice of nursing. An awareness of what constitutes malpractice and negligence will aid in the prevention of litigation.

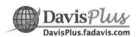

DavisPlus.fadavis.com

Critical Thinking Exercises

Consider the following case: *Thomas v. Corso* (MD 1982): The client was brought to the hospital emergency department (ED) after being involved in an automobile accident. The ED nurse assessed and recorded the client's vital signs and a complaint of numbness in his right anterior thigh. The client was able to move the right leg, and there was no discoloration or deformity. After he was given meperidine (Demerol) for his pain, his blood pressure (BP) dropped to 90/60 mm Hg, and the nurse notified the ED physician of the change. The physician ordered the nurse to arrange for admission to the hospital, which she did.

The client was transferred to a medical-surgical unit, but he could not be placed in a room because of an influenza epidemic. He was placed in the hall next to the nurses' station for close observation. A nurse checked the client's vital signs about 20 minutes after the transfer and noted that the BP was now 70/50, respiratory rate 40, and pulse 120. His skin was cool and diaphoretic, his breathing was deep and rapid, and he was asking for a drink of water. The client also complained of pain in his leg, but the nurse did not give him more pain medication because of his blood pressure.

The nurse assessed him about 30 minutes later and found his skin warmer, although he still complained of pain and thirst. The nurse also noted a strong odor of alcohol on the client's breath. An assistant supervisor also assessed the client's condition but refused to give him any water because he had obviously been drinking alcohol. She had been told about the low blood pressure by the client's nurse but attributed it to the alcohol and pain medication combination. The nurse checked his vital signs again and found a BP of 100/89. Thirty minutes later, it was 94/70, pulse 100, and respirations 28. When the nurse next assessed the client an hour later, he had a Cheyne-Stokes respiratory pattern, no pulse, and no blood pressure. She started cardiopulmonary resuscitation (CPR) and called a "code blue," but after a lengthy attempt at resuscitation, the client died.

An autopsy was performed and showed that the client had a lacerated liver and a severe fracture of the femur with bleeding into the tissues. The coroner determined that traumatic shock, secondary to the fractured femur and lacerated liver, was the cause of death. His family sued the nurses for poor judgment and the hospital for malpractice and won.

- What mistakes were made by the nurses in this case?
- What legal liability did the nurses incur by their actions?
- How can the nurses best prepare for trial in this case?
- What actions could the nurses have taken with this client to prevent a lawsuit?
- What are your feelings toward inebriated clients? Did the nurses' attitudes about inebriation affect their judgments?
- Why are clients who are drunk at higher risk for injury and poor medical outcomes than other clients?

10

How to Take and Pass Tests

Joseph T. Catalano

Learning Objectives

After completing this chapter, the reader will be able to:

- Discuss the importance of a positive attitude when taking examinations.
- Recognize the importance of careful reading of questions and answers.
- Use critical thinking in identifying the key information sought in the question stem.
- Apply key test-taking strategies to help improve examination grades when the student's knowledge may be lacking.

TEST-TAKING STRATEGIES

Knowledge First

The multiple-choice question test format is one of the most commonly used. Of course, the best way to get a good grade on any exam is to know the material. There is no substitute for knowledge. However, some individuals seem always to do well on multiple-choice question tests, whereas others seem to have problems with that test format. The individuals who always do well are not necessarily more intelligent than you; rather, they may have intuitively mastered some of the strategies or "tricks" necessary to do well on multiple-choice tests. Fortunately, once you become aware of these strategies and master them, you also will be able to improve your scores on this type of examination format.

Knowing the material is the most important determinant of your grade on an exam. However, knowing how to take a multiple-choice examination and optimizing the selection of the correct answers are skills that will help you score higher than you might otherwise have.

Strategy in Action

When mastery of test-taking skills is combined with knowledge of the key material, the probability of passing any exam, including the National Council Licensure Examination (NCLEX), increases greatly. The following section lists and describes these important test-taking strategies that can be used when taking classroom exams, the NCLEX, or certification exams. Strategies 1 to 11 work best when you know the material pretty well and you are fairly confident about the correct answer. Strategies 12 to 34 can be used when you are unsure of the material or do not have a clue about what the question is asking.

A number of sample questions throughout the chapter demonstrate how the particular test-taking strategy might help you answer the question. Try to answer the question the best you can before checking the answer at the end of the chapter.

STRATEGY 1. Think positively and reduce test anxiety. The night and morning before the exam, sit back, relax, and say the following to yourself: "I am intelligent and I will pass." "I'll show the instructor that I can do it." "I can do well on this exam." Avoid negative people; don't even talk to them! Before you read a test question, close your eyes, take three deep breaths, and say to yourself, "I'm going to nail this one!"

STRATEGY 2. Read the case study or client situation and the question stem carefully. Studies have shown that 10 percent of incorrect answers result from students' misreading the question.

Cover up the answers. Read only the case study or client situation and the question. Looking at the answers right away pulls your attention away from the question. As you read the question, try to determine what specific knowledge the question is aimed at.

Clarify the Question. Look for and make a mental note of any key words, qualifiers, or statements that may help select the correct answer or eliminate the incorrect ones. Ask yourself, "What is this question really asking?" Rephrase it in your own words. It will usually be about a nursing action in response to a disease process, client problem, symptom, or medication. Look at the details. Is it asking for a nursing action? A client response? A family response? Every word counts. If the question provides information about client age, gender, or marital status, it is probably important in selecting the correct answer, especially on the NCLEX.

Restate the Question. Ask yourself, "What information do I need to have to answer this question? Is there information in the client situation I can use to answer the question? What type of information is the question stem asking me for?" Restate the question in your own words to see if you really understand it. You will find that, in some questions, knowledge of the disease process is not critical to the answer.

Formulate Your Own Answers. Create a mental pool of answers before you look at the answers given to

> *The best way to get a good grade on any exam is to know the material. There is no substitute for knowledge.*

the question. Then see whether any of your answers are similar to those that are provided. The given answer that is closest to the answer you thought up is probably correct.

One Question at a Time. On the NCLEX in particular, treat each question individually. In answering, use only the information that is provided for that particular question. Even though client situations somewhere else in the examination may be similar to the one you are currently working on, avoid returning mentally to these previous items for help.

Do Not Read Into the Question. You should also be careful about reading into a question information that is not actually provided. Avoid making clients in the questions sicker than they already are. Avoid recalling exceptions or unusual clients that you may have encountered in your clinical rotations when trying to answer questions.

Remember that there are no staffing shortages or lack of equipment in the NCLEX hospital. If the question mentions a piece of equipment, you can use it in the answer. By and large, questions on the NCLEX ask for "textbook" levels of knowledge of the material. Instructors will often give you study guides that outline the type of material they will include on their tests.

Let's practice restating the question and figuring out what knowledge is required:

1. A client is admitted with sudden acute respiratory syndrome (SARS). Which statement made by the client indicates that additional teaching is required?
2. A postpartum client is being sent home with a prescription for methylergonovine (Methergine) 0.4 mg. What should the nurse include in the discharge teaching plan?

STRATEGY 3. Uncover the answers one by one and ask yourself, "Does it answer the question?" Eliminate the incorrect answers and then leave them alone. Read *all* the answers carefully. Priority-type questions may have more than one correct answer. Many mistakes are made on this type of examination because the person taking the test did not read all parts of the question carefully. Look for the most specific answer to the question.

Restate this question, figure out what knowledge is needed, and then make a mental pool of answers before looking at the answers given:

3. Identify the nursing action that is most effective in preventing autonomic dysreflexia in a client with a spinal cord injury.
   a. Give the client a prn dose of oxazepam (Serax) before PT (possible)
   b. Keep the client in the sitting position as much as possible (no)
   c. Encourage a fluid intake of at least 1000 mL per day (no)
   d. Maintain the patency of the urinary catheter (possible)

4. A 22-year-old woman is brought into the emergency department (ED) for a fractured radius by her boyfriend, who says she fell off the sofa when napping. The nurse finds new injuries on top of old injuries on exam. How should the nurse chart these findings?
   a. Three new and four old ecchymotic areas located on right and left arms (possible)
   b. Many injuries on arms from physical abuse (no)
   c. Ecchymotic areas on both arms from unknown reasons (possible)
   d. Several injuries on arms from what looks like a baseball bat (no)

Avoid making clients in the questions sicker than they already are. Avoid recalling exceptions or unusual clients that you may have encountered in your clinical rotations when trying to answer questions.

STRATEGY 4. Make sure you are actually "seeing" the words in the question and the answers. Picture what the words are saying about the question and examine the root words, suffixes, and prefixes. A large percentage of mistakes are made because test takers misread the question.

5. A client who was in an automobile crash has been in skeletal traction for 10 days. Identify the complication the nurse will anticipate for this client.
   a. Orthostatic hypotension
   b. Diarrhea
   c. Muscular hypertrophy
   d. Decreased level of consciousness

STRATEGY 5. Take the time to do the test well the first time. After you select an answer, go back and reread the question to make sure the question and answer match. On your class tests, do *not* go back at the end and reread all the questions and answers. Mark the ones you are unsure of as you go through the first time and then go back and look only at those. You cannot do this on the NCLEX because once an answer is selected, the question cannot be accessed again.

6. Select the nursing action that is most helpful in relieving the pain from an episiotomy in a 1-day postpartum client.
   a. Increase fluid intake to 2000 to 3000 mL per day.
   b. Encourage the client to breastfeed the infant every 3 hours or on demand.
   c. Apply cold compresses to the perineum every 2 hours.
   d. Administer methylergonovine (Methergine) as prescribed prn.

STRATEGY 6. Don't spend a lot of time on questions you don't know. Manage your time wisely, but don't rush—use all the available time. Generally allow 1 minute per question. If you are spending more than 2 minutes on any question, put an answer down and move on to the next question if you are taking the NCLEX or, on classroom tests, put a mark by the question and come back to it later.

Although the NCLEX examination, strictly speaking, is not timed, the graduate is never sure how many questions will need to be answered. If you plan on taking all 265 questions in 6 hours, you will need approximately 80 seconds per question. Actually, most individuals who take this type of test average approximately 45 seconds per question; thus, it is likely that you will be finished well before the time limit is reached. Take a watch along to the examination. Theoretically, you could sit in front of the computer screen for 6 hours with the same question. There is a mandatory 10-minute break at 2½ hours and another optional break at 4 hours. Of course, breaks can be taken any time during the exam, but that time is lost from the total allowed time.

STRATEGY 7. Don't change your answers! Trust your intuition. When a question and the answers are read for the first time, an intuitive connection is made between the right and left hemispheres of the brain. The end result is that the first answer selected is usually the best choice. Educational psychologists have shown that test takers change the wrong answer to the correct answer only about 1 percent of the time. Most of the time they change the correct answer to the wrong answer or one wrong answer to another wrong answer.

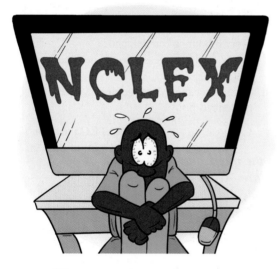

When you read a question too many times, you may start to read into it elements that are really not there. On the NCLEX, once an answer is selected, it cannot be changed, but on class tests, change answers only when you are 100 percent sure that the answer you are changing to is correct. If there is any doubt at all, don't change your answer.

STRATEGY 8. Pay attention to where the client is in the disease–recovery process. One-day postoperative clients have different needs than 4-day postop clients. The assessments of clients who have been on antibiotics for a week will be different from those of clients who were just started on antibiotics. A client newly diagnosed with diabetes will require different care than a 10-year diabetic client.

7. Identify the assessment of a client who had a neuroblastoma removed 3 hours ago that would require immediate intervention by the nurse.
   a. Diminished appetite
   b. Pinkish-tinged urine
   c. Temperature of 99.8¼°F
   d. Dressing saturated with bright red blood

STRATEGY 9. Look for priority or qualifying words in the question stem. Some important words can help determine what type of information is being elicited in the answer. Some of these words are:

First   Better
Best   Fastest
Most   Highest priority
Initial

When words like these appear in the question stem, it is an indication that more than one of the choices are correct and perhaps that all four of them are correct. The task then becomes selecting the one answer that should be first or the answer that ought to receive the highest priority. Remember Maslow's hierarchy of needs (physiological and safety needs have highest priority), the ABCs (airway, breathing, circulation) of cardiopulmonary resuscitation (CPR), and the nursing process. The first step in the nursing process is always assessment, so if you have a question asking what the nurse should do first, look for the answer with an assessment in it. Remember to always assess the client before the equipment.

8. A client is admitted with the symptoms of anthrax infection, including fever of 102°F, severe dyspnea, tachypnea, and chest pain. Which nursing diagnosis has highest priority?
   a. Anxiety related to fear of death
   b. Pain related to pressure on the sternum
   c. Hyperthermia related to bacterial infection
   d. Ineffective airway clearance related to retained respiratory secretions

9. A 62-year-old client who has a history of coronary artery disease is brought into the emergency department (ED) complaining of chest pain. What action should the nurse take first?
   a. Give the client nitroglycerin grain 1/150 sublingual now.
   b. Call the client's cardiologist about his admission.
   c. Check his blood pressure and note the location and degree of chest pain.
   d. Place the client in an elevated Fowler's position after loosening his shirt collar.

10. A client diagnosed with sickle cell disease is admitted in acute crisis. Which action by the nurse has highest priority?
    a. Open the airway and begin high-flow oxygen therapy.
    b. Administer prescribed narcotic pain medications.
    c. Establish a strong therapeutic relationship.
    d. Begin prescribed rehydration with intravenous (IV) fluids.

STRATEGY 10. For delegation questions, match the activity with the person.

Know the person's skill level and education.
Know the job description.
Evaluate the client's status (acute = not appropriate vs. chronic = OK to assign; unstable = not appropriate vs. stable = OK to assign).

LPNs can do most skills, but for the NCLEX:

- **Cannot** perform admission assessments
- **Cannot** give IV push medications
- **Cannot** write nursing diagnoses
- **Cannot** do most teaching
- **Cannot** do complex skills
- **Cannot** take care of clients with acute conditions
- **Cannot** take care of unstable clients

For unlicensed assistive personnel (UAPs), certified nursing assistants (CNAs), and aides on the NCLEX:

- Look for the lowest level of skill required for the task.
- Look for the most uncomplicated task.
- Look for the most stable client.
- Look for the client with the chronic illness.

In the real world of health care, these individuals often perform functions beyond their legal scope of practice, but for the NCLEX, these are the general limitations.

11. Identify the task that the registered nurse (RN) may delegate to a (license practical nurse (LPN) if all of the clients are stable
    a. Adding potassium (KCl) to a bag of D_5W that is already hanging
    b. Developing a nursing diagnosis for a newly admitted client with diarrhea
    c. Teaching a newly diagnosed diabetic client how to self-administer insulin
    d. Turning a comatose client with a head injury from side to side every 2 hours

12. Which client would be most appropriate for the charge RN to assign to an LPN?
    a. A ventilator-dependent client with chronic obstructive pulmonary disease (COPD)
    b. A client with dementia who is clutching her chest
    c. A client with a history of head trauma transferred from the intensive care unit (ICU) 1 hr ago
    d. A newly admitted client who is vomiting bright red blood

13. The medical unit is staffed today with three RNs and one LPN. To which client would it be appropriate to assign the LPN?
    a. A man with tuberculosis (TB) who is being discharged today
    b. A woman who fell and is now in skeletal traction
    c. A woman who is scheduled for an esophagogastroduodenoscopy (EGD)
    d. A man newly diagnosed with gout

14. Select the task that is most appropriate for the RN to delegate to a CNA.
    a. Suction a client with a new tracheostomy.
    b. Change a sterile dressing on a 60-year-old man with fresh skin grafts.
    c. Complete the initial postoperative assessment on a client just returned from the recovery room.
    d. Obtain the temperature of a 29-year-old woman who is receiving the final 30 minutes of a whole blood transfusion.

STRATEGY 11. Once you realize something is seriously wrong with the client, do NOT delay care! Serious conditions require immediate treatment. Delaying action only allows the client to die slowly rather than quickly.

15. While the labor and delivery nurse is administering IV oxytocin (Pitocin) to augment labor, he or she notices that the fetal monitor is showing late decelerations and loss of beat-to-beat variability. What is the initial action the nurse should take?
    a. Reassess the fetal heart tone (FHT) in 15 minutes.
    b. Call the physician immediately.
    c. Increase the rate of the primary IV.
    d. Turn off the medication.

What if you are unfamiliar with the material and really don't know the answer? Don't panic! Use the rest of these strategies to help you figure out the answer or at least increase your odds of answering it correctly.

STRATEGY 12. An educated guess is better than no answer at all. There is no penalty for guessing on the NCLEX, and you have to put an answer down to move on to the next question. On both the NCLEX and classroom tests, if you are unable to make any decision at all about the correct answer, you should just select one and move on. There is at least a one-in-four chance of choosing the correct answer. However, studies have shown that answer 3 (c) has the highest probability (30%), answer 2 (b) the next highest, answer 4 (d) the third highest, and answer 1 (a) the lowest probability of being the correct answer. Wild guessing for large numbers of questions, of course, will have a negative effect on the total score.

STRATEGY 13. If you know the other three answers are wrong, the one that is left is correct. Use the process of elimination to select the correct answer. Usually, one or more of the answers can easily be identified as being incorrect. By eliminating these from the possible choices, you will be better able to focus attention on the answers that have been identified as having some chance of being correct. Go back and read the stem question again to try to determine exactly what type of information is being asked. If you are still unable to decide which of the remaining two answers is correct, select one and move on. Using this method increases the probability of choosing the correct answer to 50–50.

66 *What if you are unfamiliar with the material and really don't know the answer? Don't panic! Use the rest of these strategies to help you figure out the answer or at least increase your odds of answering it correctly.* 99

16. What action by the nurse has the highest priority for a client who is developing Stevens-Johnson syndrome?
    a. Place tight tourniquets in the antecubital spaces of both arms.
    b. Give all medications through the client's arterial line.
    c. Hold the client's next dose of Bactrim and notify the physician.
    d. Inform the family that the client will die within 24 hours.

STRATEGY 14. If part of the answer is incorrect, the whole answer is incorrect. One incorrect part of a multipart answer makes the whole answer incorrect.

17. Identify the side effects a nurse should evaluate for a client who is receiving oral prednisone (Deltasone).
    a. Edema, hypotension, mood swings
    b. Dehydration, hyperglycemia, hirsutism
    c. Unstable moods, moon face, hypoglycemia
    d. Euphoria, hyperglycemia, hypertension

STRATEGY 15. Look for the answer that has the broader focus. Another method that may be used when the choices have been narrowed down to two is to examine the answers and try to determine whether one answer may include the other. The answer that is broader, is more inclusive, or includes the other answer is usually the correct one. The most nearly complete answer leaves the least room for error.

18. Select the finding by the nurse that best identifies when a 10-year-old child with acting-out behavior requires help.
    a. Child has frequent fights with peers.
    b. Multiple aspects of the child's life are affected.
    c. Grades start to decline.
    d. Relationships with siblings and parents are stressful.

19. Identify the best instructions for the RN to give to the CNA for ambulating a client who has been on bedrest for 3 days.
    a. Put nonskid shoes on the client before ambulating.
    b. Ambulate the client 50 feet and notify me if there are any problems.
    c. Ambulate the client only as far as she can go without becoming tired.
    d. Ambulate the client to the nurses' station and back and return her to bed if she becomes tired.

STRATEGY 16. Watch for similarities in the content of the options. When answers are grouped by similar concepts, activities, or situations, select the one that is different. If three of the four choices have some common element that makes them similar, and the fourth answer lacks this element, the different answer is probably correct.

20. How can the nurse best help a 7-year-old boy diagnosed with acute lymphoblastic leukemia cope with the fear of dying?
    a. Instruct the parents to avoid bringing up the subject of death.
    b. Redirect the child's questions to safe topics when he mentions death.
    c. Answer the child's questions at the level of his understanding.
    d. Emphasize that nurses are not allowed to make prognosis about death.
21. A woman has been treated for severe chronic emphysema for several years using bronchodilators and relatively high doses of prednisone (Deltasone). Select the activity that would pose the least risk for this client in relation to the side effects of prednisone therapy.
    a. Shopping at the mall on Saturday afternoon
    b. Spring-cleaning her two-story house
    c. Attending Sunday morning church services
    d. Serving refreshments at her 6-year-old son's school play party

STRATEGY 17. Look for negatives in the question stem. Although there are very few negative questions on the NCLEX, negative words or prefixes in the question stem change how the correct answer is selected. Some common negatives include:

Least	Except
Unlikely	Inconsistent
Inappropriate	Untoward
Unrealistic	All but
Lowest priority	Atypical
Contraindicated	Incorrect
False	Not

In general, when a negative question is asked, it indicates that three of the choices are correct and one is incorrect. The incorrect choice is the answer. When a negative question appears, the test taker needs to ask: "What is it they don't want me to do in this situation?" or "What is the wrong statement?" On the NCLEX, negative questions are often disguised so that you have to read them carefully to figure out what they are asking. Questions such as "What indicates the need for more teaching?" are really telling you that one of these statements the client made is incorrect—which is it? The negative word is often at the end of the question like a hook on a fishing line. If you don't read the whole question, you'll miss it!

22. Identify the client statement about taking aspirin at home for arthritis that requires further discharge instructions.
    a. "I need to take it with food or milk."
    b. "A small amount of blood in my urine is normal."
    c. "I should call the clinic if I develop large black-and-blue areas on my body."
    d. "Ringing in my ears may mean that I am taking too much medication."
23. Identify a side effect of a benzodiazepine-class medication that would be considered atypical.
    a. Syncope
    b. Depression
    c. Tremor
    d. Excitement

STRATEGY 18. Do not panic if a totally unfamiliar question is encountered. Some standardized diagnostic examinations and the NCLEX are designed so that no one gets a 100 percent. As a result, there are questions that are very complex, dealing with disease processes, medications, and laboratory tests that may be unfamiliar to the test taker. Questions like this may be encountered no matter how much review or study has been done. Often the "A+" students have the most difficulty with this type of test because they are not used to seeing questions they don't have a clue about answering.

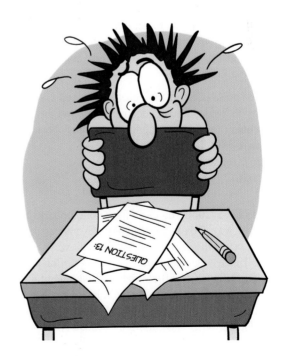

Remember, nobody knows everything! When you encounter these types of questions, it is important not to panic. Take a few deep breaths and think to yourself, "I can answer this question!" It is just one question out of many. Use some of the strategies already discussed in this chapter to select the best answer. Remember that nursing care is very similar in many situations even though the disease processes may be quite different. Select the answer that seems logical and involves good general nursing care. Common sense can go a long way in dealing with these types of questions.

24. What is the best action for the nurse to take when she or he discovers that a 9-year-old girl has a positive Rovsing's sign?
    a. Have the child rest quietly and assess the vital signs.
    b. Call a code blue and begin CPR.
    c. Inform the child's parents that she only has 3 months to live.
    d. Confront the child about which adult member of the family had been sexually molesting her recently.

> *In general, when a negative question is asked, it indicates that three of the choices are correct and one is incorrect. The incorrect choice is the answer.*

STRATEGY 19. Remember, if you have never heard of it, probably no one else ever has either! Don't select answers that are totally unfamiliar. Stick with the things you know.

25. The nurse is caring for a client diagnosed with Smith-Strang disease. Identify the lab test the nurse would consider most significant for this client.
    a. α-5 ST 1
    b. CA 155 antigen
    c. ICD
    d. UA

STRATEGY 20. If you can't figure out the answer any other way, look at the length of the answers. This is not a very reliable method, but it might work sometimes. The average-length answer is most often correct. The NCLEX is difficult because the material itself is difficult, but the examination is not designed to be tricky or difficult for the sake of confusing the test taker. On the other hand, the test question writers are not going to make the correct answer obvious. There-

fore, if one answer is much longer or shorter than the other three, it is probably not the correct choice.

Be wary of answers that sound as if they are trying to rationalize the correct choice by using a lot of explanation, particularly when the other answers do not have lengthy explanations. Such answers are probably incorrect. You should also avoid answers that are different from the other three because of measurements or the way in which they are presented.

26. How can the nurse best administer tetracycline oral liquid suspension to an 8-year-old child?
    a. Quickly
    b. Through a drinking straw
    c. With milk or antacid to prevent stomach irritation and vomiting
    d. Hidden in the child's food so that the bitter taste will be disguised and the child will complete the full course of treatment

STRATEGY 21. If there is a lengthy client situation or case study, read the stem question before reading the case study. Reading the question first will help you focus on the information you will need to obtain from the case study. This is a way to save a little time. On the NCLEX, the amount of space for the client situation is limited to half the computer screen, so this will not be a problem.

STRATEGY 22. Avoid automatically passing the decision or intervention to the physician. Class tests, as well as the NCLEX, are for nurses and deal with conditions and problems that nurses should be able to resolve independently. Often a nursing action can and should be taken before notifying the physician. However, it is an important element of nursing knowledge and judgment to know when notifying the physician is appropriate, but do so only when there is nothing else the nurse can do to help the client.

27. A postlobectomy client pulls out his chest tube while going to the rest room. What is the appropriate initial nursing action?
    a. Call the physician immediately.
    b. Position the client on the operative side.
    c. Insert a new sterile chest tube and reconnect it to underwater seal drainage.

d. Cover the insertion site with an occlusive dressing.

STRATEGY 23. Avoid answers that focus on medical knowledge or are a medical action. It is unlikely that questions on class tests or the NCLEX would require a medical action as an answer. The NCLEX in particular focuses on information to measure competency as a nurse. Remember that nurses cannot legally initiate medical actions independently. There are two exceptions to this rule. One exception is when standing protocols exist, but unless the question tells you there are standing orders or protocols, do NOT assume they exist. The second exception is when a treatment or medication is causing immediate harm to the client. These should be stopped immediately and the physician notified.

28. Which nursing action has the highest priority when the nurse notes late fetal heart rate decelerations in a pregnant client who is in labor?
    a. Insert a urinary catheter to relieve pressure on the fetus.
    b. Begin oxygen by non-rebreather mask at 10 L/min to decrease fetal hypoxia.
    c. Initiate a magnesium sulfate IV drip at 1 g/hour.
    d. Position the client on her left side.

STRATEGY 24. Avoid selecting answers that have absolutes in them. Answers that contain absolutes are almost always incorrect choices. Some absolute words to be aware of include:

Always	All
Every	Never
Only	None

Humans are very complex biochemical entities. Every person is different and almost every rule will have an exception.

29. Which factor should the nurse include in the teaching plan of a client with a home prescription for reserpine (Serpalan)?
    a. Walk 2 miles every day.
    b. Never eat any candy or ice cream.

c. The physician is the only one who can cut your toenails to prevent bleeding.
d. Try to take the medication at the same time each day.

STRATEGY 25. Avoid answers that make the client seem inferior, immoral, unworthy, or ignorant. Nurses are obligated by the code of ethics to treat all clients equally, regardless of race, gender, lifestyle preferences, disease process, or economic status. Be careful of cultural differences and biases that can color the way the nurse interacts with a client. Also be particularly cautious in situations that are emotionally charged, such as child abuse, drug or alcohol addiction, spousal abuse, teen pregnancy, HIV, sexually transmitted disease (STD), or homosexuality.

30. Identify the most therapeutic statement by the nurse to a 14-year-old girl who admits she is sexually active and has just been informed that she has gonorrhea and is 3 months pregnant.
    a. "You obviously lack the intelligence to understand how to use the birth control pills and condoms you were given at the clinic at your last visit."
    b. "Tell me how you think your pregnancy will affect your life."
    c. "I hope you now understand the consequences of your lack of moral standards."
    d. "Tell me how you feel when your classmates call you a slut behind your back."

STRATEGY 26. Look for answers that have words identical or similar to those in the question stem. If there is no other way to determine the correct answer, similarities to the stem may act as a clue to the correct answer, but this will require careful reading of both the stem and answers. With therapeutic communication questions, look for the answer that reflects or restates the emotions the client is expressing and ask open ended questions.

31. Which assessments indicate to the nurse that a client was developing steal syndrome after the insertion of an arteriovenous (AV) graft in the left forearm?
    a. Hypotension and irregular pulse

> *The NCLEX is difficult because the material itself is difficult, but the examination is not designed to be tricky or difficult for the sake of confusing the test taker.*

b. Weak radial pulses and mottled fingers of the left hand

c. Elevated temperature and purulent urinary drainage

d. Bruit and thrill over the surgical site

32. Select the most therapeutic response when a client says to the nurse, "That stupid doctor of mine makes me so mad I could spit nails! I want to leave this dump now!"
   a. "You seem very angry. Tell me why you want to leave."
   b. "If you sign the AMA sheet, you can go home now."
   c. "It is your right to change to a new physician if you are not satisfied with your care."
   d. "If there is no one to care for you at home, legally the hospital cannot release you."

STRATEGY 27. Watch for grammatical clues that may be a tip-off to the correct answer. All the options should be grammatically consistent with the question stem; however, question writers tend to pay more attention to this detail with the correct answer. Answers that grammatically do not match the stem or disagree in number (singular/plural) are usually incorrect. When the stem is an incomplete statement, the options should complete the sentence in a grammatically correct manner.

33. Identify the assessments that would lead the nurse to suspect that a newly admitted client was developing Kugelberg-Welander disease.
   a. Compression fracture of L4
   b. Blood-tinged urine
   c. Muscle atrophy and twitching of the extremities
   d. Grade 3 pansystolic murmur over the point of maximal impulse (PMI)

34. An important therapeutic measure for the nurse to take when treating a client with a *Dracunculus medinensis* is to:
   a. Maintain a steady traction by winding around a small object like a pencil
   b. Keeping the client on strict bedrest throughout the treatment period
   c. Soaking the affected area in warm bath water several times a day
   d. Active and passive range of motion every 4 hours

STRATEGY 28. Look for qualifiers in the answers. The answer that includes a qualifying word when the others do not is often the correct answer. Qualifying words include:

Generally	Might
Tends to	About
Usually	Approximately
Often	Most
May	Many

35. What is the most accurate information for the nurse to provide to the parents of an infant with gray syndrome?
   a. Gray syndrome is always caused by a genetic defect.
   b. You can take the baby home after 2 weeks' treatment with antibiotics.
   c. The baby will require open-heart surgery to live past age 3.
   d. Approximately 40% of newborns with gray syndrome die by the 5th day of life.

STRATEGY 29. When two of the answers are opposites, one of them is usually correct. Look for answers that, when considered, cover all the possibilities of action. One of the answers must be correct, and you will have improved your odds to 50–50.

36. What should the nurse conclude when she or he finds a positive scarf sign while assessing a newborn infant?
   a. The infant was born after 30 weeks' gestation.
   b. The mother of the infant used cocaine during her pregnancy.
   c. There is a genetic predisposition for sickle cell disease.
   d. The infant was born before 30 weeks' gestation.

STRATEGY 30. When the question asks about numerical values or dates, the answer in the middle range is more often correct. Numerical ranges can be from large to small or small to large. Dates can range from present to past or past to present. Extremes in numerical values or dates are usually incorrect.

37. Identify the serum medication level that indicates to the nurse that a client with seizure disorder was taking his or her clonazepam (Klonopin) as prescribed.
   a. 142 ng/mL
   b. 112 ng/mL
   c. 72 ng/mL
   d. 12 ng/mL

STRATEGY 31. Avoid looking for a pattern in the selection of answers. Although you may be able to detect a pattern in your teacher-made exams, the questions and answers on the NCLEX are arranged by the computer in a random fashion without any particular pattern.

If something appears to be in a pattern, ignore it. Any pattern is just coincidental. For example, if question 6 had answer 1, question 7 had answer 2, question 8 had answer 3, question 9 had answer 4, question 10 had answer 1, and question 11 had answer 2, you might expect that question 12 would require answer 3. This is probably not the case.

Here is another example of a pattern-type situation that sometimes occurs with answers on this type of test. Questions 22 to 29 all have 3 (c) as their correct answers. The answer to question 30 also seems to be 3, but the tendency may be not to select it because of all the other choice 3 answers on the previous questions. The correct answer may very well be 3, and if that is the best choice, go ahead and select it. It is important that each question be treated individually.

STRATEGY 32. If you don't have a clue about what the question is asking, select the answer that has the most serious or worst client outcome if no action were to be taken by the nurse.

38. Which complications can the nurse anticipate a client diagnosed with antiphospholipid antibody syndrome (AAS) to develop?
    a. Ecchymotic areas on the trunk and back
    b. Osteoporosis and hirsutism
    c. Weakness of the legs
    d. Cerebrovascular accident (CVA) and pulmonary emboli (PE)

STRATEGY 33. Avoid answers that leave the client or family alone. Only on very rare occasions should clients or family be left alone. To have effective therapeutic communication, the nurse must interact with the client and family.

39. Select the best action for the nurse to take when a client in the ICU dies and his distraught family is present.
    a. Allow the family grieving time alone with their deceased loved one.
    b. Contact the client's religious leader by phone.
    c. Provide a quiet space apart from the unit for grieving.
    d. Stay at the bedside to answer questions.

STRATEGY 34. Be positive about the examination. Motivational research has shown that people who have a positive attitude about an examination score higher than people who are negative about it. Believe in yourself. Think positive thoughts all the time. Not only will you do better on tests, but you will also be a happier and friendlier person!

GENERAL STUDY TIPS

Study Using Images. Most people remember pictures better than words. Outline the pictures in your books with magic marker, highlighter, crayon, lipstick, or whatever. Color in the pictures in the book or draw your own pictures. Try to visualize what is being taught. If you can see it in a picture, you understand it and are more likely to remember it.

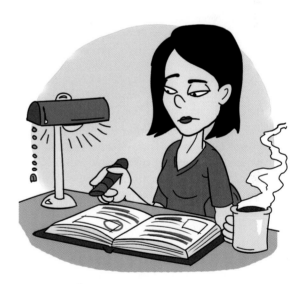

Act out situations (role-play) when you group-study. The more senses involved, the better the learning; connect situations with an emotion—humor, anger, fear. Your best teachers will often tell a funny story to demonstrate a point. They are connecting the learning with an emotion so you can remember it better. You can do this yourself (Box 10.1).

Don't Cram! Don't Cram! Don't Cram! Don't Cram! Don't Cram! If you always do what you've always done, you will always get what you always got! The day before the next class, review the notes from the last class at a rate of 15 minutes per 1 hour

Box 10.1

ABCs for Success in Nursing School

A: Apply yourself to the task at hand. Learn all that you can about everything. This is the profession that you have chosen. To be successful, you must give it all that you've got.

B: Be organized. Set up a three-ring binder or notebook with a calendar and dividers for each subject.

C: Children do NOT belong in the classroom. If you have children, make care arrangements with a backup plan for unexpected illnesses or child care call-ins.

D: Dress for success. Make sure you follow the dress code policy for the clinical rotations. Prepare for your clinical days the night before by washing and ironing your uniform.

E: Exercise regularly. It is a great stress reducer. Start it before you need it.

F: Front of the class is where it's at! Students who sit up front can see better, can hear better, and are less distracted.

G: Group-study. It helps reinforce learning. Follow the rules for group-study.

H: Healthy habits will keep you physically and mentally fit for nursing school. Eat right: stay away from fatty foods, and eat lots of fruits and vegetables. Rest. Nursing school is physically and mentally demanding.

I: Introduce yourself to the course instructors and your advisor early on. They are there to help you.

J: Journal your experiences in nursing school. You will be surprised by how much you have learned from month to month.

K: Keep all your books and notes until you pass the NCLEX. They make good references and you may need them in other classes later on.

L: Look up procedures and skills in designated books before doing the skill with the instructor in lab or clinic.

M: Make your own flash cards from index cards to study while waiting at stop lights or other places.

N: Network with students who have gone before you. The information they give you about courses and instructors will be helpful.

O: Ooze enthusiasm! Look forward to each new learning experience; volunteer for activities; join your student nursing association and encourage other students. Strive to be the kind of nurse you would want caring for your family members.

P: Practice test-taking. The more test questions you practice answering, the less test anxiety you will experience.

Q: Question things you don't understand or think are incorrect. Don't administer a medication if you have any question about it.

R: Research, used correctly, is an important tool. Learn how to look things up before you do them. Help in research projects if asked.

S: Study skills are essential for success. Develop some. Find out what works for you. Repetition is the best teacher: listen, read, write, and talk about it.

T: Teach others what you have learned. You will really have to know and understand a topic to teach it and you will remember it forever.

U: Unwind after a day in class or clinical. Find things to do that will take your mind off school and clinicals for a while. Meditate, listen to music, exercise, take a hot bath, dance, take up a hobby, play a computer game, and so on.

V: Vent your emotions. Have a designated sounding board (friend, spouse, parent) who is willing to listen to you without criticizing or trying to solve the problem. Keeping emotions inside can lead to high blood pressure and ulcers.

W: Watch out for information on the Internet when doing papers. Not all of the information is of high quality.

X: Excuses don't cut it in nursing school. Your instructors have heard them all before. It is better to just say "I don't know" than to try to bluff your way through.

Y: You can if you think you can! Think positively all the time. What you truly believe, you can achieve.

Z: Zap negative thoughts! Think positively all the time. Stay away from negative people; they will bring you down and add to your stress level. Seek out positive people who want you to be successful in school and your career.

of class; it increases memory by 30 to 50 percent. Ask questions during class; it reinforces memory.

Play "stump the professor." Try to find a question in the book you are pretty sure the teacher doesn't know the answer to. You'll remember it forever.

Set Group Study Rules. These few simple rules will make the study session much more effective:

1. Be selective of the members—four to six maximum; including too many people makes the group hard to control and limits each member's participation. The more you participate, the more you will learn! Study with people you like and with whom you feel comfortable. Don't ask the class clown or gossip to participate in the group. Avoid negative classmates like the plague.
2. Prepare before the group meets: assign topics or content to prevent the "what are we going to study tonight" syndrome. The goal of group study is for the members of the group to help each other learn. If someone doesn't know anything, that person is not going to be much use to the other members of the group.
3. Limit the length of the sessions. Most people can usually concentrate for only 60 to 90 minutes maximum. Sessions that go longer start to get off track, and people will start to become negative.
4. Use role-playing to reinforce information. It adds a visual and emotional (usually humorous) element that reinforces memory.
5. Remain positive. You can never be too positive.
6. Relax; have fun, but don't turn it into a party. It's OK to have some light snacks and drinks, but don't overdo it. You can really party AFTER you pass the test.

Practice Doing Questions Like the Ones the Professor Asks on Exams. After the first test, try to formulate your own questions about the material you study. Get a review book that has a lot of questions in it and practice taking those questions. When you do test reviews in class, try to understand why you missed the questions you missed. Was it due to lack of knowledge? Failure to think critically? Not reading the question carefully? Changing the answer?

Make Notes About Key Concepts When You Read or During Class. Create your own flash cards (e.g., med name on the front, side effects on the back; or disease on the front, symptoms on the back). Summarize what you have read and **think,**

think, think about it. Don't just memorize. Try to become interested in the material. If you find a topic boring, try to relate it to something that interests you.

Over-Learn the Material. Everyone forgets stuff. You can improve the chance of remembering if you continue to review and relearn material. Go back over material you are unsure of or have questions about.

Never Leave a Class if You Do Not Clearly Understand the Content that Was Covered. The teacher is getting paid to explain the material so that you can understand it. If you don't understand it, the teacher is not earning his or her salary. Keep asking questions until the material is explained in a way that is clear to you. Especially ask "why" questions. Some teachers don't like these questions, but your best teachers will ask you "why" questions during the presentation of material. This is important because when you understand "why," you are using critical thinking. Then you won't have to memorize the material because you'll understand it.

If you are still having problems after class, make an appointment with the teacher to see whether the material can be explained more clearly.

Get Rid of Negative Thoughts. If you think any of the following, you are guilty of negative thoughts:

- "I have to get a perfect score."
- "I'm always anxious during a test."
- "I'm a loser because I didn't remember that answer."
- "If he/she asks about_____, I'm dead."
- "I don't know what I'll do if I fail the exam."
- "My family will think I'm stupid if I fail."
- "My classmates will think I'm stupid if I fail."
- "I'll think I'm stupid if I fail."
- "No one ever understands what this teacher is talking about."
- "I just know I won't know the answers during the exam."
- "Everyone knows I can't get an A, so why even try?"
- "I'm not smart enough to be a nurse."
- "The teacher asks such tricky questions that it doesn't matter if I study or not."
- "I'll be happy if I can make a C-minus."
- "The information just flies out of my head when I sit down to take an exam."

Think Positively! Think Positively! Think Positively! Oh, and if you are having a really bad time on a test, THINK POSITIVELY some more!

Conclusion

Mastering test-taking and study skills is like mastering any other skills. It takes some concentration and practice. The test-taking and study skills outlined earlier can be used to prepare for both classroom exams and the NCLEX. Although nothing is as effective for passing an examination as paying attention in class, good note-taking, and thorough studying, mastering these test-taking skills may improve your scores.

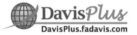

DavisPlus
DavisPlus.fadavis.com

ANSWERS TO THE QUESTIONS IN CHAPTER 10

1. **Restatement of the question:** What type of disease is SARS? Which statement is incorrect (wrong) about SARS? (what are possible answers?)
2. **Restatement of the question**: What is Methergine? Which statement about Methergine is **correct?** (What are possible answers?)
3. What is autonomic dysreflexia? What triggers it? What can the nurse do to prevent autonomic dysreflexia? **Correct answer: d.** Autonomic dys-reflexia is a condition found in clients with spinal cord injuries in which a localized stimulus, like a distended bladder or impaction, causes a systemic response.
4. What information should the nurse include when charting? What is good charting? **Correct answer: a.** Good charting is specific, detailed, and descriptive. It should never include judg-ments, opinions, or suppositions.
5. **Correct answer: a.** If you selected answer *c,* you probably were thinking "atrophy," which is the decrease in size of a muscle when it is not used for a long period of time. The word "hypertrophy" means the enlargement of something, which would not occur in this client.
6. **Correct answer: c.** Although the other answers may be appropriate nursing measures, they do not address the problem of pain relief.
7. **Correct answer: d.** The client is freshly postop-erative, and one of the important assessments the nurse must make is the condition of the dressing. A dressing saturated with blood indicates a prob-lem that needs attention. The other assessments are to be expected in a recent postoperative client.
8. **Correct answer: d.** Airway-related nursing diagnoses have highest priority (ABCs of CPR).
9. **Correct answer: d.** The first step in the nursing process is assessment. Always look for an assessment-type answer when asked what to do first.
10. **Correct answer: d.** Rehydration dilutes the blood cells and prevents the clumping and clot formation that cause permanent damage from sickle cell crisis. Answer *a* may seem correct except for the fact that high-flow oxygen will

make the crisis worse. Also, a closed airway is not a problem in sickle cell.
11. **Correct answer: d.** *a.* IV med: no; *b.* nursing Dx: no; *c.* teaching: no. The client in *d* is stable and chronic, and this is a procedure an LPN is qualified to do.
12. **Correct answer: a.** A ventilator-dependent client with COPD is stable with a chronic disease process. Client *b* is unstable/chronic; client *c* is unstable/chronic; client *d* is unstable/acute.
13. **Correct answer: b.** This client is stable and does not require any teaching at this point. Situations *a, c,* and *d* require teaching.
14. **Correct answer: d.** This client is stable, and the procedure is uncomplicated. *a.* Client is unstable with a complicated procedure; *b.* client is stable, but procedure is complicated; *c.* client is unstable, and procedure is complicated.
15. **Correct answer: d.** Late decelerations and loss of variability indicate fetal distress likely caused by excessively strong contractions from the medica-tion. Stopping it is the only way to save the fetus.
16. **Correct answer: c.** Stevens-Johnson syndrome is a type of erythremic edema that is commonly seen in clients who are taking Bactrim for urinary tract infections. The other three answers are things that the nurse should never do.
17. **Correct answer: d.** Prednisone causes fluid retention, resulting in hypertension and edema; raises the blood sugar, resulting in hyper-glycemia; affects the mood, causing instability; and causes abnormal fat distribution, resulting in moon face and buffalo hump.
18. **Correct answer: b.** It includes all of the other answers.
19. **Correct answer: d.** It includes all the other measures when ambulating a client and therefore offers the most complete instructions.
20. **Correct answer: d.** All the other answers try to avoid talking about death with the child.
21. **Correct answer: b.** All the other answers place the client at risk for infection by exposure to large groups of people in open public areas.
22. **Correct answer: b.** The other three answers would be considered correct for a client taking aspirin. There should never be any blood in the urine.
23. **Correct answer: d.** The negative or "hook" word is atypical. It means unexpected. Benzodi-azepine-class medications are used as antianxiety

agents and sedatives. You wouldn't expect them to cause excitement.

24. **Correct answer: a.** Rovsing's sign is an indication of appendicitis. The child should rest quietly until she can go to surgery.

25. **Correct answer: d.** Smith-Strang disease is a metabolic disease that produces methionine malabsorption syndrome leading to abnormal urine with a very strong smell. Urinalysis (UA) will show these abnormalities. The other tests are made up.

26. **Correct answer: b.** Tetracycline liquid stains the teeth and is best given to children through a straw. Note that answer *a* is very short, and answers *c* and *d* have long rationales.

27. **Correct answer: d.** Covering the site quickly is an acceptable nursing action and will prevent the pneumothorax from becoming larger. The physician can be called later.

28. **Correct answer: d.** Late decelerations are often caused by pressure on the umbilical cord, and changing position is a simple and effective way to relieve the pressure that is an independent nursing action. The other three measures are medical and would require an order.

29. **Correct answer: d.** The other three choices all have absolute words in them.

30. **Correct answer: b.** Good therapeutic communication answers reflect or explore the client's feelings. The other three answers all make judgments about the girl's moral character or intelligence.

31. **Correct answer: b.** Steal syndrome occurs when too much of the arterial blood is shunted away from the hand. Note that answer *b* is the only one with the word *left* in it, matching the stem question that has the word *left*.

32. **Correct answer: a.** Good therapeutic responses reflect the emotions and content of the client's statements.

33. **Correct answer: c.** Kugelberg-Welander disease is a neuromuscular disorder that affects primarily teenagers, leading to loss of coordination and paralysis starting in the legs. Note that answer *c* is the only plural answer matching grammatically the question that asks for "assessments."

34. **Correct answer: a.** A *Dracunculus medinensis* is a type of parasitic worm that infects the upper part of the leg. It can be removed by maintaining a slow, steady traction force on it over a period of time. Note that answer *a* is the only one of the answers that grammatically completes the open-ended statement of the stem question.

35. **Correct answer: d.** Gray syndrome occurs in infants who were treated with chloramphenicol during the newborn period and is highly lethal. Note that answer *d* is the only one with a qualifying word, *approximately.*

36. **Correct answer: d.** Scarf sign is elicited when the elbow of the infant can be drawn across the chest without resistance. It is a sign of prematurity. Note that answers *a* and *d* cover all the possible options for age.

37. **Correct answer: c.** The therapeutic range for clonazepam is 20 to 80 ng/mL. Throw out the high and low, and the answer that is closest to the middle of the extremes is answer *c.*

38. **Correct answer: d.** AAS is a disease process that causes blood clot formation. CVA and PE are caused by blood clots and are the most serious of the conditions listed in the answers.

39. **Correct answer: d.** Staying at the bedside and answering questions is the best way to use therapeutic communications. All the other answers take the nurse away from the family.

11

NCLEX: What You Need to Know

Joseph T. Catalano

Joseph T. Catalano

Learning Objectives

After completing this chapter, the reader will be able to:

- Describe the NCLEX-RN, CAT test plan.
- Discuss the NCLEX-RN, CAT test format.
- Analyze and identify the different types of questions used on the NCLEX-RN, CAT.
- Select the most appropriate means for preparing for the NCLEX-RN, CAT.

I DON'T WANT TO TAKE THIS EXAM!

The primary purpose of licensure examinations is to protect the public from unsafe or uneducated practitioners of a profession. When you pass the National Council Licensure Examination (NCLEX), it indicates that you have the minimal level of knowledge or competency deemed necessary by the state to practice nursing without injury to clients. Licensure is a legal requirement for all professions that deal with public health, welfare, or safety.

Most people have varying levels of anxiety before taking an exam. The more important the examination, the higher the anxiety levels. Anxiety is sometimes defined as fear of the unknown. This chapter presents key information about the NCLEX test plan to better help you understand and anticipate what you will encounter when you take the exam. It also includes some suggestions for study for the NCLEX and do's and don'ts for the exam itself. This information should help lower your anxiety levels about the NCLEX. Sample practice questions throughout the chapter give you an idea of how the NCLEX asks about different types of nursing information. Try to answer these questions as you read. The answers and rationales are found at the end of the chapter.

NCLEX TEST PLAN

The NCLEX is a computerized, **criterion-referenced examination** that you take after you graduate from a school of nursing. Unlike a **norm-referenced examination,** which bases a passing score on the scores of others who took the exam, criterion-referenced examinations compare your knowledge to a pre-established standard. If you meet or exceed the standard, you pass. The NCLEX measures nursing knowledge of a wide range of subject matter, but mostly measures your ability to think critically and make good sound judgments about nursing care. With computerized adaptive tests such as the NCLEX, the computer selects questions in accordance with the examination plan and how you answered the previous questions.

Changes in the Test Plan

Every 3 years the National Council of State Boards of Nursing (NCSBN) undertakes an analysis of current nursing practice, with the most recent changes in 2010. An expert panel of nine nurses conduct a survey that asks approximately 12,000 newly licensed nurses about the frequency and importance of performing the 15 NCLEX-RN test plan nursing care activities. These activities are then analyzed in relation to the frequency of performance, impact on maintaining client safety, and client care settings where the activities are performed. Two changes based on the results of the survey indicate that new graduates are using increased critical thinking:

2009: Evaluate and document responses to procedures and treatments.
2010: Recognize trends and changes in client condition and intervene appropriately
The 2009 standard was stated: Assess client's vital signs.
The 2010 standard is stated: Assess and respond to changes in client's vital signs.

Because the findings of the NCSBN survey indicated an increase in the complexity of care, the difficulty level required to pass was increased by 0.05 logits (from minus 0.21 logits in 2009 to minus 0.16 logits in spring 2010). In the past, when the criterion difficulty level has been increased, the national average pass rate has decreased between 3 and 5 percent.

Questions Distributed by Category

In the past, the numbers of questions from each of the five categories were more or less equal. This changed in 2010. Questions dealing with management and management issues have increased to 22 percent of the exam, the highest percentage of any single type of question. Pharmacology-related questions have increased to 19 percent. Both of these increases reflect issues found in current nursing practice.

The NCLEX Computerized Adaptive Testing for Registered Nurses (NCLEX-RN, CAT) test plan is organized into three primary components: (1) client needs, (2) level of cognitive ability, and (3) integrated concepts and processes. The third component was expanded to include nursing process, caring, communication, cultural awareness, documentation, self-care, and teaching and learning. Alternative-format questions are now being used, and the length of time allowed to complete the exam was increased from 5 to 6 hours.

Client Health Needs

The NCLEX asks questions about four general groups of material called client health needs:

- Safe and effective care environment
- Physiological integrity
- Psychosocial integrity
- Health promotion and maintenance needs

Safe and Effective Care Environment (21 to 33 percent)

a. Management of care: 13 to 19 percent of NCLEX questions
b. Safety and infection control: 8 to 14 percent of NCLEX questions

The questions in this category make up between 21 and 33 percent of the total questions on the NCLEX. These questions deal with overt safety issues in client care (such as use of restraints), medication administration, safety measures to prevent injuries (such as putting up side rails), prevention of infections, isolation precautions, safety measures with pediatric clients, and special safety needs of clients with psychiatric problems.

This needs category also includes questions about laboratory tests, their results, and any special nursing measures associated with them; legal and ethical issues in nursing; a small amount of nursing management; and quality assurance issues. Questions on these issues are interspersed with other questions throughout the examination.

Physiological Integrity (43 to 67 percent)

a. Basic care and comfort: 6 to 12 percent of NCLEX questions

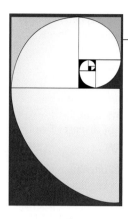

Issues Now

Handling Your Anxiety

First, it is perfectly reasonable to be slightly anxious about taking the NCLEX. You have expended plenty of blood, sweat, and tears to come to this point. As one diploma grad told me, "I was in debt up to my ears and running out of money fast when I took the NCLEX. Passing was literally my meal ticket." Even if you're not in such dire financial straits, it's no small thing to be tested on years of accumulated knowledge. You would have to be comatose not to feel butterflies in your stomach at this point. Do not be anxious about being anxious.

Because you cannot go back and change answers, treat each question as an exam in itself; once you hit the "N" next button, immediately turn your attention to the next question. Tell yourself not to be surprised by anything. You are at a psychological disadvantage if you expect the computer to turn off at a certain number and it doesn't. So if you can, avoid looking at the question number as you answer each question.

If you are distracted by the clicking of other people's computers or other such annoying sounds, you can ask for earplugs. The testing service provides them; they are disposable and not entirely unattractive.

Finally, there are going to be other people close to you or next to you who may sit down at the computer at the same time as you do. They may get up before you, but ignore them. The testing centers administer many different tests, so you can realistically tell yourself that the person next to you who finished in 45 minutes was not even taking the NCLEX. Even if they were taking the NCLEX, you do not need to think about it. A little denial in this situation can go a long way.

Source: Dunham, KS: How to Survive and Maybe Even Love Nursing School. Philadelphia, FA Davis, 2008, pp. 101–115, with permission.

b. Pharmacological and parenteral therapies: 13 to 19 percent of NCLEX questions

c. Reduction of risk potential: 13 to 19 percent of NCLEX questions

d. Physiological adaptation: 11 to 17 percent of NCLEX questions

The physiological integrity needs are concerned with adult medical and surgical nursing care, pediatrics, and **gerontology.** This category comprises the largest groups of questions, with about 43 to 67 percent of the total number of questions on the NCLEX. The more common health-care problems, both acute and chronic conditions, that nurses deal with on a daily basis include:

- Diabetes
- Cardiovascular disorders
- Neurological disorders
- Renal diseases
- Respiratory diseases
- Traumatic injuries
- Immunological disorders
- Skin and infective diseases

There are also questions about nursing care of the pediatric client, including such topics as:

- Growth and development
- Congenital abnormalities
- Child abuse
- Burn injury
- Fractures and cast and traction care
- Common infective diseases in children
- Common childhood trauma such as eye injuries

Psychosocial Integrity (6 to 12 percent)

a. Coping and adaptation: 5 to 11 percent of NCLEX questions

b. Psychosocial adaptation: 5 to 11 percent of NCLEX questions

Psychosocial integrity needs are health-care issues that revolve around the client with psychiatric problems. This material also deals with coping mechanisms for high-stress situations such as acute illness and life-threatening diseases or trauma. These clients do not necessarily have any psychiatric disorders. This category constitutes at most 12 percent of the examination and includes questions about the care of clients with eating disorders, personality disorders, anxiety disorders, depression, schizophrenia, and organic mental disease. Also included in the psychosocial

needs section are questions about therapeutic communication, crisis intervention, and substance abuse.

Health Promotion and Maintenance (6 to 12 percent)

a. Life span growth and development: 7 to 12 percent of NCLEX questions

b. Prevention and early detection of disease: 5 to 11 percent of NCLEX questions

Health promotion and maintenance needs deal with birth control measures, pregnancy, labor and delivery, the care of the newborn infant, growth and development, and contagious diseases, particularly sexually transmitted diseases. This section constitutes approximately 12 percent of the total examination. Teaching and counseling are important parts of the nurse's care during pregnancy, and knowledge of diet, signs and symptoms of complications, fetal development, and testing used during pregnancy is necessary.

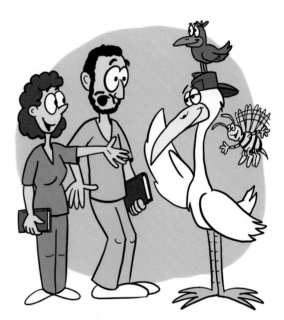

"THESE ARE MY HEALTH PROMOTION TUTORS."

Levels of Cognitive Ability

The level of cognitive ability is a component of the NCLEX that measures how information has been learned and how it can be used by the nurse. For the NCLEX, knowledge is tested at three different levels.

Level 1

Level 1 consists of knowledge and comprehension questions. Fewer than 10 percent of the questions are at this level, and there is a good chance that you may not even see a level 1 question. These questions involve recalling specific facts and the ability to understand those facts in relation to a pathophysiological condition. They cover knowledge of specific anatomy and physiology, medication dosage and side effects, signs and symptoms of diseases, laboratory test results, and the elements of certain treatments and interventions.

Being able to remember and understand information is the most basic way of learning. Although this type of knowledge is important and underlies the other levels of knowledge, it is not sufficient to ensure safe nursing care. An example of a level 1 question is:

1. A client is admitted to the medical unit with respiratory failure. Identify the normal range for the Po_2.
   a. 10–30 mm Hg
   b. 35–55 mm Hg
   c. 10–20 cm H_2O
   d. 70–100 mm Hg

Level 2

Level 2 questions add an additional step to the answering process. These questions presume that you have the basic information memorized and then ask you to analyze, interpret, and apply information to specific situations. Analysis and application questions are more difficult to answer because they require you to do more than simply repeat the information you have read or heard in class. Analysis requires the ability to separate information into its basic parts, decide which of those parts are important, and then make a decision about what the information is telling you. Application requires that you be able to use that information in client-care decisions.

Some examples of this type of question involve interpreting electrocardiographic (ECG) strips, interpreting blood gas values, making a nursing diagnosis based on a set of symptoms, or deciding on a treatment plan. These questions provide a better indication of your ability to safely care for clients. An example of a level 2 question is:

Being able to remember and understand information is the most basic way of learning. Although this type of knowledge is important and underlies the other levels of knowledge, it is not sufficient to ensure safe nursing care.

2. A client is becoming progressively short of breath. The results of his arterial blood gas (ABG) tests are pH, 7.13; Po_2, 48; Pco_2, 53; and HCO_3, 26. What do these values indicate?
   a. Metabolic acidosis
   b. Respiratory alkalosis
   c. Respiratory acidosis
   d. Metabolic alkalosis

Level 3

Level 3—synthesis, judgment, and evaluation— takes the process a step further. More than 95 percent of the questions on the NCLEX are at either level 2 or level 3. Questions at the synthesis and judgment level ask you to process information on more than one fact; apply rules, methods, principles, or theories to a situation; *and* make judgments and decisions about client care. You can identify these higher-level questions by recognizing that they require you to *process two or more* facts, concepts, theories, rules, or principles of care before you can answer the question.

One factor that adds to the difficulty of answering level 3–type questions is that there is often more than one correct answer. You may be asked to choose the best, or highest-priority, answer from among several correct answers. Questions at this level often ask about the priority of care to be given, the priority of nursing diagnosis formulated, how to best evaluate the effectiveness of care you are giving, and the most appropriate nursing action to be taken. Your ability to make decisions about nursing care at these higher levels is the best indication of your critical thinking ability and best demonstrates the ability to provide safe nursing care. Three examples of level 3 questions are:

3. A client is becoming progressively short of breath. The results of his arterial blood gas (ABG) tests are pH, 7.13; Po_2, 48; Pco_2, 53; and HCO_3, 26. What action should the nurse take first?
   a. Call a code blue and begin cardiopulmonary resuscitation.
   b. Call the physician and report the condition.

c. Make sure the client's airway is open and begin supplemental oxygen.
d. Give the ordered dose of 200 mg amino-phylline intravenous piggyback (IVPB) now.

4. After receiving shift report at 0645, identify the client the nurse should assess first.
   a. 65-year-old man with stable angina
   b. 37-year-old woman with possible GI bleeding; vital signs stable
   c. 56-year-old woman with COPD and an oxygen saturation of 89%
   d. 19-year-old man with type 1 diabetes and a fasting blood sugar of 55 mg/dL

5. The nurse assesses a 7-month-old hospitalized girl and finds that the infant has a positive tonic neck reflex. What intervention would be most important for the nurse to include in the child's nursing care plan?
   a. Daily head circumference measurements
   b. Measure intake and weigh all diapers
   c. Position the infant on her back for naps
   d. Assess neuro/developmental levels each shift

Integrated Concepts and Processes

The integrated concepts and processes component includes the following:

- Nursing process
- Concepts of caring
- Therapeutic communication
- Cultural awareness
- Documentation
- Self-care
- Teaching and learning

These concepts are integrated throughout the examination and are included as elements in the four needs categories.

Nursing Process

The nursing process has traditionally been a very important part of the NCLEX. The NCLEX-RN, CAT uses the five-step nursing process: assessment, analysis, planning, intervention and implementation, and evaluation. Each of the questions you will be asked on the NCLEX falls into one of these five categories.

It is important that you keep in mind the steps of the nursing process when answering questions. Often questions that ask, "What should the nurse do first?" are looking for an assessment-type answer because that is the first step in the nursing process. Questions on the nursing process are no longer equally divided on the examination. Recent analysis has shown a higher percentage of questions in the implementation phase of the nursing process.

Assessment

The **assessment** phase primarily establishes the database on which the rest of the nursing process is built. Some components of the assessment phase include both subjective and objective data about the client, significant history, history of the present illness, signs and symptoms, environmental elements, laboratory values, and vital signs. Often the examination will ask you to distinguish between appropriate and inappropriate assessment factors. An example of an assessment phase question is:

6. What would be the most important information for the nurse to obtain when a client is admitted for evaluation of recurrent episodes of Stokes-Adams syndrome?
   a. Ability to perform aerobic exercises for 15 minutes
   b. Bradycardia and increases in blood pressure
   c. Changes in level of consciousness
   d. Ability to discuss fat and sodium diet restrictions

Analysis

The analysis phase of the nursing process involves developing and using nursing diagnosis for the care of the client. The NCLEX uses the North American Nursing Diagnosis Association (NANDA) nursing diagnosis system. Questions concerning nursing diagnosis will often ask you to prioritize the diagnoses. (See Chapter 10 for information about prioritization). An example of an analysis phase question is:

7. A client is admitted to the unit with a diagnosis of bronchitis, congestive heart failure, and fever. The nurse assesses him as having a temperature of 101.8°F, peripheral edema, dyspnea, and rhonchi. The following nursing diagnoses are all appropriate, but which one has the highest priority?
   a. Anxiety related to fear of hospitalization
   b. Ineffective airway clearance related to retained secretions
   c. Fluid volume excess related to third spacing of fluid (edema)
   d. Ineffective thermoregulation related to fever

Planning

The planning phase of the nursing process primarily involves setting goals for the client. Included in the planning phase are such factors as determining expected outcomes, setting priorities for goals, and anticipating client needs based on the assessment. These questions may ask you to identify the most appropriate goal or may ask you to identify the highest-priority goal from several appropriate goals. You can prioritize goals the same way you did the nursing diagnosis. Remember that a good goal is measurable, client centered, time limited, and realistic. An example of a planning phase question is:

8. A client is found to be in respiratory failure and is placed on oxygen. Which goal has the highest priority for this client?
   a. Walk the length of the hall twice during a nurse's shift.
   b. Complete his bath and morning care before breakfast.
   c. Maintain an oxygen saturation of 90% throughout the shift.
   d. Keep the head of the bed elevated to promote proper ventilation.

Intervention and Implementation

The intervention and implementation phase of the nursing process involves identifying nursing actions that are required to meet the goals stated in the planning phase. Some of the material in the **intervention** and **implementation** phase includes:

- Provision of nursing care based on the client's goals
- Prevention of injury or spread of disease
- Therapy with medications and their administration
- Giving treatments
- Carrying out procedures
- Charting and record keeping
- Teaching about health care
- Monitoring changes in condition

An example of an intervention and implementation phase question is:

9. When the nurse ambulates a client who has been on bed rest for 3 days, he suddenly becomes very restless, displays extreme dyspnea, and complains of chest pain. Select the most appropriate nursing action.
   a. Call a code blue.
   b. Continue to help the client walk, but at a slower pace.
   c. Give the client an injection of his ordered pain medication.
   d. Return the client to bed and evaluate his vital signs and lung sounds.

Evaluation

The **evaluation** phase of the nursing process determines whether or not the goals stated in the planning phase have been met through the interventions. The evaluation phase also ties the nursing process together and makes it cyclic. If the goals have been achieved, it is an indication that the plan and implementation were effective, and new goals need to be established. If the goals were not met, then you have to go back and find the difficulty. Were the assessment data inadequate? Were the goals defective? Was there a deficiency in the implementation?

Evaluation is a continuous process. Material in the evaluation phase includes comparison of actual outcomes with expected outcomes, verification of assessment data, evaluation of nursing actions and client responses, and evaluation of the client's level of knowledge and understanding. Evaluation questions are often worded very similarly and are relatively easy to identify after you have experienced a few of them. An example of an evaluation question is:

10. A client is being prepared for discharge. He is to take theophylline by mouth at home for his lung disease. Which statement by the client indicates to the nurse that her teaching concerning theophylline medications has been effective?
    a. "I can stop taking this medication when I feel better."
    b. "If I have difficulty swallowing the time-released capsules, I can crush them or chew them."
    c. "If I have a lot of nausea and vomiting or become restless and can't sleep, I need to call my physician."
    d. "I need to drink more coffee and cola while I am on these medications."

> *Contrary to rumor, no graduates are randomly selected to take all 265 questions.*

NCLEX FORMAT

You will take the NCLEX examination on a personal computer at a Pearson Professional Center (Fig. 11.1). The majority of the questions are in a multiple-choice format and are constructed similarly. They include a client situation, a question stem, and four answers, or distractors, like the sample questions you have seen so far in this chapter.

All the multiple-choice questions on the NCLEX stand alone, although a similar situation may be repeated. Occasionally a single question may be included without a case situation.

Choosing the Right Answer

For the multiple-choice questions, you are asked to select the one best answer from among the four possible choices. No partial credit is given for a "close" answer; there is only one correct answer for any particular question. The questions are totally integrated from the content areas that were previously discussed along with the approximate percentages that were identified. Each question carries an equal weight or value toward the final score.

When the question appears on the screen, read the question and answers using the process described in Chapter 10. When you decide what the correct answer is, place the cursor in the circle in front of the answer, and click (Fig. 11.1). This selects the answer. If you decide to change the answer (not a good idea; see Chapter 10), place the cursor on the answer you selected and click again. It will remove the indicator and you can move the cursor to another answer.

When you are sure you have selected the correct answer, click the "N" next button on the button bar at the bottom of the screen. That question will disappear and a new one will appear. You cannot go back and change an answer after you click the "N" next button.

Alternative Format Questions

In 2004, alternative format questions were first added to the exam; in 2010, three new types of alternative format questions were added. The latest information is that between 2 and 10 percent of the total number of questions will be alternative format and that each graduate will have at least two of them on the exam. There are several types of these questions. They are scored like the multiple-choice questions in that they are either correct or incorrect (no partial credit). They are also given a difficulty rating based on the same criteria as the multiple-choice questions. If you want to practice these types of questions, go to www.ncsb.org/testing, where you will find several examples, or obtain one of several books that contain alternative format questions. Most of the NCLEX review books now have samples of these questions for students to practice.

Fill in the Blank
These alternative format questions may ask for a range of information. They may be calculation questions or may ask for knowledge. After you read the questions, you need to type the answer in the box provided (Fig. 11.2). If it is a calculation question, you may use the pop-up calculator, accessible by clicking the cursor on the "C" calculator button on the button bar (Fig. 11.3). After you have typed in

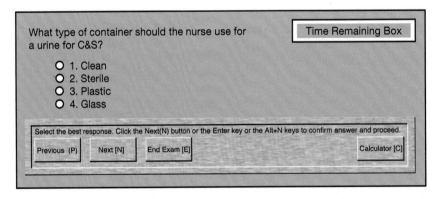

Figure 11.1 Sample multiple-choice question. Select the answer by placing the cursor in the circle and click or type in the answer. Change the answer by placing the cursor in a new circle and click. Move to the next question by clicking on the "Next (N)" button at the bottom of the screen.

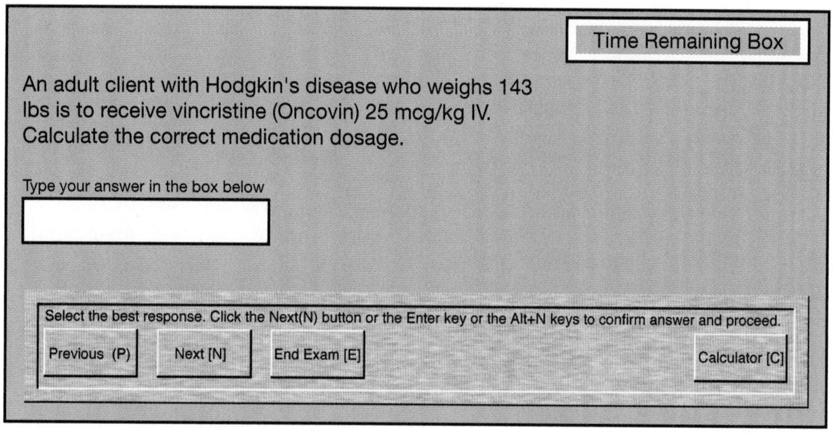

Figure 11.2 Alternative format question. Fill in the blank by clicking on the "Calculator (C)" button at the lower right corner of the bar.

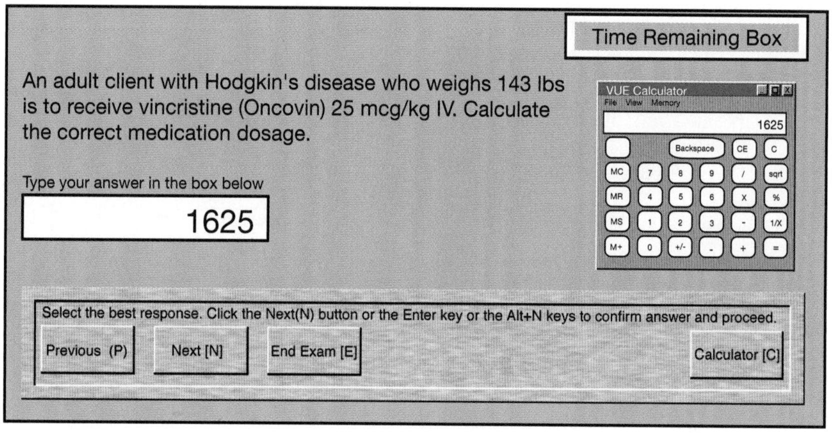

Figure 11.3 Alternative format question. Fill in the blank by using the calculator to click on number buttons. Then type in the answer box. Do *not* use spaces or commas in the answer. Close the calculator by clicking on the "X" button on the calculator screen.

your answer, you can go back and change it. Once you have decided that it is correct, click on the "N" next button and a new question will appear.

Multiple Answers

With the multiple-answer format questions, you are given a list of options or answers and must select all that are correct. You must get them all correct in order to get credit for the question. To select the options you think are correct, place the cursor in the circle or box before the option and click (Fig. 11.4). If you decide that one of the options is not really the one you want, you can click on the circle again and it will be removed. When you decide you have the

options you want, click on the "N" next button and the next question will appear on the screen.

Sequencing Items

Sequencing format questions provide you with a question and then four or more options (items) that are related to the question. Your task with this type of question is to place them in the proper sequence (Fig. 11.5). You do this by selecting the circle or box in front of the option you think is number one and typing in "1." Then move to the option you believe is number two and type that number in, and so forth. You can change the numbering by clicking on the boxes to remove the numbers.

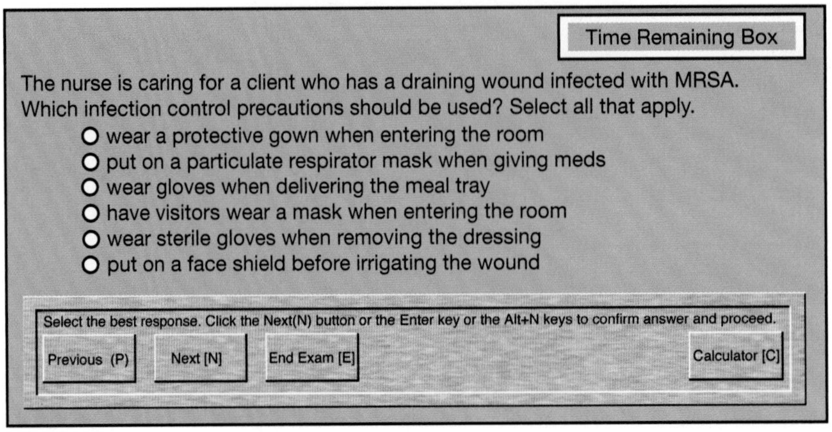

Figure 11.4 Alternative format question—multiple answer.

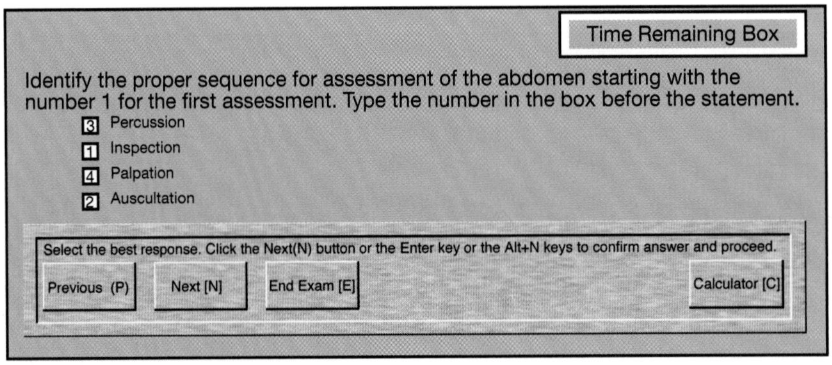

Figure 11.5 Alternative format question—sequencing items.

A variation on this type of question uses the "drag and drop" format. With drag and drop, you will be given a series of items in a box on the left side of the screen. You will be asked to sequence them by clicking on them one at a time and putting them in the proper order in a box on the right side of the screen. When you have the options sequenced the way you think they should be, click on the "N" next button on the button bar and a new question will appear on the screen.

Identify the Area (or Hot Spot)

These types of questions provide you with a picture or diagram and then ask you to identify an area or a structure on the picture (Fig. 11.6). You place the cursor on the area that you think is correct and click. An "X" will appear. If you decide that is not where you really want the "X," you can click on the "X" again to remove it and then place the cursor in a new

spot and click again. Once you decide that you have it where you want it, click on the "N" next button, and the next question will appear on the screen.

Chart/Exhibit Items (Type 1)

A chart or exhibit item will present you with a chart, graph, or some other picture or graphic item, or with a series of charts, graphs, or other pictures. You will need to be able to read the chart, graph, or picture to obtain the information to answer the question. Then you will be asked to select the correct answer from four or more options by using the information you gleaned from the chart, graph, or picture.

Exhibit Items (Type 2) (Added in 2010)

With this type of question, you are presented with either a question or a problem. To answer the question or solve the problem, you must click on an "Exhibit Button." Each exhibit contains three tabs

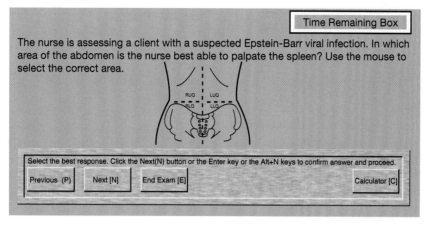

Figure 11.6 Alternative format question—identify area. With this type of question, you are given a diagram or picture and asked to locate a structure or area. Place the cursor on the area you think is correct and click. An "X" will appear in that area. To deselect the answer, click on the "X" and move the cursor to the new area. When finished, click on "Next (N)."

with drop-downs; you must click on each tab and read the information. The question will ask you to find some data provided by one of the tabs. Once you determine which tab has the correct information, you must select the one corresponding correct item from the four options provided. Then you click on the "N" next button and move on to the next question.

Exhibit item questions test your ability to use information correctly. This type of question responds to the increase in the use of evidence-based practice in the health-care setting. If a nurse cannot understand and interpret research findings correctly, the safety of clients becomes an issue.

Audio Items (Added in 2010)

This type of question requires the use of a headset. When the question comes up, you will initially see what looks like the audio bar from a DVD with the usual symbols for play, pause, forward, stop, and reverse:

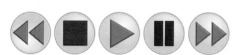

There will be four options (answer choices) underneath the bar. You must put on the headset and click on the arrow-shaped play button to listen to the audio clip. The volume can be adjusted using the volume slide bar. After listening to the clip, you must select the one correct option related to it. You can

repeat the clip as often as you want, stop it, or pause it by clicking on the appropriate audio bar symbols. After selecting your answer, click the "N" next button to move on to the next question.

The NCSBN has not indicated what you might find on these audio clips. Logically, it would seem that anything a nurse usually "hears" in the course of a day's work could be included: heart sounds, breath sounds, bruits, and even client statements (is this client depressed, angry, anxious, or expressing echolalia?). These might be difficult.

Graphic Items (Added in 2010)

These questions are similar to the traditional multiple-choice questions in that there is a written question. However, the question presents four pictures or graphics, not written options, as answer selections. As with the audio items, the NCSBN has not provided any indication of the types of graphics you might encounter. They could be charts of disease frequencies, pictures of rashes or wounds, ECG strips, types of syringes, medication labels on bottles, or just about anything a nurse might see during a work shift.

How Many Questions?

You may take between 75 and 265 questions, depending on how you answer. Of the first 75 questions, only 60 count. The other 15 are "trial" questions that will be used on future examinations, but you don't know which ones do not count, so you need to do the best you can on all of them. The NCSBN is attempting to establish reliability and validity data on the new trial questions.

If you seem to be getting a lot of questions in a particular category, for example, pediatrics, it may mean one of two things. The NCSBN may be testing pediatric questions on your exam, so you are receiving a lot of them, or it may mean that you are having some problems answering pediatric questions correctly. The computer will continue to give you questions in a particular content area until you meet the requirements of the test plan. The computer randomly draws the questions you are seeing from a pool of more than 4000 questions.

The NCSBN, which is responsible for designing the test, publicly states that no graduates are randomly selected by the computer to take all 265 questions. You can pass or fail the test with either 75 or 265 questions or any number in between. The average number of questions taken over the past 5 years is 119, and the average time is just over 2 hours.

How Long It Takes

There is a maximum time limit of 6 hours for the entire examination, although there is no minimum time limit. There is a mandatory break when the computer "locks up" about 2½ hours into the test. For 10 minutes, you will not be able to answer any questions. There is another optional break at about 4 hours into the test, although the computer will not lock up at this time. You can take breaks at any time during the exam if you need to use the restroom, but remember that you will lose this time off your total time for the exam.

The exam is not really timed except for the overall time limit. Theoretically you could sit at the computer for the full 6 hours with question number 1 on the screen. The computer does not make you take questions at any particular rate. Most people can answer a multiple-choice question in about 45 seconds. As a rule of thumb, if you are spending more than 2 minutes on any single question, put an answer down and move on to the next question.

If you calculate that you are going to take 265 questions in 6 hours, it comes out to about 80 seconds per question. Some of the alternative-format questions may take a little longer to answer, although some may take less time than the multiple-choice questions. Take a watch along and keep an eye on the "Time Remaining" box at the top of the screen.

How It's Graded

The NCLEX is graded on a statistical model that compares your responses with a pre-established standard. If you can demonstrate a knowledge level consistently above the standard, you will pass the examination.

Because the NCLEX-RN examination is given by computerized adaptive testing (CAT), increases in the passing standard do not necessarily require you to answer a higher number of items correctly. However, the new passing standard does require that you answer questions correctly at a slightly higher difficulty level than the previous year's graduates. Questions are assigned a difficulty value on a seven-logit (unit) scale called the NCLEX-RN logistic scale, ranging from the easiest (–3), which all graduates should answer correctly, to the most difficult (3), which almost all graduates would be expected to miss (Box 11.1). It is important to keep in mind that a "logit" is not a percentage point, nor does it have anything to do with percentages. The current pass criterion is almost in the middle of the seven-point logit scale.

So What Is a Logit?

The term "logit" is an abbreviation for "log odds units." It was originally developed for use in mathematical probability calculations in which different-sized units of data are analyzed as if they were all the same size. On the NCLEX, ranking the questions to logit levels compares the difficulty of items (criterion referencing) rather than the answers different graduates might give (norm referencing). This establishes a more objective standard for passing the

Box 11.1

NCLEX-RN Logistic Scale

Logits	
3	Most difficult
2	
1	
0	Approximate pass level
–1	
–2	
–3	Least difficult

exam. So what percentage must you answer correctly to pass? It doesn't really matter. You must answer enough questions ranked above the pass criteria to demonstrate that you can practice nursing safely. If you do that, you pass the NCLEX.

Level of Difficulty

The difficulty level of the questions is determined by the writers and question reviewers. It is based on such factors as when the material is usually presented in nursing programs (material presented earlier is considered less difficult) and the complexity of the material. To you, the test taker, difficulty level is somewhat relative. If you know the answer to a question, then it will seem relatively easy to you even if it is classified by the test writers as a higher difficulty–level question. Similarly, if you do not know the answer, that question will be difficult for you even if it is determined to be at a relatively low difficulty level.

No Happy Questions

Keep in mind also that there are no "happy" questions on the NCLEX. There is always something wrong, and if there is a problem in the question, you need to worry about it. Also, as a general guiding principle, anything you know really well from your classes will NOT be on the NCLEX, so anticipate difficult questions.

> *Keep in mind that the NCLEX is designed so that no one can answer all the questions correctly. Even your most knowledgeable nursing instructor would not be able to answer some of the questions on the exam.*

After you finish the mandatory tutorial on the use of the computer, the first real question you will see will be at a medium difficulty level, probably a little above or a little below the pass criteria. If you answer it correctly, the next question will be a little more difficult. If you answer that one correctly, the next question will also increase in difficulty, and so forth, until you start missing questions. Then the computer will give you slightly less difficult questions until you start answering them correctly. The computer is trying to establish your "zone of knowledge." If that zone is above the pass standard, then you will pass the exam.

Your Zone of Knowledge

If you miss the first question, and many graduates do because of anxiety, the computer will give you a slightly easier question for number 2. If you answer that one correctly, the next one will increase in difficulty level, and so forth, until you start missing questions. If the computer can clearly determine your zone of knowledge within the first 75 questions, it will stop the test and ask you to complete a short survey. The reason many graduates take more than 75 questions is because the computer is having difficulty establishing a clear zone of knowledge above or below the pass standard. It will keep giving questions until a clear determination is made. Graduates who take all 265 questions have answered questions above and below the pass standard throughout the whole exam. If you do have to take all 265 questions, it does not necessarily mean you failed.

Example: Low Difficulty Level

11. What blood test does the nurse evaluate as the best measure of a client's long-term control of diabetes mellitus?
    a. Fasting blood sugar
    b. Arterial blood gases
    c. Glucose tolerance test (GTT)
    d. Glycosylated hemo globin (Hgb A_1C)

Example: Mid-Difficulty Level (Pass Criteria)

12. While evaluating the results of a pulmonary function test, the nurse notes that an adult man who is short of breath has a vital capacity of 2800 mL, a tidal volume of 375 mL, and a residual volume of 2200 mL. Select the action the nurse should avoid implementing for this client.
    a. Position the client with the head of the bed elevated 45 degrees.
    b. Encourage fluid intake of 2 to 3 liters per 24 hours.
    c. Begin oxygen by non-rebreather mask.
    d. Encourage the client to cough and to breathe deeply every hour during the shift.

Example: High Difficulty Level

13. While monitoring a client with a pulmonary artery catheter, the nurse notes catheter fling artifact on the pressure tracing. Identify the

nursing measure that best compensates for this problem.

    a. Record only mean pressures.

    b. Ask the physician to reposition the catheter.

    c. Irrigate the catheter forcefully with heparinized saline solution.

    d. Level and zero the transducer before taking readings.

Remember that it is probably a good sign that you are getting difficult questions. It means that you are answering questions above the pass standard. You do not want a lot of easy questions on the NCLEX. Also keep in mind that the NCLEX is designed so that no one can answer all the questions correctly. Even your most knowledgeable nursing instructor would not be able to answer some of the questions on the exam.

However, the NCLEX asks entry-level–type questions that tend to be very "textbookish." When you are answering NCLEX questions, look for the expected textbook-type knowledge. Don't look for exceptions. Each examination is different and unique to the person taking it because future questions depend on how you answered previous questions.

NCLEX BACKGROUND INFORMATION

Test Vendor and Logistics

The test vendor for the NCLEX is VUE, a subsidiary of NCS Pearson Professional Centers. The tests are given at Pearson Professional Centers. The test items and the format of the examination always stay the same, even if vendors change, because the exam is owned by the NCSBN, which contracts with vendors to administer the examination.

After you graduate from your nursing program, you must apply to the state board of nursing for permission to take the NCLEX. Once you have been approved by the State Board, that information is sent on to the NCSBN, which sends you an "authorization to test" card or document. You will receive your authorization document more quickly if you select the "e-mail" option on the application form for the examination.

You then call for an appointment at the center where you wish to take the test. Appointments are made on a first-come, first-served basis. The centers are required to schedule the examination within 30 days from the time you apply. Each state establishes its own maximum time interval for the graduate to take the exam after graduation, usually 1 year.

There are both morning and afternoon sessions of 6 hours' duration. Depending on the size of the center, between 8 and 15 graduates may be taking the test at the same time. There may be other people at the center taking examinations in other disciplines at the same time as the nursing graduates.

Testing by Computer

The computer skills required are minimal. The mouse is used for most of the examination, with minimal typing required. A digital picture is taken at the time you enter the examination room, and that picture, along with your information, appears on one of the computer screens in the room. A digital thumbprint and signature are also obtained when you enter the exam center.

You sit at the computer with your picture on it and complete a tutorial on the use of the mouse and computer. You have two attempts at completing the tutorial successfully. If you are unable to do so after the second try, a person who is working at the testing center will come and help you. After the examination is completed, you will be asked to complete a short computerized personal data questionnaire and an evaluation of the examination site.

Questions appear one at a time on the computer screen, with a button bar on the bottom of the screen and a "time remaining" box in the upper corner. After you select an answer, the question is replaced with another question and answers. No question is ever repeated, nor are you able to change the answer once you have clicked on the "N" next button.

An on-screen pop-up calculator is available for answering dosage and other questions that require calculations. Because of the increased emphasis on pharmacology and the concern about medication errors, it is probably safe to assume that the difficulty level of future calculation questions will increase markedly.

Security

Security is very tight at the examination sites. All exam sessions are videotaped, and there is a proctor in the room monitoring all the test takers. Although cheating on the NCLEX is virtually impossible— every examination is different—it is important to not even look as if you are attempting to cheat. Do not talk to the person next to you. Keep your eyes on your own computer. Do not take out any papers or electronic devices during the exam. Magic slates are generally provided for use as "scrap paper," so you will not need any paper or pens during the exam. Lockers are provided and you must leave all your personal belongings at the door, so do not bring a lot of things with you to the examination site.

How the Test Is Graded

The NCLEX is graded on a pass–fail basis. If the graduate has failed, the entire examination must be taken again. The NCSBN requires a 45-day waiting period before repeating the examination, and first-time takers are given preference over those who are repeating the examination. A number of states have restricted the number of times the graduate can retake the test, usually to three. Check with your state board of nursing for the particular regulations.

When the computer shuts off, it knows if you passed or failed, but it will not give you that information at that time. At the end of the day, after the last testing session, results are downloaded electronically to NCSBN in Chicago. The next business day, NCSBN notifies the state board of nursing electronically and sends hard copy; then it is up to the state board of nursing to notify you.

The exam results may be sent to you by mail, usually within 7 to 10 days after the exam has been completed, although this time frame varies from state to state. Most states now offer online results within 72 hours after the exam. Check with your state board of nursing to make sure they offer this service and to find out how to access the site. The NCSBN offers a service that allows you to obtain unofficial results by telephone 3 days after you take the examination. The telephone number is 900-225-6000; the cost for the call is $7.95. You can also access the NCSBN on the Web at www.pearsonvue.com/nclex and sign in with your user name and password. Cost is $7.95. Not all states participate in the service, and your employment agency may or may not accept the results.

NCLEX STUDY STRATEGIES

There are several ways to prepare for examinations, including the NCLEX. To attempt to take the examination with an attitude of "If I don't know it by now, I never will" is to court failure. Carefully directed study and preparation will considerably increase the chances of passing the examination. Review

Chapter 10 for general tips on how to study for and take exams. Below is some specific information for preparation for the NCLEX.

The NCSBN Website

You can access the NCBSN website at www.ncsbn.org. This website can provide significant help as you prepare to take the NCLEX. It provides the most recent information on any changes in the test, has a sample tutorial about the exam, and even has some sample questions. You can also access sample examination questions at http://www.vue.com/nclex. The more you learn about the exam before you have to take it, the lower your anxiety and the better you will do.

Review Books

The material covered by review books is the key material found on the NCLEX. These books usually follow the NCLEX Test Plan very closely. A review book is, however, just that; it reviews the material that you should already know. Reviewing is important to reinforce learning and recall of information you may not have used in a year or more.

What Do You Think?

When was the last time you sat in on a group study session? List three of the problems you encountered at the session. How could they be solved?

Review books are not really designed to present any new information about key material. If you are totally unfamiliar with the material in a particular section of the review book, reading a more comprehensive textbook on that particular subject area will be necessary.

Another important function of a review book is to point out areas of weakness. If you find a section that seems to contain "new" material, it is important to investigate that section in more detail. If you find most of the material familiar and easy to grasp, you are probably well on your way to success on the NCLEX.

Group Study

Group study can be an effective method of preparation for an examination such as the NCLEX. To optimize the results of group study sessions, several rules should be followed.

Rule 1. *Be very selective when choosing the members of the study group.* They should have a similar frame of mind and orientation toward studying. They should be graduates who are also going to be taking the NCLEX. The ideal size for a study group is between four and six people. Groups larger than six become difficult to organize and handle. After the group has been formed and has begun its study sessions, it may be necessary to ask an individual to leave the group for not participating or for being disruptive to the study process or displaying negative attitudes about the examination.

Rule 2. *Have each individual prepare a particular section for each group study session.* Study groups generally meet once or twice a week. For example, if next week the group is going to study the endocrine system, assign group member 1 the anatomy and physiology of the system, member 2 the pathological conditions, member 3 the medications used for treatment, and member 4 the key elements of nursing care. When the group comes together, have each individual present his or her prepared section. This type of preparation prevents the "What are we going to study tonight?" syndrome that often plagues group study sessions.

Following this process organizes the study group and allows for more in-depth coverage of the topic. It also permits the members of the group to ask questions of the other members, thereby reinforcing the information being discussed.

Rule 3. *Limit the length of the study session.* No single study session should be longer than between 60 and 90 minutes. Sessions that go longer tend to get off the topic and foster a negative attitude about the examination. Try to avoid making group study sessions into party time. A few snacks and refreshments may be helpful to maintain the group's energy level, but a real party atmosphere will detract significantly from the effectiveness of the study session.

Rule 4. *Use role playing to reinforce information.* The more senses you can involve in the learning process, the better the learning.

Rule 5. *Remain positive.* Although group study times should not be party times, relax and have some fun with the study.

Individual Study Tips

No matter what other study and preparation methods are used, individual preparation for the NCLEX is a necessity. This preparation can take several forms.

Tip 1. As previously discussed, use of a review book is valuable to indicate areas of deficient knowledge. Reading and studying the appropriate textbooks and study guides can be helpful if it is approached correctly. It is important that the graduate mentally organize the information being read into a format similar to that found in the NCLEX. After reading each page of a textbook or study guide, the graduate should be able to ask three or four multiple-choice questions about that information. These questions can be asked silently or written out and should answer the question, "How might the NCLEX test my knowledge of this material?"

> *No matter what other study and preparation methods are used, individual preparation for the NCLEX is a necessity.*

Tip 2. Take practice exams on the computer. Practice answering questions similar to those found on the exam you are going to take or the NCLEX itself. Most of the review books come with a CD that has practice questions on it. It will help alleviate some of the unknowns, particularly if you have not had a lot of experience with computer-based exams.

Learning the Format. Experts recommend that you take between 3000 and 5000 practice questions before you take the NCLEX. Try to take at least 1000 questions using a computerized format and alternative format questions. Obviously, starting early in this process (6 months) is important, along with some planning and time management. Don't try to take 1000 questions at a time! For maximum learning, take 50 to 100 at a sitting and review the answers to understand why you missed the ones you missed.

When practice questions are answered, the following important mental processes occur:

Getting Comfortable. First, you are becoming more familiar with and therefore more comfortable with the format of the examination. In research, this process is termed the practice effect; it must be accounted for when analyzing the results from pretest/post-test types of research projects. Individuals will have better results after a test, even without any type of intervention, because of having practiced answering questions on the pretest. Similarly, your score on the NCLEX may increase by as much as 10 percent through answering practice questions.

Reinforcing Information. A second result of answering practice questions is that it reinforces the information already studied. Although it is unlikely that a question on the NCLEX examination will be identical to a practice question, there are many similarities. Realistically, only a limited number of questions can be asked about any given subject. After a while, the questions will begin to sound very similar.

Identifying Weak Spots. A third advantage of answering practice questions is that it quickly reveals subject areas that you will need to study. It is relatively easy to say, "I understand the renal system pretty well." It is quite another to answer correctly 10 or 15 questions about that system. If you answer the questions correctly, you can move on to the next topic. If you miss the majority of the questions, however, further review is required.

After you have answered the questions, you need to review them and compare your answers with the answers provided in the study book. You should also look at the rationales and the categories into which the questions fall. Try to understand why you missed the questions you did. Was it lack of knowledge? Didn't read the question carefully? Didn't use critical thinking?

Tip 3. Complete a 265-item test in one sitting in 6 hours. Many websites provide testing materials and sample examinations. One is http://passneclex.mcphu.eduwww.sjsu.edu/depts/itl/graphics/main.html.

Tip 4. Take the NCLEX as soon as possible after you graduate. The NCSBN has done some studies that show the following:

- The NCLEX taken less than 26 days after graduation has an 89 percent average pass rate.
- The NCLEX taken between 27 and 39 days after graduation has an 80 percent average pass rate.
- The NCLEX taken between 40 and 62 days after graduation has a 72 percent average pass rate.
- The NCLEX taken more than 62 days after graduation has a 45 percent average pass rate.

Formal NCLEX Reviews

The NCSBN does not endorse or sponsor any review courses for the NCLEX directly, but many companies offer reviews shortly after graduation. An online comprehensive review course for the NCLEX-RN examination on the NCSBN website is offered by an independent company (www.learningext.com). These review courses range from 2 to 5 days and basically cover the information found in review books. They are rather expensive, and the quality of NCLEX reviews varies. In general, they are only as good as the people who are presenting the material. Also, look at the reported pass rate of the graduates after they take the review. Courses with higher pass rates are probably better.

> *Experts recommend that you take between 3000 and 5000 practice questions before you take the NCLEX. Obviously, starting early in this process is important, along with some planning and time management.*

PREPARING FOR THE BIG DAY

Several Months to One Week Before the Exam

1. Get mentally and physically prepared. Eat a good healthy diet; emphasize foods with protein, vitamin K, and calcium. These foods have been shown to help control long-term stress.

   Exercise regularly. Drink lots of water (64 ounces per day) to rid your body of accumulated toxins. Avoid alcohol, street drugs, and even over-the-counter medications like antihistamines that can affect your ability to concentrate and think. Ease off on the caffeine and stop smoking.
2. Practice doing NCLEX type questions—lots of them!
3. Avoid major life-altering activities, such as buying a car or planning a wedding, major vacation, or baby shower!

The Day Before the Exam

1. Don't work. Most employers understand that the NCLEX produces anxiety and are willing to let you have the day off. If your stress levels are high, it may be difficult for you to concentrate on your work, possibly compromising the health and well-being of your clients.
2. Do something fun and relaxing, but don't overdo it. Activities that involve some moderate exercise will help with anxiety levels.
3. Eat citrus fruits or drink liquids with vitamin C. Vitamin C has been shown to decrease short-term stress.
4. If you are unfamiliar with the area where the test center is located, drive to the test site. Note parking facilities and places where you can get a meal. This preparation will save you from getting lost the next day and help you be on time.

The Night Before the Exam

1. Make sure you have all the materials you will need for the exam, including two forms of picture ID, authorization to test card, and Social Security card.
2. Review formulas, common medications, and information that can be summarized in tables or on cards and lists. It is probably not a good time to pull out all your old textbooks and notes and try to read them. Concentrate on things that are visual and may have caused you some problems in the past, like the list of cranial nerves or the glands and hormones in the endocrine system. Don't try to study everything. The "If I don't know it now, I never will" attitude is a negative thought process. You can always learn something.
3. Avoid strange or exotic foods that you have never eaten before. This can be a real temptation if you have to travel away from home and stay in a hotel the night before the exam. Stick to your usual diet. New or unusual foods may cause some gastrointestinal consequences that can be very distracting during the exam.
4. Go to bed at a reasonable hour. It is probably best to stick to your normal schedule. Staying up all night trying to study is counterproductive. You will be nervous and may have some problems sleeping, but stay away from sleep aids. They will interfere with your decision-making ability on the exam.

Even if you are not sound asleep, the fact that you are resting will be helpful.

The Day of the Exam

1. Stick to your regular schedule and routine as much as possible. Avoid drinking excessive amounts of caffeine or sugary beverages to try to stay awake. They will only make you nervous and may increase the amount of time you need to spend on breaks in the restroom.
2. Eat breakfast, especially if you are scheduled for the morning session. Eat something with some glucose for a quick start (bread with jelly) and something with protein to get you through the morning (cereal and milk; egg and bacon). Drink some cinnamon tea, eat some lemon drop candies, or chew some peppermint gum. These flavors have been reported to enhance learning and sharpen thought processes! If you are taking the exam in the afternoon, eat lunch, but avoid a large meal with a lot of greasy food. It will make you sleepy and sit in your stomach like a lump.
3. Don't let the security at the site fluster you. They will take a digital picture, thumbprint, and signature. They will make you leave all your belongings in lockers at the door. Someone will be walking around the room during the exam. Just concentrate on your computer and answer the questions and you will do fine (see "Issues Now" box).

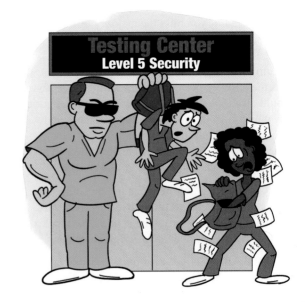

4. Wear comfortable clothes. You don't get extra points on the NCLEX for looking like a fashion model. Dress appropriately for the season, but keep in mind that some buildings are cool in the summer because of air conditioning and hot in the winter because of heating systems. Wear something you have worn before. Sweat clothes are a good choice, particularly because you can dress in layers. If you feel too warm, you can take a jacket off; if you feel cold, you can leave it on.

5. Think positively! If you truly believe you will do well, you will do well. If you go into the exam with an "I'm never going to pass this—I'm too dumb" attitude, you probably are not going to do as well.

Conclusion

Taking and passing the NCLEX-RN, CAT is a necessary step in the process of becoming a professional registered nurse. Like all licensure examinations, its purpose is to protect the public from undereducated or unsafe practitioners. The examination is comprehensive and includes material from all areas of the graduate's nursing education. Although most graduates have some anxiety about taking this examination, knowledge about its format and content and strategies for taking the examination can lower anxiety to an acceptable level.

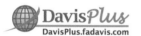

DavisPlus.fadavis.com

Critical Thinking Exercises

- Obtain an NCLEX-RN, CAT review book. Analyze the questions in the practice examination for type, cognitive level, and level of difficulty.
- Identify three to five other students in your class with whom you would feel comfortable working in a study group. Organize a study group session before the next major course examination.
- When you get the results of your next course examination, identify why you missed the questions you missed and what strategies might have been used to answer those questions correctly.

ANSWERS TO QUESTIONS IN CHAPTER 11

1. **Correct answer: d.** You either have or do not have the knowledge for this particular laboratory test.

2. **Correct answer: c.** Not only do you need to know the normal values for each of the blood gas components given, you must also be able to use that information in determining the underlying condition.

3. **Best answer: c.** Choices *b* and *d* are also actions that should be carried out, but at this time, opening the airway and oxygenating the client must receive highest priority. Not only does this question require that you know the normal values and be able to interpret them, but it also requires that a decision be made about the seriousness of the condition (analysis) and a selection of the type of care to be given from several correct options (judgment).

4. **Correct answer: d.** This question measures critical thinking and decision-making ability by asking you which of these clients is the sickest or least stable. Type 1 diabetic patients may have symptoms of hypoglycemia even when their blood glucoses are normal. This one is below normal, and all the other clients are stable.

5. **Correct answer: d.** This question requires you to know what a tonic neck reflex is and its significance. It is present in the newborn because of immaturity of the central nervous system and usually is gone by 1 month. If a child at 7 months still has it, it indicates a delay in neurological development.

6. **Correct answer: c.** Stokes-Adams syndrome is a suddenly occurring episode of asystole. The client becomes unconscious quickly.

7. **Correct answer: b.** Nursing diagnoses that deal with the airway always have highest priority.

8. **Correct answer: c.** Choice *a* is unrealistic for this client; choice *b* is not client-centered; choice *d* is a nursing intervention, not a goal. Maintaining an oxygen saturation of 90 percent is realistic, measurable, and within normal limits.

9. **Correct answer: d.** These are symptoms of a pulmonary embolism, which is a common complication of prolonged bed rest.

10. **Correct answer: c.** Answer *c* lists some side effects of theophylline medications that may indicate the onset of toxicity. The physician needs to know about these so that the theophylline level can be determined and the dosage adjusted accordingly. Other instructions that the client could be given when taking theophylline medications include to avoid excessive amounts of caffeine, never to suddenly stop taking the medication, to take it with a full glass of water and a small amount of food, and to watch for interactions with over-the-counter (OTC) medications.

11. **Correct answer: d.** Laboratory tests and their significance are considered basic knowledge and are taught in the early part of most nursing programs.

12. **Correct answer: c.** The pulmonary function test (PFT) indicates that the client has chronic obstructive pulmonary disease (COPD). High levels of oxygen that can be delivered by a nonrebreather mask can put the client into respiratory arrest.

13. **Correct answer: a.** The question asks about how to compensate for the problem, not correct it. Invasive hemodynamic monitoring is considered advanced medical-surgical nursing and is usually presented during the last year of nursing school.

Figure 11.1 (computer screen). Correct answer: 4. Kayser-Fleischer rings are caused by the deposition of a golden-brown pigment from an increased copper level secondary to hepatolenticular disease, a familial disorder of abnormal copper metabolism. The liver is damaged, and the tests related to the liver are abnormally high. Other symptoms include dysphasia, dysarthria, rigidity, and coarse resting tremors (wing-beating tremors).

12

Reality Shock in the Workplace

Joseph T. Catalano

Learning Objectives

After completing this chapter, the reader will be able to:

- Describe the concept of reality shock.
- Describe appropriate documents and procedures for job interviews.
- List evidential artifacts used to develop professional nursing portfolios.
- Define burnout and list its major symptoms.
- Discuss the key factors that produce burnout.
- List the important elements in personal time management.
- Analyze how the nurse's humanity affects nursing practice.
- List at least four health-care practices nurses can use to prevent burnout and to improve their professional performance.

WHAT IS REALITY SHOCK?

"That is not how we do it in the real world." How many times do students and new graduate nurses hear that sentence? In many ways, that sentence is correct: in nursing school, students are instructed in the ideal theoretical, research-based, and instructor-supervised practice. Although demanding physically, mentally, and emotionally, nursing school shelters students from the realities of the real world, where nursing practice consists of not only theory and research but also heuristic practice, human emotion and response, policies, regulations, and the push and pull of life responsibilities. Things are different in the real world. The transition from nursing student to registered nurse is referred to as **reality shock (transition shock).**

MAKING THE TRANSITION FROM STUDENT TO NURSE

At any point in their lives, most people fulfill several different roles simultaneously. Sometimes, role conflict occurs. Role conflict exists when a person is unable to integrate the three distinct aspects of a given role: *ideal, perceived,* and *performed role images.* For nursing students, a significant role conflict may occur when they transition from the role of student to that of registered nurse.

Ideal Role
In the academic setting, the student is generally presented with the ideal of what a nurse should be. The ideal role projects society's expectations of a nurse. It clearly delineates obligations and responsibilities as well as the rights and privileges that those in the role can claim. Although the ideal role presents a clear image of what is

expected, it is often somewhat unrealistic to believe that everyone in this role will follow this pattern of behaviors.

An Angel of Mercy. The ideal role of the nurse might require someone with superhuman physical strength and ability and unlimited stamina who possesses superior intelligence and decision-making ability, yet remains kind, gentle, caring, and altruistic, not concerned about money. This perfect nurse can communicate with any client at any time and is able to function independently and know more than even the physician. This angel of mercy is able to prevent grievous errors in client care while continuing to always be responsive to clients' needs and requests and carry out the physician's orders with accuracy and absolute obedience. Perceptive students soon begin to suspect that this ideal role of nurse does not exist anywhere in the real world.

Perceived Role

The perceived role is an individual's own definition of the role, often more realistic than the ideal role. When individuals define their own roles, they may reject or modify some of the norms and expectations of society that were used to establish the ideal role. Intentionally or unintentionally, though, the ideal role is often used as the intellectual yardstick against which the perceived role is measured.

After a minimal amount of clinical experience, nursing students may realize that nurses do not possess extraordinary physical strength or intellectual ability but may continue to accept unconditionally, as part of their perceived role, that nurses must be kind, gentle, and understanding at all times with all clients and other health-care staff. The perceived role is the role with which the nursing student often graduates.

Performed Role

The performed role is defined as what the practitioner of the role actually does. Reality shock occurs when the ideal or perceived role comes into conflict with the performed role. Many new graduate nurses soon realize that the accomplishment of role expectations depends on many factors other than their perception

The Department of Health and Human Services currently projects a shortfall of up to 800,000 registered nurses by the year 2020.

and beliefs about how nursing should be performed. The environment has a great deal to do with how the obligations of the role are met.

In nursing school, where students are assigned to care for one or two clients at a time, there is plenty of time to practice therapeutic communication techniques; to provide completely for the physical, mental, educational, emotional, and spiritual needs of the client; and to develop an insightful care plan. The realities of the workplace may dictate that a nurse be assigned to care for six to eight clients at a time. In this situation, the perceived role of the nurse may have to be set aside for the more realistic performed role, from communicator to task organizer. Meeting all of the client's physical, psychological, social, and spiritual needs becomes less possible, and the care plan becomes more brief and to the point.

Cognitive Dissonance. Such situations can produce what is called cognitive dissonance in many new graduate nurses. They know what they should do and how they should do it, yet the circumstances do not allow them to carry it out. The end result is increased anxiety. High levels of anxiety, left unrecognized or unresolved, can lead to various physical and emotional symptoms. When these symptoms become severe enough, a condition called burnout may result. In today's health-care climate and with the current nursing shortage, it is important that health-care agencies retain high-quality nurses and that nursing schools prepare graduates for their transition from student to nurse.

A NURSING SHORTAGE

A lack of qualified nurses has been present in the health-care system for so long that the term *nursing shortage* has become a truism. However, as recent history has demonstrated, the demand for nurses increases and decreases with changes in the health-care system. In addition, the demand for nurses is to some extent regional. Some areas of the country have a higher demand for registered nurses, and others may have fewer available jobs. However, studies about employment opportunities project that there will continue to be a shortage of nurses well into this century.[1]

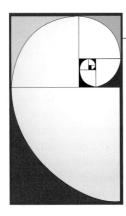

Issues in Practice

Nurses as They Are Portrayed on Television—Really?

I was so excited when I heard that several new fictional television shows were planned for the new television season in the fall of 2009 that featured nurses. One of these actually had the nurse's name and RN in the title. I sincerely hoped these dramas would more accurately portray real-life nursing care. I, once again, was extremely disappointed. After years of not watching medical dramas such as "House," "Grey's Anatomy," and the last several years of "ER," I was looking forward to a drama that depicted more accurately the role of the nurse. I guess it is not meant to be this season.

Why are many current shows depicting nurses as handmaidens to physicians or sex objects? Why are nurses seldom seen on many of these shows? Why do physicians on these shows perform nursing responsibilities? In some shows, a nurse may never been seen unless she or he is being reprimanded because a doctor deemed it so. Why do the nurses in the show, if seen at all, say, "I am just a nurse" or "because the doctor said so"? Why are these shows displaying doctors saying, "I am the doctor, and you are just a nurse" or "you take orders only and are not paid to think." I even had a student tell me she wanted to be a nurse so she could meet and marry a cute doctor like the ones on "Grey's Anatomy."

I had great hope for one of the new television shows. However, I was disappointed in the first 15 minutes when the "nurse" worked with a psychotic patient, found a newborn baby outside the door of the emergency department, started a scalp intravenous line on an infant, worked with a patient in oncology, and made certain policies and procedures were followed. All in the first 15 minutes! I came to three conclusions in these first 15 minutes: (1) the show must be a comedy; (2) this was one "super nurse"; or (3) I have been sorely lacking in organizational skills for the past 30 years. I was exhausted just watching this super nurse.

I decided to watch another new fictional medical drama. Within the first 13 minutes, the "nurse" hit a patient with her fist, worked in several departments, and then kissed one of the "doctors." Needless to say, I turned this show off immediately as well.

Over the past several years, I have tried to watch television shows that accurately depicted the role of the nurse. "ER" did a fairly good job during the first few years, but it even drifted more to a show about physicians and delegated the role of the nurses to the background.

Instead of constantly complaining about the shows, I have tried writing the major television studios, producers, and directors of these shows. None of my letters has ever received a reply. So I do what I can and boycott the shows. This is one act I can do to voice my displeasure.

However, sometimes when I need a break, I may turn on these television medical dramas (or comedies) just to laugh. They can be entertaining even if they are not accurate. Sometimes, they are just good for a laugh, and I do believe laughter is good for the body, mind, and soul.

So if you feel these shows do not accurately depict the role of nurses, make your concerns known to the studios, writers, and producers. Consider not watching except when you need a good laugh.

Issues in Practice   continued

I would like to see a show about real nurses. Let a camera crew follow a real critical-care nurse and record his or her actions during a routine shift. This would truly be an eye-opening experience for the viewing public.

Now on to another subject.

Happy National Nurses Week! Remember, you are a key and essential active participant in health care and in the care of your critically ill patients. Celebrate your profession. Tell people what nurses really do in their chosen profession. Thank a mentor or a colleague. Send a thank-you note to a teacher who made a significant difference in your career. Show those fake "nurses" on television what real nurses do every day.

So, in closing, thank you for all you do for your profession. I appreciate everything you do, and I hope you will continue if you practice for a long time. Moreover, if I am ever one of your patients, I want one of you to be my nurse, not one of those "super nurses" on television.

Respectfully submitted:

Vickie A. Miracle, EdD, RN, CCRN, CCNS, CCRC Editor, DCCN, and Lecturer Bellarmine University School of Nursing Louisville, KY vmiracle@aol.com

Reprinted with permission: Dimensions of Critical Care Nursing, 29(3), 156, 2010.

What Do You Think?

Is there a nursing shortage in your region? Does it affect the health care that you can obtain at your local hospital? How can the nursing shortage be "fixed"?

Nurses in Demand

The demand for nurses is finally being recognized by high school counselors and employment agencies. They are now encouraging young people to enter nursing schools, and enrollment is up. After several years of declines in nursing school enrollments that reduced the number of graduates by almost 30 percent nationally, nursing schools are starting to see dramatic increases in enrollment. Drops in enrollment tend to occur when the economy is strong.

In short, when the economy is strong, there are more opportunities outside of the traditional female employment areas for young women to pursue. Also, overall enrollment in higher education decreases during periods of strong economic growth and increases when the economy takes a downturn.

> *Preceptorships allow students to experience a more realistic employment situation before they graduate.*

There are several reasons for the increased demand for registered nurses. One of the primary reasons is the ever-increasing demand for health care. As the population of the United States continues to age, and there is a recognition that an older population has increased health-care needs, the demand for well-educated, highly skilled nurses will continue to increase. It is also important to note that a high percentage of the currently working registered nurses will retire within the next 10 years and therefore will not be an active part of the workforce. The Department of Health and Human Services currently projects a shortfall of up to 800,000 registered nurses by the year 2020.[2]

During the past several years, some facilities have tried to cut costs by reducing the number of their most expensive personnel, the registered nurses. Most of these facilities have recognized that, although a reduction in registered nurse positions may reduce the costs in the short term, the long-term effects on the quality of health care are devastating. It is obvious that exchanging qualified nurses for lower-paid unlicensed technicians will eventually affect the quality of client care. Hospitals and other health-care facilities are experiencing the results of personnel cutting practices in a reduced number of clients seeking care at these facilities as well as units being closed and revenue being lost.

Decentralized Care

Certain groups of nurses are in higher demand than ever; these include nurses who can practice independently in several different settings, multiskilled practitioners, home care nurses, community nurses, and hospice nurses.[3] A major trend in health care today is to move the care out of the hospital and into the community and home settings. Provision of nursing services in these settings often requires that a nurse have at least a bachelor's degree or even higher education. Fewer than 50 percent of all new graduate nurses today are graduating from bachelor's degree programs.[4]

Although most nurse practitioners are currently based in community clinics, there is an ever-expanding opportunity for them to become involved in the care of hospitalized clients. A key element in many proposed health-care reform plans is that clients must be evaluated by a primary health-care provider before they can be referred to secondary health-care providers or specialists. The advanced-practice education of nurse practitioners would make them eminently qualified to fill this role of primary health-care provider.

Certain specialty areas (e.g., intensive care, neonatal, and burn units) are always seeking nurses. As with community nurses, nurses who provide care in specialty units must be able to work independently and to draw from a large base of theoretical knowledge.

The nursing profession and nursing educators need to increase their vigilance during nursing shortages to maintain the high standards of the profession, to recruit high-quality students, and to retain professional nurses.

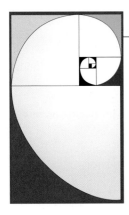

Issues in Practice

The Nursing Shortage: An International Problem

Most of the major nursing organizations in the United States, including the American Nurses Association (ANA), have for many years taken a position against the importing of large numbers of foreign nurses into the United States. Intended to relieve the nursing shortage in this country, this practice is considered bad for the nursing profession and client care. The primary basis for this position is the inconsistent quality of foreign-educated nurses and the lack of control over their practice. Most schemes to use foreign nurses employ some type of institutional licensure, which professional nursing has opposed for more than 60 years (see Chapter 3).

Despite strong opposition from the nursing profession, legislators continue trying to get foreign nurses into the United States. Under the current immigration laws, up to 14,000 nurses can immigrate to the United States each year on employment visas. After working here for 1 year, they can bring their families into the country and obtain green cards. Senator Sam Brownback (R—Kansas) has sponsored a little-noticed proposal in the immigration bill that would raise the floodgates on foreign nurses. He is supported by the American Hospital Association, which wants to fill vacant nursing positions at any cost.

Senator Brownback projected that few nurses from African countries would make the transit, but that the influx of nurses from the Philippines and India, which already send thousands of nurses here each year, would probably increase. His proposal is a Senate-only provision and would remain in effect until 2014. Legislators paid little attention because there were no financial provisions attached. The proposal was tabled, and no action was taken.

Health officials in developing countries were enraged when they learned of the proposal. They believe that removing the restrictions on immigration of nurses into the United States would further deplete their already low supply. In particular, officials in the Philippines view this proposal as contributing to the continued deterioration of their health-care system. Tens of thousands of nurses have moved to the United States in recent years, pulled by the promise of higher wages and better living conditions. In addition, many underpaid physicians in the Philippines have abandoned their medical practices to work as nurses in the United States.

The ANA continues to oppose this practice. They believe that a flood of foreign nurses would negatively affect health care in both the United States and the nurses' countries of origin. One ongoing issue is the effect on the multibillion-dollar effort by the United States to control the worldwide epidemic of AIDS and the resurgence of malaria. If key health-care providers are removed from the countries where these diseases are epidemic, it will become impossible to control their spread.

The ANA maintains the position that Congress should increase appropriations for domestic nursing programs rather than outsourcing nursing education to Third World countries. One significant factor limiting the numbers of nurses educated in the United States is the shortage of nursing faculty. Nurses have little incentive to go into education when professors often earn less than the new nurses they just graduated. Another limiting factor is the access to clinical sites. Hospitals

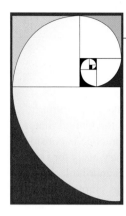

Issues in Practice

are making it increasingly difficult to get students into the various units for clinical practice.

Currently the nursing importation provision is stalled along with the immigration bill. However, it is important that nurses make their position on this issue known to their legislators.

Sources: Brush, BL: International nurse migration: Lessons from the Philippines. Policy, Politics & Nursing Practice 8(1):37–46, 2007.
Carbery, S: Working with international nurses. Healthcare Traveler 14(10):16, 18, 2007.
Dugger, C: U.S. plan to lure nurses may hurt poor nations. New York Times May 24, 2006.
Lumby, J: Solving the global nursing workforce shortage problem. Nursing 8(1):16, 2007.

A POSITIVE TRANSITION TO PROFESSIONAL NURSING

The reality shock that new graduates often experience can be reduced to some extent. Some schools of nursing have instituted preceptor clinical experiences during the last semester of the senior year. The main goal of this type of clinical experience, which occurs just before graduation, is to help the student feel more comfortable in the role of registered nurse.

Preceptorships allow students to experience a more realistic employment situation before they graduate.

A student who works with a preceptor is assigned to one registered nurse for supervision for most of the semester. The student experiences the role of the RN by working the same hours and on the same unit as the nurse to whom he or she is assigned. As the student absorbs the role expectations of the workplace during the preceptor experience, the student's perceived role expectations also change, allowing movement from the student role to that of practicing professional with less anxiety and stress.

Another experience that lessens role transition shock may be called an internship or externship depending on the name used by the hospital. Internships or externships are available to students between the junior and senior years at some hospitals. These experiences allow students to work in a hospital setting as nurses' aides while permitting them to practice, with a few restrictions, at their level of nursing education. These experiences are invaluable for gaining practice in skills and for becoming socialized into the professional role.

Employment in Today's Job Market

Although the health-care industry is in dire need of registered nurses, employers are still looking for the best of the best for the positions they have available.

What Do You Think?

Have you ever been on a job interview? What were some of the mistakes you made? How can you correct these mistakes in the future?

Initial Strategies

Employers are looking for graduates who can function independently, require little retraining or orientation, and can supervise a variety of less-educated and unlicensed employees. The ability to use critical thinking skills in making sound clinical judgments is a necessity in today's fast-paced, complicated, and highly technical health-care systems.

Although these requirements may seem daunting, some strategies can be used to increase the chance of being hired. Students should take advantage of preceptor and intern or extern experiences in their junior and senior years and should attempt to meet their clinical obligations in the institution where they want to be employed. In this way, the student can evaluate the hospital closely and observe its working conditions and the type of care provided to clients.

The hospital, on its part, has the opportunity to examine closely the student's knowledge, skills, personality, and ability to relate to clients and staff. The hospital benefits by getting employees who are familiar with the hospital before employment starts, thus decreasing the overall time of paid adjustment (referred to as "orientation").

The Resume

In today's job market, the **resume** is often the institution's first contact with the nurse seeking employment, and it has a substantial effect on the whole hiring process (Box 12.1). First impressions are important. Preparing a neat, thorough, and professional-looking resume is worth the time and effort. If you have access to a computer, a good-looking resume can be prepared at almost no cost. If a computer is not available, it is a good idea to spend a few dollars to have the resume professionally prepared and reproduced.

Box 12.1
Sample Resume

Mary P. Oak
100 Wood Lane, Nicetown, PA 22222 Telephone (333) 555-1234 (H) e-mail: moak@aol.com

Objectives
Obtain an entry-level position as a Registered Nurse; deliver high-quality nursing care; continue my professional development.

Skills
- Good organizational and time management skills
- Communication and supervisory ability
- Sensitivity to cultural diversity

Education
Mountain University, Nicetown, PA
Bachelor of Science in Nursing, May, 2011

Experience
Supercare Hospital, Hilltown, PA
Nursing Assistant, 2009 to present
    Responsibilities: Direct client care, including bathing, ambulation, daily activities, feeding paralyzed clients, assisting nurses with procedures, charting vital signs, and entering orders on the computer.
Big Bob's Burgers, Hilltown, PA
Assistant Manager, 2004–2009
    Responsibilities: Supervised work of six employees; counted cash-register receipts at end of shift; inventoried and ordered supplies.

Awards
Nursing Student of the Year, 2010
Mountain University, Nicetown, PA
Pine Tree Festival Queen, 2004
Hilltown High School, Hilltown, PA

Professional Membership
National Student Nurses Association, 2010 to present
Mountain University, Nicetown, PA

A Complete Picture

The goal of a resume is to provide the hospital with a complete picture of the prospective employee in as little space as possible. It should be easy to read and visually appealing and have flawless grammar and spelling. Although various formats may be used, all resumes should contain the same information. Each area of information should have a separate heading (see Box 12.1).

Many books available in local bookstores can serve as a guide in organizing the information in a resume. Many new computers now come from the factory loaded with software for the preparation of resumes in different formats. Keep an electronic copy of the resume for future use or reference. The required information includes the following:

- Full name, current address (or address where the person can always be reached), and a telephone number (including area code) and e-mail address.
- Educational background (all degrees), starting with the most recent, naming the institution, location, dates of attendance, and degrees awarded. Usually high school graduation information is not necessary.
- Former employers, again starting with the most recent. Give dates of employment, title of position, name of immediate supervisor, supervisor's telephone number, and a short description of the job responsibilities. Should non–health-care-related work be included? Very basic jobs, for example, cooking hamburgers at Big Bob's Burgers, could probably be omitted unless it fills in a large gap in your employment history. However, if the job required supervision of other employees or demonstrated some higher degree of responsibility such as developing budgets, handling money, or preparing work schedules, it should be included and described.
- Describe any scholarships, achievements, awards, or honors that have been received, along with any professional development activities in which you participated, starting with the most recent.
- List professional memberships, offices held, and date of memberships.
- List any publications. If both books and journal articles were published, list the books separately, starting with the most recent.
- Include an "Other" category to describe any unpublished materials produced (e.g., an internal hospital booklet for use by clients), research projects, **fellowships,** grants, and so forth.
- Provide professional license number and annual number for all states where licensed, along with the date of license and expiration date.

References

References should be included on a separate sheet of paper. Most institutions require three references. After obtaining permission from the individuals listed as references, the nurse preparing the resume should make sure to have current and accurate titles, addresses, e-mail addresses, and telephone numbers.

An individual selected for a reference must know the applicant well in either a professional or a personal capacity, have something positive to say about the applicant, and be in some position of authority. The director of the nursing program, esteemed nursing faculty, supervisory-level personnel at a health-care facility, and even a physician make good references. It is best not to list relatives, unless the hospital is asking specifically for a personal reference.

Do not obtain letters of reference until the facility asks for them. Many facilities are now using e-mail or phone references in place of letters as a time-saving method.

> *First impressions are important. Preparing a neat, thorough, and professional-looking resume is worth the time and effort.*

Online Resumes

Creating a Personal Website Summary

By the time students have completed their nursing education, they have looked at enough websites to know which ones grab their attention and which ones they quickly skip over. There are some general principles that all personal websites should follow, although creativity has a place as long as it is not too far out there! Then when the job applicant e-mails a prospective employer, a link can be attached to the site. Remember that first impressions count.

What to include in a Web page:

1. A professional photo of the applicant on the first page. Grainy cell-phone shots with red eyes do not make a good initial impression. Each page should

have a different, related photo. A resume page should have a candid photo of you in a work setting. A personal page should have a tasteful photo of you at play.

2. On the first page, use creative graphics or background photos that say something positive about you. A picture of a field of wildflowers behind the individual indicates a calm, attractive personality. A picture of a waterfall projects an image of power and direction.

3. Give a short summary of your personality and strengths on the home page. Use third-person descriptions. For example: "Julie's passion is to provide high-quality care to the most vulnerable of the population—premature infants and abused children." This page should also summarize your background. How did you become interested in nursing—through a specific event (e.g., a parent having cancer) or a person who inspired you? Did you have to overcome any particularly difficult circumstances in nursing school? This page can also demonstrate your writing skills. Make sure an experienced writer or editor reviews it before you post it.

> *Harassing the personnel director or director of nursing about a job is not usually an effective employment strategy.*

4. Write a career objective page. This page is like a resume, but it can be longer and is in paragraph form. You can include portfolio images of your work to demonstrate your accomplishments visually—show pictures from that in-service presentation you gave as part of the leadership class assignment. Make sure you include information about your education, employment history, and a description of what you would consider the "perfect career." Describe in a few sentences what your dream job would be like and why. Describe your professional objectives and why they are important to you. Do you want to go back to school to become a nurse practitioner at some point in the future? Why?

5. Include a resume page. This page should use the standard resume format for professional resumes. It should be no longer than one page. Make sure you update the information on this page as it changes. You will be sending the hard copy of this page to employers.

6. Include a contact page with all your contact information: address, phone numbers, and e-mail addresses. Make sure these are kept current. Include a link to the site you created, just in case the prospective employer is not adept at previewing job candidates electronically. Also include a link to the personal website.

Where to Post It?

Several websites are generally recognized as locations for professional resumes. Web-savvy employers will often search these first. They include:

1. www.linkedin.com. This site contains more than 5 million professional resumes and is often used by professionals to track each other. Employers can use it for finding potential employees in specific fields of expertise.

2. www.blogger.com. Probably the easiest of the sites to use. It takes the user through the step-by-step process of setting up a blog in less than 30 minutes.

3. www.moveabletype.com. This corporate communications site for professionals is a little more complicated than the others. It features copyediting and proofreading services that may be useful for beginning bloggers.

4. www.wordpress.com. This site is generally used by top-level professionals, although anyone can post on it. It has some advanced features in design and content generation.[5]

The Cover Letter

A cover letter should be sent with every mailed resume (Box 12.2). Like the resume, it should be neatly typed without errors and should be short and to the point. Although a friendly, rambling letter might provide insight into a prospective employee's underlying personality, most personnel directors or directors of nursing are too busy to read through the whole document. The letter should be written in a business letter format, be centered on the page, and include the name and title of the person who will receive the letter. Letters beginning with "To Whom It May Concern" do not make as favorable an impression.

Box 12.2

Sample Cover Letter

Mary P. Oak
100 Wood Lane
Nicetown, PA 22222

May 25, 2011

Mr. Robert L. Pine
Director of Personnel
Doctors Hospital
Gully City, PA 44444

Dear Mr. Pine:

I am interested in applying for the Registered Nurse position in the General Medical/Surgical Unit. I have 5 years of experience in providing care for a variety of clients with medical/surgical health-care problems as a nursing assistant. I completed my baccalaureate degree in nursing on May 9, and am scheduled to take the NCLEX examination on June 3. Enclosed find my resume.

I believe that my organizational and time management skills will be a great asset to your fine health-care facility. I work well with all types of staff personnel, and having been a nursing assistant for the past 5 years, I can appreciate the problems involved in their supervision.

Thank you very much for consideration of my resume and application. I will call you within the next few days to arrange a date and time for an interview. Feel free to call me at home anytime (333) 555-1234 or contact me by e-mail: moak@ol.com.

Sincerely,

Mary P. Oak

Organizing the Letter

The statement of interest and name of the position should constitute the opening paragraph of the letter. The prospective employee should mention where he or she heard about the position. This information should be included in the first paragraph as well as a date when the applicant would be able to begin working.

The second paragraph should give a brief summary of any work experience or education that qualifies the applicant for this position. Newly graduated nurses will have some difficulty with this part, but they should include their graduation date, the name of the school they graduated from, the prospective date for taking the NCLEX, and the name of the director of the program. This paragraph should also state which shifts the applicant is willing to work.

The third paragraph should be very short. It should express thanks for consideration of the nurse's resume, a telephone number, and an e-mail address. Both the letter and resume should be sent by first-class mail in a 9- by 12-inch envelope so that the resume will remain unfolded, thus making it easier to handle and read.

Will They Ever Answer?

Waiting for a reply can be the most difficult part of the process. Resist the urge to call the hospital too soon. Because most health-care institutions recognize the high anxiety levels of new graduates, they attempt to return calls within 1 to 2 weeks after receipt of the application. If no response is given after 3 weeks, the nurse should call the hospital to see whether the application was received. Mail does get lost. If the application has been received, the applicant should make no further telephone calls. Harassing the personnel director or director of nursing about a job is not usually an effective employment strategy.

The Portfolio

Today's current work climate requires recruiters to interview, screen, and hire the most qualified person for the job in a short amount of time. The nursing shortage and a workforce that embraces career portability have created the need to often recruit and hire nurses on a moment's notice.

Evidence of Positive Outcomes

Professional portfolios are being looked at closely by many nonartist professions to document skill qualifications, continued competency, accountability for professional development, and credible evidence to support employment claims during an interview. Nursing is one of the professions embracing this concept, and if the trend continues, student nurses of today will become the next generation of the 2.6 million registered nurses in the United States who use portfolios instead of resumes to interview for jobs, become certified, maintain certifications, and demonstrate competency.

Health-care employers today are looking for nurses who believe that high-quality performance on the job is more important than just having a job. Professional nurses can apply the nursing process to their own personal development, and evidence of positive outcomes is placed in the portfolio.

Constructing a portfolio requires looking at a career as a collection of experiences, which can be grouped and reordered to match the changing direction of one's career journey. A portfolio also offers an opportunity for nurses to evaluate their experiences, create new goals, create and implement a plan, and then evaluate it. The portfolio supports the life-long process of self and career development.[6]

Assembling a Portfolio

Once a student has decided to initiate a portfolio as a professional vehicle for showcasing his or her experiences, education, skill set, accomplishments, and potential for achievement, it will require time and effort to create it. The effort, however, is well worth it in the long run.

The initial development of a portfolio may be somewhat time consuming, but once it is developed, keeping it current should become part of a professional's routine activities. Many books are available that describe the format and organization of a portfolio; an example is also discussed here.

Use a Binder. One format that many experts agree on is a three-ring binder. This should include a table of contents, and the various sections should be separated by dividers.

Ask Yourself Questions. Questions to ask while you prepare to gather materials for your portfolio include, What do I want to do next in my career? Why do I think I am qualified for this job? What do I want to tell the employer about myself? Why should my employer promote me?

Interview a Professional. Once a decision has been made on an employment area of interest, it is helpful to discuss the needed skills and education with someone who is currently employed in that work setting. Personal interviews can provide information about what skills or education is required. It is a good idea to show a draft of the portfolio to the nurse being interviewed to see if it reflects the required knowledge or if there is a need to pursue further education or skill development.

> *Portfolios are an excellent way to impress potential employers, reach a larger employment pool, and put the Internet to work for a prospective employee.*

Showcase Your Education. Box 12.3 lists work samples that can be included in the portfolio. Box 12.4 lists basic categories for organizing the portfolio. Remember, these are just examples, and each nurse needs to use a format that will best showcase his or her education, work experience, skill set, and accomplishments.

Use the Internet. Creating a Web version of the portfolio can enhance the application process (see earlier). Links can be created to digitized versions of portfolio information, examples of presentations, or photos of accomplishments or events. Portfolios are only limited by the nurse's imagination and access to space on the Web. Portfolios are an excellent way to impress potential employers, reach a larger employment pool, and put the Internet to work for a prospective employee. Even if the nurse has a Web version, it is a good idea to bring the portfolio to an interview.

Box 1 2.3

Examples to Collect for a Professional Portfolio

1. Education and training examples
2. General work performance examples
3. Examples regarding using data or nursing informatics
4. Examples pertaining to people skills
5. Examples demonstrating skills with equipment
   Items that may be collected to support these areas include, but are not limited to, the following:

Articles	Awards
Brochures	College transcripts and degrees
Drawings and designs	Forms
Flyers	Grants
Letters of commendation	Letters of reference
Manuals and handbooks	Merit reviews
Photographs	Military service and awards
Presentations	PowerPoint presentations
Proposals	Professional memberships
Resumes	Research
Technical bulletins	Scholarships
Videos	Training certificates

Box 1 2.4

Categories to Organize Your Professional Portfolio

1. **Career Goals:** Where do you see yourself in 2–5 years?
2. **Professional Philosophy/Mission Statement:** What are your guiding principles?
3. **Traditional Resume:** Concise summary of education, work experience, achievements.
4. **Skills, Abilities, and Marketable Qualities:** Examples that support skill area, performance, knowledge, or personal traits that contribute to your success and ability to apply that skill.
5. **List of Accomplishments:** Examples that highlight the major accomplishments in your career to date.
6. **Samples of Your Work:** See Box 12.3; you can also include CD-ROMs.
7. **Research, Publications, Reports:** Include examples of your written communication abilities.
8. **Letters of Recommendation:** A collection of any kudos you have received, including clients, past employers, professors, etc.
9. **Awards and Honors:** Certificates of award, honor, or scholarship.
10. **Continuing Education:** Certificates from conferences, seminars, workshops, etc.
11. **Formal Education:** Transcripts, degrees, licenses, and certifications.
12. **Professional Development Activities:** Professional associations, professional conferences, offices held.
13. **Military Records, Awards, and Badges:** Evidence of military service, if applicable.
14. **Community/Volunteer Service:** Examples of volunteer work, especially as it may relate to your career.
15. **References:** A list of three to five people who are willing to speak about your strengths, abilities, and experience; prepared letters from same.

As discussed in the previous section, a resume is an excellent tool for allowing the prospective health-care recruiter or employer to receive a concise overview of a potential employee in as little space as possible, and it will serve as a frame of reference once the interview process is complete. A nurse who offers to share a portfolio during the interview process provides tangible evidence of skills, accomplishments, and future potential. Showing a well-prepared portfolio leaves a positive lasting impression with the interviewer and provides a foundation to build on as the nurse's career develops into the future.

Interviews

The next important step in the process is the interview. The interview allows the institution to obtain a firsthand look at the applicant, as well as providing an opportunity for the applicant to obtain important information about the institution and position requirements. The interview often produces high levels of anxiety in new graduates who are interviewing for what might be their first real job.

Make a Good Impression

Again, first impressions are important (Box 12.5). The interview starts the moment the applicant enters the office. Conservative business clothes that are clean, neat, and well pressed are an absolute necessity. Similarly, a conservative hairstyle and a limited amount of accessories, jewelry, and makeup produce the best impression. Smoking, chewing gum, biting fingernails, or pacing nervously does not make a good first impression. The interviewer recognizes that interviews are stress producing and will make allowances for certain stress-related behaviors, but do try to avoid the mistakes listed in Box 12.6.

Box 12.5
Fashion Do's and Don'ts of Interviews

The Do List
Men
1. Do shave or trim facial hair closely.
2. Do use aftershave and/or cologne sparingly (a little goes a long way).
3. Do carry a money clip or leather wallet, and a small, plain functional briefcase.
4. Do wear leather shoes that are polished and in good repair. Lace-up or slip-on shoes are best.
5. Do wear calf-length dark socks.
6. Do wear a tailored suit (blue, gray, beige are best) with a dress shirt (lighter in color than the suit). Do wear a conservative tie.
7. Do shut off your cell phone or beeper.

Women
1. Do apply perfume or cologne sparingly (a little goes a long way).
2. Do invest in a good haircut/perm. Clean, neat, and conservative is best.
3. Do wear shoes that are polished and in good repair. Plain pumps with medium heels are best.
4. Do carry a briefcase or simple (small) handbag that matches your shoes.
5. Do wear hose that coordinate in color, style, and texture with your shoes and outfit. Do take an extra pair for emergencies.
6. Do apply makeup lightly and carefully.
7. Do apply conservatively colored nail polish carefully.
8. Do dress conservatively.
9. Do wear colors that make a strong statement, such as shades of gray in medium to charcoal, or blue in a medium to navy.
10. Do wear small, conservative earrings.
11. Do shut off your cell phone and beeper.

Continued

Box 12.5

Fashion Do's and Don'ts of Interviews—cont'd

The Don't List

Men

1. Don't overstuff wallet, money clip, or briefcase.
2. Don't carry a can of smokeless tobacco in your back pocket or pack of cigarettes in a shirt pocket.
3. Don't wear sandals, running shoes, or cowboy boots.
4. Don't wear socks that are a lighter color than your trousers.
5. Don't wear green or flashy colors.

Women

1. Don't wear sneakers, sandals, cowboy boots, or heels more than $1\frac{1}{2}$ inches high.
2. Don't overstuff your handbag or briefcase.
3. Don't apply makeup so that it looks artificial and heavy.
4. Don't use black or bright or dramatically colored nail polish.
5. Don't wear skimpy or low-cut outfits, leather, or fringed apparel.
6. Don't wear large, dangling earrings or have other body piercings, such as nose rings, lip rings, tongue rings, or multiple earrings.

Sources: Iacono, M: The selection process: Interview tips for nurse managers. Journal of Perianesthesia Nursing 19(5):345–347, 2004.

Puetz, B: The winning job interview: Do your homework. American Journal of Nursing 2005 Career Guide 30–32, 34–35, 2005.

Arriving a few minutes early allows time for last-minute touch-ups of hair and clothes and gives the applicant a chance to calm down. Carrying a small briefcase with a copy of the resume, cover letter, references, and information about the hospital also makes a favorable impression.

Come Prepared

Mental preparation is as important to a successful interview as physical preparation. Most interviewers will start with some "small talk" to attempt to put the interviewee at ease. Resist the temptation to launch into a long and rambling account of personal experiences. Next, the interviewer will usually ask about the resume or portfolio, if one is used. A quick review just before the interview is helpful so that the person being interviewed can avoid appearing ignorant about what information is contained in the resume or portfolio.

Expect questions about positions held for only a short time (less than 1 year), gaps in the employment record (longer than 6 months), employment outside the field of nursing (e.g., waitress, clerk), educational experiences outside the nursing program, or unusual activities outside the employment setting.

Answer the questions honestly but briefly. Most personnel directors or directors of nursing are busy and do not appreciate long, detailed, chatty answers. Applicants can anticipate being asked:

- Why do you want this position?
- Why have you selected this particular facility?
- Why do you think that you are qualified for the position?
- What unique qualifications do you bring to the job to make you more desirable than other applicants?
- Where do you see yourself 5 years from now? Ten years from now?

Using the portfolio will help answer some of these questions. By showing tangible examples of qualifications and accomplishments, the interviewee can help the busy interviewer discern between actual performance and mere rehearsed answers.

Forbidden Topics

Because of the emphasis placed on political correctness and discrimination issues in recent years, there are a number of areas that prospective employers are not supposed to discuss, but sometimes do anyway.

Box 12.6
Twenty Worst Job Interview Mistakes

1. Arriving late
2. Arriving too early (10–15 minutes is OK)
3. Dressing wrong (see Box 12.5)
4. Having your cell phone or beeper go off during the interview (and answering it)
5. Drinking alcohol or smoking before the interview
6. Chewing gum and/or blowing bubbles
7. Bringing along a friend, relative, or children
8. Not being prepared—not having an interview "dress rehearsal"
9. Calling the interviewer by his or her first name
10. Not knowing your strengths and weaknesses
11. Asking too many questions of the interviewer (a few are OK)
12. Not asking any questions at all
13. Asking about pay and vacation as the first questions
14. Accusing the interviewer of discrimination
15. Bad-mouthing your present or former boss or employer
16. Name-dropping to impress the interviewer
17. Appearing lethargic and unenthusiastic
18. Weak, "dead fish," or bone-crusher handshake
19. Looking at your watch during the interview
20. Losing your cool or arguing with the interviewer

Sources: Chun J: Questions to ask during a job interview. Nursing Review 13(26):472, 2010.
Cotton C: Career clinic. Should I bring up pay and conditions issues during the job interview? Community Care 9(1765):32, 2009.
Marriott P: Quality in practice … get the best out of job hunting: Polish your CV and shine at interview. Community Care 4(1808):34, 2010.
Smith LS: Are you ready for your job interview? Nursing 40(4):52–54, 2010.
Strzelecki MV: "I got the job!" How to shine in an interview—and on the job. Occupational Therapy Practice 14(16):9–10, 12, 2009
Yale JW, Mullett S: Nailing the interview for your dream job. Career Search 13–15, 2009.

These include questions about sexual preferences or habits, age, race, plans for a family, personal living arrangements, **significant others,** and religious or political beliefs.

If these questions are asked, the applicant needs to consider the implications of not answering them. Although there is no legal obligation for the applicant to answer, refusal to do so or pointing out that the question should not have been asked in the first place may be unwise. If the graduate answers these personal questions, which violate an individual's right to privacy or seem discriminatory, and then is not hired for the position, there may be grounds for some type of legal action based on discrimination.

Ask Your Own Questions

At some point in the interview, usually toward the end, applicants are asked whether they have any questions. Although most do have questions, many applicants are afraid to ask. In fact, asking questions can be seen as a demonstration of independence, initiative, and intellectual curiosity—all traits that are highly valued by health-care providers. It is important that the first questions are not about salary, vacations, and other benefits. Questions that indicate interest in the institution are included in Box 12.7.

After these questions have been answered, the applicant may want to ask about salary, raises, vacations, and other benefits. It would also be wise to inform the interviewer of the dates scheduled for the

Box 12.7

Questions Interviewees Should Ask

- What are the responsibilities involved in the position?
- Who are the other staff or personnel working on this unit?
- What is the typical client-to-staff ratio for the unit?
- Are there any mandatory rotating shifts, weekend obligations, overtime, or floating?
- Does the hospital offer opportunities for continuing education, clinical ladder, advancement, or movement to other departments?
- Please describe the facility's policies for employee health and safety.

National Council Licensure Examination (NCLEX) so that arrangements can be made for time off. The applicant should also ask for written material on the nurse's contract with the institution, including benefits and job descriptions. Often the interviewer will provide this information without being asked in the course of answering some of the other questions.

It is appropriate to close the interview by asking for a tour of the facility. A tour allows first-hand evaluation of the workplace and a chance to observe the staff and clients in a real work setting. The interviewer may not be able to provide a tour at that time and so may ask another individual (e.g., a secretary) to take the applicant on the tour.

Beware of the Internet
Nothing is Private

Savvy employers almost always Google the name of a prospective employee before an interview. Some employers go even further to find out about the candidate; often they can electronically locate unflattering pictures or video sequences, ill-advised comments or tirades, and even financial information. Although somewhat slow to catch on in the healthcare arena, this trend is taking hold. The following scenario is an example of what happened during one candidate's interview for a job.

The job applicant had successfully fielded all the usual interview questions: "Why do you want this job?," "What are your qualifications?," "Why should I select you over other candidates?" Then the interviewer asked the question that all job applicants hate: "What do you consider your major weakness?"

The applicant's idea of the "right" answer was "I tend to be a perfectionist and spend too much time trying to get things perfect." After hearing this statement, the interviewer replied, "I found a video segment of you on MySpace.com that was shot about 2 years ago showing you at a party with very few clothes on. Would you mind commenting about that?"

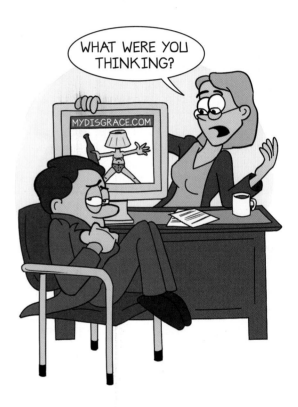

It Never Goes Away

As a candidate for a job, especially as a new graduate, you need to be aware that the person sitting across from you at the interview desk may well have run your name through an electronic search engine. Personal blogs can be deleted and after a time will become harder to access. However, the truth is that once something goes electronic, it never completely goes away. Search engines have improved to such a point that they can find information that is 5 or more years old.

Although you can use the Internet to your advantage, it can also be a tool of your own demise in the job market. You may feel secure and private in a chat room with your "friends," but in reality, anything you post on the Internet can end up on MySpace, Facebook, YouTube, Xanda, or one of the other blog websites. You may feel safe using a pseudonym or password protection, but these are only as trustworthy as the people who have access to your information. A jilted boyfriend or girl-friend, a friend who thinks what you said was funny, someone with a large circle of electronic friends: all have the power to reveal your most private information.[7]

You can offset negative information about yourself by generating as much positive information as possible. Eventually, the positive information will get more hits, and the negative information will be pushed to the end of the site, where people are less likely to see it. Remember, nobody is perfect, and all people have information they would prefer to keep secret. If negative information about you does exist online, you can try to control it by spinning it in the best way possible.

Business Cards—Old School?

In some circles, business cards are considered old school. Some experts recommend that, instead of sending out piles of resumes and waiting for a call back, modern job seekers send out Web-based summaries of themselves. These summaries, icons, or branded bios go by the name of "thlogs."

Follow-Up

As with the resume, making frequent calls about the results of the interview is unwise. It is, however, appropriate for the applicant to send a letter within 1 week after the interview to thank the interviewer for his or her time and express appreciation for being considered for the position (Box 12.8). The applicant should also acknowledge how much it would mean to him or her to become a member of the staff at such a high-quality agency or hospital, but avoid overdoing the compliments.

If the position is offered, a formal letter of acceptance or refusal should be sent to the institution. Health-care facilities will not hold positions

Box 12.8
Sample Follow-up Letter

Mary P. Oak
100 Wood Lane
Nicetown, PA 22222

June 20, 2011

Mr. Robert L. Pine
Director of Personnel
Doctors Hospital
Gully City, PA 44444

Dear Mr. Pine:

Thank you very much for considering my resume and for the interview on June 3, 20116. I learned a great deal from the interview and from my tour of the hospital after the interview.

I am writing to let you know that I am still interested in the position and was wondering about the status of my application. If at all possible, I would appreciate it if you could either call me or write a note relating to my potential employment at your facility.

Feel free to call me at home any time (333) 555-1234, or contact me by e-mail: moak@aol.com

Sincerely,

Mary P. Oak

indefinitely, and failure to accept the position formally in a timely manner may result in their offering the position to someone else.

WHEN NURSES BURN OUT

The **burnout syndrome** has existed for many years and has been recognized as a problem that can be reduced or even prevented. A widely accepted definition of burnout is a state of emotional exhaustion that results from the accumulative **stress** of an individual's life, including work, personal, and family responsibilities. Although the term is not often applied to students, many of the symptoms of burnout can be observed in these aspiring nurses.[8]

Who Burns Out?

The people who are most likely to experience burnout tend to be more intelligent than average, hard working, idealistic, and perfectionist. There are certain categories of jobs and careers that tend to produce a higher incidence of burnout: situations and positions in which there is a demand for consistently high-quality performance, unclear or unrealistic expectations, little control over the work situation, and inadequate financial rewards. These jobs or careers tend to be very demanding and stressful, with little recognition or appreciation of what is being done. Also, jobs in which there is constant contact with people (i.e., customers, clients, students, or criminals) rank high on the burnout list.

Even with the most superficial knowledge of nursing, it is easy to see that many of these elements are present in the nurse's work situation. It is possible to recognize nurses who are in the early stages of burnout by identifying some classic behaviors (Box 12.9).

How It Starts

One of the earliest indications of burnout is the attitude that work is something to be tolerated rather than eagerly anticipated. Nurses in the early stages of burnout often are irritable, impatient, cynical, pessimistic, whiny, or callous toward coworkers and clients. These nurses take frequent sick days, are chronically late for their shifts, drink too much, eat too much, and often are not able to sleep.

Box 12.9

Symptoms of Burnout

- Extreme fatigue
- Exhaustion
- Frequent illness
- Overeating
- Headaches
- Sleeping problems
- Physical complaints
- Alcohol abuse
- Mood swings
- Emotional displays
- Anxiety
- Poor-quality work
- Anger
- Guilt
- Depression

Eventually, as their idealism erodes, their work suffers. They become careless in the performance of their duties, uncooperative with their colleagues, and unable to concentrate on what they are doing, and they display a general attitude of boredom and **apathy.** If allowed to continue, burnout may lead to feelings of helplessness, powerlessness, purposelessness, and guilt.[9]

Avoiding Burnout

Despite this bleak picture, nurses do not have to fall victim to the burnout syndrome. Many nurses practice their profession for many years, manage to deal with the stress, and find great personal satisfaction in what they do. These satisfied and motivated nurses have developed ways to deal with the stress of their careers while maintaining their goals and purpose as nurses.

The first step in dealing with burnout is to be able to recognize its signs. Many nurses who are burning out use denial and rationalization to block recognition of burnout because it is just too painful for them to think they put so much time, money, and effort into preparing for a career they no longer want or enjoy. It is important to realize that it is not the career that is producing the burnout, but rather the difficulty in coping with the stresses the career is producing. Although it may not be possible to change the requirements of the profession significantly, it is possible to learn how to cope more effectively with stress.

Manage Stress and Time

Although there are many schools of thought about stress- and time-management techniques, several common threads run through many of these theories. These views include setting personal goals, identifying problems, and using strategies for problem solving.

Set Personal Goals

Goals and goal setting are an important part of client care. Nursing students—and, by extension, practicing nurses—are highly proficient in the planning stage of the nursing process, in which goal setting is the primary task. Nurses know that a good set of goals should be client centered, time oriented, and measurable and that they should write these goals with every care plan they prepare.

In their personal lives, however, these nurses may rush full tilt into one erratic day after another, subordinating their own needs to the needs of others and working long, hard hours, but without accomplishing very much and feeling frustrated about it. What is the problem here? Very simply, nurses can prepare realistic, beneficial goals for their clients, but they seem to be unable to do the same for themselves.

" Health-care employers today are looking for nurses who believe that high-quality performance on the job is more important than just having a job. Professional nurses can apply the nursing process to their own personal development, and the evidence of positive outcomes is placed in the portfolio. "

Long-Term Goals

Personal goals should include both long-term and short-term goals. Typically, personal long-term goals look into the future at least 10 years and include a statement about what the nurse wants to achieve during his or her lifetime. Some examples are going back to school to obtain an advanced degree, becoming a director of nursing, or even writing a book about nursing.

Practicing nurses who are caught up in the whirlwind of everyday life find it difficult to formulate statements about the future. One other important characteristic of long-term goals is that they need to be flexible. As life circumstances change, modifications are required.

Short-Term Goals

Short-term goals are those that the nurse expects to accomplish in 6 months to 2 years. These goals should be aimed primarily at making the nurse's professional or personal life more satisfying and fulfilling. Like long-term goals, they do not need to be related to work. Perhaps visiting a foreign country, going on a skiing trip in the mountains, and even learning how to paint a picture or play the piano may be achievable in a relatively short time. In the professional realm, joining a professional organization, becoming a head nurse, or changing an outdated hospital policy are goals that can be achieved in a short time. The fact that everyone ages over time cannot be altered, but that time can also be used to achieve personal satisfaction in life and increase knowledge and accomplishments.

An End Achieved

Although goal setting is an important first step in dealing with the stress that leads to burnout, any good nurse recognizes that a plan without implementation is useless. As difficult as goal setting may be for nurses, carrying it out may be even more difficult. Although goal achievement requires a degree of hard work and personal sacrifice, when people are working toward something they really want, the effort that it takes to achieve the end actually becomes enjoyable. At first glance, this process may seem like a lot of work (and it is), but it becomes an exciting adventure in its own right.

Identifying Problems

Another important step in dealing with burnout is to identify the problems that are producing the stress. Again, nurses are taught as students that they need to identify client problems so that they can work toward solving them.

Self-Diagnosis

Formulation of a nursing diagnosis is nothing more than precisely stating a client's problem. One thing nurses realize early in the learning process is that what may appear to be an obvious problem may in reality not be a problem at all. Conversely, something that a client only mentions in passing may turn out to be the real source of the client's nursing needs. Perhaps nurses should look at their own lives and attempt to formulate nursing diagnoses that deal with their stress-related problems (setting the North American Nursing Diagnosis Association list aside).

What Do You Think?

List three tasks that you have put off today. Why did you avoid doing these? How can you get them done sooner?

For example, a new graduate has just completed a shift during which he was assigned to eight complete-care clients. He has had to supervise two badly prepared nurses' aides and has put in 55 minutes of overtime (for which he will not be paid) to complete the charting. This nurse is feeling tired, frustrated, and even a little bit guilty because of an inability to provide the type of care that he was taught in nursing school.

> *It is important to realize that it is not the career that is producing the burnout, but rather the difficulty in coping with the stresses the career is producing.*

What is the problem? A possible nursing diagnosis might be: Alterations in personal satisfaction related to excessive workload, evidenced by sore feet, headache, shaky hands, feelings of guilt, frustration, and a small paycheck.

Goals and Interventions

Now that the problem has been identified, goals and interventions can be introduced to solve the problem. The goals may range from organizing time better to refusing to take care of so many complete-care clients. Interventions, depending on the goals, can include activities such as attending a time-management seminar, talking to the head nurse, or changing a policy in the policy and procedure book.

RESPONDING TO MAJOR STRESSFUL EVENTS

Crisis Intervention

Although nurses often learn how to deal with the stresses routinely found in their daily work, major traumatic events that produce overwhelming stress, such as the devastation of the World Trade Center Towers or Hurricane Katrina, may leave nurses with a sense of horror, helplessness, and powerlessness in addition to the normal stress responses of shock, disbelief, anger, and grief. Nurses do have a number of skills that help them deal with traumatic events in their workplace; however, they are not super-people and should not expect that they can handle all stressful events without help. The end result may well be a complex of symptoms similar to burnout syndrome, including physical symptoms, depression, and chronic anxiety.

In response to major tragedies in recent years, the critical incident stress debriefing (CISD) process was developed to help health-care providers deal with major acts of violence and traumatic disasters. The American Red Cross has been instrumental in training and providing resources for local CISD teams. These are made up of mental health professionals specially trained in crisis intervention, stress management, and treating post-traumatic stress disorder (PTSD).

To be most effective, the CISD teams need to be on site within 2 to 3 days after serious events, ranging from the death of coworkers to acts of terrorism and natural disasters such as tornadoes. The goal of the team is to encourage the participants to verbalize their feelings and thoughts, identify and develop their coping skills, and generally lower overall grief and anxiety levels. They provide an intensive stress management course compressed into a few hours or few days.

Post-Traumatic Stress Disorder

One of the keys to working with nurses is to help them recognize that they are not expected to be able to handle all situations and can appropriately ask for help. Although nurses study the stress response and grieving process in school, it is sometimes hard for them to apply information about normal stress reactions to themselves. When nurses do not recognize their own problems in responding to traumatic stress, they increase their risk for developing long-term stress reactions. When they do not seek help, they can develop the symptoms of PTSD anywhere from a few days to as long as 6 months after the event.

Warning signs of PTSD include:

1. Recurring nightmares and inability to sleep
2. Intrusive and vivid flashbacks
3. Prolonged depression
4. High levels of anxiety
5. Maladaptive coping behaviors, such as drug and alcohol abuse

The CISD session generally requires up to 3 hours. Sessions can be longer or shorter depending on the nature of the event and number of people affected. Besides having an opportunity to express emotions and feeling, the participants are educated in some ways about reducing anxiety and promoting mental and physical health. Advice includes:

1. Not watching televised replays of the event over and over
2. Staying with friends as much as possible
3. Avoiding unhealthy, high-fat diets
4. Engaging in regular aerobic exercise as much as possible
5. Avoiding excessive dependence on alcohol and drugs for sleep
6. Getting back to a comfortable routine as soon as possible
7. Feeling comfortable seeking professional help when it is needed

During the CISD sessions, nurses are asked for their input about the process. If the team feels it is necessary, additional referrals for long-term treatment may be recommended.

STRATEGIES FOR PROBLEM SOLVING

Nurses already know the nursing process as a client problem-solving technique. Why not apply the same knowledge and skills to personal problems? The stress level only increases if problems are left unsolved.

Although specific problems may require specific solutions, several widely accepted methods exist to deal with the general stresses produced by everyday work and personal life. Included in these methods are activities such as recognizing that nurses are only human, improving time-management skills, practicing what is preached, and decompressing.

Time-Management Skills
In modern life there is often not enough time to do everything that needs to be done. The key to time management is setting priorities. In the world of nursing and client care, nurses are often required to do many tasks. Multitasking, the process of doing several tasks at the same time, tends to fragment the nurse's attention and concentration.

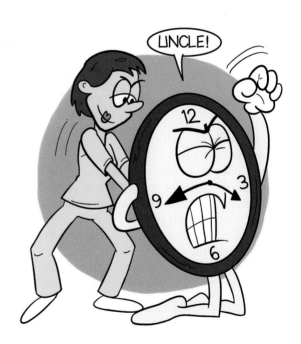

Nurses need to recognize that only some nursing activities are essential to the safety and well-being of clients. These include performing thorough assessment and ensuring that the clients get their medications on time, that their comfort needs are met, and that accidental injuries are prevented. Beyond these actions, nurses really have a great deal of discretion in what they can do when providing care to clients.

Make Room for Fulfillment

Burnout results mainly from personal and professional dissatisfaction. If nurses feel fulfilled in what they are doing, burnout is much less likely to occur. Activities that may increase nurses' satisfaction include spending time talking with clients, learning new skills, and decreasing the anxiety of families through teaching and listening. After such activities have been identified, time should be set aside for them during the shift. The real secret in using time management to prevent burnout is for the nurse to use the time left for those nursing activities that bring the most professional and personal satisfaction.

Several skills need to be developed to allow time during a shift for these preferred activities. First, the nurse must learn to delegate by letting the licensed practical nurses (LPNs) or aides do those tasks they are supposed to be able to do. Many nurses graduate from nursing school with the attitude that if you want it done right, you need to do it yourself. After becoming familiar with the LPN's and nurse's aide job descriptions, nurses need to give others a chance to prove themselves.[10]

> *Tension must be released, or it will eventually cause a major explosion or (if turned inward) produce anxiety.*

Overcome Procrastination

Another necessary skill is overcoming procrastination. Most people have a natural tendency toward procrastination, particularly when unpleasant or difficult tasks are involved. The primary reasons people postpone or delay doing something are that they either do not want to begin or do not know where to begin the task. More time and energy are expended in inventing excuses for putting off tasks than would be taken in doing the tasks.

The Most Distasteful Task. The best way to overcome procrastination is by starting the task, even if it is only a small step. An effective method is to select the most distasteful task to be done that day and to commit just 5 minutes to it. After 5 minutes are over, the task can be either set aside or continued. It is very likely that once the task is started and momentum builds, the task will be carried out to completion.

Tasks can be prioritized by listing them in three categories. Category A tasks (e.g., assessments, passing out medications, treatments, and dressing changes) are important and need to be completed on time. Category B tasks (e.g., baths, linen changes, lunch breaks, charting) are important, but can be postponed until later in the shift. Category C tasks (e.g., cleaning up, organizing the supply room) are tasks that can either be delegated or wait until the next day.

Problems Don't Solve Themselves. For daily tasks, both pleasant and unpleasant, the best time to do them is immediately. If achievement of the plan requires delegation, it needs to be done at the beginning of the shift, not at the middle or end of the shift. Often nurses have a built-in fear of taking chances. As a result, they avoid doing things if there is a chance of failure, in the hope that somehow the problem will resolve itself.

Any time an important decision is made, there is a chance that someone will disagree or that the decision will be incorrect. These types of situations need to be viewed as a challenge or an opportunity rather than a life-altering risk to be avoided. Although mistakes in health care do have the potential to be fatal, learning from mistakes is one of the most fundamental ways of increasing knowledge.

Time management, like other skills, requires some practice. Once a nurse masters this skill, his or her life becomes more satisfying.

Practicing What You Preach

Because nursing is oriented toward keeping people healthy as well as curing illness, nurses spend a large amount of their time teaching clients about eating well; getting enough sleep; going for regular dental, eye, and physical examinations; avoiding too much drinking and smoking; and exercising regularly. It might make an interesting student research project to have nurses rank themselves on how well they have incorporated these health maintenance activities in their own lives. The results would probably indicate a low overall score on the "practice what you preach" scale.

Nurses know all about the food pyramid, but they do not translate that knowledge into feeding themselves properly. In reality, there are going to be some busy days when it is impossible to eat right, but it should be possible, on a regular basis, to follow a diet that will promote health and reduce the buildup of fat plaques in the arteries.

It is important to get enough sleep to avoid chronic fatigue. People can adjust to a state of fatigue, but it tends to decrease the enjoyment that they find in life, as well as make them irritable, careless, and inefficient. Most people need between 5 and 8 hours of good sleep each night. It also probably would not hurt for nurses to take a short nap during the afternoon on their days off.

The Right Kind of Exercise
Many nurses feel they get enough exercise during their busy shifts, and, in truth, the average staff nurse walks between 2 and 5 miles during each 8-hour shift. Unfortunately, this type of walking does not qualify as the type of aerobic exercise recommended for an improved cardiovascular condition. Exercise, in order to be beneficial, must be done consistently and must raise the heart rate above the normal range for an extended period. The short sprint-type walking involved in client care does not accomplish this goal. Walking 1 to 2 miles a day outside of work is a beneficial, simple exercise that will improve health. Nurses can also use a wide variety of exercise equipment for those days when walking outside is undesirable. The important requirement is that the exercise be done consistently and frequently. Regular exercise not only improves the cardiovascular system but also helps improve stamina, raise self-image, and promote a general sense of well-being.

Decompression Time
The profession of nursing is stressful, even under ideal circumstances. Nurses are required to deal with other people constantly and to carry out numerous tasks that are potentially dangerous. At the end of any shift, even the most skilled and best-organized nurse has a sense of internal tension. This tension must be released, or it will eventually cause a major explosion or (if turned inward) produce anxiety.

Establish a Daily Decompression Routine
It may take a little time to discover, through trial and error, what works to reduce the tension built up during the shift. Some effective techniques include setting aside approximately 30 minutes of private, quiet time to dream and reflect about the day's activities. Perhaps relaxing in a tub of hot soapy water or sitting in a favorite reclining chair might meet the need for decompression. Relaxation activities, such as swimming, shopping, or even going for a drive, can help reduce tension and act as a time for decompression. Of course, stress-management techniques learned at seminars (e.g., self-hypnosis or meditation) can be used by those who have developed these skills. Finally, meeting with a nurse support group can help the nurse vent feelings and make constructive plans for solving problems.

Conclusion

Although transition shock and burnout are realities of the nursing profession, they can be reduced or even avoided altogether. Nurses should be able to recognize the causes and early symptoms of transition shock and burnout to prevent them from developing into a problem. Therefore, nurses should use techniques to prevent these disorders from becoming insurmountable obstacles. In doing so, nurses will be able to practice their profession proficiently and gain the satisfaction that only nursing can provide.

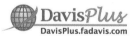
DavisPlus.fadavis.com

Critical Thinking Exercises

- Make a list of the characteristics that would be found in the "perfect nurse." Make a second list of characteristics found in nurses observed in actual practice. Discuss how and why these lists differ.
- Outline a plan for implementing a preceptor clinical experience for the senior class of a nursing program. Make sure to include how many hours of practice are required, criteria for the selection of preceptors, student objectives from the experience, and methods of evaluation.
- Write at least three long-term and five short-term personal or professional goals. Develop a realistic plan and time frame for achieving these goals. Make sure to include what is required to achieve these goals.
- Complete this statement, using as many examples as possible: "I feel most satisfied when I am done with my shift in knowing that . . ." Analyze these answers and discuss how they can be implemented in everyday practice.
- Think of at least three situations in which you were asked to do something that you really did not want to do. How did you handle these situations? How could they be handled in a more assertive manner?

3

Leading and Managing

13

Principles of Leadership and Management

Joseph T. Catalano

Learning Objectives

After completing this chapter, the reader will be able to:

- Identify and discuss the three major theories used to explain leadership.
- Define and distinguish among the three styles of leadership.
- Discuss the relationship of transformational and situational theories to leadership style.d
- Identify the key behaviors and qualities of effective leaders.
- Distinguish the differences between management and leadership.
- Identify and discuss the two major theories of management.

In today's health-care system, even new graduates who have an "RN" after their name will be placed quickly in positions of leadership and management.

LEADERSHIP

The old saying that "leaders are born, not made" implies that at birth a person either is a leader or is forever relegated to the rank of follower. Not many agree with this statement. Although some people may have an easier time filling the leadership role than others, most experts believe that almost everyone can develop leadership skills.

Many definitions of leadership refer to the ability of an individual to influence the behavior of others. When nurses exert leadership, they inspire other health-care workers to work toward one or more of several goals that include providing high-quality client care, maintaining a safe working environment, developing new policies and procedures, and increasing the power of the profession.

Some leadership theories try to explain why some people are leaders and others are not, but as yet none covers all the possibilities. That may be because leadership requirements differ according to the situation. In the intensive care unit (ICU), for example, where quick decisions are a matter of life and death, the leader is the nurse with highly developed critical thinking and analytical skills and the confidence to make decisions under pressure. In quality management, where the problems are often long term and complicated, the leader tends to be well organized and can methodically sift through a mountain of information and statistics to develop a policy that covers the widest range of possibilities. Several of the better-known leadership theories are discussed here.

Trait Theory

The trait theory identifies qualities that are common to effective leaders (Box 13.1). Trait theory by itself is limited because it focuses only on the traits of the individual and does not take into account how the person

Box 13.1

Leadership Traits

- High level of intelligence and skill
- Self-motivation and initiative
- Ability to communicate well
- Self-confidence and assertiveness
- Creativity
- Persistence
- Stress tolerance
- Willingness to take risks
- Ability to accept criticism

acts in specific situations. The question left unanswered is why everyone who has these traits is not a leader.[1]

Leadership-Style Theory

One of the best-known theories of leadership looks at three leadership styles:

1. Laissez-faire
2. Democratic
3. Authoritarian

Although these theories are discussed separately, they are a continuum of leadership style ranging from a mostly passive approach to a highly controlling one (Table 13.1).

The Laissez-Faire Style

The **laissez-faire** (French for "leave it alone") leadership style is also described as permissive, nondirective, or passive. The laissez-faire style leader allows the group he or she is leading to determine their own goals and the methods to achieve them. There is little planning, minimal decision making, and a lack of involvement by the leader. This style works well in only a few settings, for example, in a research laboratory that is staffed by self-motivated scientists who know what they want to achieve and are familiar with the means of achieving it.

The laissez-faire style works best when the members of the group have the same level of education as the leader and the leader performs the same tasks as the group members. In most situations, however, the laissez-faire leadership style can leave people feeling lost and frustrated because of the lack of direction by the leader. When they do try to achieve some goal, often the only input from the leader is that they are doing it incorrectly. When faced with a difficult decision, laissez-faire leaders usually avoid making a decision in the hopes that the problem will resolve itself.

The Democratic Style

In the **democratic** (also called supportive or participative) leadership style, all aspects of the process of achieving a goal, from planning and goal setting to implementing and taking credit for the success of the project, are shared by the group.

The democratic leadership style is based on four beliefs:

1. Every member of the group needs to participate in all decision making.
2. Within the limits established by the group, freedom of expression is allowed to maximize creativity.
3. Individuals in the group accept responsibility for themselves and for the welfare of the whole group.

Table 13.1 Comparison of Authoritarian, Democratic, and Laissez-Faire Theories

	Authoritarian	Democratic	Laissez-Faire
Degree of freedom	Little freedom	Moderate freedom	Much freedom
Degree of control	High control	Moderate control	Little control
Decision making	Leader only	Leader and group	Group or no one
Leader activity level	High	High	Minimal
Responsibility	Leader	Leader and group	Abdicated
Quality of output	High quality	High quality/creative	Variable
Efficiency	Very efficient	Moderately efficient	Variable

Source: Whitehead, DK, Weiss, SA, Tappen, RM: Essentials of Nursing Leadership and Management (5th ed). Philadelphia, F. A. Davis, 2010, p. 6

4. Each member must respect all the other members of the group as unique and valuable contributors.[2]

    The leader using the democratic style provides guidance to the group, and all members share control. This style works best with groups whose members have a relatively equal status and who know each other well because they have worked together for an extended period. In its purist form, democratic leadership can be time consuming and inefficient in some situations, particularly when group members disagree strongly, but in the end, when a goal is achieved or a decision made, there is a strong sense of ownership and achievement by the whole group. Many leaders are uncomfortable with this style of leadership because of the minimal control they have over the group. Participative leadership allows the leader more control over the final decision. After considering all the opinions of the group, the leader makes the final decision based on what is best to achieve the goal.

The Authoritarian Style

The leader with an **authoritarian** (also called controlling, directive, or autocratic) style maintains strong control over all aspects of the group and its activities. Authoritarian leaders provide direction by giving orders that the group is expected to carry out without question. The final decision-making authority rests with the leader alone, although input from the group may be considered.

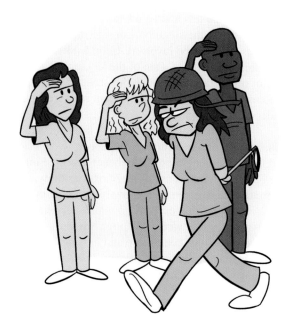

The Dictator

A leader using a dictatorial authoritarian style has no regard for the feelings and needs of the group members. Achieving the goal is the only thing that matters, and the leader will use any means, including harsh criticism, to do so. A military mission to destroy a terrorist group by a Delta Force assault team is an example of this type of leadership.

What Do You Think?

Have you ever had to be a leader in a group? What type of leadership style did you use? How successful was the outcome of the group work?

The Benevolent Leader

The benevolent authoritarian leader uses a more paternalistic approach to achieving the goal. That leader attempts to include the group's feelings and concerns in the final decision, but ultimately the leader makes the decision. Some group members may feel that the benevolent leader is condescending and patronizing.

    The authoritarian leadership style works best in emergency situations, when clear directions are required to save a life or prevent injury, or in situations in which it is necessary to organize a large group of individuals. Although highly efficient in achieving goals and completing tasks, authoritarian leadership suppresses the creativity of the group members and may reduce the long-term effectiveness of the group. Authoritarian leadership also reduces the motivation levels of the group and may lead to passive–aggressive behavior by the members that will further reduce the effectiveness of the group. Although some people can accept the need for the total control exerted by an authoritarian leader, most people in a long-term work relationship with this type of leader will become frustrated and even rebellious at some point.

    In reality, few leaders use only one style. Most leaders use multiple leadership styles that depend on the situation. Many factors may influence what type of leadership style is used at any given time, including external regulations and requirements, the ability of the group members, the work setting, and the problem being solved. For example, a nurse manager on a hospital unit may use a highly democratic style in most of the routine activities of the unit, but when a client goes into cardiac arrest, she may revert to a highly authoritarian style while directing the staff through a code.

Relationship–Task Orientation
High Relationship–Low Task

Another commonly used theory rates leaders on whether they are oriented more toward establishing relationships or achieving assigned tasks and resolving problems. Leaders with high relationship–low task orientations are usually well liked by their groups because of their acceptance of the group members as individuals, consideration of their feelings, encouragement, and promotion of good feelings among all the group members.

> *The old saying that 'leaders are born, not made' implies that at birth a person either is a leader or is forever relegated to the rank of follower.*

However, this kind of leader often sacrifices the achievement of the task or resolution of a problem when it conflicts with the feelings or good will of the group. This leader often allows the group to make its own decisions without regard to the task at hand and ultimately may not achieve the goals the group was organized for in the first place.

High Task–Low Relationship

The opposite extreme is the leader with a low relationship–high task orientation. This form of leadership is similar to the authoritarian style, where the leader does all the planning with little regard to the input or feelings of the group, gives orders, and expects them to be carried out without question. Various forms of punishment are used by this leader, ranging from verbal put-downs to poor performance evaluations that are used to determine pay raises.

Both Extremes

The worst leader is the person with a low relationship–low task orientation. This leadership style simulates the laissez-faire style, in which the leader is uninvolved, does no planning, has little concern for the group members' feelings, and accomplishes little. On the other hand, the best leader is the one with a high relationship–high task orientation. This leader combines the best of both worlds: he or she is open to input and actively communicates with the group members, provides constructive direction, quickly resolves conflicts, and ultimately achieves creative and effective solutions to problems.

Certainly, perfect leaders are difficult to find. Most use a combination of styles and adjust them to the circumstances surrounding the problem. Again, think of the nurse manager who uses a high relationship–high task orientation for managing the unit in most day-to-day operations. In the cardiac arrest situation, this nurse manager may quickly change her or his orientation to one of low relationship–high task until the crisis is resolved.

RECENT THEORIES OF LEADERSHIP

Although the behavior and trait theories remain popular, researchers have come to the conclusion that leadership is really a more complex process. The situational theory recognizes that no one approach works in all situations. A leader needs to acknowledge this and adjust the leadership style and behavior to the situation, considering the many variables that may be involved. Good leaders seem to do this instinctively. One of the key factors is the type of organization in which the group is located. The environment is always important in exercising leadership.

The transformational theory takes the situational theory one step further. This theory recognizes that multiple intangibles exist whenever people interact. Factors such as sense of meaning, creativity, inspiration, and vision all are involved in creating a sense of mission that exceeds good interpersonal relationships and rewards. Although this is true in most work settings, health care and nursing, in which care of human beings is the primary goal, require that nurses do something positive. In many health-care facilities, nursing leaders are expected to inspire excitement and commitment in nurses, who often must provide care to very ill clients in less than ideal circumstances.

KEY LEADERSHIP BEHAVIORS

Traits are characteristics that an individual possesses. Traits may or may not lead to the actions or behaviors that are required for successful leadership. It is also possible to lack leadership traits, yet be able to carry out successful leadership behaviors.

Critical Thinking. The ability to think critically is a multistep process similar to the nursing process. Critical thinkers must be able to analyze data, organize and plan, and use creativity in the resolution of problems (see Chapter 6). Leaders must often make important decisions on the basis of incomplete data.

Problem Solving. Being able to use the problem-solving process effectively is essential to effective leadership. Leaders in the health-care setting face problems that arise from many sources, including staffing and personnel, scheduling, and administrative, budget, and client demands.

Acknowledgment and Respect for Individual Differences. Personality is the sum total of people's experiences. Because no two people have identical experiences, each one has different needs, feelings, and orientations. The effective leader recognizes these differences and is able to direct people to their highest level of achievement given their varying orientations.

Active Listening. To be effective, leaders must be able not only to hear the words that the person is saying but also to observe the body language and its underlying emotions and meaning. The experts tell us that only 7 percent of communication is verbal; 93 percent is all the other nonverbal content. Leaders often fail in their leadership roles when they do not listen to the full message of the individuals they are attempting to lead.

Skillful Communication. Communication is a complex process that involves an exchange of information and feedback (see Chapter 14). Mistakes happen

> *The authoritarian leadership style works best in emergency situations, when clear directions are required to save a life or prevent injury, or in situations in which it is necessary to organize a large group of individuals.*

on both sides when the information being shared is incomplete or confusing. Providing frequent and positive feedback is one of the best methods for leaders to determine how well they are communicating and how open the communication channels remain. It also can boost morale and improve the working environment. Effective leaders should also be able to give and use negative feedback to improve performance. If negative feedback is given in a nonthreatening and encouraging manner, the person receiving it will often appreciate the chance to improve his or her skills.

Establishment of Clear Goals and Outcomes. The old question, "How do you know when you've arrived if you don't know where you are going?" is a truism that all leaders must address at some point by establishing clear goals and outcomes for the group. Groups who lack clear goals often feel frustrated and lost. Initially, leaders must clearly identify their goals. Then they must identify the goals shared by the group and use them to motivate the group. Successful outcome is often a thoughtful melding of the vision of the leader and that of the group.

Continued Personal and Professional Development. One of the most valuable lessons that nursing students can learn while in school is that education does not end when they graduate—it just begins. One of the primary goals of the nursing education process should be to teach the student how to learn. Lifelong learning is a goal that effective leaders seek not only for themselves but also for those whom they are leading. Leaders can function as teachers in certain settings, but a more effective means of encouraging others to continue to learn is to set a good example. It is important to recognize that learning takes place not only in a formal school-like setting but also in all those encounters and situations that affect attitudes, beliefs, and behavior.

KEY LEADERSHIP QUALITIES

No matter what style a leader favors, successful leaders have common qualities (Box 13.2).

Box 13.2
Keys to Leadership

Key Qualities
- Integrity
- Courage
- Initiative
- Energy
- Optimism
- Perseverance
- Well-roundedness
- Coping skills
- Self-knowledge

Key Behaviors
- Critical thinking
- Problem solving
- Acknowledgment of and respect for individual differences
- Active listening
- Skillful communication
- Establishment of clear goals and outcomes
- Continued personal and professional development

Source: Adapted from Tappen, RM, et al.: Essentials of Nursing Leadership and Management (5th ed). Philadelphia, F. A. Davis, 2010, p. 8.

Integrity. For many years, nursing has been ranked number one as the most trusted and respected profession in the annual Gallup Poll. One of the keys to this trust and respect is the integrity of the profession as it is perceived by clients and their families. The public expects nurses, as a group, to be honest, trustworthy, ethical, moral, and professional. The American Nurses Association (ANA) Code of Ethics for Nurses (see Chapter 7) is directed toward promoting and maintaining the integrity of the profession. If a group observes less than complete integrity in their leader, that person's ability to lead is markedly diminished.

Courage. Although all leaders must have the courage to maintain their convictions in the face of adversity, certain leadership positions may require a higher degree of courage. Nurses in middle management positions, such as unit managers, house supervisors, or quality control coordinators, often find themselves caught in a no-man's land between two opposing

worlds.[3] For example, higher management may be attempting to implement a plan or procedure that the staff nurses strongly object to, or the staff nurses may be complaining about some issue, such as staffing, that the middle manager has little control over. The leader in this situation may need to risk offending one or the other of the groups to resolve a difficult problem.

Initiative. Effective leadership demands that the leader be a "self-starter" and have the ability to start projects without pressure from above. Often the group relies on the leader to begin the process of completing a task or resolving a problem.

Energy. Energy refers not only to the ability to do work but also to the display of that energy in the form of enthusiasm for the work. Energy and enthusiasm are contagious. Charismatic leaders are the ones who are the most energetic and enthusiastic. The group needs to see that the leader is willing to work as hard as they are being asked to work. However, energy has to be rationed carefully to maintain the optimum levels. It is easy for a leader to burn out, particularly when the expenditure of energy seems to produce little or no tangible result.

Optimism. A positive attitude is also contagious. Conversely, so is a negative attitude, which often leads to discouragement and failure (Table 13.2). A leader who has an overall positive attitude and views new problems as opportunities for success will be much more successful than the leader who constantly complains about each new crisis.

Table 13.2 Winner or Whiner—Which One Are You?

A Winner Says . . .	A Whiner Says . . .
We have a real challenge here.	This is a big problem.
I'll do my best.	Do I have to do this?
That's great!	That's nice, I guess.
We can do it.	It can't be done, it's impossible.
Yes.	Maybe, when I have some time.

Source: Whitehead, DK, Weiss, SA, Tappen, RM: Essentials of Nursing Leadership and Management (5th ed). Philadelphia, F. A. Davis, 2010, p. 8.

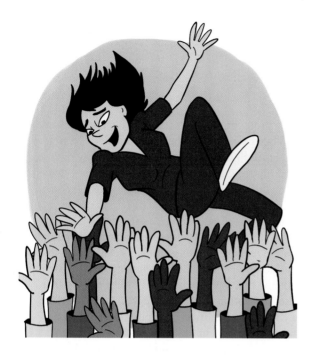

Self-Knowledge. Leaders who do not know and understand themselves are less able to understand those who are working for them. Self-awareness is the beginning of self-acceptance as a thinking, feeling person who interacts with other thinking, feeling persons. Unless leaders understand and accept their motivations, biases, and perceptions, they will not be able to understand why they feel and react in certain ways to certain individuals and situations.

MANAGEMENT

Unlike the development of leadership theory, which primarily focused on the leader, the early study of management was aimed toward influencing employees to be as productive as was humanly possible. Two schools of thought address and define management.

Time–Motion Theory

Time–motion theory developed out of the early industrial age, in which theorists concentrated on ways to complete a task most easily and efficiently. Often their efforts resulted in increased productivity but decreased employee satisfaction. From this viewpoint, management can be defined as planning, organizing, commanding, coordinating, and controlling the work of any particular group of employees. In the time–motion approach, providing the right incentives, primarily money, is expected to increase employee productivity. Although the weaknesses of this approach make it less desirable in today's society, variations of it served as the harbingers of many of the business techniques currently in use.

Human Interaction Theory

Early in the study of management, the limits of the time–motion approach became evident. Researchers observed that some lower-paid employee groups had higher levels of productivity than others with higher pay who were doing the same jobs. It appeared that factors such as employees' attitudes, fears, hopes, personal problems, social status in the group, and visions strongly influenced how they worked. From this perspective, management can be defined as the ability to elicit from employees their commitment, loyalty, creativity, productivity, and continuous improvement.

Perseverance. Leaders need to be able to continue to work through difficult problems in difficult circumstances, even when others feel like quitting. Again, if the leader sets the example for the group with a "there's more than one way to skin a cat" attitude, the group will be encouraged to find new and creative solutions.

Well-Roundedness. Leaders, as well as those they are leading, live multifaceted lives. It is important to develop and foster nonwork relationships with friends and family. Time at work should be balanced with recreational, spiritual, social, and cultural activities that complete the person and round out the personality. Time must also be invested in maintaining good health through proper nutrition and regular exercise, which will help prevent burnout (see Chapter 12).

Coping Skills. All jobs have some degree of stress, although people in leadership positions often experience higher levels. Stress can be handled in two ways: unconsciously, through defense mechanisms, or consciously, by bringing learned coping skills into play. A more productive way to deal with stress is to use coping skills developed in dealing with past stressors to promote a positive and healthy resolution to the stress. Some people learn how to use the stress they experience to motivate them and to tap into the energy it generates to achieve at a higher level of functioning.

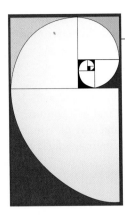

Issues Now

Leadership/Management Case Study

Resolving Staffing Issues

On a busy medical-surgical unit, a group of staff nurses were concerned about the process of making assignments. They believed that the usual practice of assigning nurses to a different group of clients each day eliminated any continuity of care, decreasing the quality of care and lowering morale among the staff. They agreed to meet with the nurse manager as a group to discuss ways of resolving the issues.

The meeting soon became confrontational. The staff nurses expressed a feeling of having very little autonomy in the selection of assignments. The nurse manager expressed the opinion that the nurses were being uncooperative and didn't understand the problems involved in making client assignments. She stated that her primary responsibility was to ensure provision of the best nursing care possible to all clients. The staff nurses countered that the current system wasn't doing that.

The staff nurses proposed a solution: After shift report, they would be allowed to select the clients they felt most qualified to care for, with the same clients reassigned to them on subsequent days until the clients were discharged. The initial response by the nurse manager was that it would be impossible to use this method in a fair and equitable manner. She also wondered what would happen if no one wanted to care for a very difficult client, and how continuity would be maintained on the nurses' days off.

QUESTIONS FOR THOUGHT

1. How would a nurse manager who used an authoritarian system of management resolve this issue?

2. How would a nurse manager who used a laissez-faire system resolve this issue?

3. How would a nurse manager who used a participative system resolve this issue?

4. What initial mistake did the nurse manager make in dealing with this problem?

(Answers are found at the end of the chapter.)

Managers who favored the human interaction theory were required to develop a different set of management skills, including understanding human behavior, counseling effectively, increasing motivation, using effective leadership skills, and maintaining productive communication. Just being a "nice guy" was not enough to guarantee employee cooperation and commitment. To be effective, management needed to be able to recognize and respond to employee concerns and needs, gain acceptance, and protect workers from pressures from higher administration.

It is also important to keep in mind that different management forms are necessary for different work settings. A predominantly time–motion approach may still work best in an area such as manufacturing of automobiles or washing machines. Using the same approach would be inappropriate and probably ineffective for managing a group of registered nurses (RNs) working in an ICU of a busy city hospital.

Motivational Theory

Motivational theory can be defined as the ability to influence the choices people make among a number of possible choices open to them. For example, what factors would motivate a new graduate nurse to work at one hospital when there are four facilities offering her or him a job? Are the pay and benefits better? Maybe it is closer to home. Perhaps the shifts are better and the facility does not require mandatory overtime.

Several theorists have attempted to explain this phenomenon. Probably the best known is Abraham Maslow, who developed the Hierarchy of Needs Theory. Although nursing students are taught and use this theory to deal with client needs, the theory also has applications in the realm of leadership and management. Maslow believes that human needs are arranged in a hierarchy from the most basic and essential to the more complex. Most basic are the physiological and safety needs, and until these are met in at least a satisfactory fashion, the person is less likely to deal with the higher needs such as social relationships, self-esteem, and self-actualization.[4]

For example, if a nurse was not being paid a salary that would meet the needs for food, housing, and clothing, those needs would become the nurse's

Charismatic leaders are the ones who are the most energetic and enthusiastic. The group needs to see that the leader is willing to work as hard as they are being asked to work.

primary concern rather than delivering high-quality client care. Realistically, needs are never fully met, but they have to be accommodated to a degree to which the person feels comfortable enough to move up in the hierarchy.

Motivation–Hygiene Theory

Another theory that has become popular is Herzberg's Motivation–Hygiene Theory. Although there are some similarities between Maslow's and Herzberg's theories, particularly in their applications, Herzberg believes that people have two different categories of needs that are fundamentally different from each other.[5]

Hygiene Factors

The first category is referred to as needs dissatisfiers, or hygiene factors. According to Herzberg, if these needs are not met, the person feels dissatisfied with his or her job and focuses more on the environment than the work that is supposed to be performed. Hygiene factors are related to the work environment and include, for example, salary and benefits, job security, status in the organization, work conditions, policies, and relationships with coworkers.

Hygiene factors are related to the conditions under which the work is performed and not to the work itself. They only serve as negative motivators—when they are not met, work productivity is reduced. However, if they are satisfied, there is no guarantee that increased productivity and higher-quality performance will result.

Needs Motivators

The second category of needs, according to Herzberg, is called satisfiers, or needs motivators. Unlike the hygiene factors, satisfiers focus primarily on the work. Some of the more important satisfiers that have been identified include elements that expand the work challenges and scope, such as career advancement, increased responsibility, recognition for achievements, and opportunities for professional growth. The satisfiers can have both a positive and a negative motivation effect. If they are satisfied, they can motivate workers to increased productivity and higher-quality work. If they are not satisfied, they often have the opposite effect.

Motivation in the Hospital Setting

Herzberg concludes that employers must satisfy the hygiene factors as a minimum requirement before there can be any increase in productivity. Programs to promote job enrichment will be effective in upgrading the achievement, roles, and satisfaction of employees. In the hospital setting, career or clinical ladder programs provide nurses with the recognition for achievement and opportunity for advancement, along with financial rewards (hygiene factor), and allow them to remain in direct client care.

It is important for RNs to understand and be able to use motivation techniques, even if they are not in a designated management role. The ability to motivate is one of the keys to success in delegation at any level, and the success of RNs is often assessed by the job performance of people on the health-care team they are supervising. Successful motivation is the door to successful leadership because these are the people who can make things happen in an organization.

> *The ability to motivate is one of the keys to success in delegation at any level, and the success of RNs is often assessed by how well people on the health-care team they are supervising perform their jobs.*

MAKING CHANGES SUCCESSFULLY

Motivating people to change is one of the most challenging and most important functions of leadership. Simply stated, change is the process of transforming, altering, or becoming different from what was before.[6] Although change is a constant in health care and nursing, it is surprising how resistant nurses can be to even minor changes in their work environment.

Internal or External?

Two primary forces bring about change: external forces that originate from outside the person or organization, and internal forces that start from within the individual or organization. A primary example of external change is what happens when government agencies pass down new rules and regulations, such as the HIPAA legislation, that affect health care. An example of internal change would be a hospital increasing salaries or eliminating mandatory overtime from the work action of a group of nurses.

Planned or Unplanned?

Change can be planned or unplanned. Planned change is more productive and occurs when there is a directed and designed implementation of some element within the organization. Change can affect all aspects of an organization, including policies, goals, organizational philosophy, work environment, and even structure. Planned change can be used for all sorts of projects, ranging from the minor to the most complex.

Unplanned change, sometimes called reactive change, occurs when a problem forces a person or organization into a situation in which it must respond. These changes are often minor but sometimes can involve projects that are large in scope and complexity. Examples in nursing include changes in staffing because of nurses who call in sick, clients who experience cardiac arrest, or even equipment failures, such as when the electricity fails or a water main breaks.

A Driving Force for Change

Nurses often take on the role of the change agent, that is, the one who brings about the change (Box 13.3). All change requires the ability to overcome resistance to change (called restraining forces) by a driving force that pushes toward change. When the driving and restraining forces are equal, no change occurs, and the status quo is maintained.

Change can occur only when the driving force is greater than the restraining force. Those who want to change have a tendency to push, but those who are being asked to change tend to push back to maintain things as they are. It is important when attempting to implement change to identify the restraining forces and ways to overcome them. Habit, comfort, and inertia are the three most common restraining forces.

Box 13.3

Characteristics of an Effective Change Agent

- Is well organized
- Identifies restraining forces
- Is able to motivate
- Demonstrates and maintains commitment to change
- Develops trusting relationships
- Responds to feedback and negotiation
- Is goal directed
- Communicates well
- Maintains optimistic attitude

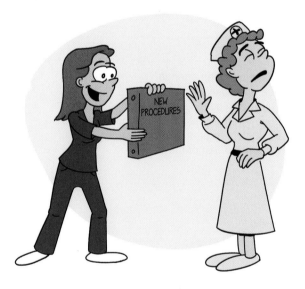

Planned change works best when it is well organized, proceeds at a steady pace, and has a definite date for achievement. There is a level of excitement that raises energy levels when a change is near completion, but postponing the date for the change can drain that energy and lead to disappointment.

GROUP DYNAMICS

A Common Goal

All successful leaders and managers understand and are able to use the principles of group dynamics. A group exists when three or more people interact and are held together by a common bond or interests. Groups are open systems that interact with the environment to achieve a goal (see Chapter 4). The individuals who make up the group are its subsystems and interact with each other as well as with the environment. Group dynamics provides the principles that underlie team building, which is essential to the success of nursing units. Establishing and sharing common goals is the starting point for successful team building.

When the common goal is to help one another, effective team building results. Members of the team respond most positively when they feel included in the decision making and when they realize that their input is valued by the other team members. It is important that the leader always ask team members for their ideas about the goal that the team is working toward. A strong team spirit is crucial to the success of the team.

A Common Understanding

Similarly, the team will only function smoothly when the members understand their roles and the roles of the other members. Their roles identify their places on the team and establish what is expected from each member. To be successful, the leader must establish the belief that all the roles are of equal importance in achieving the goals or purposes of the group.

Mutual Support. Team members need to realize they are not merely responsible for their own roles but also must support the roles of the other members. Although the leader establishes the goals to be achieved, it is important that the team members be allowed to achieve their tasks in ways that are most appropriate for them, particularly in the case of self-motivated professionals such as nurses.[7]

Reward for Achievement. Ongoing or complicated projects require a long-term commitment that is sometimes difficult to maintain. Effective team leaders are good at finding accomplishments along the way that the team can celebrate and enjoy. It allows the team members to feel good about what they have achieved to this point and motivates them to accomplish more in the future. A good leader also recognizes the accomplishments of others and rewards them appropriately. Often even simple statements of praise can be effective.

Identity and Trust. Finally, establishing a sense of team identity and trust completes the group dynamic and team-building process. Some degree of creativity may be required for establishing team identity, ranging from similar uniforms to buttons or pins. Trust allows the team members to be more open to communications from other members and more willing to take risks. Trust empowers the members, allowing them to make independent decisions and promoting the smooth functioning of the team (Table 13.3).

CARE DELIVERY MODELS

Nowhere are the elements of group dynamics reflected better than in the nursing units of a hospital or health-care facility. The organizational structure found in the nursing units of a facility reflects how the nursing department interacts with coworkers and participates in the delivery of client care. Various models may be used in the delivery of nursing care. Many health-care facilities have made a transition from one model to another and may even incorporate several different models at the same time. The nurse must recognize which model is being used as well as its strengths and weaknesses. These models include functional nursing, team nursing, primary care nursing, and modular nursing (Table 13.4).

Functional Nursing

Functional nursing has as its foundation a task-oriented philosophy: each person performs a specific job that is narrowly defined according to the needs of the unit. The medication nurse, for example, focuses

Table 13.3   Do's and Don'ts of Effective Change Agents

Do's	Don'ts
Do develop a sense of trust.	Don't have a hidden agenda.
Do establish common goals.	Don't be unpredictable.
Do facilitate effective communication.	Don't miss or reschedule meetings frequently.
Do establish a strong team identity.	Don't use threats or bluffs to manipulate members.
Do contribute as much as possible.	Don't volunteer to be the record keeper.
Do find reasons to celebrate and recognize accomplishments.	Don't follow the rest of the crowd.

Table 13.4   Comparison of Common Client-Care Models

Model	Nurses Are Called	Description	Where Model Is Used
Functional	Charge nurse Medical nurse Treatment nurse	Nurses are assigned to specific tasks rather than specific clients.	Hospitals Nursing homes Nurse consultants Operating rooms
Team	Team leader Team member	Nursing staff members are divided into small groups responsible for the total care of a given number of clients.	Hospitals Nursing homes Home care Hospice
Primary care	Primary nurse Associate nurse	Nurses are designated either as the primary nurse responsible for clients' care or as the associate nurse who assists in carrying out the care.	Hospitals Specialty units Dialysis Home care
Modular	Care pair	Nurses are paired with less-trained caregivers. Generally involves cross-training of personnel.	Hospitals Home health care Transport teams

on administering and documenting medications for the assigned group of clients.

In this organizational unit, the nurse manager is called the charge nurse, whose main responsibility is to oversee the various workers. Charge nurses are also appointed for each shift to manage the care during that time. This model relies on ancillary health workers, such as nurses' aides and orderlies. Some believe this model fragments care too much. Because many people have specific tasks, coordination can be difficult, and the holistic perspective may be lost.[8]

Team Nursing

Team nursing has a more unified approach to client care, with team members functioning together to achieve client goals. The team leader functions as the person ultimately responsible for the clients' well-being. More cohesiveness is present among the members of the team than is found in the functional model. Rather than having a narrow task to accomplish, team members focus on team goals under the coordination of the team leader. The team conference provides for effective communication and follow-up among team members and is the key to successful team nursing.

Primary Care Nursing

The primary care nursing model gives nurses the opportunity to focus on the whole person. The **primary care nurse** provides and is responsible for all of the client's nursing needs. The nurse manager in this model becomes a facilitator for the primary care nurses. Primary care nurses are self-directed and concerned with consistency of care. The primary care model is similar to the case management model, which has one nurse providing total care for one or more clients. Many home health-care agencies use this method of assigning an RN to work with an individual or family for the duration of the services rendered.

Modular Nursing
A Response to Downsizing

Modular nursing, also called client-focused care, is one model that was developed in response to professional nursing personnel shortages and to the downsizing of professional nursing staffs. This model is based on a decentralized organizational system that emphasizes close interdisciplinary collaboration. Redesigning the method of nursing care delivery takes much planning and input from the various departments involved, such as nursing, respiratory therapy, physical therapy, radiology, laboratory, and dietary.

Important aspects of modular nursing include relying on unlicensed assistive personnel (UAPs), also called unit service assistants, for the provision of direct care, grouping clients with similar needs, developing relative intensity measures, and emphasizing team concepts in small groups that remain constant.

Strong, Explicit Leadership

Cross-training of personnel is another important aspect of modular nursing. For example, using this system, respiratory therapists do not just provide respiratory treatments but also help clients to the bathroom and turn bedridden clients. Nurse managers in this system are responsible for providing explicit job descriptions, maintaining the work group's cohesiveness, carefully monitoring each staff person's abilities, delegating tasks as appropriate, and evaluating the effectiveness of care.

The role of UAPs is one area of the client-focused care model that needs more definition, particularly in relation to the RN's accountability and responsibilities in supervising these workers. State boards of nursing across the country are considering possible changes in nurse practice acts necessitated by the use of UAPs.

Benefits of this care delivery model include decreased staffing cost and greater autonomy of cross-trained personnel. The nurse manager must be a strong leader for this model of care delivery to succeed. Consistent collaboration between the nurse manager and physician is of utmost importance in planning client care.

> *Leadership can be exerted either formally or informally. Often the most effective leaders in a group are not the ones who are officially designated as the leaders.*

LEADERSHIP VERSUS MANAGEMENT

Several questions arise when people speak about leadership and management.

Are They the Same Thing?

Leadership can be exerted either formally or informally. Often the most effective leaders in a group are not the ones who are officially designated as the leaders. On the other hand, managers are given the title by some higher authority and have formally designated authority to supervise a group of employees in the achievement of a task. Similarly, managers can be held formally responsible for the quality, quantity, and cost of the work that the supervised employees produce.

Do Managers Need Good Leadership Skills?

The most effective managers will have highly developed leadership skills. However, by virtue of their title and position, even managers with poor leadership skills are still the official authority, although their effectiveness is reduced. Often, in groups in which the manager is not a good leader, unofficial leaders emerge and exert either a strong positive or a negative influence on the group. If the unofficial leader is generally supportive of the manager's and administration's goals, the work group can be highly productive, and the organization's goals will be achieved. Conversely, if the unofficial leader's goals are opposed to those of the manager and administration, productivity may decrease to a point at which higher-level management asks the manager to leave the position.

Are Leaders Always Good Managers?

A person who has leadership ability may not have good management skills. This phenomenon is often seen in the nursing profession when a highly effective and skilled staff nurse who functions as the unofficial unit leader is taken out of that role and promoted to an official management position. Some do well; others may require additional training in management principles and skills. Some never quite master the skills needed for management.

Management and leadership skills complement each other. As with all skills, they can be learned and require practice and experience to be developed fully. Even new graduate nurses can be effective leaders within their new nursing roles. As they gain experience and develop new skills, their ability and opportunities to provide leadership will also increase. Learning and improving skills in one area will increase the ability in the other.

FUNCTIONS OF THE NURSE MANAGER

Nurse managers often find themselves located on the organizational chart between employees and upper-level management. The functions and duties of nurse managers depend to a great degree on how the institution defines the role. One of the first activities of a new nurse manager is to make sure he or she understands the job description, responsibilities, and level of authority the position has in the institution where he or she is employed. Some of the tasks that have been identified as being a regular part of a nurse manager's position are listed in Box 13.4.

In today's health-care system, nurse managers continue to follow the trend of moving away from close supervision of the staff nurses' work to helping them complete their work safely and effectively. As this role continues to evolve, the emphasis will shift from traditional management functions to highly supportive functions, such as are seen in the leadership role.[9]

Box 13.4

Common Tasks for Nurse Managers

- Conduct orientation of new staff
- Evaluate staff
- Terminate employees with unsatisfactory work performance
- Develop time schedules that cover the unit safely
- Make team and staff assignments
- Develop a realistic budget for the unit
- Justify the number of nursing hours used by the unit
- Call in nurses on their days off when staffing falls short
- Attend nursing management meetings
- Hold regular meetings with unit staff to resolve problems and implement new policies and procedures
- Set unit goals for staff
- Contribute to facility goals
- Communicate regularly with physicians about unit problems
- Conduct quality assurance studies
- Provide rewards for high-quality care

Conclusion

Over the years, there has been one constant in the changing health-care system: the registered nurse is still expected to provide leadership and management skills to direct and ensure the high quality of the health care given to clients. Both leadership and management require sets of skills that can be learned. Nurses who learn these skills will become successful managers and the leaders of the health-care system in the future.

Successful leaders and managers understand and often combine the best aspects of the many theories that deal with leadership and management. Knowledge of one's strengths and weaknesses provides the basis for successful management. Developing effective leadership and management skills is a lifelong, ongoing process. Learning from books and articles, as well as from other successful nurse managers, presents an opportunity for professional and personal growth.

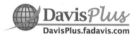

DavisPlus.fadavis.com

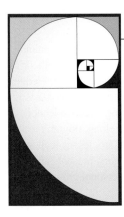

Issues in Practice

Jill, a registered nurse, was recently appointed as the evening charge nurse on a busy postsurgical unit. She has been an active participant in the hospital's quality assurance committee for the past 2 years since her graduation. One of the issues the committee identified as a problem was the higher-than-average surgical wound infection rate on Jill's unit. After some research, Jill determined that a major component of the high infection rate was the procedures that were used when changing postoperative dressings.

After obtaining permission from the unit manager and hospital education director, Jill developed a new procedure for dressing changes, incorporating the most current research. She presented the changes in a short in-service program to the unit personnel, and explained the changes several times to each of the three shifts to make sure that all the nurses and staff on the unit were familiar with the new changes. The expectation was that there would be a 25 percent reduction in wound infections after the new procedures had been used for 1 month.

At the end of the first month of using the new dressing change procedures, the postoperative wound infection rate showed no improvement over the previous month's rate. At the monthly staff meeting, Jill discovered that the licensed practical nurses (LPNs) on the unit were refusing to use the new procedures because they "took too much time" and had reverted to the procedures they had always used before.

Answers to Case Study Questions

Issues Now: Leadership/Management Case Study (page 264)

1. A nurse manager who uses the authoritarian system would maintain her position that the proposed plan was unworkable. Relying on her position of authority, she would insist that the nurses continue to use the established system of assignment. Any staff nurse who felt she or he could not work under this system could seek reassignment to another unit.
2. A nurse manager using the laissez-faire system would allow the nurses to try out the proposed system as they wanted. If any problems resulted from it, they would have to figure out how to resolve the problems themselves.
3. A nurse manager using the participative system would recognize that there is always some common ground between herself and the staff nurses. It is important to identify the common points and then work toward resolving the areas of disagreement. For example, the nurse manager could work with the staff nurses to develop a set of criteria for assignments that would be agreeable to all parties and ensure the quality of client care. The nurse manager would then retain the ability to assign clients, but would be using criteria that were developed by the staff. In the end, staff cooperation and morale would increase, as would the continuity and quality of care being provided by the unit.
4. The initial mistake the nurse manager made was meeting with the staff nurses as a group. The staff nurses would have done better to select one or two representatives to bring their issues to the nurse manager. Using this approach eliminates the "mob mentality" that sometimes develops with large groups. It also forces the staff nurses to identify the specific issues they want to resolve.

Source: Whitehead, DK, Weiss, SA, Tappen, RM: Essentials of Nursing Leadership and Management (4th ed). Philadelphia, F. A. Davis, 2006.

Critical Thinking Questions

- What was the style of leadership and management that Jill used when attempting to initiate the dressing procedure change?
- Other than the stated reason, why do you think the LPNs did not want to use the new procedures?
- How can Jill increase the level of compliance by the LPNs on the unit?
- What is the role of the unit manager in initiating the new dressing change procedures?

14

Communicating Successfully

Joseph T. Catalano

Learning Objectives

After completing this chapter, the reader will be able to:

- Explain the importance of understanding human behaviors.
- Describe conflict resolution and relationship tools.
- Identify communication styles.
- Analyze and apply problem-solving and conflict-resolution tools.
- Discuss the use of the nursing process in conflict resolution.
- Formulate coping strategies to handle difficult people.

THE NURSE AS COMMUNICATOR

Good communication skills are often advertised as the answer to many of the problems encountered in everyday life. Television personalities, instructors, and psychologists promote improved communication skills as the answer to parental, marital, financial, and work-related problems. The nursing profession recognizes communication as one of the cornerstones of its practice. Nurses must be able to communicate with clients, family members, physicians, peers, and associates in an effective and constructive manner to achieve their goals of high-quality care. Good communication is essential for good leadership and management.

In today's rapidly evolving health-care system, registered nurses (RNs) are called on to supervise a growing number of assistive and unlicensed personnel. One of the keys to good supervision is the ability to communicate to people what they must do to provide the required care and, often, how the care should be given. It is not always easy. Many of the people whom nurses supervise have limited training, lack the theoretical and technical knowledge base of the nurse, and may display attitudes that make them resistant to direction. However, nurse supervisors can be and often are held legally responsible for the actions of those individuals who work under their direction.

FACTORS THAT AFFECT COMMUNICATION

Change

Change is one of the few absolute certainties in today's health-care system. Change can produce many emotions, ranging from excitement and anticipation to stress, fear, and anxiety. How people deal with change can affect how they respond to the environment and communicate with others.

At minimum, change makes most people feel uncomfortable. Any change can be simultaneously positive and negative. During the process of learning new skills, treatments, or techniques, most people feel a sense of accomplishment at the same time that they feel afraid of making mistakes, being judged by others, or being labeled as "slow learners."

Fear of the Unknown

Imagine a new graduate nurse starting his or her first day at work, very excited about the new experience and the potential for career development. However, at the same time the nurse is worried about being accepted into the group, being able to practice what was learned in nursing school, and being able to learn the new skills required by the unit. Almost everyone has a sense of dread when moving away from activities with which they have become comfortable. Setting realistic personal goals and time lines for learning new information helps reduce fear and stress when making major changes.

Change affects communication in various ways. People may be afraid to ask questions about new procedures or policies because they fear that they might appear "stupid" in front of their colleagues. Fear of being criticized closes individuals off to positive suggestions and new ideas. Others may hesitate in sharing ideas because they are afraid of being labeled as confrontational.

> *People may be afraid to ask questions about new procedures or policies because they fear that they might appear 'stupid' in front of their colleagues.*

For example, a nurse is reassigned from the medical-surgical unit to the intensive care unit (ICU). This nurse will initially be somewhat fearful in the new environment with the highly trained and assertive expert unit nurses who always seem to be in control. A more positive approach would be for the new nurse to take advantage of the unit nurses' expertise and learn from their examples. The new nurse needs to remember that everyone on that unit was a novice at one time. In the current health-care system, almost everyone is fearful much of the time of making mistakes and of falling short of the high standards of the profession.

The Need to Take Risks

Change can have both positive and negative effects. Often a staff who initially resist a change and fight to prevent it, once they have gone through the process, would never go back to the old way of doing things. All change involves some risk taking, and some people are better at risk taking than are others. Consider the following case study:

> After analyzing the needs of the clients and the nursing workload of a busy medical unit, the unit manager decided to change the work shift times. In addition to the standard 7 a.m. to 3 p.m., 3 p.m. to 11 p.m., and 11 p.m. to 7 a.m. shifts, she decided to add a 5 a.m. to 1 p.m. shift to increase coverage during the busiest period of the shift. The registered nurse (RN) assigned to the new shift recognized the benefits to the unit and clients; thus, she accepted and supported the change with few objections. Also, the change in shift times allowed her to alter her personal schedule so that she could take extra courses toward her master's degree at a local college. For the RN, the change in shifts was a positive experience.
>
> However, the licensed practical nurse (LPN) assigned to this new shift was upset with the change. She was a "late sleeper" and did not want to come in so early. She liked the shifts the way they were and did not see any advantages to changing things needlessly.
>
> After the new shift was initiated, the LPN was usually 15 to 30 minutes late, called in sick frequently, and was "grumpy" and hard to talk to when she did come in to work. For this LPN, the change was negative and unacceptable.

Grief Stages

Nurses need to keep in mind that the communication abilities of clients experiencing change will be affected in much the same way as those of nurses experiencing change. As a result of disease, trauma, or surgery, many clients face sudden and major alterations in their bodies, as well as changes in their ability to function and carry out daily self-care activities. For example, a client with a new colostomy must adapt to major physiological, psychological, and emotional changes.

Most clients who have surgical procedures that result in major body function alterations go through the stages of the grief process: denial, anger, guilt, depression, and resolution. Communication with a client in the anger stage, who is hostile, critical of his care, and verbally abusive, will be very different from communication with a client in the depression stage, who is withdrawn, reticent, and sleeps most of the time. Recognition of the communication behaviors of each of the grief stages is essential to understanding why clients are acting in a particular way. A decision must then be made regarding the most effective communication technique to use when providing care.

Stress

Stress is produced by many factors and always affects an individual's ability to communicate. Some common causes of stress for health-care workers include institutional restructuring, group interaction and dynamics, unilateral management decisions, and personal issues and experiences. Regardless of the source, stress usually decreases people's ability to interact and communicate and increases the demands on their coping mechanisms.

A Destructive Circle

When people are unable to cope with a stressful situation successfully, they may experience an increased state of tension or anxiety. They may develop physiological symptoms, such as nausea, stomach cramps, diarrhea, or palpitations; in extreme cases, they may even become paranoid or psychotic. Uncontrolled high levels of stress on a nursing unit may lead to competition among the nurses that affects their teamwork, productivity, and the quality of the care given.

Physicians who are stressed by worry about a severely ill client, or threats to their autonomy, practice, and income from changes in reimbursement policies, may become tense and highly critical of or even verbally abusive toward nurses. The hospital management may also experience increased stress owing to the escalating responsibility of maintaining high-quality services with ever-shrinking revenues. Management often deals with its stress by becoming more autocratic, making increased demands on the nursing staff while reducing the control that nurses have over their practice and becoming closed off to input from nurses and physicians.

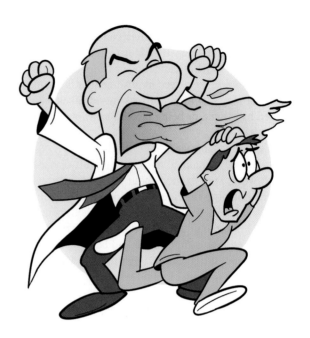

At some point, one group's stress always affects the stress level of another group, whose stress in turn increases another group's stress. The process becomes a destructive circle of cause-and-effect responses that increase the stress levels for everyone in the facility.

What Do You Think?

List four factors or situations that have produced high levels of stress for you in the hospital or health-care setting. Why did these incidents produce stress? How did you deal with the stress?

Clients Under Stress

Stress in the health-care environment is not just experienced by health-care providers. Stress for clients starts when they first come into contact with the health-care system; peaks when they have to undergo physical examinations, surgery, or invasive treatments; and continues throughout the recovery period. The fear that a nurse may not respond to clients' needs increases clients' stress levels, and they sometimes become more demanding of care, which in turn increases the nurse's stress levels. If the nursing staff is experiencing high stress levels, clients

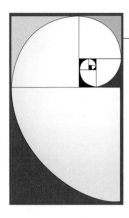

Issues in Practice

Managing Change

The busy nonacute outpatient unit at a large hospital had become disorganized. It consistently received evaluations of "poor" when clients were asked about the care being provided. They often complained about the long waits to be evaluated and treated. The staff also recognized the problems with the care they were providing but didn't have any solutions.

In an attempt to improve the evaluations, the administration replaced the current director with a new director from an even larger facility across town. She was charged with the task of improving client care and was promised that she would have whatever resources she needed.

Within 6 months, the new director completely reorganized the staffing patterns and modernized all the information systems using the latest software. She replaced old equipment with new models and bought additional equipment that the unit had never used before. She also managed to expand and brighten up the unit by remodeling extensively and by securing unused space from the radiology department, which occupied adjacent rooms. She increased the salaries of the nursing staff, hired new nurses, and expanded the hours of service. She implemented a "management by objectives" model for evaluation that allowed the staff nurses increased input into their working conditions and evaluations.

Client surveys indicated an increase in overall satisfaction with the care being provided; the wait time had been decreased to a point at which there were hardly any complaints. However, approximately half the experienced nurses on the unit resigned, and the rest of the nurses began the process of organizing into a collective bargaining unit for the first time in the history of the nonacute outpatient unit.

QUESTIONS FOR THOUGHT

1. What was the underlying issue that led to the nurses' responses to the changes?

2. What could the director have done to increase the staff's acceptance of change?

(Answers are found at the end of the chapter.)

often sense this subconsciously, and as a result, clients' stress levels also increase.

Several techniques can be used to reduce clients' stress levels so that they can better communicate and become more receptive to teaching. Stress reduction techniques range from very simple measures that everyone can use, such as distraction with music or simple activities, exercise, or reduction in stimuli, to more advanced techniques such as meditation, **biofeedback,** and even antianxiety medications.

Eliminate the Situation

Nurses need to be able to identify situations that produce stress, recognize the symptoms shown by someone in a stressful situation, know how to reduce stress, and be able to use appropriate communication techniques with someone under stress. Of course, if possible, the best way to reduce stress is to eliminate the stressful situation. Consider the following case:

The hospital management has just sent a memo to all the hospital units that a new client assessment form they have developed is to be implemented next week. This new form is in addition to the ones that the nurses already fill out each day. The new form is to be completed by RNs only and must be done each shift on every client and then sent to the house supervisor so that management can track acuity. Because of recent facility restructuring and changes in staffing patterns, often there is only one RN on the 3 p.m. to 11 p.m. and 11 p.m. to 7 a.m. shifts to cover a 42-bed unit. This extra, time-consuming, and seemingly redundant paperwork increases the stress of the staff RNs to an unacceptable level.

They meet as a group with management and propose that the assessment forms they are already using be modified to include the data that management wants on the new forms. Photocopies of the revised form could then be made by the unit clerk for each shift and given to the supervisors, thus eliminating the new form. Management notes the high stress levels

of the RNs, recognizes that increased stress lowers the quality of care, and decides to follow the RNs' proposal, thus eliminating the primary source of the RNs' stress.

Although all sources of stress cannot be eliminated completely, in most situations they can be reduced to a manageable level. However, high stress levels should never be used as an excuse for destructive anger and behaviors, failure of communication, or abuse of individuals.

Anger

In addition to being one of the stages of the grief process, anger can be a symptom of personal frustration, lack of control, fear of change, or feelings of hopelessness. Anger is one of the strong primitive natural emotions that help individuals protect themselves against a variety of external threats. Although everyone experiences anger, how it is expressed often depends on a person's family and ethnic background, life experiences, and personal values. In some cultures, loud and physically expressive outbursts are the norm for the expression of anger, whereas in other cultures, anger is internalized and expressed only as a "controlled rage."

> *At some point, one group's stress always affects the stress level of another group, whose stress in turn increases another group's stress. The process becomes a destructive circle of cause-and-effect responses that increases the stress levels for everyone in the facility.*

Positive or Negative Expression

As with most of the other factors that affect communication, anger can be either positive or negative. When anger is used in a positive, productive manner, it can promote change and release tension. Anger can be used positively to increase others' attention, initiate communication, problem-solve, and energize the change process. Sensitivity to internal anger can warn individuals that something is wrong either within themselves or with someone or something in the external environment.

Many individuals have difficulty expressing and using their anger in a positive manner. Anger that is used negatively is very destructive. It hinders communication, makes coworkers fearful, and erodes relationships with others. Anger expressed by abusive behaviors, such as pounding on nursing station counters, throwing charts or surgical instruments, verbal outbursts, or even violent physical contact, is never acceptable and may lead to civil or criminal action against the perpetrator.

The negative expression of anger may cause the person who is the object of the anger to retaliate or seek revenge, but probably the most destructive form that negative anger can take is when it is internalized and suppressed. Long-term, suppressed anger has been associated with a number of physiological and psychological problems ranging from gastric ulcers and hypertension to myocardial infarctions, strokes, and even psychotic rage episodes.

What Sets People Off

Nurses who understand what makes both themselves and others angry are better able to either avoid anger-producing situations or cope effectively with their own anger or with that of others. For example, even new graduate nurses soon learn that some situations will almost always evoke an angry response from hospitalized clients. These include serving meals that are cold or poorly cooked, not answering call lights in a timely manner, waking up soundly sleeping clients at midnight to give them a sleeping pill, or taking 10 attempts to start an intravenous (IV) line.

Similarly, unit managers and hospital administrators quickly learn that some of the things they do will almost always produce angry responses from the staff. These actions include unilateral changes in the work schedule, additional paperwork, reduction in staffing levels, or refusal of requests for vacation or time off.

It is important that nurses understand that anger is a normal human emotion. Once it is recognized, it should be dealt with and then let go. Sometimes situations are not going to change, no matter how angry the person becomes, and sometimes no amount of anger will prevent changes from occurring.

GROUP DYNAMICS

The power of the group over an individual's behavior should never be underestimated. Groups establish and exert their power through a set of unique behaviors or norms that their members are expected to follow. These norms may be formal or informal, written or unwritten, promulgated or merely understood. Unfortunately, in most nursing units the norms are often not clearly expressed, yet they may be used as judgment tools or standards for evaluating work behaviors. When new nurses begin work on a particular unit, they must quickly learn the unwritten unit norms and identify the informal leaders to function effectively.

Unwritten Rules

As with most elements in communication, group dynamics may be positive or negative. Nurses who do not learn and fail to display the expected group behaviors may be ostracized from the group, thus making the work environment psychologically uncomfortable and perhaps even physically difficult. For example, nonconforming nurses may find that there is no one around when they need help ambulating an unsteady client. A particular nursing unit staff may have a strong team approach. If the new nurse is highly independent and prefers to work alone, he or she may not "fit in" and may experience hostility or sarcasm from the other nurses on the unit.

Going Against the Group

Consider the following scenario demonstrating group dynamics:

The ICU is responsible for on-call coverage in the recovery room for unscheduled postoperative clients on the evening shifts, night shifts, and all of the weekend shifts. There is no formal written policy, but coverage has traditionally been handled on a voluntary, rotating basis.

Because it is "voluntary," one of the ICU nurses has decided that he does not want to take call any more. He is the only member of the ICU staff who does not take call. Soon after he announces his decision, he begins to sense anger and experience alienation from his peers. He is very knowledgeable, has highly developed nursing skills, and provides consistently high-quality care to assigned clients on his regular shifts. However, on his semiannual peer evaluation, he receives low ratings from his coworkers on the basis of the informal call coverage standard and expectations. The unit nurses feel that he is no longer a team player.

The nurse becomes angry because he feels that the use of unclear, unwritten standards is an unfair way to evaluate his ability as a nurse. He soon finds that the other ICU nurses accidentally "forget" to invite him to group functions. He also seems to be assigned the most difficult and largest number of clients during any given shift, seemingly to compensate for not taking call.

Group dynamics involves many factors, including methods of communication, professional behaviors, professional growth, flexibility, problem-solving, participation, and competition. The ability to understand and use the elements of group dynamics has a direct relationship to the behaviors, cooperation, and effectiveness of the team. Often, when a team labels an individual member as "difficult," it most likely means that the individual is not following one or more of the informal, unwritten group norms.

COMPETITION

Competition can be a very powerful element in group dynamics and communication. Depending on how it is channeled, expressed, and used, competition can be a positive or negative force within the group. The various forms of competition can be individual, team, or unit focused.

Peer Evaluation. A common expression of competition in the group setting is peer evaluations. For peer evaluations to be a positive form of competition, the unit must decide ahead of time on the norms and expectations that they value and then design an objective measurement tool to evaluate whether the individual is meeting the norms. Each individual being evaluated must be aware of the criteria before the evaluation is conducted. The evaluation team must be educated on evaluation techniques and must be as objective and professional as possible.

In the health-care setting, it is important for all professionals, unit groups, and management to promote competition in a positive, progressive, and supportive environment. When competition is channeled positively, it leads to new and creative ideas,

> *The ability to understand and use the elements of group dynamics has a direct relationship on the behaviors, cooperation, and effectiveness of the team.*

better programs, increased growth, more productive interactions, and higher-quality client care. When the competition is negative, it often produces failures, depression, sabotage, unit turf conflicts, decreased productivity, and lower-quality care. Consider the following case:

The competition on a nursing unit turned negative: the nurses on the 7 a.m. to 3 p.m. shift began competing with the nurses on the 3 p.m. to 11 p.m. shift in order to appear more knowledgeable about client care to the nurse manager. To "look better," the nurses on the 7 a.m. to 3 p.m. shift intentionally withheld selected client laboratory test results during shift report.

As a result of this action, several tests scheduled for the 3 p.m. to 11 p.m. shift were not done, angering the physicians, potentially threatening the safety of the clients, and making the nurses on the 3 p.m. to 11 p.m. shift appear incompetent. In addition, the nurses on that shift had to complete several incident reports on the errors that occurred on their shift.

One informal component the unit manager uses to evaluate the staff nurses' performance is the number of incident reports that a nurse must file. The more incident reports, the poorer will be the nurse's performance evaluation. To the unit manager, the nurses on the 7 a.m. to 3 p.m. shift appeared to be more competent because of the seemingly poor care, indicated by a large number of incident reports, that is being given on the 3 p.m. to 11 p.m. shift. However, when the nurses on the 3 p.m. to 11 p.m. shift discovered what had really happened, they devised several ways to "get even" with the nurses on the 7 a.m. to 3 p.m. shift.

WORKING ENVIRONMENT

Health care reform is raising many questions about the health-care system and the delivery of care. The model remains largely fee-for-service, but as the elements of the reform are implemented over the next decade, the managed care model will likely become dominant. Health-care reform also promotes the shift from acute inpatient care to long-term outpatient care and from being illness based to a prevention and wellness focus. The changes produced by these transitions will create a high degree of stress at all levels of the health-care system. As discussed earlier, both change and stress are major barriers to effective communication.

Active Involvement in Change

One measure that can be taken to both alleviate some of the stress caused by the current changes in health care and improve unit communication is to encourage all members of the health-care team to participate in the renovation of their work environment. Through active participation, workers can have an impact on and direct the changes that are being made. Some people mistakenly believe that if they do not become involved, the changes will not happen. Unfortunately, when people are not actively involved in the restructuring process, others who are probably less qualified will make the changes anyway.

Increased fear, high stress levels, angry outbursts, and feelings of insecurity all are potential results of a work environment in which the workers do not participate in the change process. Difficult behaviors resulting in unclear communication become more evident during times of change and stress. Ugly rumors, feelings of resentment, and increased insecurity often result when intergroup communications are not clear. An open, interactive work environment increases the probability of successful communication and adaptation to change.

Coping With Difficult Behavior

Understanding what motivates a person's behavior permits the individual to design a plan or develop coping mechanisms for communication based on sound interpersonal techniques. When individuals are able to separate themselves from the difficult situation, they are less likely to take things personally and more likely to begin to focus on the underlying issues causing the problems than on the other person's difficult behavior. The interaction becomes less judgmental and threatening to the other person. However, understanding the other person's motives never excuses unacceptable behaviors such as sarcasm,

angry outbursts, and abusive language. Rather, it allows for direct confrontation of the behavior in a more controlled and less emotional way.

What Do You Think?

Have you ever been in a situation in which others have intentionally sabotaged your work? What was the situation? How did you feel? How did you deal with it? Did you try to retaliate?

All professional nurses need to develop coping mechanisms to deal with difficult people. The very nature of the profession exposes nurses to a large number of people who are experiencing change, are under stress, and have a wide range of backgrounds and values as well as varying expectations. By understanding communication, using **behavior modification,** developing **assertiveness,** avoiding submissive and aggressive behaviors, and appreciating diversity, the nurse can develop the coping skills required for problem-solving, handling conflict in the work setting, and confronting the unacceptable behaviors of difficult people.

UNDERSTANDING COMMUNICATION

Encoding and Decoding

Communication is an interactive sharing of information. It requires a sender, a message, and a receiver. After the sender sends the message, the receiver has a responsibility to listen to, process, and understand (encode) the information and then to respond to the sender by giving feedback (decoding). The encoding process occurs when the receiver thinks about the information, understands it, and forms an idea based on the message.

Several factors can interfere with the encoding process. On the sender's side, these can be factors such as unclear speech, monotone voice, poor sentence structure, inappropriate use of terminology or jargon, or lack of knowledge about the topic. On the receiver's side, factors that may interfere with encoding include lack of attention, prejudice and bias, preoccupation with another problem, or even physical factors such as pain, drowsiness, or impairment of the senses.

For example, a staff nurse is in a mandatory meeting where the unit manager is discussing a new policy that will be starting the next month. However, the nurse is thinking about an important heart medication that her client is to receive in 5 minutes. The nurse's primary concern is to get out of the meeting in time to give the medication. After the meeting, the nurse has only a minimal recollection of what was said because she did not encode the information well. The following month, when the new policy is started, the staff nurse is confused about what she should do and makes several errors in relation to the policy.

Verbal or Nonverbal?

There are two primary methods of communication: verbal and nonverbal. **Verbal** communication is either written or spoken and constitutes only about 7 percent of the communicated message. **Nonverbal** communication, which makes up the other 93 percent of communication, is everything else, including body language, facial expressions, gestures, physical appearance, touch, vocal cues (tone, pauses), and spatial territory (personal space). When the verbal and nonverbal messages are congruent, the message is more easily encoded and clearly understood. If the verbal and nonverbal messages are conflicting, the nonverbal message is probably the most reliable. It is relatively easy for people to lie with words, but nonverbal communication tends to be unconscious and more difficult to control.

For example, the nurse suspects that the mother of a newborn infant may be experiencing postpartum depression. The nurse asks the mother how she feels about her new baby. The mother responds in a low-volume, very slow monotone, "I'm so happy I have this baby," while looking down at her feet in a slouched-over posture. The message from the mother is conflicting. The words are saying she is happy, but all the nonverbal signs indicate that she is depressed. The observant nurse concludes that more assessment for depression is required.

Effective communication requires understanding that the perceptions, emotions, and participation of both parties are interactive and have an effect on the transmission of the message. Nurses often encounter situations that require clarification of the information for accuracy and encoding. The following is an example of client teaching requiring a return demonstration:

A nurse gave a teaching session to a client who was being sent home with a T-tube after surgical removal of gallstones from the common bile duct. After the nurse finished, she asked the client whether he understood how to empty the drainage bottle and measure the drainage. The client looked very confused, but mumbled "Yes" while shaking his head back and forth. The nurse recognized that although the verbal response was positive, the nonverbal responses indicated that he really did not understand. The nurse surmised that further explanation or demonstration was required for this client to encode the message properly.

> *Through active participation, workers have an opportunity to have an impact on and direct the changes that are being made. Some people mistakenly believe that if they do not become involved, the changes will not happen.*

Nurses should recognize the many barriers to clear communication as well as the benefits of clear communication. Once the barriers to communication are identified, they can be overcome, and the benefits of clear communication will follow. These barriers and the benefits that result when they are overcome are outlined in Box 14.1.

COMMUNICATION STYLES

There are two predominant styles of communication: assertive and nonassertive. Nonassertive communication can be either submissive or aggressive. Individuals develop their communication styles over the course of their lives in response to many personal factors. Although most people have one predominant style of communication, they can and often do switch or combine styles depending on the situation in which they find themselves. For example, a unit manager who uses an assertive communication style when supervising the staff on her unit may revert to a submissive style when called into the nursing director's office for her annual evaluation. Recognizing

Box 14.1

Barriers to and Benefits of Clear Communication

Barriers	Benefits
• Unclear or unexpressed expectations	• Clear expectations
• Confusion	• Understanding
• Retaliation	• Forgiveness
• Desire for power	• Recognized leadership
• Control of others	• Companionship
• Negative reputation	• Respect
• Manipulation	• Independence
• Low self-esteem	• Realistic self-image
• Biased perceptions	• Acceptance
• Inattention	• Clear direction
• Mistrust	• Trusting relations
• Anger	• Self-control
• Fear or anxiety	• Comfort
• Stress	• Motivation or energy
• Insecurity	• Security
• Prejudice	• Increased tolerance
• Interruptions	• Increased knowledge
• Preoccupation	• Concentration

which communication style a person is using at any given time, as well as a person's own style, is important in making communication clear and effective.

Assertive Communication

Assertive communication involves interpersonal behaviors that permit people to defend and maintain their legitimate rights in a respectful manner that does not violate the rights of others. Assertive communication is honest and direct and accurately expresses the person's feelings, beliefs, ideas, and opinions. Respect for self and others constitutes both the basis for and the result of assertive communication. It encourages trust and teamwork by communicating to others that they have the right to and are encouraged to express their opinions in an open and respectful atmosphere. Disagreement and discussion are considered to be a healthy part of the communication process, and

negotiation is the positive mechanism for problem-solving, learning, and personal growth.

Assertive communication always implies that the individual has the choice to voice an opinion, sometimes forcefully, as well as to not say anything at all. One of the keys to assertive communication is that the individual is in control of the communication and is not merely reacting to another's emotions.

What Do You Think?

Consider the health-care providers with whom you have worked in the recent past. What were their communication styles? How did those styles affect the way you communicated with them?

Assessing Self-Assertiveness

Answer the following questions to assess your self-assertiveness:

• Who am I and what do I want?
• Do I believe I have the right to want it?
• How do I get it?
• Do I believe I can get it?
• Have I tried to be assertive with a person I am having difficulty communicating with?
• Am I letting my fears and perceptions cloud my interactions?
• What is the worst that can happen if we communicate?
• Can I live with the worst?
• Will communications have a long-term effect?
• How does it feel to be in constant fear of alienation or rejection?

Rules for Assertiveness

Anyone can learn to use an assertive communication style and develop assertiveness. When first developing this skill, people often feel frightened and overwhelmed. However, once individuals become comfortable with assertiveness, it helps reinforce their self-concepts and becomes an effective tool for communication. There are a few rules to keep in mind while developing assertiveness along with an assertive communication style:

• It is a learned skill.
• It takes practice.

- It requires a desire and motivation to change.
- It requires a willingness to take risks.
- It requires a willingness to make mistakes and try again.
- It requires an understanding that not every outcome sought will be obtained.
- It requires strong self-esteem.
- Self-reward for change and a positive outcome is essential.
- Listening to self is necessary for identifying needs.
- Constant reexamination of outcomes helps assess progress.
- Role-playing with a friend before the interaction builds skill and confidence.
- Goals for assertiveness growth need to be established beforehand.
- Assertiveness requires recognition that change is a gradual process.
- Others should be allowed to make mistakes.

Personal Risks of Assertive Communication

There are always personal risks involved in learning any new skills or in attempting to change behavior. Learning assertive communication is no exception. People often fear that they may not choose the "perfect" assertive response. However, even seasoned assertive communicators may err from time to time because every encounter is unique, involving different people and situations. The person who is new to assertive communication needs to recognize that it is a skill that takes practice.

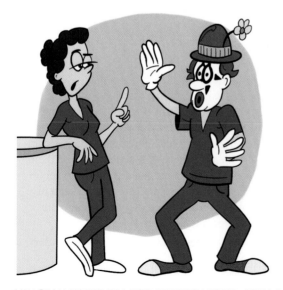

"YOU REALLY NEED TO WORK ON YOUR VERBAL SKILLS."

I Win, You Win

Assertiveness does not mean that a person will always get his or her way in every situation, and it is likely the individual will handle some situations better than others. Remember that the goal of assertive communication is not to have an "I win, you lose" situation, but rather an "I win, you win" outcome. A win-win goal is achieved when both parties have the ability and willingness to negotiate even though they do not get all they want. However, there may be situations when personal goals are not achieved. Some questions to consider when this occurs are:

- How do I feel about losing?
- Did I express my opinion clearly? Why not? How could I make it more clear?
- Did I do the best I could do? How could I have done better?
- Was I in control when responding to the situation? When did I lose control? What should I have done to regain control?
- Did I stay focused on the issues? What side issues distracted me? How could I have avoided distractions?
- Did I allow the situation to get personal? Did the other person initiate the personal attack? How could I have redirected it away from the personal?
- Was what I asked for under my control? If not, why did I ask for it? What would have been more realistic?

Reviewing these questions and analyzing the answers will help when you attempt to be assertive in future communications. For example, if the answer to the second-to-last question was yes, then during the next communication, a special effort can be focused on avoiding personal attacks during the encounter. Learning to communicate assertively is a process of continual improvement.

Familiar Barriers to Change

Another risk factor that quickly becomes evident when changing to an assertive communication style is the impact that it has on those who know the person best. Sometimes family, friends, peers, and coworkers become barriers to change. As was mentioned earlier, change always produces some degree of stress. Those individuals who are closest to the person trying to initiate changes may feel uncomfortable because they have become accustomed to the old communication styles and behaviors over a long time. They can no longer anticipate and depend on the person's responding and reacting in the usual way. In addition, they will have to develop new communication patterns of their own to match the changes caused by assertive communication.

Sometimes family, friends, peers, and coworkers become so uncomfortable that they may try to sabotage the person's attempts at assertive communication. It is important to recognize why and when these sabotage efforts occur and also to remember that assertiveness is an internal, personal process. Everyone has a right to change, and it must be respectfully communicated to others that their support for these changes is important.

It is also important to know and periodically review the rights and responsibilities of assertiveness to help reinforce the assertive communication process. The rights and responsibilities of assertiveness are listed in Box 14.2.

Practice and reinforcement of assertiveness skills may be required, especially when preparing for an anticipated conflict negotiation or a confrontational meeting with another. Although a confrontational situation always produces anxiety, rather than being feared, it should be recognized as having the potential to be highly productive. Box 14.3 lists several

Box 14.2
Rights and Responsibilities of Assertiveness

- To act in a way that promotes your dignity and self-respect
- To be treated with respect
- To experience and express your thoughts and feelings
- To slow down and make conscious decisions before you act
- To ask for what you want
- To say "No"
- To change your mind
- To make mistakes
- To not be perfect
- To feel important and good about yourself
- To be treated as an individual with special values, skills, and needs
- To be unique
- To have your own feelings and opinions
- To say "I don't know"
- To feel angry, hurt, and frustrated
- To make decisions regarding your life
- To recognize that your needs are as important as others'

Box 14.3
Conflict Resolution Tips

In nursing practice, good communication and conflict management skills are essential. The following tips may help resolve communication problems:

Improve Your Conflict Management Skills
- Seminars
- Books
- Mentors

Change Your Paradigm
- Focus on the positive, not the negative.
- Realize that appropriate confrontation is a risk-taking activity for:

Achieve Better Communication
- Improved relationships
- Improved teamwork
- Mentoring

Understand Your Values
- Focus on a win-win.
- Be willing to negotiate and compromise.
- Be direct and honest.
- Focus on the issues.
- Do not attack the person.
- Do not make judgments.
- Do not become the third person; encourage peers to go direct.
- Do not spread rumors.

Set Personal Guidelines
- Confront in private, never in front of anyone else.
- Confront the individual; do not report him or her to the supervisor first.
- Do not confront when you are angry.
- Start with an "I" message.
- Express your feelings and opinions.
- Allow the other person to talk without interruptions.
- Listen attentively.
- Set goals and future plans of action.
- Let it go.
- Keep it private and confidential.

behaviors that, if practiced and used, will help increase confidence and assertiveness skills during anticipated confrontational meetings.

You can use the checklist in Box 14.4 to determine your own degree of assertiveness.

Nonassertive Communication

Two types of interpersonal behavior are considered to be nonassertive: submissive and aggressive behaviors.

Submissive Communication

When people display submissive behavior or use a submissive communication style, they allow their rights to be violated by others. When people use submissive behavior or submissive communication, they surrender to the requests and demands of others without regard to their own feelings and needs. Many experts believe that submissive behavior and communication patterns are a protective mechanism that helps insecure persons maintain their self-esteem

---

Box 14.4
Assertiveness Self-Assessment

Statement	Communication Behavior
1. I didn't say what I really wanted to say at the last staff meeting.	_____
2. I always express my opinion because it is better than everyone else's.	_____
3. I have the courage to speak up almost all the time.	_____
4. I wish someone else would speak up at the meetings besides me.	_____
5. I am not intimidated by the high-pressure tactics of supervisors, physicians, and/or teachers.	
6. I have trouble stating my true feelings to those in authority.	_____
7. I really put that know-it-all aide in her place last shift.	_____
8. After the last meeting with my unit director, I felt hopeless, resentful, and angry.	_____
9. I speak up in meetings without feeling defensive.	_____
10. When I need to confront someone, I avoid the problem because it will usually resolve itself.	_____
11. When I need to confront individuals, I address them directly.	_____
12. When I confront individuals, I let them know in no uncertain terms that they are wrong and need to change their behavior.	_____
13. When I'm reprimanded, I keep silent even though I'm seething inside.	_____
14. The last time I was asked to stay over for another shift, I said "no" and didn't feel guilty.	_____

by avoiding negative criticism and disagreement from others. In other situations, it may be a means of manipulation through type of passive–aggressive behavior.

What Do You Think?

Recall a recent exchange with someone (e.g., friend, instructor, parent, physician) where you felt you "lost" the exchange. How did you feel? How did you respond? How could using an assertive communication style have helped?

Because of their great fear of displeasing others, personal rejection, or future retaliation, submissive communicators dismiss their own feelings as being unimportant. However, at a deeper level, submissive behavior and communication merely reinforce negative feelings of powerlessness, helplessness, and decreased self-worth. Rather than being in control of the communication or relationship, the person is trading his or her ability to choose what is best for the avoidance of conflict. Every communication by a submissive person becomes an "I lose, you win" situation. However, subconsciously it is more of "You may think you win, but I really am winning because I'm getting what I want or need."

Aggressive Communication

Sometimes there is only a very fine line separating assertiveness from aggressive behavior and communication. Whereas assertive communication permits individuals to honestly express their ideas and opinions while respecting the rights, ideas, and opinions of others, aggressive communication strongly asserts the person's legitimate rights and opinions with little regard or respect for the rights and opinions of others.

Aggressive communication—used to humiliate, dominate, control, or embarrass the other person or lower that person's self-esteem—creates an "I win, you lose" situation. The other person may perceive aggressive behavior or communication as a personal attack. Aggressive behavior and communication are viewed by some psychologists as a protective mechanism that compensates for a person's own insecurities. By demeaning someone else, aggressive behavior allows the person to feel superior and helps inflate his or her self-esteem.

Aggressive communication can take several different forms, including screaming, sarcasm, rudeness, belittling jokes, and even direct personal insults. It is an expression of the negative feelings of power, domination, and low self-esteem. Although aggressive persons may seem outwardly to be in control, in reality they are merely reacting to the situation to protect their self-esteem.

DIVERSITY

Diversity is a multifaceted issue that involves many areas of people's lives, including culture, values, life experiences, instinctual responses, learned behaviors, personal strengths and weaknesses, and native abilities or skills. Each time two people interact, they bring the sum total of all these elements into their communication. To communicate effectively, both parties need to first recognize that the other person is different, then understand how these differences affect the communication, and finally accept and build on these differences.

Building on Differences

Rather than being divisive, diversity, when recognized and used correctly, can promote teamwork, improve communication, and increase productivity. Recognizing diversity helps people better understand each other as well as themselves. The ultimate goal of diversity recognition is to use each individual's strengths, rather than emphasizing the weaknesses, to build a stronger, more self-confident, and productive environment. For example, consider the following scenario:

Anne B, RN, is a nurse in your unit who has a reputation for being a "nitpicker." She is constantly judging her peers and criticizing their actions on the basis of her own personal standards. Her judgments of others are not well accepted by her coworkers, who try to avoid her as much as possible.

Betty A, RN, another nurse on the unit, always seems to be coming up with ideas for changing things in the unit, but then avoids joining the committees that are formed to put the ideas into practice. When she does join a committee, she quickly gets bored and does not follow through on her responsibilities. The other committee members become angry and frustrated by Betty's behavior. They feel that because it was her idea in the first place, she should work as hard as everyone else to make the change.

You have been selected as the chairperson for a committee that has been formed to design a new client care documentation tool. Both Anne and Betty are on the committee. The other committee members are upset because Anne and Betty are on the committee. Everyone knows about Anne's and Betty's personality quirks. As chairperson of the team, you need to draw on everyone's strengths while recognizing their diversities to develop a new, comprehensive, yet easy-to-use form. If you perform well in your chairmanship role, each team member's self-esteem should be enhanced, and the morale of the group should improve.

At first glance, these may not seem like diversity issues. However, Anne is a detail-oriented person, whereas Betty is a visionary. Although their interests and abilities are very diverse, neither one is right or wrong. Persons who are preoccupied with details are left-brain dominant; creative, visionary individuals are usually right-brain dominant.

Two primary tasks are required to complete the project:

Task 1. Conduct brainstorming sessions with staff members, physicians, and ancillary personnel to develop a general concept of what the documentation should include and how the form should look.
Task 2. Work with the print shop to design the specific layout and content of the final form.

Plan

Task 1. It would be most appropriate to include Betty in the group that directs the brainstorming efforts and collects different ideas. She probably has no preconceived form in mind before starting the process and will feel comfortable investigating

> *Rather than being divisive, diversity, when recognized and used correctly, can promote teamwork, improve communication, and increase productivity.*

and researching a variety of different possibilities. Anne would have difficulty with this task. The lack of structure of the brainstorming process would make her feel out of control and would probably frustrate her urge to consider all the details of the project. Anne would most likely already have a good idea of the form she wanted.

Task 2. Anne would be much better at this task because of her orientation to structure and detail. Working with the print shop, she could focus her attention on each item on the form and decide where it should be placed, how much room it should be given, and how it flows in the document. She would make sure the form met all the standards and regulatory requirements of The Joint Commission as well as ensuring it was error free. Betty, on the other hand, would very quickly become bored with this aspect of the project. To her, all the attention given to the details would seem like a waste of time, and she would probably start recommending changes in other unit forms.

Placing people in the working environments that correspond with their strengths will ensure success for the project. The project will be a successful experience for the nurses and will promote positive changes in peer relationships.

A Focus on Strength

For many people, working with diversity can be difficult, especially when individuals feel insecure about their skills or abilities. When people feel insecure, they may revert to submissive or aggressive behavior or communication styles to hide their weaknesses or differences.

Because assertive persons recognize that everyone, including themselves, has both strengths and weaknesses, they feel comfortable with diversity and are more likely to accept and support others by recognizing and using their strengths. Focusing on people's strengths provides them with positive feedback and helps them grow personally and professionally. Focusing on weaknesses and differences tears down an individual's self-esteem, creates an uncomfortable work atmosphere, and makes people defensive and sometimes hostile.

PROBLEM-SOLVING

Problem-solving is a process that everyone uses all the time. For example, on the way to work, a tire goes flat on a person's car. That is a problem. How the person solves the problem depends partially on critical thinking skills, partially on past experiences, and partially on physical abilities. If the person with the flat tire is a 250-lb, 33-year-old male construction worker in good health, he most likely has changed tires before and will probably be physically able to remove the flat tire and put on the spare without difficulty. However, if the person with the flat tire is a 90-lb, 67-year-old female church organist who is unable to distinguish a lug nut from a tire valve, her solution to the problem will likely be different. She will probably call the automobile association and have someone come and change the flat for her.

One of the primary activities for nurses in the work setting is problem-solving using the nursing process. It really does not matter whether the problem is client centered, management oriented, or an interpersonal issue; the nursing process is an excellent framework for problem resolution. It focuses on the goals of mutual interaction and communication to establish trust and respect. Using the process of assessment, analysis, planning, implementation, and evaluation helps the nurse organize and structure interpersonal interactions in a way that will produce an "I win, you win" situation.

The basic problem-solving steps of the nursing process form the framework for successful conflict management. Nurses who are good problem-solvers using the nursing process also tend to be good at conflict resolution, and nurses who are good at conflict resolution tend to be excellent problem-solvers. Rather than being avoided in the work setting, conflict should be considered an opportunity to practice and grow in the use of problem-solving skills.

CONFLICT MANAGEMENT

Many people experience less anxiety when practicing personal problem-solving than when they are involved in conflict management. Problem-solving is often perceived as less emotional and more structured, whereas conflict management is considered to be more emotionally charged, with the potential to produce hostility. However, the steps of conflict management are almost identical to those of the nursing process. The one additional element that must be included in conflict resolution is the ability to use assertive behaviors and communication when discussing the issues.

Conflict on the Job

Everyone experiences conflict at one time or another as a part of daily life. Often people feel more comfortable addressing the conflict that arises in their personal lives than the professional conflicts that arise in the job setting.

A common situation that causes conflict is the nurse's feeling of being overworked or overwhelmed by assignments. The overloaded nurse might say something like "I have such a heavy load today, why isn't anyone helping me?" rather than asking a particular individual for help. When the person who is expected to help fails to comply with the implied request, the overworked nurse becomes angry and resentful. The other person may not understand where this anger is coming from and often avoids addressing the angry person for fear of making him or her angrier. This type of poor communication and lack of direct, respectful conflict management produces tension among workers, deterioration of working relationships, decreased efficiency, and, ultimately, poor client care.

Individuals are uncomfortable handling or addressing conflict for many reasons, including:

- Fear of retaliation
- Fear of ridicule
- Fear of alienating others
- Mistaken belief that they are unable to handle the conflict situation
- Feeling that they do not have the right to speak up
- Past negative experiences with conflict situations
- Family background and experiences
- Lack of education and skills in conflict resolution

> *Everyone experiences conflict at one time or another as a part of daily life. Often people feel more comfortable addressing the conflict that arises in their personal lives than the professional conflicts that arise in the job setting.*

Conflict Resolution

Several different strategies can be used to resolve workplace conflicts. Depending on a person's communication style and personality traits, different outcomes may occur.

Strategy 1: Ignore the Conflict

- Submissive personality: Person avoids bringing the issue to the other through fear of retaliation or ridicule if he or she confronts and expresses honest feelings or opinions.
- Aggressive personality: Person has decided not to pursue the conflict because the other person is "too stupid to understand" or it would just be a "waste of my time."

Strategy 2: Confront the Conflict

- Submissive personality: Person does not handle the situation directly but refers the problem to a supervisor or to another person for resolution.
- Assertive personality: Person sets up a time and place for a one-on-one meeting. At the meeting, the two parties focus on the issues that caused the conflict and negotiate to define goals and problem-solve.
- Aggressive personality: Person confronts the other loudly, in front of an audience, and attacks the other's personality rather than the issue. Person either walks away before the other can speak or keeps talking without stopping and does not allow the other person to respond. The communication is strictly one-sided and very negative.

Strategy 3: Postpone the Conflict

- Submissive personality: Person keeps track of the issues until they reach a critical point, then dumps all the issues at one time on the offender in a highly aggressive manner. The other person generally has no idea why he or she is being attacked and may respond with anger or submission.
- Aggressive personality: Person waits until he or she can either use the incident as a threat or blackmail or express the conflict in front of an audience.

> *Keep in mind that unresolved conflicts never really go away. Ignoring a conflict situation may postpone it, sometimes for a long time, but it will not resolve the issue.*

Professional nurses need to be assertive and feel comfortable when handling conflict situations and confronting others. The conflict situations that nurses may encounter range from uncooperative clients and lazy coworkers to hostile, insecure, but influential physicians and administrators. Practicing assertiveness skills during confrontational situations helps increase the nurse's confidence in handling daily work-related conflicts and allows the honest but respectful expression of opinion and ideas. Keep in mind that unresolved conflicts never really go away. Ignoring a conflict situation may postpone it, sometimes for a long time, but it will not resolve the issue. Unresolved conflicts often fester until they either reach the boiling point or are manifested in negative behaviors or feelings. Some of the feelings and behaviors that are symptoms of unresolved conflicts include:

- Tension and anxiety manifested as sudden angry outbursts
- Generalized distrust among the staff members
- Gossiping and rumor spreading
- Intentional work sabotage
- Backstabbing and lack of cooperation
- Isolation of certain staff members
- Division and polarization of the staff
- Low-rated peer evaluation reports

Improved Communication Skills

Often, when conflict is handled appropriately, it produces much less anxiety than was initially anticipated. An individual who prepares for a confrontational meeting by expecting the worst-case scenario may be pleasantly surprised when the meeting and discussion take place. Many conflicts turn out to be merely errors in perception, simple misunderstandings, or misquotes of something that was said. If a situation is cleared up at an early stage, this prevents the development of the symptoms of unresolved conflict (listed earlier) and improves staff relationships. Individuals feel more confident and have better self-esteem when they resolve the conflicts in an adult and productive manner.

Another advantage of good conflict management is the improvement in communication skills.

As with any skills, the more these skills are practiced, the easier they will become to use. A conflict situation is illustrated in the second Issues in Practice box at the end of the chapter.

DIFFICULT PEOPLE

Identifying the Problem

All nurses recognize that obtaining a thorough history and understanding the underlying disease processes better prepare them for the care of their clients. Similarly, in working with difficult people, a knowledge of their backgrounds and understanding of the underlying personality traits better prepare the individual to deal with the important issues. It would seem that nurses should be better at handling conflict and difficult people: an understanding of cause and effect and the intricacies of human nature are skills used daily in the care of clients.

Shifting the communication paradigm from one of instinctual or reflex "knee-jerk" response to one that uses the nurse's relationship skills should make dealing with difficult people a much less difficult task. Remember that the behavior displayed by a difficult person is really a symptom of a deeper problem, just as an assessment of shortness of breath is a symptom of a respiratory disease. Identifying the cause of the problem permits the nurse to treat the disease rather than just the symptoms. The problem will not be cured by merely ignoring it or dealing only with the symptoms. In the long term, that usually only makes things worse.

Identifying Difficult People

Most of the time, it is easy to identify when a person is being "difficult." However, some behaviors of difficult people may not be evident at first glance. Each type of difficult person requires a different strategy for dealing with his or her behaviors.

There are four basic behavioral pattern types of communication: (1) in control and responsive, (2) in control but unresponsive, (3) uncontrolled and responsive, (4) uncontrolled and unresponsive.

Anyone who has been employed in or even associated with the health-care setting for any length of time soon becomes aware of a variety of personality types among the staff members. These personality types can be identified by their predominant behaviors and require different strategies for communication. Keep in mind that these are stereotypes that tend to batch individuals into groups on the basis of predetermined characteristics. In reality, people may have combinations of or overlapping characteristics that may require combining the listed strategies for communication (Box 14.5). The various types of characterizations, behavioral patterns, and stereotypes all are interrelated and based on individual communication styles. An increased awareness of the various identifying characteristics and communication strategies will help develop the coping skills and communication techniques necessary for communicating with difficult people.

DEVELOPMENT OF COPING SKILLS

Building on Existing Skills

Just as developing communication skills requires a willingness to change and a lot of practice, so does the development of coping skills. Coping skills can be used to resolve crisis situations, deal with anxiety, and resolve difficult issues of communication. Everyone has at least a fundamental set of coping skills that they have developed during their lives, and these can be used as the foundation for adding to or

Box 14.5

Assertive Communication Suggestions

- Maintain eye contact.
- Convey empathy; stating your feelings does not mean sympathy or agreement.
- Keep your body position erect, shoulders and back straight.
- Speak clearly and audibly; be direct and descriptive.
- Be comfortable with silence.
- Use gestures and facial expressions for emphasis.
- Use appropriate location.
- Use appropriate timing.
- Focus on behaviors and issues; do not attack the person.

building new coping skills for future problems. Presented here are some strategies that will help in the development of coping skills to use in communicating with difficult people.

Avoid Personal Attacks

First, separate the person from the problem by focusing on the issues without attacking the person. Having the facts about the situation makes people much more receptive to resolution of the problem than attacking their personality does. When situations are made into personal attacks, people feel defensive, responsible, or persecuted, and communication is either blocked or closed off.

One way to avoid turning a conversation into a personal attack is to use "I" rather than "you" messages. Avoid starting a conversation by saying, "You made a mistake," or "You said this about me," or especially "You always do this" or "You know what your problem is?" People are less likely to perceive a communication as a personal attack when the conversation begins with an explanation of a personal view of the situation or even how feelings were affected. Statements such as "I thought it was done this way," or "I heard something the other day," or even "I feel hurt when people judge me" are more productive ways to begin an exchange of ideas and information. For example:

> During shift report on a particular client, the 11 p.m. to 7 a.m. nurse forgot to tell the 7 a.m. to 3 p.m. charge nurse, Gail L, RN, that the client had fallen out of bed during the night shift. Later in the day, both the client's physician and family confronted Gail to find out what had happened and why the client was not placed on "fall protocols." Later, when Gail confronts the night nurse about the omission, she has two options for initiating the discussion of the incident with the responsible night nurse. Which approach would the night nurse probably take as a personal attack?

Option 1. Gail: "I was taken off guard and unprepared when the family and physician asked me about this client's fall, and I felt unprepared to explain the problem or a solution to them. My lack of knowledge about the fall really made me feel incompetent."

Option 2. Gail: "You failed to tell me about his fall last night. Because of you, I was not aware of the incident and was not prepared to answer questions. You always make me look like a fool!"

Another way to avoid making issues into personal attacks is to avoid judging what a person should have done by a personal standard. This type of statement becomes an arbitrary judgment call. Instead, ask the person for his or her ideas on how the situation could have been handled differently or what other options were available. Especially, avoid becoming personally or verbally abusive.

> *Shifting the communication paradigm from one of instinctual or reflex 'knee-jerk' response to one that uses the nurse's relationship skills should make dealing with difficult people a much less difficult task.*

Listen Actively

A second important strategy for developing communication-related coping skills is to be willing to listen actively to and respect the other person's perspectives, ideas, or opinions. Active listening can help minimize the misunderstandings or erroneous perceptions that cause much of the tension seen on nursing units. As mentioned earlier, active listening involves "listening" not only to the words but also to the body language to hear the real meaning of the communication and understand the underlying message.

A person who is focused on communication is not preoccupied with other issues or mentally preparing a response or a defense. Allowing the other person to say all he or she has to say without interruption before responding creates an atmosphere in which honest and open communication can occur. In some situations, merely allowing a person to ventilate emotions by using active listening reduces the levels of anger and animosity and sometimes even solves the conflict situation. Also, when intelligent people are allowed to speak openly and freely, they may be able to develop a new solution to the problem that they had not considered previously.

Before responding to a person, it is important to ask clarifying questions that validate the person's concerns, feelings, and perceptions. Validating will help ensure that the responses address the real issues. Also, avoid reflex-type reactions to hostile or aggressive statements. It is a human instinct to become defensive when attacked and to attack back. However, this behavior only escalates the anger and tension and blocks effective communication.

Ignore Trivia

A third strategy that is useful in developing communication coping skills is always to make a conscious decision about the importance of the issue that needs to be discussed. When individuals can identify the issues that really matter and focus their efforts on them, they gain credibility among their peers and develop a reputation for caring and realism. Again, it is a very human tendency to become preoccupied with trivial and unimportant issues. If people spend large portions of their energy dealing with trivia, they will have little energy left to deal with major issues when they come along. By establishing and analyzing the outcomes to be attained and by being open to negotiations and compromise, both parties will leave the confrontation with a sense of accomplishment and fair resolution even if they did not get everything they wanted.

Setting the Stage

After a decision is made to deal with a difficult issue or person, it is important to set the stage for a positive experience. The location for the exchange should be private. The format of the meeting needs to be established ahead of time, including an explanation to the other person that both parties will take turns expressing their opinions and feelings without interruption.

> *It is a very human tendency to become preoccupied with trivial and unimportant issues. If people spend large portions of their energy dealing with trivia, they will have little energy left to deal with major issues when they come along.*

Establishing Trust

An important issue in conflict negotiations is the establishment of trust. Trust can be established by a show of respect for the other person's opinions and ideas and by talking first and directly to the person about the problem rather than to everyone else on the unit. Being talked about behind one's back makes people resentful and defensive.

You can reinforce trust by making it known that all you want is to resolve the issue and then move on. When the threat of retaliation is removed, people are more likely to express themselves honestly, as well as becoming more open to the other side's ideas. Once two people begin to trust each other, even if they disagree about some of the issues, they are much more likely to come to a satisfactory resolution of the problem.

The Exchange

When the exchange takes place, it is important to avoid "I" language and to be direct by focusing on the facts and issues. Remember that active listening is a two-way street. A person's body language, tone of voice, and eye contact can say much more than the words spoken. Showing the other person that his or her opinion is respected, even if not agreed with, helps develop that important sense of trust between the two parties (Box 14.6).

After both people have had a chance to express themselves and validate the communication, they begin to address the issues and develop a solution for the problem. Sometimes there is a need to set goals for, or at least agree on, how the issues are to be approached and settled. It is fairly common that some issues will remain unresolved after the first meeting. A decision about when and where the second meeting will take place needs to be made before the first meeting ends. Also, before leaving the first meeting, both parties should summarize what they agreed to and how they felt about the

Box 14.6

Seven Principles of Communication

1. Information giving is not communication.
2. The sender is responsible for clarity.
3. Use simple and exact language.
4. Feedback should be encouraged.
5. The sender must have credibility.
6. Acknowledgment of others is essential.
7. Direct channels of communication are best.

Source: Adapted from Whitehead, DK, Weiss, SA, Tappen, RM: Essentials of Nursing Leadership and Management (4th ed). Philadelphia, F. A. Davis, 2006.

exchange. This summary will help clarify any miscommunications and give each party one last chance to introduce any issues that remain unresolved.

Dealing with difficult people and resolving conflict are never pleasant undertakings. However, like most skills, the more they are practiced, the more comfortable you will become using the communication techniques discussed. The importance of handling problematic situations in a timely, honest, and caring manner is self-evident. The anxiety and fear provoked by confrontation are part of the price that nurses must pay to do their jobs well and provide high-quality client care.

Conclusion

A person's professional and personal life is influenced by communication styles and behavioral patterns. The ability to analyze personal strengths, weaknesses, and communication behaviors is particularly important in dealing with difficult people.

Certain specific communication qualities and skills are essential for interacting with difficult people. First, it is important to develop the skill of assertive communication, which allows people to express themselves openly and honestly while respecting other people's opinions and ideas. Being able to identify submissive and aggressive behavior is also essential in trying to resolve problems, as well as recognizing issues of diversity, which underlie many problems in communication. Difficult situations are ultimately resolved through the practice of conflict management. Because it is an outgrowth and extension of the problem-solving method, nurses should be able to quickly grasp its structure and master its use.

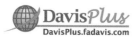

DavisPlus
DavisPlus.fadavis.com

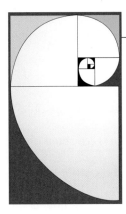

Issues in Practice

Julie H, RN, has been working the 7 p.m. to 7 a.m. shift in a busy, 32-bed surgical unit of a large university hospital since her graduation from a small bachelor of science in nursing (BSN) program 6 months ago. Although Julie was told by the unit director when she was hired that she would have at least a full year of training before she had to work as charge nurse, tonight the other two RNs who usually work the shift called in sick, and Julie was left in charge. The 7 p.m. to 7 a.m. shift is always busy because the unit has to discharge clients who are ready to go home after surgery, as well as admit clients who are coming in for surgery the next day. Hospital policy requires that the RN make and sign both the discharge and admission assessments.

Although Julie is nervous about this new role as charge nurse, she feels that she can handle the responsibility if she has some additional help. Normal staffing for the unit on this shift is three RNs, three LPNs, and three unlicensed assistive personnel (UAPs). Julie calls the house supervisor to see if she can get some help. The only place in the hospital that is not busy that night is the obstetrics (OB) unit, so the supervisor sends two of the OB unit's UAPs to the surgical unit to help Julie.

It was not the help Julie really wanted, but she feels that she can handle the responsibility. However, when Julie begins to make assignments, the older of the OB unit UAPs, Hanna J, informs Julie that for the past 15 years she has worked only in the newborn nursery and does not know anything about the care of adult clients who have had surgery. In addition, Hanna states that she has a bad back and cannot lift or turn adult clients. She is also afraid that she might catch some disease from the adults that she would take back to the babies. Julie asks Hanna, "What do you feel you are qualified to do on the surgical unit?" In response, Hanna crosses her legs, folds her arms across her chest, puts her head down, and mumbles under her breath, "A lot more than a new know-it-all RN like you."

Answers to Case Study Questions

Issues in Practice: Managing Change (page 277)

1. The underlying problem was that there was too much change too quickly. Even though the staff recognized that change was needed, there is always a built-in resistance to change. Sudden, unpredictable change creates the most anxiety and therefore the most resistance. It also can produce a great deal of cohesion among those being asked to change when it is viewed as a threat. This last point is borne out by the nurses seeking to organize into a collective bargaining unit.

2. The director of the unit could have decreased resistance by having the staff "buy into" the changes, allowing them to participate in decision making from the beginning. Also, the whole process of change could have been slowed down—perhaps spread over 1 year to 18 months. A slower process would have given the nurses a chance to adjust to one change before another was implemented.

Sources: Sources Whitehead, DK, Weiss, SA, Tappen, RM: Essentials of Nursing Leadership and Management (5th ed). Philadelphia, F. A. Davis, 2010.

Yu, M: Employees' perception of organizational change: The mediating effects of stress management strategies. Public Personnel Management 38(1):17-32, 2009.

Critical Thinking Exercises

- What messages, both verbal and nonverbal, are being communicated? How should Julie respond to this comment? What should she do to rectify the situation?
- Using what you learned in this chapter, identify the personality type of each of the persons involved in the situation.
- How can the RN best communicate with this UAP? What were some of the communication mistakes the RN made?
- What background, cultural, and diversity factors played a part in this situation? Develop a strategy for resolution of this conflict.
- Make a list of your values and where they came from. Describe how each value affects your work ethic and life.
- List your communication strengths and weaknesses. Rank them on a scale of 1 to 10 (10 being the highest). Determine which weaknesses you want to change and create an improvement plan.
- Identify your primary communication style and character type.
- Complete this statement, using as many situations or statements as possible: "In a conflict situation, I have difficulty saying _____." Analyze reasons that prevent you from saying it. What would have been the worst thing that could have happened to you if you had said it? Create a phrase that you feel comfortable with that you could use the next time you want to say something difficult to the members of your team.
- Identify the communication and behavior characteristics of your work group or team. List areas of diversity for each member, including yourself. Identify their strengths and weaknesses. Identify methods for using the team members' diversity to enhance the team.

15

Incivility: The Antithesis of Caring

Cheryl Taylor
Sharon Bator
Edna Hull
Jacqueline J. Hill
Wanda Spurlock

Learning Objectives

After completing this chapter, the reader will be able to:

- Define caring in the context of civility: the importance of caring relationships.
- Define incivility and related concepts in academia (among faculty and students) and in the workplace.
- Discuss the ethical codes violated by incivility in the profession.
- Describe behaviors that are considered uncivil and civil in the academic and clinical settings.
- Discuss professional boundaries, use of social media, and other factors that are contributing to the rise in incivility in nursing.
- Discuss intervention strategies for eliminating incivility from academia and the workplace.
- Describe interventions that could help overcome incivility in different settings.
- Clarify mentors' and tormentors' roles with nursing students.

INTRODUCTION

What Is Civility?

The nursing profession today is filled with complaints about "incivility" in academia and the workplace. Everyone has an understanding of what civility is and is not, but few actually can define it. Civility is often thought of simply as good manners; however, its meaning is much broader. Civility implies taking actions that fight injustice and oppression while at the same time respecting others. Civility, therefore, is based on recognizing that all human beings are important. The Civil Rights Act of 1964 provides that all individuals have equal protection under the law and that human beings matter equally, regardless of race, color, religion, gender, national origin, or disability.[1]

Civility, in many respects, is the opposite of discrimination. Outright discrimination in society is not as obvious as in the past; however, more subtle and chronic forms are still a reality for certain groups. An analysis of existing research shows that even perceived discrimination can produce negative mental and physical health outcomes through stress responses and destructive health behaviors. Protection can be found in social support, active coping styles, and group identification.[2]

Civility in Nursing

In nursing, civility is one of the underpinnings of caring and can even be considered a moral imperative.[3-5] Professional nursing journals and textbooks link civility with client advocacy, relationship-centered care, and scholarly inquiry into caring. An example of the caring–civility link in nursing is the use of thoughtful and committed scholarly research in overcoming health-care disparities.[6] Providing interventions for the vulnerable is another example of civility.

Civility in the profession enables nurses to participate fully in making caring a moral imperative (see Chapter 1). Being civil to each other, to students, to colleagues, and to clients promotes emotional health and creates a positive environment for learning and for the promotion of healing. It also develops emotional intelligence in nurses.[1]

Communication and Civility

In Watson's nursing theory, caring can be demonstrated and practiced interpersonally (Box 15.1). The consideration of others within interpersonal relationships is a key aspect of civility.[7] The rise of incivility in nursing seems to contradict its primary moral imperative to care for clients and to be a caring person. The reasons can be found in a closer examination of relationships and of workplace and learning environments that may foster incivility.

The health and well-being of clients are predicated on excellence in communication and civility. The Institute of Medicine report, *Crossing the Quality Chasm: A New Health System for the 21st Century*, notes that finding new strategies to improve communications is critical. Further, intimidation, even when subtle, results in harmful outcomes of psychological abuse, horizontal and lateral violence, bullying, relationship aggression, workplace incivility, and mobbing. However, ethical codes and values in society affirm civility as the antidote to incivility. The Golden Rule, stated simply, is the practice of

> " *To learn how to be happy we must learn how to live well with others, and civility is a key to that. Through civility we develop thoughtfulness, foster effective self-expression and communication, and widen the range of our benign responses. Practicing civility means that we are doing more than outwardly manifesting politeness. Being civil is using and developing our emotional intelligence."*
> Sophie Sparrow

decency or the consideration of others within interpersonal relationships.

Relationships fostering incivility need to be addressed, defused, and overcome. These relationships can be found among faculty, students, administrators, nurses and other health-care providers, and clients. Obstacles to civility within these relationships sometimes relate to the historically hierarchical nature of the nursing profession, which emphasizes discipline, authority, punishment, and adherence to rigid procedures. Clearly, better interpersonal capacities are needed in stressful working circumstances.

What Is Incivility?

Incivility is an enduring human problem, and tools of civility are needed to mitigate it. It can generally be defined as any type of speech or behavior that disrupts the harmony of the work or educational environment. Many professionals agree that civility has declined in society, but they are hopeful that behavior and relationship education will result in more harmony and productivity and will improve society.[7] When people are under stress, lapses into incivility become more common and can escalate into outright violence if left unchecked.[8]

Incivility and intimidation in the academic and workplace environments are not new. However, technology has made them even more toxic, widely distributed, and damaging. Research indicates that cyber-harassment, vicious anonymous e-mails, text messaging, hate mail, acts of rudeness, and social rejection are forms of incivility that can be considered violent. Students targeted in this way experience more fear, anxiety, and avoidant behaviors than if they were victims of theft or attack.[7]

Incivility in the health-care setting is not a new problem. It has been discussed under a variety of labels: "nurses eating their young," the "doctor–nurse game," "assertive versus aggressive or passive

Box 15.1

Watson Model of Human Caring

"Caring Science is the starting point for nursing (in) relational ontology that honors the fact that we are all connected and belong to Source."

Source: Watson J: Nursing: The Philosophy and Science of Caring (revised ed). Boulder, CO, The University Press of Colorado, 2008.

communication," and "workplace violence," to name a few. The ultimate consequence of incivility and intimidation is to jeopardize client safety. Incivility has been linked to increased medical errors and the creation of hostile academic and workplace environments. Such negative environments can create situations that end in loss of health or even life. Fatal campus violence was seen in 2002, 2007, and 2008 at the University of Arizona, Virginia Tech, and Northern Illinois University, respectively. Could it have been prevented?

A Desensitized World

Current newspaper, television, and Internet reports indicate that callousness is increasing in the world. It sometimes seems that continual violence and its reporting in the media have desensitized people to the point of threatening the bonds of humanity. For years, the effect of technological changes on caring and relating have created a tension in which the scientific and technical sides are overstressed while the environment and other aspects of education are neglected.[9] Technology and caring must become balanced so that they can work together synergistically.

Of the nine human response patterns used as a conceptual basis for classifying nursing diagnoses, one is relating and the other eight are exchanging, communicating, valuing, choosing, moving, perceiving, feeling, and knowing.[10] Perhaps nursing needs to create a new diagnosis: "Risk for alteration in the bonding process for humanity." The new diagnosis might task the nursing profession with maintaining civility by establishing interpersonal bonds in all settings. Bonding provides individuals or groups with a reason to feel that they have a duty to each other. The source of bonding

within interpersonal relationships comes from the moral capacity to care deeply in mind–body–spirit with another in the lived moment.[3] A key role of nursing is to help all clients to achieve maximal well-being within their potential.

INCIVILITY IN NURSING EDUCATION

In its broadest sense, academic incivility is any speech or action that disrupts the harmony of the teaching or learning environment.[11]

The classroom experience reflects the larger society, with inequities as well as humanitarian qualities such as caring. Academic incivility is an interactive and dynamic process in which individuals or groups make the choice to behave uncivilly. Within nursing education, the two parties or groups who need to take primary responsibility for the disruptive atmosphere are faculty and students.[12]

Student-to-Faculty Incivility
An Escalating Problem

Some nursing faculty are too embarrassed to admit that incivility exists in higher education, particularly in their own classrooms, despite a documented increase in student hostility, insubordination, and even intimidation.[13,14] High levels of student classroom incivility directly relate to low levels of attention, poor note-taking corresponding with low levels of teacher enthusiasm, lack of clarity and organization, and discomfort with expressions of empathy. Faculty may be perceived as being unapproachable. It is painful for students to endure boring teachers. Other factors that promote incivility include extending class times past their designated endpoint.[14]

Student incivility is also demoralizing for faculty. Hence, the reciprocal behaviors of faculty and students exacerbate the problem. When faculty have more immediacy with students, they are less likely to be perceived as uncaring or incompetent.

Inappropriate behavior by students typically includes missing classes, cheating, refusing to participate in class activities, coming unprepared, and distracting teachers and other students. These behaviors are found throughout higher education—but to what extent do they reflect what is occurring in nursing classrooms? In a recent survey with 504 respondents from 41 states, including 194 nursing faculty and 306 nursing students, academic incivility was rated as a significant problem. Common uncivil student behaviors included cell phone use during class, talking out of turn, making demeaning remarks about other students and the professor, and using one's higher rank to diminish another.[15]

It is critical for nursing faculty to deal constructively with angry students. The most common cause of angry behavior among nursing students is their perception that faculty are unreasonable. Incidents at the University of Arizona College of Nursing and especially the Appalachian School of Law, where fatal violence was caused by angry students, make it clear that the issue of addressing incivility is critical to preventing its escalation into violence. Incivility sets a stage for decreased learning and increased stress for everyone. Uncorrected incivility in the educational setting often carries over into the workplace, where failure to deal with anger can erupt into violence.[14]

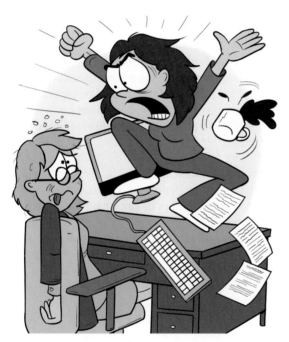

INCIVILITY CAN CREATE A TOXIC CLASSROOM

When students' rude and disruptive behavior is not addressed, it may turn into aggression or violence.[12] Most nursing students recognize the importance of treating others respectfully, studying diligently, disagreeing gracefully, and listening attentively. However, when stress levels are high, they may struggle to remain civil.[1] Studies show a correlation between increased student stress and student incivility, resulting in some faculty doubting their abilities as educators or even having concerns for their personal safety. The key to effective education lies in the quality of the interpersonal relationship between student and teacher.[16]

What can nursing educators do to promote the positive interpersonal relationships that encourage civility? The National League of Nurses (NLN) faculty development program includes strategies to manage incivility and offers a program of cosponsorship for those interested (http://dev.nln.org).

The Student's Perspective

Although many schools of nursing actively engage in curriculum and program improvement measures, few examine the impact of incivility on student learning (Box 15.2). Examples of incivility in nursing education range from minor insults, delivered either electronically or face to face, to full-blown acts of physical violence. Violent acts in the work environment often take the form of horizontal violence, which can be vicious, mean, and often covert.[17] Regarding the rise of incivility in nursing education, two questions have dominated the literature in recent years: (1) What factors are contributing to it? (2) What measures can be taken to minimize its impact on student learning?

Contributing Factors

Nursing students reported that several faculty behaviors seem to display incivility. These faculty actions included rigid attitudes, unfair treatment of students, expectation of too much conformity, and discrimination.[18] It is well known that nursing students have major challenges that cause increased stress levels. Identified stressors include juggling multiple roles, such as meeting the demands of work, study, and family responsibilities; financial pressures; time management; lack of support; faculty incivility; and their own mental health problems.[19]

One study reported that other contributing factors to incivility included student developmental issues caused by isolation from professional role models and reduced exposure to decisions made by them. Other nursing students did not believe in the social hierarchical structure of nursing school but rather that everyone was a peer. For them, the chain of command did not exist, and there were no boundaries in the lines of communication between students and faculty.[19]

Faculty-to-Faculty Incivility
Colleagues as Targets

In recent years, faculty have become less civil to one another (Box 15.3).[20] On the receiving end, many faculty report being the target of negative remarks, insinuations, and harassment, all of which are counterproductive to their work as well as their credibility. Some faculty dismiss the behaviors as "part of the job" and look the other way. Others note the rise in incivility and report anger, disappointment, and embarrassment as the result of colleagues' actions.

By its definition as any speech or actions that are discourteous, rude, or impolite, incivility would certainly seem to be commonplace in U.S. society. Incivility can also imply the persistent demeaning and downgrading of humans through vicious words and cruel acts. When applied to the academic setting, incivility can extend to any action that interferes with the teaching–learning process.

Faculty-to-faculty incivility encompasses a wide range of behaviors. These include aggressive behavior that is often expressed as, but not limited to, remarks made during faculty committee meetings and in the presence of students.

Any discussion on the topic of faculty-to-faculty incivility requires examination of workplace incivility. Expressed in many different forms, workplace incivility can include horizontal violence, toxic environment, workplace violence, and bullying. The result is a workplace setting that fosters hostility, is impersonalizing, and at times results in aggression. More specifically, if an administrator is responsible for the actions, the work environment becomes highly toxic and leads to an atmosphere in which incivility becomes the norm, with everyone too fearful to question it. Serious problems are often covered up or denied, and the turnover rate is high.

Box 15.2
A Student's Perspective on Bullying

"Wow, I feel as if I'm being kicked to the curb by a faculty member that I trusted. I will know better in the future," came the message from the student. Angry because he had failed a nursing course, he shared his concerns with a nursing administrator and lodged a grievance against the instructor of the course he had failed. Ignoring relationship boundaries, he delivered an angry e-mail retaliation to his being ineligible to advance in the program. Many words included in the message fitted the descriptions in the academic literature of uncivil acts committed by students: aggression; anger; rude, disruptive, violent behaviors. Shocked at the student's approach in managing his academic failure, the administrator began longing for the old days, when, despite the disappointment of a failed course, most students were humble when petitioning for an academic appeal to repeat a course and requesting reinstatement.

Box 15.3
The Pecking Order

I chose to teach in a program with a long-standing faculty. I was the "new kid on the block" but had many years of experience and came as an associate professor. I was told by a fellow faculty member that there was a decision to be made and that only senior faculty could make the decision. I asked what the definition of senior faculty was and was informed that it meant "associate professors only." I informed her that I was a senior faculty member by that definition. She looked shocked and quickly recovered and said, "You're not invited."

Source: Heinrich K: Joy stealing: 10 Mean games faculty play and how to stop the gaming. Nurse Educator 32(1):34–38, 2007.

The Rise of Incivility

The increase in incivility in nursing education has several causes. For many nonacademics, the university setting is believed to be a purely intellectual environment. In reality, the academic culture is often controlling and driven by faculty insecurities and competitiveness. Historically, the education and preparation of nurses began in the hospital setting but moved into the academic setting in the 1980s, joining other male-dominated professions such as medicine and engineering.[21]

Nursing remains a female-dominated profession. Many nurse faculty faced a chilly climate as they stepped into the educational setting that had been traditionally designed, controlled, and administered by men. The outcome of this move has left nursing faculty feeling subservient after years of male dominance both in academia and in the clinical practice setting. In this climate of inequality and exclusion, tension and control in decision-making surfaced as nursing faculty fought to participate in the decision-making process.[14]

Many nursing faculty stepped into their teaching role underprepared. On-the-job training became the norm as nursing faculty adapted to the academic setting with its triple requirements of teaching, research, and service. Underpreparation for a job can lead to conflicts. Nursing faculty felt marginalized and subordinated. As subordinates, they often found themselves victims of uncivil behaviors and bullying through unequal, often overtly supervisory relationships or discrepancies in faculty status and rank.[21]

Violators and Tormentors

Violators are faculty members who inflict uncivil acts on other faculty. Such acts can include alienation, divulging confidential information, belittling the opinions of others, manipulating those who are powerless, and openly criticizing other faculty.

In the past, nursing faculty were poorly prepared for their work as academicians. Because of the lack of preparation, nursing faculty often felt inferior, leading to compensating behaviors that included bullying and manipulation of others. Because violators still seek the approval of others and want to be liked by both students and faculty, they often prey on faculty less vocal or weaker than themselves. In many cases, they were the object of bullying themselves early in their careers.

A vicious circle of bullying behavior takes place when faculty members bullied in the past become the bullies to new faculty. Oppression theory notes that marginalization is a key contributing factor to incivility and bullying. Nurses often use horizontal violence to attack one another as a means of venting their frustrations and anger against a larger system.[15]

Violators have some of the qualities identified in individuals who mentor but who are not helpful and become tormentors. Their energy and attitudes are negative, and they often display codependence, self-absorption, rigid behavior, manipulation, and control of access to information.

Tormentors help those they are mentoring (mentees) remember what they did incorrectly by using a punitive interpretation of the errors. Although potentially charming on the outside, the tormentor will often keep a score card, be a "know-it-all," and generally make the mentee feel inferior. This way of relating also may make the mentee feel like a victim.[22]

Victims

Victims are faculty who are the targets of uncivil behavior. Victims of incivility are often unrecognized and feel powerless. With a lack of status, victims can easily attract violators. For example, victims report that by simply speaking up in a meeting to offer their opinion, they can provoke retaliation from the violators or tormentors. Retaliation in academia can take many forms, including silence or workload increases. Such acts can result in effects ranging from self-doubt to resignation.[21]

Because academia is a competitive work environment, many faculty are hired by a selective process. Advertisements and calls are made for individuals meeting predetermined qualifications to teach. Although the interview process may be well intended, it rarely ensures that the final selection is someone who supports the institution's overall mission as well as having the teaching and subject matter qualifications. The end result is the hiring of a faculty member who may be out of step and alienated when he or she questions the status quo.

Normally, nursing faculty operate in a highly interactive social system.[23] Most of the day-to-day operations of classes and committees require working closely with other nursing faculty. In some cases, when faculty members disagree strongly with policies, procedures, or lines of authority, they may develop feelings of exclusion or alienation.

The nursing profession is based on a long history of strong traditions. Although nursing educators recognize that challenging the status quo is essential for the growth of the profession, it still is often resisted. Challenging faculty can be silenced and sometimes even shunned by colleagues when they attempt to take a contradictory stand on an important decision.[21] This is most noticeable when an experienced nurse faculty member is hired and then is expected to blend seamlessly into the group.

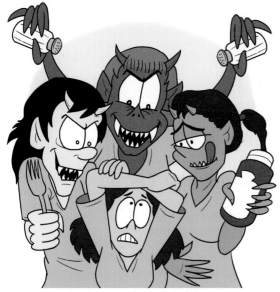

NURSES ARE KNOWN FOR EATING THEIR YOUNG

Many nursing faculty can relate to these situations from their experiences in higher education. One example is the ongoing debate between the doctorate in nursing science (DNS) and the research-oriented PhD as the terminal academic degree. Another example is the issue of nursing specialist (e.g., maternal–child health) versus generalist (medical–surgical nursing) preparation for faculty.

High-quality mentoring for new nurses and new faculty can build healthier relationships. Constructive mentor relationships include respectful listening, focused thinking, maturity, wisdom, and positive energy, all of which help those being mentored correct mistakes and accomplish goals.[24]

College Administrators

College leaders can be both violators and victims of incivility. As violators, academic leaders can actually be bullies or, more commonly, can ignore and deny that incivility exists at their institutions. To ignore incivility communicates tolerance of the problem, which also increases it. "That's the way it's always done here" may work in the short run; however, denial of problems often leads to bigger and more severe problems down the road. Lack of action from administrators often triggers feelings and actions related to a sense of automatic defeat. It is far better to take precautionary measures to prevent incivility and stop it as soon as it starts. Once incivility is allowed to become the status quo, it becomes almost impossible to stop without radical action.[24]

Solutions to Academic Incivility
A Degree of Improvement

The situation has improved somewhat over the past decade. As an alternative to on-the-job training, universities are now offering master's degrees in Nursing Education that teach students how to teach and the political ins and outs of the academic setting. Graduates come to the field of education with an understanding of curriculum development, evaluation, testing, course preparation, and many other aspects of surviving in higher education. They are taught to be more assertive and to express their opinions with a reasonable lack of fear.

In recent years, the nursing profession has emphasized the importance of not "eating our young." This consideration applies both to the workplace setting and to nursing education. Senior nursing educators are much more sensitive to the needs of new faculty and have a strong incentive to nurture them and help them develop into high-quality educators.[25]

A Model for Civility

A recently developed model allows faculty and students to promote civility in the academic setting. Although the model does not include administrators, their responsibilities, or their perceptions about incivility, it emphasizes the critical importance of the climate and infrastructure established by administrators. It is called the Conceptual Model for Fostering Civility in Nursing Education (Fig. 15.1).[26] The model depicts how, as stress levels increase for both students and faculty, student attitudes of entitlement and faculty attitudes of condescending superiority can lead to incivility.

The positive or negative attitude of administrators can determine whether these stressful situations

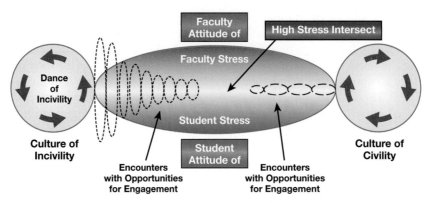

Figure 15.1 Conceptual model for fostering civility in nursing education. (Reprinted with permission from SLACK Incorporated: Clark, C. M., & Springer, P. J. (2010). Academic nurse leaders' role in fostering a culture of civility in nursing education. *Journal of Nursing Education, 49*(6), 319–325, doi: 10.3928/01484834-20100224-01. Epub 2010 Jun 3.)

are addressed. Unaddressed, the culture of incivility permeates, but when constructive problem-solving and respectful encounters are the norm, a culture of civility can prevail. A civil climate enhances both teaching and learning.

The Conceptual Model provides a basis for creating a culture of civility by focusing on the levels of stress for nursing faculty and students. Possible research questions include the following:

1. What do you perceive to be the biggest stressors for nursing students?
2. What uncivil behaviors do you see nursing students displaying?
3. What do you perceive to be the biggest stressors for nursing faculty?
4. What uncivil behaviors do you see nursing faculty displaying?
5. What is the role of nursing leadership in addressing incivility?[27]

These questions were asked of 126 academic nurse leaders in attendance at a Western statewide conference. The responses emphasized in particular the importance of accepting individual responsibility for negative behaviors and providing mentoring and rewards for civility. They also made the point that students and faculty must have opportunities for stress reduction, counseling when required, and new policies to reduce stress and improve communication. Respondents felt that civility should become a part of the curriculum and that civility consultants should be part of the faculty.

Incivility was shown as harmful to educators, students, clients, and the future work environment of new graduates.[27]

ETHICAL PROHIBITIONS TO INCIVILITY

A Guide for Caring
The Joint Commission notes:

"Intimidating and disruptive behaviors can foster medical errors, contribute to poor patient satisfaction and to preventable adverse outcomes, increase the cost of care, and cause qualified clinicians, administrators, and managers to seek new positions in more professional environments. Safety and quality of patient care is dependent on teamwork, communication, and a collaborative work environment. To assure quality and to promote a culture of safety, health care organizations must address the problem of behaviors that threaten the performance of the health care team."[28]

The American Nurses Association (ANA) Code of Ethics (see Chapter 7) also has principles that support ethical, civil, caring relationships. It was developed as a guide for carrying out nursing responsibilities in a manner consistent with quality in nursing care and the ethical obligations of the profession. The NLN website gives high priority to the Code of Ethics and to faculty responsibility as a way of dealing with student behavioral problems. The specific parts of the ANA Code of Ethics that relate to incivility are as follows:

1. "The nurse, in all professional relationships, practices with compassion and respect for the inherent dignity, worth, and uniqueness of every individual...."
1.5 Principles of respect extend to all encounters, including colleagues. "This standard of conduct precludes any and all prejudicial actions, any form of harassment or threatening behavior, or disregard for the effect of one's actions on others"
3.5 "Nurse educators have a responsibility to ... promote a commitment to professional practice prior to entry of an individual into practice."[29]

The Joint Commission, the ANA, and the NLN make it clear that underlying attitudes of caring and respect are essential expectations of those who enter the profession of nursing. It is essential for nurses to learn and internalize these attitudes. A caring attitude is *not* transmitted from generation to generation by genes—it is transmitted by the culture of a society.[3] The ANA has had a Task Force on Workplace Violence for several years. It developed a website that assists nurses in understanding more about this problem (http://www.nursingworld.org/ workplaceviolence).

Ethical behaviors in nursing school correlate with ethical behaviors in professional practice.[27] The American Association of Colleges of Nursing (AACN) stresses the importance of professional standards including the development and acquisition of an appropriate set of values and an ethical framework. It stresses that incivility is unethical and notes that nursing faculty have a "moral imperative" to deter incivility.[19] The AACN reinforces the moral imperative to care, suggesting that educators try to determine the presence of incivility before students enter a program.[27]

Codes of Conduct

Some universities and colleges have instituted honor codes. Academic settings with an honor code have less cheating. One type of honor code for students and faculty is called HIRRE, which stands for "honesty, integrity, respect, responsibility, and ethics." In HIRRE, students sign a pledge promising not to cheat or plagiarize.[27] Faculty and students can use a reporting system to identify violations of the honor code. Enforcement by faculty, directors, or the dean can include expulsion for honor code infractions.[11]

The Internet Society has an established Code of Conduct that is used as a guide for responsible behavior of Internet operators. It is important to remember that the Internet relies on the good conduct of those who use it.[13] However, because of recent misuses that have led to teenage suicides, ethical codes are continuing to evolve.

> *Once a tipping point is passed, the potential for violence increases dramatically. Interrupting the spiral with positive interventions and communication before that tipping point is important in defusing the anger.*

WORKPLACE INCIVILITY

Workplace Violence

Workplace incivility is blamed for the deaths of more than 1000 people a year in the United States. When the uncivil behavior is directed toward harming someone, it is no longer ambiguous and is labeled workplace violence. The estimated cost of workplace violence in the United States is $4.2 billion per year. Whether in the form of mere workplace incivility or full-blown workplace violence, these behaviors result in negative outcomes for clients as well as health-care workers.[22]

Workplace violence in the health-care setting is a growing problem. It is important to be able to recognize characteristics in a person that may indicate escalating cycles of violence. Institutions need a comprehensive plan to deal with violence, including client violence toward health-care workers. Disrespect and unresolved conflict can spiral out of control and eventually lead to violence without appropriate interventions.[17]

The incivility spiral (Fig. 15.2) depicts uncivil behavior between two people or two groups. The behavior can escalate, or those involved can let go of their resentment and stop the incivility from progressing. The path chosen depends largely on communication, both at the beginning of the conflict and during its progress. Conflict resolution interventions are essential to the process.

The higher up the spiral the uncivil behavior advances, the more coercive behavior is displayed and the greater is the desire for revenge. The victim of the incivility experiences loss of face, increasing anger, and a desire for disproportionate revenge. Once a tipping point is passed, the potential for violence increases dramatically. Interrupting the spiral with positive interventions and communication before that tipping point is important in defusing the anger.

Incivility within the health-care setting is a leading reason nurses leave the field and has been linked to male faculty leaving nursing education.[12]

Solutions to Incivility in the Workplace
A Positive Environment

Alertness is essential to defusing incivility in the work setting. Listening to fellow-workers' accounts of incivility is a first step and should be followed by reflection and development of an action plan. Ignoring the problem never solves it and often escalates the frequency and intensity of the incivility. To break the cycle, it is necessary to be proactive about incivility incidents and to see them as signs of potentially more dangerous problems.

The Nursing Organizations Alliance recommends eight actions to help build a positive workplace environment and overcome incivility[26]:

1. Building a collaborative culture that includes respectful communication and behavior
2. Establishing a communication-rich culture that emphasizes trust and respect

Sample Incivility Spiral

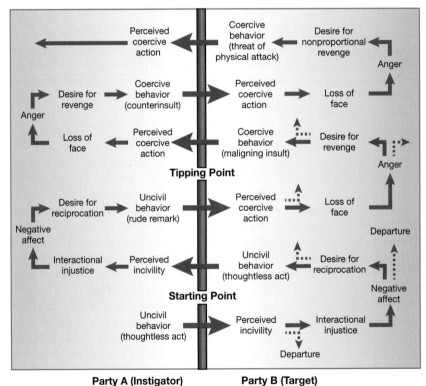

Figure 15.2 The incivility spiral. (From Anderson LM, Pearson CM: Tit for tat? The spiraling effect of incivility in the workplace. The Academy of Management Review, 24(3): 453–471, Jul. 1999. http//www.jstor.org/stable/259136, with permission.)

3. Making accountability central to the culture with clearly defined role expectations
4. Maintaining an adequate work force
5. Training competent leaders
6. Sharing decision-making
7. Continuously developing employee skills and knowledge
8. Recognizing and rewarding employees' contributions

Leadership for Job Satisfaction

Healthy workplace environments that empower nurses are critical to the success of the profession. Nurses must be vigilant for acts of incivility that are less obvious but affect the work of nurses in all settings. Healthy workplace environments are supported by the Magnet Hospital Designation (Agency for Healthcare Research and Quality [AHRQ], 2008). A healthy workplace decreases absenteeism, increases productivity, and dramatically reduces turnover rates.

Mentoring is a proven way to become an effective nurse. Mentoring partnerships and increasing cultural competence enhance job satisfaction with expanded and updated educational input.

Transformational leadership (TL) is essential to reversing incivility in the academic or workplace environment. TL acts as a lens through which leaders can reflect and change inequalities.[30] TL as an intervention requires an extraordinary capacity for self-restraint, self-reflection, and deep consciousness of the inner sense of responsibility. In addition, TL plays an important role in implementing needed changes in present and future practices.[31] Box 15.4 lists 13 transformational leadership qualities that would all be assets to improved civility.

Box 15.4
Thirteen Qualities of Transformational Leaders

1. You hold a vision for the organization that is intellectually rich, stimulating and rings true.
2. You are honest and empathic. People feel emotionally safe and trust that you have their interests at heart.
3. Your character is well developed, without the prominent dark side of ego power.
4. You set aside your own interests in looking good and getting strokes, instead making others look good and giving others power and credit.
5. You evince a concern for the whole (not just your own organization), reflected in your passionate and ethical voice being heard when necessary.
6. Your natural tendency is to help others engage, deepen their perspectives, and be effective.
7. You can share power with others—you believe sharing power is the best way to tap talent, engage others, and get work done in optimal fashion.
8. You risk, experiment, and learn. Information is never complete.
9. You have a true passion for work and the vision. It shows in your time commitment, attention to detail, and ability to renew your energy.
10. You communicate effectively both in listening and in speaking.
11. You understand and appreciate management and administration. They appreciate that you move toward shared success without sacrifice.
12. You celebrate the now. At meetings or anywhere else, you sincerely acknowledge accomplishment, staying in the moment before moving on.
13. You persist in hard times. That means you have the courage to move ahead when you are tired, conflicted, and getting mixed signals.

Source: Johns C: Becoming a transformational leader through reflection. Reflections on Nursing Leadership 30(2):24–26, 2004.

Conclusion

Incivility violates trust and undermines the moral imperative to care. It creates insecurity and hostility and degrades learning, collaboration, and performance in all institutions where it is found. In all settings, relationships are adversely affected by incivility. Research and active efforts to deal with the problem will help to ensure better client care. TL qualities can transform incivility into civility and caring. TL can stop upward-spiraling incivility and help with spotting, intervening in, and overcoming incivility. Constructive mentor–mentee rather than tormentor–mentee relationships will promote professional growth in nurses and improve both the academic environment and the health-care setting. Emotional intelligence arising from the practice of civility is essential and basic to the practice of nursing.

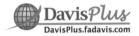

DavisPlus.fadavis.com

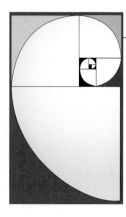

Issues Now

Promoting Civility through Reflection on Your Personal Qualities

Job satisfaction is important to the attitude brought to the workplace. The likelihood of workplace incivility being present is high. Job satisfaction helps to deal with incivility.

Likewise, the Department of Labor also lists preferred qualities for different career choices (http://www.onetcenter.org/content.html). These are not personality tests, but rather are measures of qualities that meet common core expectations. It is hypothesized that a match between your qualities and those of your chosen career helps job satisfaction.

As you prepare for employment or further professional development, reflect on your own qualities. Identifying them will provide a lens through which to preview your chosen field. Be prepared to have them tested as you progress in your healthcare career, reflecting on the assets and competencies that you bring to the world.

What Do You Think?

How do you think incivility compares with child abuse or elder abuse?
Are the measures to overcome child or elder abuse similar to those required to overcome workplace violence?

16

Delegation in Nursing

Joseph T. Catalano

Learning Objectives

After completing this chapter, the reader will be able to:

- Apply the principles of delegation to nursing practice.
- Analyze and identify situations in which delegation is used improperly.
- Discuss the legal implications of delegation in the current health-care setting.
- Distinguish between delegation and assignment.

AN ESSENTIAL SKILL

Delegation is an essential component of client care and management of nursing units in today's health-care system. It allows health-care managers to maximize the use of caregivers who are educated at multiple levels in a variety of programs. Delegation, if performed properly, permits nurses to meet the requirements of high-quality care for all clients and is a basic skill that registered nurses (RNs) must learn. However, the skill set required to delegate safely is one of the most complex that nurses must master, requiring the ability to make high-level clinical judgments. The goal of delegation is to meet the increased demands for services as they intersect with the shrinking resources of the health-care system.[1]

Look to All These Things

The concept of delegation has been a part of health care since the time of Florence Nightingale, when she instructed the nurses she educated ". . . to look to all these things yourself does not mean to do them yourself."[2] As far back as 1991, the American Nurses Association (ANA) initially addressed and defined delegation when it was beginning to become a more widespread practice in health care. They further refined the definition in 1997. The National Council of State Boards of Nursing (NCSBN) also addressed delegation in 1995 and periodically since then. Although some minor revisions have occurred since then, the basic concepts and basic principles of delegation remain essentially unchanged.

DELEGATION OR ASSIGNMENT?

Although delegation and assignment are closely related concepts, they are different. **Delegation** is recognized as designating ancillary personnel for the responsibility of carrying out a specific group of nursing tasks in the care of certain clients. Delegation includes the understanding that the authorized person is acting in the place of the RN and will be carrying out tasks that generally fall under *the RN's scope of practice*. However, the person taking on the RN-level task must be qualified to perform the task within the nurse's state practice act.[3]

Assignment, on the other hand, is designating tasks for ancillary personnel that fall under their *own level of practice* according to facility policies, position descriptions, and if applicable, state practice act. In the everyday work setting, RNs usually both make assignments and delegate tasks, often to the same individuals. It can be confusing; however, clarifying the difference can be helpful in reducing the level of confusion. In either case, the concepts of supervision, authority, responsibility, and accountability are key to successful client care. Supervision is required by the RN in both delegation and assignment.[4]

When nurses delegate nursing tasks to non-nurses, the RNs must always supervise those individuals to ensure that the care given meets the standards of care. However, if the facility, the state board of nursing, or some other official body has a predesignated list of tasks that non-nursing personnel may undertake in the care of clients, the RN is responsible only for supervising them to make sure the tasks are carried out safely.

Legally, the authority or power to delegate is restricted to professionals who are licensed and governed by a statutory practice act. RNs are considered professionals, with state-sanctioned licenses governed by a nurse practice act, and therefore are authorized to delegate independent nursing functions to other personnel. However, not all RN functions can be delegated to assistive personnel because of restrictions in the nurse practice act and institutional policies. For example, performing admission assessments, developing care plans, and making nursing diagnoses are activities generally restricted to RNs only.

RESPONSIBILITY AND ACCOUNTABILITY IN DELEGATING

The ANA defines delegation as "the transfer of responsibility for the performance of an activity from one individual to another while retaining accountability for the outcome."[5] The ANA stresses the belief that, even though the leader or manager delegates a task to another employee, he or she remains accountable for the care that is provided.

Nurses often can be heard saying, "If I delegate, then that person is practicing on my license and I don't want the responsibility." This statement implies that responsibility has legal liability attached to it. In reality, it does have liability attached, but only with the performance of duties in the specific role. When they accept a delegated task, assistive personnel accept the responsibility attached to it. Delegatees do not practice on the RN's license. They practice on their own license (if licensed practical nurses [LPNs] and licensed vocational nurses [LVNs]) or, if unlicensed, within their own level of education. Assistive personnel, when they agree to accept the delegated task, are responsible for their own actions in performance of the task.[6]

When the RNs accept responsibility for delegating an assignment appropriately, they become accountable for the delegation process. **Accountability** looks to see if the RN used his or her nursing knowledge, critical thinking, and clinical judgment skills in delegating a task. For example, suppose an RN delegates a task to assistive personnel that is appropriate for the person's educational level and skill set. If the person accepts it, then totally botches the task, leading to the death of the client, the RN has met the requirements of accountability, and the responsibility for the client's death rests on the assistive personnel. On the other hand, if the RN delegates inappropriately to a person who is clearly *not* qualified, and the client dies, the RN and the assistive personnel could both be held liable. So how does the RN make the decision to delegate or not delegate? The steps outlined below are a guide to the decision-making process.

Guidelines for Delegation
Assess the Client
Before delegating any task, RNs should give careful consideration to the condition of the client and the client's health-care needs. Assessing clients is a designated **responsibility** of RNs. Without a thorough assessment, it is likely that critical needs will remain unidentified by less trained personnel, leading to potential errors in care. Clients who are relatively stable and not likely to experience drastic changes in health-care status are the most suitable for delegation. Also,

the tasks being delegated must be relatively uncomplicated and routine, must be performed without variation from policy or procedure, and should not require the use of nursing judgment while being performed. Delegation of repetitive tasks produces higher efficiency because the time and skills of the RN are used more effectively.

What Do You Think?

Is delegation used in the facility where you have clinical rotations? Who does the delegation on the unit? Does it work well?

Know Staff Availability

The delegating nurse needs to know the availability of staff and the education and competency levels of the personnel to be delegated. These factors must be matched with the level of care required by the client. Key information to obtain is how often the delegatee has performed the required tasks or cared for this type of client, what units the delegatee has worked on and feels comfortable in, and his or her organizational abilities. It is important to keep the team informed of who is delegated what tasks and when changes are made.

Know the Job Description

One large group of health-care workers to whom RNs delegate is generally called unlicensed assistive personnel (UAP). This group includes individuals who have been through some type of training program ranging from a few hours up to several months (Box 16.1). They may receive a certificate of completion, but they do not have any type of licensure and therefore do not have legal status.

The RN needs to know the institution's official position description for the UAP as well as the individual UAP's abilities. For example, the position description may state that the UAP can care for postoperative clients who have multiple wound drains. However, when the RN assigns a specific UAP to such a postoperative client, the nurse discovers that the UAP has worked only in the newborn nursery for the past 5 years and has no knowledge of how to care for adult postoperative clients. If the RN delegates this UAP to care for complicated postoperative clients and a major complication develops because of the UAP's lack of competence (even though the

Box 16.1

Other Names for Unlicensed Assistive Personnel

Certified nurse assistant (CNA)
Nurse's aide
Home health aide
Registered nurse assistant (RNA)
Nurse technician (NT)
Medication technician (MT)
Nursing assistant
Patient care assistant (PCA)
Orderly
Client attendant
Psychiatric attendant

position description states that this is an appropriate function for the UAP), the RN will also be held legally liable for the poor outcome. When the RN determines that the client's needs match the skills and abilities of the UAP or LPN, only then should that person be assigned.

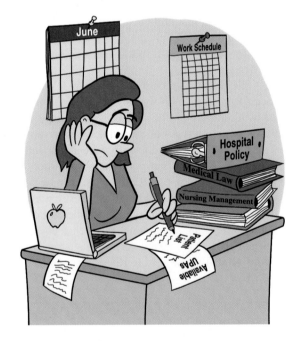

Educate the Staff Member

RNs who delegate are also responsible for educating the UAP about the task to be done. If the UAP is unfamiliar with the task, the RN is required to demonstrate how the task or procedure is performed and then document the training. Education also includes telling the UAP what is expected in the completion of the task and what complications to watch for and report to the RN. The ANA suggests that the RN watch the UAP perform the designated task at least initially, then make periodic observations throughout the shift to ensure safe and competent care for the client.[7] Furthermore, the RN must always be available to answer questions and help the UAP whenever assistance is required.

Consider the following situation:

Elsie Humber, RN, is the evening charge nurse on a busy oncology unit of the county hospital. On one particularly busy evening, she discovers during shift report that one of the scheduled LPNs has called in sick and no other LPNs are available to take her place. Ms. Humber assigns the LPN's duties and clients, including a heat lamp treatment for a decubitus ulcer, to a UAP who has worked on the unit for several months. The UAP protests the assignment, but Ms. Humber rebukes her, saying, "I have no one else. If you don't care for these clients, they won't get any care this shift." In setting up the heat lamp treatment, the UAP knocks the lamp over and burns the client. Because of his suppressed immune system from chemo-therapy and generally debilitated condition, the burn does not heal and develops into an infection. The client later sues the hospital for malpractice. The hospital in turn attempts to shift the legal responsibility for the burn to Ms. Humber. Who is legally responsible for the incident? Does the client have grounds for a successful case?

Predictable and Uncomplicated

When a nurse delegates tasks, the outcomes of tasks should be clear and predictable. For example, when a UAP is assigned the task of feeding a client who has suffered a stroke and has hemiplegia, the predicted outcome will be that the client will eat and not choke on the food. The task should not require excessive supervision, complex decision making, or detailed assessment during its performance. If any of these elements are required, it needs to be reassigned to an RN.

It is important to remember that when nurses delegate nursing tasks, they are *not* delegating nursing. Professional nursing practice is both a science, based on a unique body of knowledge, and an art, guided by the nursing process. It is not merely a collection of tasks. Of all health-care workers, professional nurses are the most qualified to provide holistic care of the client by promoting health and treating disease. Nurses' education and experience provide them with the skills and knowledge to coordinate and supervise nursing care and to delegate specific tasks to others.

Although mastering delegation skills can seem like a daunting task, a nurse can take several common-sense steps to attain this skill (Box 16.2). Nursing students often have tasks delegated to them by the RNs on the units where they are having clinical rotations. It is easy to identify the RNs who have developed good delegation skills and those who still need to work on those skills.

Box 16.2
Five "Rights" of Delegation

- Right task
  Do the tasks delegated follow written policy guidelines?
- Right person
  Does the person have the proper qualifications for the tasks?
- Right direction or communication
  Are the instructions and outcomes clearly stated? When should the person report changes?
- Right supervision or feedback
  How can the delegation process be improved? Are the client goals for care being achieved?
- Right circumstances
  Are the tasks that are being delegated possible without independent nursing judgments?

Sources: Corazzini KN, Anderson RA, Rapp CG, Mueller C, McConnell ES, Lekan D: Delegation in long-term care: Scope of practice or job description? Online Journal of Issues in Nursing 15(2):4, 2010.

Whitehead, DK, Weiss, SA, Tappen, RM: Essentials of Nursing Leadership and Management (5th ed). Philadelphia, F. A. Davis, 2010.

Weydt A: Developing delegation skills. Online Journal of Issues in Nursing 14(2):10, 2010.

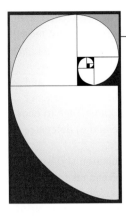

Issues in Practice

Leadership/Management Case Study: Poor Staff Performance

Angela is the emergency department (ED) Nurse Manager in a small rural hospital. Hiring qualified RNs for her staff had become more of a challenge as the nursing shortage worsened. For 8 months, a full-time evening RN position had gone unfilled. During this time, the position was filled by cross-training nurses from other departments, paying bonus shifts and overtime, contracting with agencies, and hiring available nurses from other hospitals. These nurses were excellent, but the continuity of regular staffing was lacking in the ED. Angela believed the lack of continuity was negatively affecting morale and efficiency in the department.

At this hospital, the Vice President of Nursing Services (VPNS) made all the final decisions about hiring new staff after consulting with the nurse managers. The VPNS suggested an employee who was interested in the position but did not have the experience of the nurses usually hired for the ED. Ted, who had been an LPN in a long-term care facility, had gone back to nursing school and received his BS in nursing 6 months earlier. His most recent experience after graduating was working in a physician's office. Although his combined health-care experience was more than 10 years, he had never worked in an acute care setting.

When Angela interviewed Ted, he appeared highly motivated, intelligent, a self-starter, and well groomed. Because of the nursing shortage, it had become fairly common practice to let new graduates work in specialty areas, such as EDs or intensive care units, without the traditional mandatory year of medical-surgical experience. Angela believed that Ted could, over time, learn the ED routines. He would have an experienced RN working with him for at least a year. Also, at this hospital, 90 percent of ED visits were nonurgent, office-type visits. Ted's experience of coordinating and moving clients through a busy office practice would be an asset.

Angela started by giving Ted a thorough and extended orientation to the ED. She consulted with each nurse he would be working with and asked for support in mentoring him. She encouraged the nurses to begin by letting Ted care for the more routine cases and then gradually allow him to care for clients with more acute conditions. During the orientation, Ted seemed to master the assessment and documentation aspects of the job well. Ted was also studying for ACLS certification. Obviously, he was unfamiliar with many of the medications routinely used in the ED. Angela encouraged him to ask questions and use the unit's medication reference books.

However, despite all the efforts at orientation, Ted made four serious medication errors during his first 2 months in the ED. Fortunately, they were discovered early enough so that no serious harm came to the clients. Ted was counseled by the hospital's Nurse Educator, who worked with him on a medication review. He completed the course of study successfully and passed the medication exam.

Angela began receiving feedback from the other ED staff members who had been working with Ted. They expressed insecurity about the quality of the care he was giving, and some believed he was not "carrying his load" during busy times. He would manipulate client assignments and shift work to other nurses. A personality conflict had also arisen between Ted and some of the nurses. They had begun watching his every move and documenting what he was doing or not doing.

Issues in Practice   continued

Some observed that he would leave the ED for unscheduled long breaks without notifying anyone. Others remarked that he was not monitoring clients with cardiac problems as closely as they thought he should. Angela noted that Ted seemed to have lost the support of his coworkers and that the overall morale of the unit was deteriorating.

Angela met with Ted and suggested that he attend a Certified Emergency-Room Nurse review course to improve his knowledge and skills in emergency nursing. He did attend the course. Angela also met with him several times to develop plans for improving his work. Each time he would complete the requirements of the plan, and the situation would improve for a while. After a week or two, however, he would slip back into his previous behaviors.

As the morale of the unit continued to decline, Angela began feeling depressed and under stress. She sensed that she was losing the credibility and respect of her staff. One day she overheard one of the staff nurses say, "At this hospital, any warm body can have a job!," implying that the standards and quality of care were poor. On the other hand, Angela felt responsible for placing Ted in a situation in which he could not succeed.

QUESTIONS FOR THOUGHT

1. Identify the erroneous assumptions used in the initial hiring of Ted.

2. What other measures could Angela have taken to help Ted in his adjustment to the ED?

3. What can Angela do now about the situation?

(Answers are found at the end of the chapter.)

DEVELOPING DELEGATION SKILLS

Clear Communication

In the process of developing delegation skills, students should try to emulate the good delegators. Develop good communication and interpersonal relationship skills. Make eye contact with the other person, be pleasant, and ask for suggestions. However, avoid allowing the person to whom the tasks are being delegated to control the exchange by intimidation or resistance.

After a nurse delegates a task, it's a good idea to make a written list of the responsibilities that are expected from the person, if one does not already exist. The list will help clarify what is expected and head off possible misunderstandings. It is also important to be flexible. Clients' conditions change, new clients may be admitted, and other clients may be discharged. The original assignments may have to be modified in response to changes in the environment.[8]

Simulation Exercises

Both nursing education and nursing service can increase the knowledge and skill required for effective delegation through practice scenarios that reflect daily practice. There is an increasing emphasis on simulation in nursing education, and delegation scenarios can be used alongside clinical practice ones. For students, these scenarios can be an introduction to the type of critical thinking and decision-making skills required for effective delegation. For practicing RNs, delegation scenarios reinforce earlier learned skills and demonstrate the authority the RN has in the delegation process.

Simulation allows the student or RN to make mistakes and learn from the mistakes. Feedback is essential to the educational process and allows participants to self-evaluate their interpersonal, communication, and decision-making skills.[9]

Careful Supervision

Effective delegation, as well assignment of tasks, requires the RN to master supervision skills. This includes monitoring the delegatees while they are providing care and helping them when they require help. Are they doing what they should be doing? Do they understand the responsibilities involved in the client's care? Effective delegation also presumes that the delegator will teach the delegatees who demonstrate a lack of knowledge. Continual feedback throughout the shift allows both parties an opportunity for ongoing assessment. Most important, at the end of the shift, say, "Thank you. I appreciate the hard work (good job) you've done today."

Certain delegation situations may place the RN at an increased risk for liability (Boxes 16.3 and 16.4). When delegating, try to avoid the following:

- Assigning tasks that are highly invasive or have the potential to cause significant physical harm to clients
- Assigning tasks that are designated under the scope of practice or standards of care as belonging exclusively to the RN (admission assessments, care plan development)
- Assigning tasks that the person is not trained for or lacks the knowledge to complete safely
- Assigning tasks when there is inadequate time to safely monitor or evaluate the practice of the person performing the tasks[10]

Delegation has the potential to be a powerful tool in improving the quality of client care. The knowledge and judgment of the professional nurse remain essential elements in any health-care system reforms, including clinical integration, case management, outsourcing practices, **total quality management (TQM),** and **continuous quality improvement (CQI).**

What Do You Think?

What qualities have you observed in good delegators? What qualities made the poor delegators ineffective?

LEGAL ISSUES IN DELEGATION

One area of fallout from the movement to managed care is the increase in nurses' liability for lawsuits in the area of supervision and delegation. In the search for cost-effective client care, current managed-care strategies attempt to make optimal use of relatively expensive RNs by replacing them with less costly and less educated personnel. As more and more health-care facilities move toward restructuring, the use of UAPs who have minimal education and experience will continue to increase. Although RNs have always been responsible for the delegation of some

Box 16.3

Barriers to Effective Delegation

A. Internal barriers (person delegating):
1. Lack of experience delegating
2. Lack of confidence in others
3. Personal insecurity
4. Demanding perfectionism
5. Poor organizational skills
6. Indecision
7. Poor communication skills
8. Lack of confidence in self
9. Fear of not being liked by everyone
10. Micromanaging management style
B. External barriers (circumstances or person being delegated to):
1. Unclear policies about delegation
2. Policies that do not tolerate mistakes
3. Management-by-crisis model for facility
4. Unclear delineation of authority and responsibilities
5. Poor staffing
6. Lack of competence
7. Overdependence on the person delegating
8. Unwillingness to accept responsibility for one's own practice
9. Immersion in trivia and gossip
10. Work overload

Source: Whitehead, DK, Weiss, SA, Tappen, RM: Essentials of Nursing Leadership and Management (5th ed). Philadelphia, F. A. Davis, 2010.

Box 16.4

Delegation Decision Tree

1. Are there laws and rules in place supporting the rules of delegation?
2. Is the task within the scope of practice of the UAP, LPN/LVN, RN, or new graduate?
3. Has there been an assessment of the client's needs?
4. Is the UAP, LPN/LVN, RN, or new graduate competent to accept the delegation?
5. Does the ability of the caregiver match the care needs of the client?
6. Can the task be completed without requiring nursing judgments?
7. Is the result of the task somewhat predictable?
8. Can the task be safely performed according to directions?
9. Can the task be performed without repeated assessment?
10. Is appropriate supervision available?

Source: Whitehead, DK, Weiss, SA, Tappen, RM: Essentials of Nursing Leadership and Management (5th ed). Philadelphia, F. A. Davis, 2010.

tasks and the supervision of less qualified health-care providers, delegation is now one of the primary functions of RNs in today's health-care system.

Delegation does have some advantages. It is an RN extender in that it allows more care to be given to more clients than can be given by one RN. Delegation can free the RN from lower-level, time-consuming tasks so that more time can be spent planning for care and performing those skills that less prepared individuals would be unable to perform. For those to whom tasks are delegated, it can serve as an incentive to learn additional skills, increase knowledge, develop a sense of initiative, and perhaps seek further formal education. Delegation,

if performed properly, maintains accountability and decision making where they belong—with the RN.

WHO CAN DELEGATE—LEGALLY?

An Ethical Obligation

Most state practice acts do *not* give delegatory authority to **dependent practitioners** such as LPNs, LVNs, or UAPs. In addition, professionals who delegate specific tasks retain accountability for the proper and safe completion of those tasks, as well as responsibility for determining whether the assigned personnel are competent to carry out the task. One exception occurs when the person who is assigned a task also has a license and the tasks fall under that person's scope of practice.[11] Then again, the RN is responsible only for supervision of the other licensed person. These situations are often seen when LPNs or LVNs are assigned to client care.

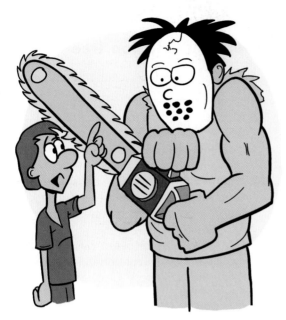

"WHY DON'T I GET SOMEONE ELSE
TO REMOVE MRS. LEMKE'S SUTURES?"

The delegation and supervision responsibilities of RNs have been and continue to be a major concern for the nursing profession, both ethically and legally. The ANA Code of Ethics for Nurses states, "The nurse is responsible and accountable for individual nursing practice and determines the appropriate delegation of tasks consistent with the nurse's obligation to provide optimum patient care" (statement 4).[12] From the ethical viewpoint, RNs have an obligation to refuse assignments that they are not competent to carry out and to refuse to delegate particular nursing tasks to individuals who they believe are unable or unprepared to perform them (Fig. 16.1).

Direct and Indirect Delegation

The legal side of the delegation issue has also been addressed by the ANA in the *ANA Basic Guide to Safe Delegation*. This document makes a distinction between direct delegation, which is a specific decision made by the RN about who can perform what tasks, and indirect delegation, which is a list of tasks that certain health-care personnel can perform that is produced by the health-care facility.[5]

The **consensus** among many experts is that *indirect* delegation is really a form of covert institutional licensure. Lists of activities from the facility allowing non-nursing personnel, who do not have the education of the RN, to carry out professional nursing functions is a de facto permission to practice nursing without a license. Indirect delegation places RNs in a precarious legal position.

Basically, indirect delegation takes away much of the authority of the RN to delegate personnel tasks, yet the RN remains accountable for the safe completion of the tasks under the doctrines of **respondeat superior** and **vicarious liability.** Although some states are beginning to address the UAP and delegation issues in their nurse practice acts, many states either have no official standards for UAP delegation or include UAP standards under the medical practice act.[13]

Delegation and the NCLEX

Because delegation is such an important issue in today's health-care system, and because decisions about delegation require considerable critical thinking skill, the number of questions about delegation on the NCLEX has been increasing steadily. It is not unusual for 10 to 25 percent of questions to deal with delegation issues. One problem graduates may encounter with these questions is that the NCLEX uses strict parameters for determining delegation. In the real world of health care, LPNs, LVNs, and UAPs often perform functions beyond their legal scope of practice. The following lists may be helpful in answering NCLEX questions about delegation.

Although LPNs and LVNs can do most skills, for the NCLEX they:

- **Cannot** do admission assessments
- **Cannot** give intravenous (IV) push medications
- **Cannot** write nursing diagnoses
- **Cannot** do most teaching
- **Cannot** do complex skills
- **Cannot** take care of clients with acute conditions
- **Cannot** take care of unstable clients

For questions concerning UAPs, CNAs, and aides on the NCLEX:

- Look for the **lowest level of skill** required for the task.
- Look for the **least complicated** task.
- Look for the **most stable** client.
- Look for the client with the **chronic illness.**

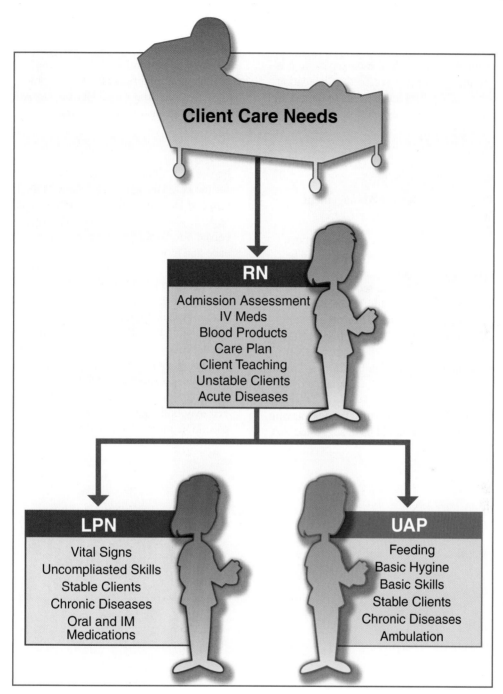

Figure 16.1 Delegation of responsibilities.

Conclusion

With the increased use of less educated and unlicensed personnel in today's health-care system, it is essential that the nurse develop effective delegation and supervision skills. The nurse needs to be mindful that the tasks that can be delegated can change on the basis of work setting, client needs, position descriptions, institutional training of personnel, and the ever-changing requirements of nurse practice acts and professional standards. Nurses also need to know when delegation is inappropriate.

Answers to Case Study Questions

Issues in Practice: Leadership/Management Case Study

1. The first erroneous assumption was that a nurse with no acute care hospital experience could be taught to provide safe care in a specialty area with only minimal orientation. The second assumption was that the other nurses would be enthusiastic about spending extra time and effort in orienting and teaching a new nurse. This group seemed to resent the imposition. The third assumption was that, because most of the care in the ED was "routine," a person with only limited experience could work there.

2. When Angela first discovered that Ted was having problems adjusting, she could have suggested that he work on a medical-surgical unit and cross-train for the ED. This approach would have given him a range of learning experiences that he could later apply to his work in the ED. After Ted had received 6 to 8 months of medical-surgical experience and cross-training, Angela and the other unit managers would have been able to better evaluate his skills and knowledge.

3. Because of the declining morale and the loss of trust in Angela by the staff, Ted needs to be removed from the ED. If his performance so indicates, he may be terminated. However, in this age of nursing shortages, a better option would be to place him on another unit and evaluate him there. Not everyone is destined to be an ED nurse, and Ted may find another unit with a more relaxed pace to be more suited to his personality and skills.

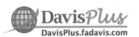

DavisPlus.fadavis.com

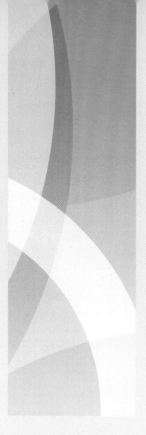

Critical Thinking Exercises

- Obtain a copy of your state's nurse practice act. Review the section that deals with delegation. Apply those criteria to the case study at the beginning of this chapter.

- As a student, you have had tasks delegated to you. Identify how delegation has changed in regard to your learning and level of skills as you have progressed through your program.

- Obtain a copy of the policy on delegation from at least two of the clinical sites where you have practiced. How do these policies differ? How are they similar? What are the reasons for the similarities and differences?

17

Governance and Collective Bargaining

Karen Tomajan
Joseph T. Catalano

Learning Objectives

After completing this chapter, the reader will be able to:

- Define governance.
- Discuss models for governance in organizations that employ nurses.
- Discuss the benefits and challenges of shared governance models.
- Analyze the professional skills necessary to participate in shared governance models.
- Define collective bargaining.
- Analyze the key issues that concern nurses in collective bargaining.
- Identify the steps in the contract negotiation process.
- Distinguish between a mediator and an arbitrator.
- Delineate the important elements in a contract.
- Analyze the effect governance has on collective bargaining.

GOVERNANCE

The term *governance* has a variety of meanings in different contexts. In general, the term describes the arrangement of the power hierarchy within an organization and how that power flows through the organization. Governance includes decision-making, resource allocation, and the development of policies and procedures.

Governance in the modern workplace has evolved over the past 100 years, during which the United States transitioned from farming to manufacturing to an information- and service-oriented economy. Over this time, the role of the worker has evolved from the brawn needed for manual labor to the brain power required of today's professional. In the manufacturing environment of the early 20th century, leadership approaches centered around what was is now called autocratic, or "command and control," styles, whereby the role of the leader was to issue orders and the responsibility of the worker was to follow commands.

By the 1960s, democratic leadership styles evolved that engaged employees in decision-making related to work and the work environment. This evolution complemented the rise in workers' education levels and increased employment of professional staff. Leaders and managers were also better trained for supervisory roles. Leadership styles evolved to incorporate participative approaches, shared governance models, or both. The model of **shared governance** provides the structure to involve employees in decisions related to work processes, resource allocation, and the work environment.

Just as businesses evolved to use and accommodate the knowledge and expertise of educated professionals in the workplace, so have health-care organizations. Health care has changed over the years, perhaps most dramatically since the late 1990s. In 1999, the Institute of Medicine released a series of reports in response to public safety concerns regarding health care in the United States. These reports have resulted in numerous fundamental changes driven by regulatory agencies, foundations, and professional groups. One of the most beneficial outcomes of this process has been a new view of the important contributions nurses and other direct-care staff make to client safety and quality outcome. Changes in governance structures are critical to the successful implementation of these changes.[1–3]

A System of Control and Coordination
Traditionally, authority is considered a type of power originating in the position that an individual holds within an organization.[4] This individual has this power only because others are willing to accept the decisions made by the person in that position. Relatively few people in the organization's hierarchy control large numbers of employees, as well as the directions and functions of the rest of the organization. In traditional organizations, power and authority, as well as decision-making boundaries, flowed from the top of the organization through management to the staff. Today, progressive health-care organizations are adopting new structures and approaches that involve employees in decision-making.[5] Generally, this interaction is accomplished through traditional organizational structures. The levels of the typical organization follow.

The Board of Directors
At the top of the governance hierarchy is the board of directors, also called the trustees or governors. The board of directors is usually composed of influential business people considered community leaders. Although they retain the ultimate legal and ethical responsibility for the operation of the organization, generally the day-to-day operation is delegated to the hospital administration. The board's main function is to set general policies and to plan for the long-range development of the organization. In addition, the board of directors holds the organization accountable for quality of care and client safety outcomes. Most boards become directly involved in the facility's operations

only when there is a crisis, such as a financial shortfall, or a major quality of care issue.

Hospital Administration
The chief executive officer (CEO) is usually the highest-ranking member of the hierarchy to be involved in the daily operation of the facility. The CEO works with the hospital administrative team, comprising the CEO and other high-level executives, who collaborate to ensure that the organization meets financial and business goals, quality and safety outcomes, and regulatory requirements. Members of the executive team include the chief financial officer, chief nursing officer, human resource executive, chief information officer, and other leaders. Members of the executive team have the education and knowledge required to direct the highly complex and technologically advanced elements that are an essential part of today's health-care system. Operational decisions are made by the executive team.

The Medical Staff
In most health-care facilities, the medical staff has an important role in the governance of the organization. The medical staff has its own internal governance structures with physician leaders and medical staff members. Traditionally, medical staff had a great deal of influence because they were not employees and operated as independent contractors, bringing their business to the facility. In recent years, with the spread of managed care, the traditional physician–institution relationship has changed remarkably. A significant portion of the physician staff in many facilities are actually salaried employees just like nurses, housekeepers, administrators, and security personnel. Their practice and productivity are monitored and evaluated, and they can be terminated for poor performance. Health-care facilities are held accountable for collaborative relationships with the medical staff to ensure high-quality outcomes and client safety.

Nurses' Role in Governance
In the past, nurses had limited voice in the governance of their facility or agency. Their traditional ideology of professionalism oriented nurses more toward loyalty and respect than toward autonomy of practice and independent decision-making about the quality of care.[6] Nurses often accepted the work hours assigned to them without question, tolerated

disrespect and abuse from physicians and administrators as part of the work environment, and were satisfied with the meager salaries paid to them because theirs was a profession of caring and dedication. This situation has changed drastically over the course of the past 30 years and will continue to change as the role of the professional nurse evolves.

Autonomy for the Nurse

As nursing responsibilities increased with advancing technology and changes in the health-care system, nurses recognized that their responsibilities far exceeded their authority to influence their practice. They embraced professional autonomy, authority, and accountability as essential elements in high-quality client care. One approach to gaining these elements was to change the organizational structure of the health-care facilities where they were employed.

Nurses challenged the traditional governance structure at a number of levels with varying amounts of success. Nursing service administrators are the leaders of the largest single group of health-care professionals in most health-care organizations—generally about 50 percent of all the employees.[4] Because of their education and experience, many nursing administrators have moved into positions of power in the health-care system and have worked to change the traditional role of the professional nurse.

Nurses in leadership roles have often been caught in the middle of conflicting expectations. For example, during a budget crisis, the chief financial officer may want to cut the budget by reducing staffing, whereas the nurses on the units recognize that they can no longer provide high-quality nursing care because the staffing levels are already too low. The chief nursing officer works with nursing directors, managers, and staff nurses to create the business case for the staffing plan. The officer also works with other members of the executive team to identify strategies for meeting budget expectations without disrupting client safety by cutting staff.

Positional Authority

Staff registered nurses (RNs) often view themselves as located at the bottom of the hierarchy with very little power. This is rarely the case. Depending on the organization of the facility, RNs have positional authority over licensed practical nurses (LPNs), nursing assistants, and individuals from the laboratory and radiology department.

Nurses have gained greater control over their practice by fostering change in the organizational structures of health-care facilities and agencies. The changes include decentralization of authority, identification of professional nurses as peers, agreement on the philosophy and goals of nursing care, and increased responsibility for directing and planning the care given to clients while they are in the facility.[7]

Nursing Administration

The nursing department is generally organized with a structure that facilitates communication and client-care coordination. The size of the facility and the complexity of the care delivery influence decisions related to structure. The current trend in nursing leadership is to maintain fairly flat organizations with fewer layers of bureaucracy. The most common organizational structure of a nursing department includes the following:

Chief Nursing Officer. The nursing division is led by a chief nursing officer or sometimes a vice president for nursing. In accredited hospitals, this individual is required be an RN with advanced education in business or hospital or nursing administration. The nursing executive is a part of the administrative team and participates in decision-making at the highest level of the organization, such as the operations council or other executive-level committees that represent the interests of the client and the nursing staff. The nurse executive reports to the hospital board of directors on nursing issues and is involved in any decision that affects client care or the nursing staff.[8]

Unit or Department Management. Each client care area has a nursing manager or clinical director with 24-hour accountability for nursing operations on that unit. This includes oversight of staffing, budgets, client care, quality outcomes, and staff satisfaction. Charge nurses or shift leaders are accountable for the unit operations on a shift-to-shift basis and work collaboratively with the nurse manager in coordinating the function of the unit. In large organizations, there are also middle managers, often with titles of administrative director, responsible for coordination of nursing functions at the division level.

Staff Nurses. In the contemporary nursing organization, the staff nurse is considered the authority on client care. The pivotal role of the staff nurse is recognized as the front line of client safety defense systems and is vital to coordinating and integrating care and services.[1] The RN's contribution to health-care outcomes can be measured and quantified.

Models for Nursing Governance

In an attempt to redistribute power and authority within health-care organizations, several alternative forms of governance have been developed. Some are used more widely than others and may be more effective, depending on the facility and the willingness of staff and managers to collaborate on ensuring a successful outcome.

Shared Governance

Shared governance is a an organizational framework for shared decision-making based on partnership, equity, accountability, and ownership at the point of service.[8] In the shared governance model, power and authority are transferred to the nursing staff rather than being seated primarily in administration. The key to shared governance is decentralization of the nursing administration structure. Its goal is to involve professional nurses in the decision-making process at all levels to ensure that their knowledge and expertise are used to deliver the highest-quality care possible.[9]

Shared governance gives the nurse autonomy in decisions about nursing practice, staffing levels, standards of care, and the work environment. It gives professional nurses the chance to be held accountable and responsible for their clinical judgment and the care they give to clients. It allows their peers a chance to recognize their knowledge and competence as true health-care professionals.

In this model, the source of power lies in clinical rather than administrative areas. Shared governance can be initiated at the unit level or across the entire nursing division; the most effective models allow staff involvement at the unit and the department levels.[10]

Councilor and Congressional Models

The councilor structure defines accountabilities for decision-making through nursing councils. In most organizations, there are five councils, which include clinical practice, quality, professional development, research, and a coordinating council.

The clinical practice council develops practice standards, policies, and procedures. The quality council handles staff credentialing and oversees quality

initiatives and clinical improvements such as fall prevention, client satisfaction, and hand hygiene initiatives. The professional development council works with the education department to assess learning needs, develop an education plan, oversee orientation, and develop training initiatives, such as in-services on new products. The research council guides the nursing department in conducting research and coordinates research and evidence-based practice projects. A coordinating council facilitates and integrates the activities of all the councils.

Direct care staff are the key decision-makers on the councils. Managers serving on councils facilitate decision-making and ensure that appropriate data and information are available to support the council's work. This model has succeeded as a springboard for expanding shared governance to embrace other disciplines within the interdisciplinary team.[10] Although this is a highly effective method to increase the autonomy of nurses, it does require a tremendous initial expenditure of time, effort, and money.[9]

Unit-Based Model

In the unit-based model, shared governance is implemented on a smaller scale. Each unit forms a council for professional practice to make decisions and address issues at the unit level. To make this model succeed, there must be a real transfer of decision-making power from the nurse manager to staff nurses. This model often is the starting point for shared governance and evolves to the councilor model over time while maintaining a unit-based process.[10]

Shared governance is an approach that places decision-making power in the hands of the nursing staff. It requires a critical mass of staff willing to participate and be actively involved at both the unit and departmental levels. It also requires managers committed to the process, willing to adopt a coaching role to champion the development of councils at the unit and division levels.

Perhaps the greatest commitment for shared governance comes from administrators willing to allocate the resources necessary to reorganize and to empower frontline staff to make decisions about client care and their work environment. More than 1000 facilities in the United States have embraced shared governance, and this number appears to be growing. In addition, a growing body of evidence is showing benefits to morale and client outcomes.[9–11]

As reported in the literature, the benefits of shared governance include increased job satisfaction, lower turnover rates, decreased job stress, and improved client outcomes. However, the evidence of these results is not consistent at this time. Additional studies are needed to fully demonstrate the value of shared governance.[12]

The challenges associated with the implementation of shared governance models revolve around the costs of establishing and maintaining councils. In addition, training is necessary to ensure that staff have the skills necessary to plan and organize council activities.

What Do You Think?

Have any of your clinical facilities had shared governance in place? What do you see as the benefits of being involved in shared governance? Do you see any drawbacks to this approach?

Other Ways to Voice Concern

Health care and health-care facilities are changing with the times. Forward-thinking, progressive facilities have identified their employees as their most important asset and have changed their operations to ensure that staff are involved in decisions affecting client care and the working environment.[2,5]

Nurses have changed as well. Nurses are well-educated individuals dedicated to high-quality client care and positive work environments. They want to be respected by their colleagues, including physicians, and valued by their leaders for their contribution to organizational outcomes. When quality of care is compromised, nurses are obligated to act to correct the situation. The American Nurses Association (ANA) Code of Ethics (see Chapter 7) clearly outlines the responsibilities of the RN to advocate for the well-being of the client.[13]

In facilities with established shared governance models, avenues are available for working with managers and administrators to address concerns. In organizations with no formalized shared governance structure, some managers have adopted an open, participative leadership style to promote staff involvement and input into decision-making. But what about situations in which staff are not involved in important decisions related to client care and the work environment? What options are there to collaborative management?

Other options do exist to initiate discussions with leaders about the resources necessary to support client care. Using the resources within the organization is one option. Working within the facility can sometimes open lines of communication. Chapter 18 describes options for using the chain of command to voice safety concerns as well as to access support departments such as safety, infection prevention, or human resources. When these approaches have not resulted in acceptable improvement, it may be time to consider seeking assistance from outside the organization.

SHOULD NURSES UNIONIZE?

The image of nursing has always been one of dedication, service to clients, and selflessness. In the past, nurses' pay and working conditions were often secondary considerations, and many nurses felt that too much emphasis on money demeaned the profession. In today's society, nurses are beginning to realize that professionals with a career should have a say in matters that affect their practice, including working conditions, staffing patterns, benefits, and income. They need to be able to express these concerns without loss of status or reputation with the general public and other health-care professionals.

As nursing continues its struggle to achieve its status as a full profession, the issue of **collective bargaining** remains important. Since the early 1960s, the number of nurses who have joined unions has increased steadily, yet the question remains: Is professionalism compatible with membership in a union? Union members still have the image of male workers in blue-collar, heavy-industry jobs. RNs are joining unions faster than all other categories of workers, with a membership in 2009 of 962,000, or 13.6 percent of the health-care workforce.[14,15]

Nursing practices have often been defined and controlled by other groups, such as physicians and hospital administrators. These groups saw the potential power of an organized, large group of well-educated and dedicated nurses and feared the time when they would become independent. Even today, in areas of the country where collective bargaining for health-care workers is not a part of the system, many hospital administrators react to any unionization attempts by nurses with hostility and resistance. As the independence, authority, and responsibility of nurses increase, they need to consider whether joining a union will help them reach their goal of full professionalism. Without a doubt, this is one of the most highly charged issues that a nurse might face in professional practice.

PERSPECTIVE ON COLLECTIVE BARGAINING

Collective bargaining is the uniting of employees to increase their ability to influence their employer and improve working conditions.[16] Collective bargaining is based on the principle that there is greater strength in large numbers. Its primary goal is to equalize the power between labor and management. The primary collective bargaining unit is the union.

Initially unions were formed to protect workers from exploitation by greedy and insensitive employers. Although confronted with much opposition, they did accomplish their goals and became very powerful entities. Over the years, unions have received a more negative image because of the use of destructive and sometimes illegal practices in the quest for additional power. The end result is that the union movement is now in a fight for survival because of decreasing membership.[17–19] For some, unions and collective bargaining arouse images of picket lines, rowdy strikes, and violence. Many professionals, including nurses, do not regard this as activity that professionals should be involved in and tend to reject the idea of union membership outright.

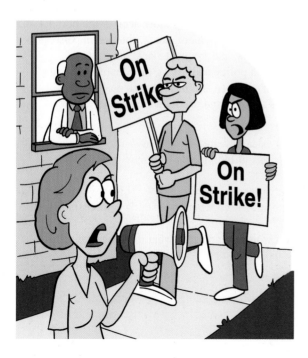

Legislative Development of Collective Bargaining
The National Labor Relations Act

Although the informal roots of collective bargaining can be traced back to the mid-1800s, formal collective bargaining in this country was first legally recognized in 1935 with passage of the National Labor Relations Act (NLRA). This act granted employees the right to organize themselves and to form, and help organizing, labor unions that could then bargain collectively through representatives. The representatives would be appointed by the union and bargain with management for the purpose of collective bargaining, mutual aid, and protection.[20] Under the NLRA, the National Labor Relations Board (NLRB) was established to supervise the implementation of the act.[21]

Originally, the NLRA did not include non-profit hospitals and other health-care providers under its authority. In its attempt to protect unions, the NLRA prevented some employers from reducing wages in hopes that higher-paid workers would spend more and decrease the severity of the Depression. One negative result of the NLRA was that many employers who did not have enough income to pay the higher wages went bankrupt.

What Do You Think?

How do you perceive unions? Do unions have any place in health care?

The Taft-Hartley Act

The NLRA was amended in 1947 by the Taft-Hartley Act, also called the Labor Management Relations Act (LMRA), with the goal of restoring equality between the unions and management. Taft-Hartley excluded nurses in nonprofit hospitals from coverage under the NLRA, legally preventing nurses from organizing collective bargaining units and going on strike. It was not until 1974 that the Taft-Hartley Act was amended to cover nurses in nonprofit hospitals, thus allowing nurses to form collective bargaining units.[22]

Bargaining Units for Hospitals

In April 1991, the U.S. Supreme Court ruled that the NLRB had the authority to define bargaining units

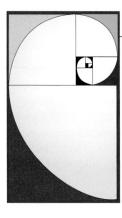

Issues in Practice

Workplace Violence in the Health-Care Setting

A person might assume that, of all the places on the planet, hospitals and other health-care facilities, dedicated to promoting wellness and curing disease, would be among the safest for workers. However, there has been a gradual but steady increase in health-care setting violence. The factors that lead to violence are also present in the health-care setting. Most violence is a result of unresolved stress that does not have an acceptable outlet. Health-care facilities are full of stress: money worries, demands of the job, short staffing, authority conflicts, and personality incompatibility.

The phenomenon of "going postal" is not isolated to the U.S. Postal Service. Study of the reasons people become violent in the workplace has demonstrated a gradual building process that occurs over many months or even many years. It is often first noted when a person begins to objectify and dehumanize coworkers and administrators. These individuals seem to have "authority issues" and often argue with those who supervise them. They may use profanity and are verbally abusive to those whom they supervise.

If such issues are not resolved early on, the behavior often becomes even more overtly threatening. Individuals caught in this escalating cycle of stress and violence often have very intense and frequent arguments with coworkers and even the clients they are caring for. They may demonstrate obvious hostility to the organization they are working for: stealing supplies, intentionally violating procedures and policies, and even making sexual or violent threats to others. They fight any attempts to change the organizational structure and react to any attempts to help them identify their problems with blatant resistance.

Left unchecked, the behavior becomes physically violent. These individuals may bring a weapon into the workplace to threaten supervisors or coworkers. They may threaten suicide. Other signs are similar to those seen in the burnout syndrome: drug or alcohol abuse, decrease in hygiene status, changes in personality, withdrawal from interactions with others, and frequent "sick" days off.

All institutions should have a policy addressing the identification of individuals who have a potential for violence and measures to deal with them early, before the problem escalates to overt and deadly actions. These policies should include:

- Zero tolerance for verbal and physical threats of violence
- Identification of early warning signs of individuals who may pose a threat to others
- Training for staff on workplace violence
- Identification of resources that can be used when a person is demonstrating an escalating cycle of violence
- An emergency response plan so workers can know what to do beforehand if a person becomes violent in the workplace

Issues in Practice continued

As unfortunate as it may be, violence in the workplace is a growing problem, even in the health-care setting. Being able to recognize persons who are manifesting characteristics that indicate an escalating cycle of violence and having a comprehensive plan for dealing with them are an essential elements in the workplace today.

Sources: Gillespie GL, Gates DM, Miller M, Howard PK: Workplace violence in healthcare settings: Risk factors and protective strategies. Rehabilitation Nursing 35(5):177–184, 2010.

Roche M, Diers D, Duffield C, Catling-Paull C: Violence toward nurses, the work environment, and patient outcomes. Journal of Nursing Scholarship, 1st Quarter 42(1):13–22, 2010.

for health-care providers in all settings, including acute care hospitals. Under this ruling, the NLRB defined eight separate bargaining units that were appropriate for use in hospitals (Box 17.1).[23]

Ultimately, this ruling by the Supreme Court permitted "all registered nurses (RNs) bargaining units" to be formed so that work issues important to professional nurses could be addressed. The current major representative for nurses is the Service Employees International Union, which represents almost 500,000 nurses and health-care providers nationwide.

The ANA has been active in the support of collective bargaining throughout its history. Although the ANA does not serve as a bargaining agent, it does support the state nurses associations (SNAs) to function as bargaining agents. As early as 1944, the ANA ruled that the SNAs could engage in collective bargaining. In response to the attempt to regulate nursing from the outside, the ANA presented a position paper in 1946. This paper stated that it was important for nursing to assume responsibility for advancing the social and economic security of its practitioners rather than leaving it to organizations outside the profession.[22] Today the SNAs represent approximately 140,000 RNs in 840 individual bargaining units across the United States, and about 20% of nurses are represented by a collective bargaining agent.

Since the ruling by the Supreme Court in 1991, there has been an increased interest in organizing additional bargaining units.[23] Several nursing unions are currently competing to serve as collective bargaining agent for nurses. The current major representatives for RNs include the Service Employees International Union, the California Nurses Association, and the United American Nurses, in addition to the SNAs.

Super Unions
Cooperation Among Unions

For many years, unions that represented nurses were competitive and almost combative. Union leaders spent almost as much time poaching members from other unions as they did negotiating for their own members. In 2009, union leaders evaluated their effectiveness in the face of the huge and ever more powerful corporate health-care institutions and decided that cooperation among the unions was a more effective tactic. They signed agreements to stop raiding each others' members and banded together in new large federations.

The Service Employees International Union (SEIU) could almost be considered a super union by itself with a membership of more than 1 million

Box 17.1
Eight Bargaining Units for Use in Hospitals

1. Nurses
2. Physicians
3. All professionals except nurses and physicians
4. All technical employees
5. All skilled maintenance employees
6. All business office clerical employees
7. All guards
8. All other nonprofessional employees

health-care workers. For many years the SEIU had a fierce rivalry with the California Nurses Association/National Nurses Organizing Committee (CAN/NNOC), which often shut down attempts by the SEIU to form new unions. The organized labor world was stunned when CAN/NNOC signed a formal truce with the SEIU in 2009. The signed agreement delineated the roles of each group in way that fostered cooperation. The SEIU focused their organizing efforts on health-care workers who were not nurses, and the CAN/NOOC limited their organizing activities to nurses only. Each organization maintains its own board of directors and identity.

The United American Nurses (UAN), a union for nurses only, began its life as part of the ANA. Although relatively small with about 40,000 members, it represents numerous states across the nation.

A Union Merger

In April 2010, three groups—the UAN, Massachusetts Nurses Association (MNA), and CAN/NNOC— approved a merger to become a single super union called the National Nurses United (NNU). It is estimated that the new group will have approximately 150,000 members in 23 states.[24] The group will maintain its affiliation with the AFL-CIO, ensuring significant muscle for negotiations with large and powerful health-care institutions.

Although the NNU is still in its formative stage, members are already seeing the benefits of belonging. The union directly represents and speaks for direct-care nurses in frontline issues such as staffing, workplace violence, and working conditions in general. New tough labor laws sponsored by the NNU make it easier for nurses to organize and protects nurses already covered by collective bargaining agreements. The union is working to create a pension plan that can be transferred from employer to employer rather than being lost when the nurse changes jobs.[25]

It remains to be seen how effective the organization will be and even if it will remain a single entity. However, health-care employers are keeping close eye

on these developments in the world of organized nurse labor. They are intimidated by the thought that other smaller nurses' unions may see how effective a super union is and begin to affiliate with the NNU.

To provide support for nurses in noncollective workplaces, the Workplace Advocacy Initiative was enacted by the ANA in 1991 to help RNs improve their work environment and gain more control over professional practice. The SNAs have been active in providing resources to assist nurses in addressing workplace issues, although the extent of support can vary from state to state. Services such as telephone consultation, leadership development programs, and tools to assist nurses in addressing staffing or mandatory overtime concerns are included in workplace advocacy approaches.

Goals of Collective Bargaining

Although the basic goal of collective bargaining is to equalize power between management and employees, the inequality of power between the two groups is not as great as it initially appears. In many organizations, management relies on employees who are near the bottom of the power structure hierarchy to carry out the work. Employees are vital to the growth, development, and even the survival of the organization. Employees also far outnumber managers. Collective bargaining takes advantage of these two factors when attempting to produce change in the organization.

> *One of the most important goals of a bargaining unit is to protect the employee against arbitrary treatment and unfair labor practices. These can be anything from working 5 weekends in a row to being fired because a physician felt the nurse was acting in an insubordinate manner.*

Collective bargaining resonates with employees who are dissatisfied with their workplace situation. Employees who are most likely to unionize generally have little power and control over their work, feel that they are not listened to, feel taken advantage of, and believe that they are not valued by management. An individual employee is highly vulnerable when attempting to force the employer to change.[16]

Basic Comforts

The main area of concern of collective bargaining is basic economic issues such as salaries and benefits.

In some hospital settings, nurses are paid less than other employees who have less education and fewer responsibilities. Collective bargaining attempts to balance these inequities.

Other concerns of collective bargaining include shift differentials, overtime pay, holidays, personal days off, the number of hours required in a work week, sick leave, maternity and paternity leave, uniform reimbursements, lunch and coffee breaks, health insurance, pension plans, and severance pay.[19,20] These elements all are found in the employment contract and may vary greatly depending on the hospital and the power of the bargaining unit.

Fair Treatment

One of the most important goals of a bargaining unit is to protect the employee against arbitrary treatment and unfair labor practices. These can be anything from working 5 weekends in a row to being fired because a physician felt the nurse was acting in an insubordinate manner. Other possible unfair labor practices include being passed over for promotion without an explanation, unreasonable staffing and scheduling policies, excessive demands for overtime, rotating shifts, unfair on-call time, transfers, layoffs, seniority rights, and failure to post job openings.

The collective bargaining unit establishes a grievance procedure by which the employee can bring a complaint against management without fear of reprisals. These grievance procedures also allow a mechanism for the employee to follow the complaint to a satisfactory conclusion.

Professional Practice

An important goal of collective bargaining is to maintain and promote professional practice. Often overlooked by management, this goal is one way nurses can keep and increase control over their own practice. For example, some nurses' bargaining units have been able to include the entire ANA Code of Ethics in the contract with the hospital. Other units have been able to address issues such as staffing, standards of care, and quality of care in the contract negotiations.

Interest-Based Bargaining

Traditionally, collective bargaining has been viewed as a struggle between two groups: one (usually employees) attempting to gain more power, and another (usually management) attempting to retain power. This type of struggle often results in hurt feelings or impasses in negotiations.

An Open Environment

Interest-based bargaining, also called mutual gains, win–win, and best-practice bargaining, is based on the idea that the way to achieve a mutually beneficial contract is to create an environment in which all parties can openly discuss all issues to the fullest extent. In interest-based bargaining, a highly structured six-step process is followed:

1. Selection of issues
2. Discussion of interests
3. Generation of options
4. Establishment of standards to measure the options
5. Measurement of the options
6. Development of solutions

This step-by-step process prevents the parties involved in bargaining from reverting to the traditional power struggle. All steps are done jointly, and even the 2-day training session that precedes negotiations requires participation by both management and labor.

The Role of the Registered Nurse

An issue that is central to the contract negotiations is ensuring that the role of the RN as the primary assessor and planner of care be maintained. The contract spells out what the RN's role will be, including activities such as assessing, planning, and evaluating the client's nursing care needs. To ensure that nursing issues are addressed adequately in contracts, RNs need to participate in facility committees that establish priorities for labor–management relations, nurse staffing, client-care standards, and health and safety policies. This partnership between nurses and hospital administrators allows for joint decision-making when issues of nursing practice and delivery of care are involved.

What Do You Think?

Who are the people who hold governing power in your clinical institution? What process can employees in health-care facilities use to affect the quality of care that they provide?

A Trend for the Future

Interest-based bargaining seems to be gaining momentum and may be the trend for the future, particularly in the health-care industry. Traditional collective bargaining methods are primarily adversarial and often leave the parties involved with deep-seated feelings of hostility toward each other. The old methods sometimes result in strikes or other types of work actions that harm the reputations of both nurses and hospitals. Interest-based bargaining allows participants to negotiate without hostility and, after negotiation of the contract, promotes the development of a more positive relationship.

NURSES' QUESTIONS ABOUT COLLECTIVE BARGAINING

Although large numbers of RNs have successfully unionized, there remain some fundamental questions about collective bargaining. These questions are at the heart of what makes collective bargaining an ethical issue for many nurses.

Is It Unprofessional?

Nurses have a great deal of difficulty in adjusting their image to that of a union member or a striker. It just does not seem professional. For many nurses it seems that there must be other ways to achieve the same goals without collective bargaining.

Organizers of collective bargaining units stress that many other professionals, such as pilots, teachers, and even physicians, are members of unions. The NLRB defines nurses as professionals because their work requires advanced and specialized education and skills. They also make critical judgments that affect the health and well-being of others. Union organizers contend that it is even less professional to accept low pay and poor working conditions than it is to join a union to improve these elements. They also feel that collective bargaining will give nurses control over their practice, which is one of the keys to professionalism.

Is It Unethical?

One of the major beliefs of nurses is the priority of the clients' health and well-being over the personal needs and gains of the health-care provider. This concern conflicts with the methods commonly used by collective bargaining units, such as strikes or work slowdowns. There is a feeling among many health-care providers that these types of actions constitute abandonment of their clients and therefore violate the code of ethics.

Those who support collective bargaining stress that poor working conditions, such as lack of qualified staff, are as much a threat to clients' health and well-being as the work actions taken to correct these conditions. The ability of nurses simply to threaten to strike, even though the strike may never materialize, is often powerful enough to bring about change.[23]

> *An issue that is central to the contract negotiations is ensuring that the role of the RN as the primary assessor and planner of care be maintained. The contract spells out what the RN's role will be, including activities such as assessing, planning, and evaluating the client's nursing care needs.*

Law requires that a 10-day notice must be given before a strike takes place. This gives the hospital a chance to prepare for the strike and to make changes to ensure client safety, such as transferring critical-care clients to another hospital, eliminating elective surgeries, and refusing to admit new clients. If the hospital fails to take appropriate measures when they have received adequate notice, the issue of client abandonment becomes their responsibility, not that of the nurses who have gone on strike.

In the few times when nurses have gone on strike, client safety and well-being have not been affected. The institutions involved were always given enough lead time to discharge or transfer the majority of the clients. The few remaining clients were cared for by management personnel, who are not covered by unions.

Is It Divisive?

Nurse Against Nurse

Does the process of collective bargaining set nurse against nurse? Collective bargaining is adversarial by nature. It sets two groups, management and employees, against each other. Although this relationship can result in conflict, it allows the staff nurses to be heard and to initiate changes that affect the practice of nursing. Nurses have been attempting for years to improve working conditions in the health-care setting and to achieve **comparable worth.** Administrators pay little attention to an individual nurse or to a small group of concerned nurses. When a collective bargaining unit speaks for all of the nurses, however, administration will listen.[19]

The CEO of a large home health-care agency in a southwestern resort area called a general staff meeting. She reported that the agency had grown rapidly and was now the largest in the area.

"Much of our success is due to the professionalism and commitment of our staff members," she said. "With growth come some problems, however. The most serious problem is the fluctuation in client census. Our census peaks in the winter months when seasonal visitors are here and troughs in the summer. In the past, when we were a small agency, we all took our vacations during the slow season. This made it possible to continue to pay everyone his or her full salary all year. However, with the pressures to reduce costs and the large number of staff members we now have, we cannot continue to do this. We are very concerned about maintaining the high quality of client care currently provided, but we have calculated that we need to reduce staff by 30 percent over the summer to survive financially."

The CEO then invited comments from the staff members. The majority of the nurses said they wanted and needed to work full-time all year. Most supported families and had to have a steady income all year around. "My rent does not go down in the summer," said one. "Neither does my mortgage or the grocery bill," said another. A small number said that they would be happy to work part-time in the summer if they could be guaranteed full-time employment from October through May. "We have friends who would love this work schedule," they added.

"That's not fair," protested the nurses who needed to work full-time all year. "You can't replace us with part-time staff." The discussion grew louder and the participants more agitated. The meeting ended without a solution to the problem. Although the CEO promised to consider all points of view before making a decision, the nurses left the meeting feeling very confused and concerned about the security of their future income. Some grumbled that they probably would begin looking for new positions "before the ax falls."

The next day, the CEO received a telephone call from the nurses' union representative. "If what I heard about the meeting yesterday is correct," said the representative, "your plan is in violation of our collective bargaining contract." The CEO reviewed the contract and found that the representative was correct. A new solution to the financial problems caused by the seasonal fluctuation in client census would have to be found.

> *The collective bargaining unit establishes a grievance procedure by means of which the employee can bring a complaint against management without fear of reprisals. These grievance procedures also provide a mechanism for the employee to follow the complaint to a satisfactory conclusion.*

Source: Whitehead, DK, Weiss, SA, Tappen, RM: Essentials of Nursing Leadership and Management (5th ed). Philadelphia, F. A. Davis, 2010, pp 106–107, with permission.)

Closed or Open Shop?

Different collective bargaining units have different membership requirements, which are often included in the negotiations. Many unions negotiate a *closed shop* or *agency shop* clause in the contract. A closed shop institution requires that all the employees pay membership dues whether they belong to the union or not. The rationale behind the closed shop approach is that because all the employees benefit from the union's negotiations, they should all pay for it. It also encourages employees to join the union because they are already paying the dues.

However, many states have *right to work* laws that make closed shop contracts illegal. In these states, the *open shop* collective bargaining model is used, and only those employees who desire to be members join the union and pay dues. There is more chance for nurse-to-nurse conflicts in open shop institutions because of the divisions between those who belong to the union and those who do not.

Collective bargaining does not have to be adversarial, and in facilities where the administration is open to change and the collective bargaining unit is realistic in its requests, the process can be very smooth and amicable.

Is There a Threat to Job Security?

Although the main goals of collective bargaining are improvement of working conditions and protection from unfair labor practices, it can itself pose a threat to job security. In some cases, employees who are active in the collective bargaining process become well known to management and may become the targets of reprisals, particularly if the collective bargaining fails. Facilities sometimes suggest that granting RNs higher wages and benefits will cause bankruptcy and closure of the facility or that the higher RN wages will at least drain the organization's resources so much that it has to cut back the number of other employees.

In reality, recent changes in contract law have resulted in some job losses. Nurses can be replaced during strikes, and even if a settlement is reached, they are hired back only after new employees leave or openings occur. If no settlement is reached, striking nurses may never be hired back.

Taking action always carries risk. Nurses involved in collective bargaining have to consider the risk-to-benefit ratio before they take action. Are the working conditions so poor and the pay so inadequate that they overshadow the risk for possible job loss? The first attempts at organizing a collective bargaining unit are usually the most dangerous in terms of job security.

Initial attempts at organizing nurses are usually made outside the hospital between representatives of the SNA and the union. This type of activity may prevent individuals from becoming targets of management's anger and makes reprisals from management more difficult for a short time. However, it is virtually impossible to keep knowledge of collective bargaining activities secret. Hospital information and rumor "grapevines" are very well developed, and at times it seems the administration hears of the activities almost before they start.

Some legal protections exist for nurses who organize collective bargaining. Grievance procedures against vengeful administrators can be initiated under the unfair labor practice rules, which vary somewhat from state to state. However, even if successful, nurses may pay a heavy financial and emotional toll terms in the process of proving they were in the right.

THE CONTRACT

Negotiation

After a collective bargaining unit has been selected, the next important step is to develop or negotiate a contract between the nurses and the hospital. The contract is a legal document that is binding for both management and the union.[16] Contracts can be very specific and include just a few items or very broad and include many. Contracts often contain requirements for union membership by the employees and set the cost of dues for that membership.

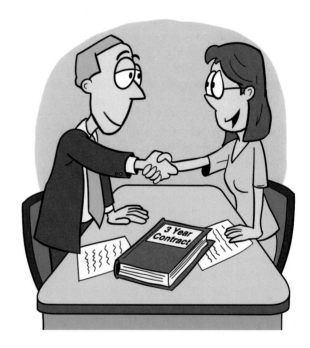

Representation

Negotiating teams are selected by both management and employee groups. One member of each of these teams is designated as the spokesperson who will be the main representative for the group. Before negotiations start, each team meets separately to decide on its position on various issues and on what they are willing to compromise. A list of demands is exchanged by the two sides; it should include everything each might possibly want.

Power and Benefits

Generally, management is reluctant to give up power or relinquish money. The employees' group tries to gain some of management's power and gain benefits for its members. Often many meetings between the two groups are required before they discover the key issues and determine where compromise is possible. Posturing and showmanship play a big part in the initial negotiations. Later, when serious issues are discussed and dealt with, final agreements may be reached behind closed doors.

Good-Faith Bargaining

The law requires that each side bargain in good faith. Good-faith bargaining requires that both parties must agree to meet at reasonable times, to send individuals to the negotiations who can make binding decisions, and to be willing to bargain with the other side.[16] A lack of willingness to negotiate is not bargaining in good faith.

Mediation or Arbitration?

Working With a Mediator

When the sides are unable to reach a settlement, a stalemate occurs. Stalemates are sometimes resolved through mediation, in which a neutral third party provided by the Federal Mediation and Conciliation Service meets with each side. After determining the nature of the conflict, the mediator brings the two sides together to attempt to work out a settlement. Both sides must work with the mediator, but they are not required to accept the mediator's recommendations.

If mediation fails, the Federal Mediation and Conciliation Service may appoint a fact-finding panel to investigate the conflict and to make recommendations. The panel's report is made public and can exert pressure on both sides to accept the recommendations of the mediator.

Binding Arbitration

In some situations, an arbitrator with binding power may be appointed. This person is a neutral third party who, like the mediator, investigates the conflict, meets with both sides, and makes a recommendation

for settlement. However, the arbitrator's recommendation, unlike that of the mediator, must be accepted by both sides. Both labor and management try to avoid binding arbitration because it limits their negotiating powers and they may lose something gained during previous negotiations.

The Prospect of a Strike

When all else fails, the final step in the contract negotiation process is work slowdowns or stoppages (strikes). Although strikes are usually the tool used by employees to gain power, management can use a form of enforced strike called a lockout, whereby employees are not permitted to enter the work facility.

The prospect of a strike is usually accompanied by more intense negotiations that may lead to a last-minute settlement. Strikes are detrimental to both sides. Employees lose pay and benefits during a strike, and management loses income. In addition, the overall public image of strikes is negative, and they have little support. Some collective bargaining units have developed alternative ways of achieving their goals without a strike. Methods such as disruption of services on a random basis or boycott of an organization can achieve the same effects as a full-blown strike without damaging the image of the union.

What Do You Think?

Did you ever sign a contract for employment? Did you read the contract? Were all the elements of a good contract present?

Ratifying the Contract

After a settlement has been reached, the contract must be ratified. The collective bargaining unit takes the contract back to the employees, who must approve it (Box 17.2). Once it is approved by a majority of the employees, the contract becomes legally binding for both management and the employees.

CONCERNS

Representation

One of the most difficult decisions that nurses have to make is who will represent them as a collective

Box 17.2

Elements of a Good Contract

- A statement outlining the objectives of both management and the employees
- A description of the official collective bargaining group
- A description of the benefits included in the contract, such as wages and salary, overtime pay, holiday pay, shift differentials, and differentials for advanced education or certifications
- A description of other benefits, such as health insurance, life insurance, retirement, and legal benefits, among others
- A description of acceptable in-house labor practices, such as transfers, promotions, seniority, layoffs, **grievance** procedures, and work schedules
- A description of the procedure to be used when employees have disciplinary problems or when there is a **breach of contract**
- A description of the grievance procedures and the due process to be followed
- A description of what is expected of the professional, including standards of care and codes of ethics

bargaining unit. It is reasonable to conclude that only a professional organization, such as the SNA, which understands the complex and varied needs of the profession, will be able to represent that profession in a collective bargaining situation.

Over the years, SNAs have developed into skilled representatives able to negotiate contracts with considerable success. However, nonprofessional unions have years of experience with negotiations and large sums of money to spend on developing skilled individuals whose only job is negotiating contracts. The union must be able to convince the group of nurses that it is able to represent their interests more effectively than the SNA.

Union groups that attempt to represent nurses soon find that nurses have difficulties forming a consensus concerning problems and issues. Individuals outside the nursing profession have difficulty understanding issues such as quality and standards of care, ethical dilemmas, or even the different levels of nursing education.

Nurses should also be concerned about the public image of the collective bargaining unit they select to represent them. Some nurses' groups have been represented by a machinists' union, a teamsters' union, or even a meat cutters' union. Although these unions are highly proficient at negotiating contracts to gain benefits for their members, some feel the image of nursing is tarnished in the process.

Nursing Supervisors: Employees or Management?

Everyone is familiar with the idea of the traditional nursing supervisor. This is the older, more experienced nurse who guides the less experienced nurses. Nursing supervisors make sure staffing is adequate for their assigned shifts, resolve problems that are beyond the skills of the staff nurse, act as mediators between physicians and nurses, and use their higher skill levels to assist the staff nurses with code blues or complicated procedures. The term *nursing supervisor* also includes nurse educators, directors of nursing, head nurses, unit supervisors, assistant head nurses, and sometimes even charge nurses on the 3 p.m. to 11 p.m. or 11 p.m. to 7 a.m. work shift.

Redefining the Supervisor

Under the 1974 amendments to the Taft-Hartley Act, a supervisor was defined as any individual with authority to hire, transfer, suspend, lay off, promote, assign, reward, or discipline another employee.[25] From this legal viewpoint, nursing supervisors were no longer employees but really members of management. Management cannot be involved in collective bargaining activities and is therefore prevented from joining unions. A careful reading of the definition of a supervisor as presented in the Taft-Hartley Act makes the category of supervisor open to interpretation. Anybody who assigns a task to another nurse could be considered a supervisor.

Management has sometimes used this provision in the Taft-Hartley Act in an attempt to control the organization and function of collective bargaining units. Management, if so inclined, can use this distinction to induce tension between nursing staff and supervisors, thus reducing the cohesion of the group. Supervisors often serve on important hospital committees to develop standards of care, foster professional recognition, and support nurse advancement.

When contracts are negotiated, the supervisors are on the opposite side of the table from the staff nurses. Often, in the heat of negotiation, things are said that foster negative feelings. After the negotiations have ended, it is difficult to re-establish that sense of unity that contributes to high-quality client care.

Some health-care institutions have attempted to categorize all of their RNs and LPNs as supervisors, thus preventing any of them from organizing into a collective bargaining unit.

A Supreme Court Decision

In 1994, in a 5 to 4 vote, the Supreme Court of the United States supported the decision that LPNs at the Heartland Nursing Home in Urbana, Ohio, should be considered supervisors because they directed the work of nurses' aides "in the interest of the employer." Under this ruling, these LPNs were not protected under the NLRA. This ruling has been of great concern to all nurses, but particularly to the ANA's Department of Labor Relations and Workplace Advocacy committee.

The implications of this decision are far-reaching and pose a direct threat to the ability of RNs to pursue collective bargaining. Employers have already begun to use this ruling to fight nurses in collective bargaining units from Alaska to Washington, DC.[26]

The ANA has been working toward developing language that would follow the description of a supervisor as found in the NLRA and the Taft-Hartley Act (see earlier discussion). Since the passage of the NLRA, nurses who provide client care have been considered to be acting within the professional nature of nursing and not in the interests of the employer (as a supervisor would primarily be).

Under the ANA's proposed revisions, the scope of the definition of supervisor would be narrowed to include only employees of health-care institutions. This change would allow the NLRB to continue to determine, on a case-by-case basis, whether nurses are supervisors or professional or technical employees. This legislation, introduced to Congress in 1996, was initially tabled. Although it was never officially acted on, recent court rulings have supported the position that not all RNs are supervisors, with resulting successful work actions and strikes nationwide.[27]

Conclusion

Although few issues elicit such strong emotions among nurses as collective bargaining, it is a reality in today's health-care system. Nurses are beginning to realize that they are not in a strictly altruistic profession, but rather one in which they use their knowledge and skills to provide high-quality services to clients. The knowledge and skills used in client care are gained at the cost of years of expensive education and dedication to an often underappreciated profession. Nurses no longer need to apologize or feel guilty about seeking payment for their work on a level commensurate with their knowledge and skills.

Negotiation is the process of give and take between groups with the goal of reaching an agreement acceptable to both sides. Negotiations may be formal or informal, hostile or friendly. A cooperative atmosphere fostered by both sides that recognizes the similarity of each side's demands will be the most productive in reaching a satisfactory contract.

Although not a new concept for nursing, collective bargaining is an issue that is still hotly debated among professional nurses. Collective bargaining is viewed by some as unprofessional, unethical, divisive, and a fundamental threat to job security. However, the goals of collective bargaining, including improvement of economic benefits, better staffing and scheduling, fair treatment for all nurses, and improved quality of care for clients, are common to all health-care providers.

In a health-care facility with a form of governance that allows nurses to have a relatively large degree of control over their practice, the issues discussed at the bargaining table are more likely to revolve around a professional agenda. In facilities with rigidly structured hierarchies of authority that give nurses little autonomy, accountability, or control over their practice, collective bargaining is more likely to center on control and power issues.

Nurses must decide at some point in their careers whether joining a collective bargaining unit will best help them to achieve these goals. This is not an easy decision to make, and each nurse should gather as much information as possible about the situation before making a decision.

(continued)

Conclusion — cont'd

Nurses need to recognize that the time has arrived to elevate the profession to a new level. Change in forms of governance is one method that nurses can use to change the health-care system. Nursing as a profession now has the opportunity to gain tremendous power and take its rightful place as an indispensable force in the health-care system. All that is required is for nurses to become educated in the issues involved and to take an aggressive stance in shaping the future.

Nurses are highly educated professionals. They recognize that they can practice autonomously and can make sound decisions about client care. They also recognize that an increased understanding of the governance process requires many of the same skills used in collective bargaining. Key elements in both processes are an understanding of negotiation, compromise, and consensus building to attain one's goals. Changes in methods of governance also will require major changes in the health-care system. Professional nurses have the power to produce those changes and the ability to deal with the future of health care successfully.

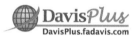

DavisPlus.fadavis.com

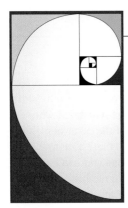

Issues Now

Nursing No Longer Recession Proof!

Often thought to be recession proof, the health-care industry is beginning to be swallowed in the whirlpool of the economic downturn. In June 2010, up to 18 major hospital systems across the eastern and central United States had begun mass layoffs of 50 or more employees. Hospital employment of all types of workers dropped by 4707 in the first 4 months of 2010. It is estimated that as many as 2000 nurses will be laid off over the next 6 months if the economy does not make a radical turnaround. This estimate is an all-time record high.

This statistic should indicate that cooperative labor relations are also at an all-time high, with unions attempting to save nursing jobs and hospital executives working to create work-friendly environments. However, cooperation between labor and management verges on becoming a street brawl. Nurses have either gone on strike or are threatening to strike at more than 14 hospitals from Minnesota to Pennsylvania to California. Issues range from staffing to wages to unpaid meal breaks.

Hospital executives have started to believe that, because they need to lay off nurses, the nursing shortage is over. They feel that with a surplus of nurses they should be able to set working conditions without interference from the unions. This is a false and misguided belief. The projections for a shortage of almost 300,000 nurse by 2015 remains accurate. The nursing population is aging: almost one third of nurses are 50 years or older, and an estimated 50 percent will retire by 2020. Nurses continue to have a high turnover rate. In many states, for every five new nurses hired, three leave for a variety of reasons, some leaving the profession altogether. Nationwide, the turnover rate ranges between 15 and 20 percent.

Sources: Bowen D: Doctors, nurses increasingly affected by mass layoffs at hospitals. June 14, 2010. Retrieved October, 2010 from http://www.fiercehealthcare.com.

Davis C: Labor unrest: Nursing strike threats, meal-break lawsuits occur amid record mass layoffs. Retrieved October, 2010 from the Healthcare Finance Group at http://www.hfgusa.com.

Suburban General warns of up to 344 layoffs in Bellevue. Pittsburgh Tribune-Review. Monday, June 14, 2010. Retrieved October, 2010 from http://www.pittsburghlive.com/.

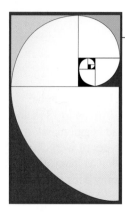

Issues in Practice

Deciding to Go on Strike

Sharon S., RN, was completing her charting on another busy 3 p.m. to 11 p.m. shift. While she was walking down the hall toward the time clock, she wondered who would be taking her place for the rest of the week. Like most of the other nurses at the medical center, she had decided to go on strike starting with the 7 a.m. to 3 p.m. shift the next day. The decision to strike had not been an easy one and had been reached only after many hours of meetings and conferences with the hospital negotiators and animated discussion among the nurses' negotiating team.

Sharon could see both positive and negative sides to a strike. On the positive side, increased salaries, better fringe benefits, and improvements in working conditions and staffing would be a plus for all the nurses and clients at the medical center. Sharon herself had felt increasingly stressed during the past year because of the hospital's measures to reorganize. From what Sharon was able to see, reorganization meant saving money by cutting professional staff and partially replacing them with less-trained, unlicensed individuals. This pattern of restaffing had led to longer hours, increased responsibilities for the RNs, and fewer support services. She also felt that the overall quality of care had decreased noticeably.

On the negative side, Sharon was experiencing a real ethical and emotional dilemma about going on strike. The quality of care was sure to deteriorate even further because of the reduced services caused by the strike. Was it really fair to decrease the services and care for clients who had nothing to do with the issues that brought on the strike? Of course, during the past 3 days, the clients who were well enough had been sent home early in anticipation of the strike. Some whose conditions were too complicated for them to be cared for at home were sent to other facilities. The hospital had severely restricted admissions, reducing the census to an all-time low.

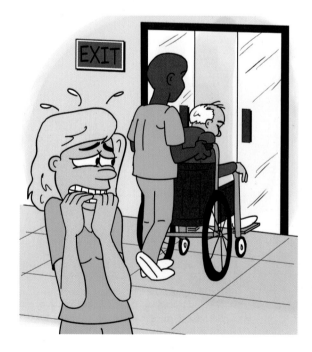

Issues in Practice   continued

Yet there were several clients who were too ill to transfer or send home. Mrs. Anderson, a 78-year-old client with renal failure, congestive heart failure, and a recent colostomy for a bowel obstruction, came to mind. Mrs. Anderson and a number of other clients like her, who had no family nearby and few resources, were highly dependent on the nursing staff to meet their needs of care. Mrs. Anderson was just beginning to be taught how to care for her colostomy. Even if she was discharged to a nursing home, there was no way to ensure that she could receive the teaching needed for her eventual self-care. Although there was to be a skeleton crew of nurses left in the facility, they would be stretched very thin in trying to care for the remaining clients.

Sharon also thought about the ANA Code of Ethics for Nurses she had been taught in nursing school, particularly the passage that stated, "the nurse participates in the profession's effort to establish and maintain conditions of employment conducive to high-quality nursing care." The reason for the strike was to bring about improved working conditions that would benefit future clients in the hospital, but should these measures be carried out when nursing services were already operating at a reduced level of care and at a minimal level of safety? Didn't that somehow contradict the first statement in the code, that "the nurse provides services with respect for human dignity"? When Mrs. Anderson had been admitted to the hospital 4 days before, she came with the expectation of the best possible care under any circumstances. The code seemed to have a split personality on strikes. While calling for service to the profession to maintain high standards and quality of care, the code also insisted that the health, welfare, and safety of the clients should be the nurse's first consideration.

What should Sharon do? Does the overall welfare of the profession ever supersede the obligation to provide client care? If Sharon does go on strike, will she be "abandoning" her clients in the legal or ethical sense of the term?

Critical Thinking Exercises

- Develop a position paper either supporting or opposing collective bargaining.
- A nurse on your unit states one day, "Membership in the state nurses' association is a waste of time and money. They can't help you make a better living!" How would you respond to this nurse?
- Develop an ideal contract for nurses. Which elements would receive the highest priority?
- Develop a plan for shared governance in a facility you are familiar with. How would the organizational process take place? What are some of the major difficulties in developing this plan?

18

Health-Care Delivery Systems

Nicole Harder

Learning Objectives

After completing this chapter, the reader will be able to:

- Discuss the implications of health-care reform on the profession of nursing.
- Analyze the evolution of the health-care delivery system in the United States.
- Analyze the evolution of the health-care delivery system in Canada.
- Evaluate the factors that influence the evolution of the health-care delivery system.
- Synthesize the concerns surrounding the uninsured in the United States.
- Analyze industry efforts to manage health-care costs.
- Evaluate the efforts being made to ensure high-quality, cost-effective health care.
- Describe and list the levels and types of health-care delivery.

HEALTH CARE REFORM

New Provisions for Health Care

In 2010, passage of the landmark Patient Protection and Affordable Care Act (PPACA) set the stage for the largest overhaul of the United States health-care system in 50 years. Now that the uproar has settled somewhat (although some of the furor continues), nurses must take the lead in implementing PPACA to move the U.S. health-care system toward becoming the best in the world for *all* its citizens.

Sometimes referred to as Health Care Reform, Obama-care, or, less frequently, Americare, the primary goal of PPACA is to provide affordable health care to U.S. citizens who before its passage were unable to pay for or obtain health insurance. Secondary goals include eliminating the insurance industry's stranglehold on the health-care system, addressing inequities in current coverage, and help struggling senior citizens. The legislative process mangled or killed several key provisions of PPACA that would have covered the almost 47 million Americans without health insurance. However, it is estimated that some 32 million additional citizens will be added to the rolls of those with health care by 2014.[1]

The detractors of PPCAC remain legion and often cite false or misleading information as their rationale for opposition. The bill does have some limitations, discussed later. The provisions of the bill will be phased in over 8 years to be less of a "change shock" to health-care providers and citizens alike.

Provisions that took place in 2010 include:

- "Doughnut hole" protection for senior citizens. They will receive a rebate from the government to supplement the $2700 limit on Medicare drug coverage. However, this fills only 50 percent of the doughnut hole for 2010; 100 percent will be filled by 2020.

- Care for all children by eliminating the preexisting conditions restrictions found in most policies.
- Access to high-risk pools for all uninsured, even adults with preexisting conditions.
- Increasing the age to 26 years for young adults to be covered on their parents' plans.
- Ending the insurance companies' ability to drop coverage for someone when he or she gets sick.
- Transparency: insurance companies must reveal how much money is spent on overhead and administrative costs.
- A customer appeals process to explain to customers how coverage determinations are made and claims are rejected.
- A 10 percent tax on indoor tanning services, with the money being used to fight skin cancer.
- Eliminating health insurance fraud and waste with a new system of inspection and checks.
- Improved quality of information on the Web. A new website makes it easier for consumers and small businesses in any state to find affordable health insurance plans.
- Improved labeling of food products for more accurate nutrient content to eliminate the confusing and sometimes fraudulent information provided by manufacturers.
- Less expensive health care plans offered to early retirees (ages 55–64 years) as part of the benefit package.

Provisions that become effective in 2011:

- Tax credits for small businesses with fewer than 50 employees to cover 50% of employee health-care premiums.
- Limited power of insurance companies to exploit small businesses; reduced out-of-pocket expenses for employees.
- A 2-year temporary credit (up to $1 billion) to encourage research into new therapies and procedures.

Provisions that become effective in 2014:

- Eliminating all preexisting illness limits for adults to obtain health insurance.
- Eliminating higher insurance premiums based on a person's gender or health status.
- No lifetime caps on the amount of insurance an individual can receive.
- Expanded Medicare payment to small rural hospitals and other health-care facilities that have a small number of Medicare clients.

- A minimum benefits package defined by the federal government including certain preventive services at no cost.
- The option of coverage that can be offered through new state-run insurance marketplaces, called "exchanges." Increased Medicare payroll taxes for high-income earners ($250,000 or more). Unearned income of $250,000 or more, now exempt from the payroll tax, would also be subject to a 3.8 percent levy.

Provisions that become effective in 2018:

- All new insurance plans to cover checkups and other preventive care without copays.

Individuals who have health insurance plans at the time of PPACA implementation can keep their plans with very little change. The plans will not be increased to match the new policies' increased benefit standards. However, as of summer 2011, no health plans will be able to set annual limits, drop individuals because of illness, drop children from parents' plans until they are 26 years old, or deny children coverage because of preexisting conditions.[2]

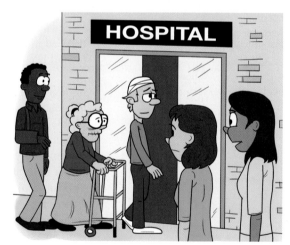

"I GUESS HEALTH-CARE REFORM MEANS JOB SECURITY!"

Concerns About Health-Care Reform

Some of the more controversial provisions in health-care reform include the anticipated gradual increase in premiums (up to 13 percent) that will be phased in from 2011 to 2016. However, most individuals and families will qualify for subsidies. These will be a sliding-scale tax break for a family of four making less than $88,000 per year. Federal insurance plans will *not* cover abortions. However, this coverage can be obtained through the state-sponsored exchange programs for an additional premium if the individual exchange plans decides to offer it. States may opt out of the abortion coverage.[3]

Another controversial aspect of PPACA is the requirement that most Americans buy health insurance or pay a penalty starting in 2014. The penalty will start out at 1 percent of income in 2014 and rise to 2.5 percent by 2016; however, the total amount will not exceed $2085 per year. Some believe this is an invasion of privacy and limits personal freedom.[4] The underlying idea is that when everyone has insurance, the rates for premiums are lower across the board. Without the requirement, people with insurance would have to pay higher premiums to cover those without insurance. This is what the health-care and insurance industries have been doing for the past 50 years.

A few groups would not be required to purchase health insurance. Most American Indians can receive health care through their tribal health-care systems. Also, those who have legitimate religious objections can avoid paying for insurance. Individuals and families with extreme financial hardship would not be penalized for inability to pay if the cheapest plan available would cost more than 8 percent of their income.[5]

Some clinicians fear that the increased number of new clients will overwhelm the health-care system, producing long waits at physicians' offices. Another concern is that the Medicare system will be inundated with a flood of new recipients and not have enough funding to cover everyone. These problems are growing pains that can be resolved along with other issues that are sure to arise.[6] New legislation always raises issues; however, reasonably intelligent people should be able to figure out the answers.

Nursing and Health Care Reform
A Goal of Maintaining Health

Nurses were at the table during the planning of the Health Care Reform Act, and nurses will have a key role as the plan moves forward. The influx of some 32 million new clients into the health-care system offers new challenges and opportunities for nurses to expand their profession and practice to the levels for which they were educated.

Sometimes overlooked or discounted in PPACA is the increased emphasis on preventive care.

All Americans can receive screening procedures such as prostate examinations, mammograms, annual physical examinations, and preventive care such as immunizations at no out-of-pocket costs. This is a major transition in emphasis from illness and disease to prevention and health promotion. One commitment that has always differentiated professional nursing from medicine is this goal of maintaining health and preventing disease.[7]

Opportunities and Challenges for Nurses

The arena where this transition will occur is primary care. During the past decade, physician training for primary care has decreased because of low reimbursement rates from insurance companies and government programs. It is unlikely that the current crop of primary physicians will be able to handle the increase in clients seeking preventive care. On the other hand, the education of nurse practitioners has increased by some 60 percent during the same decade. In addition, PPACA provides some 50 million dollars per year to develop new programs for each of the nurse practitioner roles. Also, public health will find itself on the front lines of the influx of new clients. The opportunity for nurses to lead the cutting edge of health-care reform is ripe with promise.[8]

To fulfill this promise, nurses must continue to do what they have always done, but to do it better. In the past, when demographic swings or governmental programs have created substantive changes in health care, nurses have been the leaders in developing new systems and models to accommodate the changes. Nurses are experts in increasing access to care while maintaining the quality of that care. They must work in the political arena to broaden the ability of advanced practice nurses to provide the services they were educated to provide. They must be at the table to help shape changes in health care.

As evidence-based practice becomes the norm for heath-care practice, nurses need to keep conducting the research and collecting the data that improve care. Without a solid base of research, it will be impossible to demonstrate scientific evidence of the effectiveness of preventive care and improved client outcomes. However, nurses cannot do research in a vacuum. It is essential that they collaborate with all health-care disciplines by understanding and acknowledging the importance of their roles in health-care reform. From collaborating with medical schools to providing training for patient care technicians

(PCAs), nurses can establish the trust required to work in concert with others and provided seamless, high-quality care.[9]

Health-care reform can be a double-edged sword for professional nursing. Nurses can lead the reform that will mark the success of health care for decades to come, or they can be overrun by the system and become a footnote to health care. Nurses who educate themselves about the new reforms and find the opportunities will be the leaders health care requires.

THE NEW FACE OF HEALTH CARE

Traditionally, the primary purpose of health care was to provide services to those who were ill or injured. These services were typically delivered in a hospital or clinic setting. Currently, an awareness of and interest in maintaining optimal health are resulting in a movement toward preventive and primary care as a means of promoting health. This focus has produced substantial changes to the ways in which health-care services are delivered and health-care professionals interact with these systems. As professionals, nurses need to understand health-care delivery systems. Nursing practice is influenced by political, societal, and cultural realities and needs to adapt to the changing world that affects everyday practice. Today's health-care institutions are heavily affected by the costs of delivery and of access to services and health-care professionals.

It has been long recognized that although individual health-care services in the United States are among the best in the world, the overall health-care delivery system is at best mediocre. In many key health-care indicators, such as infant mortality and chronic diseases, the United States is well behind other countries, ranking 37th out of 50.

The number of U.S. citizens who were not covered by any type of health-care insurance in 2010 was more than 47 million, about 25 percent of the population. Of the top 25 industrialized countries, the United States is the only one that does not have any type of universal health-care coverage for its citizens.[10] The PPACA is a first step to developing a system that will offer all U.S. residents the same type of health care enjoyed by members of the U.S. Congress. The new law challenges politicians to develop a system that will cover all citizens as they are covered by

their governmental health care plan. Nurses see every day the effect of lack of health care among the most vulnerable population: infants and children.

DEMOGRAPHICS AFFECTING HEALTH-CARE DELIVERY

Age
Between now and the year 2050, the number of persons 65 years or older is expected to double. By 2050, one in five people living in Canada or the United States will be elderly, and their numbers will reach an estimated 80 million.[11] Of this number, many will eventually become more dependent on the health-care delivery system as a result of chronic health problems.

Although an aging population constitutes a sizable number of persons who may require expensive long-term health care, their community activism and powerful influence at the ballot box can provide them with better access to health care than other less vocal and politically savvy groups. Additional at-risk groups consist of persons residing in urban areas with limited incomes and individuals living in remote rural areas where access to care is limited.

Chronicity
Another factor influencing the climate of health-care delivery is the long-term and expensive nature of many health problems. Although significant strides have been made in treating some acute infectious diseases, many challenges still exist in the management of health concerns such as cancer, heart disease, Alzheimer's disease, diabetes, chronic obstructive pulmonary disease, and human immunodeficiency virus (HIV). Additional concerns include environmental and occupational safety, drug abuse, and mother and child health care.

HEALTH CARE AS AN INDUSTRY

In most developed countries, health care is one of the largest industries. According to a report produced by the Kaiser Foundation, total expenditures on health accounted for 9.9 percent of the gross domestic product in Canada and 16 percent in the United States in 2005 (last year of available statistics).[12] Total expenditure was more than $2 *trillion* dollars and is expected to reach $4 trillion dollars by 2015. These numbers alone indicate the significance of health care and health-care spending to the people of these two countries.

In the United States, with the introduction of managed care, the organizations that pay for health care have the capacity to dramatically influence who provides care, how the care is furnished, and who receives compensation. The significance to the economy, along with other factors, is evident.

Health Care in the Global Context

Understanding the approach to health care in comparison with other countries is important in assessing the challenges to and potential of health-care delivery. How and why health-care systems differ is a function of multiple influences. These may include societal values and beliefs, sociocultural climate, the state of the economy, political ideologies, geographic density, international influences, historical realities, established practices and programs, and other factors. For health-care systems to develop, several factors must come into play at different points. This development is consistent throughout the world, as can be seen by examining the contexts in which various health-care systems were developed.

One way to think about system differences is to consider that Western countries provide for health care in several ways, all of which involve variable combinations of private or public funding of services and private or public delivery of services.[13] Table 18.1 shows the degree of public involvement in financing health services and the essential role envisioned for the health-care system.[14]

> *Between now and the year 2050, the number of persons 65 years of age or older is expected to double. By 2050, one in five people living in Canada or the United States will be elderly, and their numbers will reach an estimated 80 million.*

Type I Systems

In type I health-care system, private approaches to health services predominate. Physicians, other caregivers (such as midwives), and clients have maximum autonomy. In this plan, individuals who can afford private health insurance, or who simply can pay for their health care, choose their care providers and receive health services. Those who cannot pay do not have choice or benefit.

In the pure form of the type 1 system, there would be no option other than to pay for service. In reality, most countries have adopted a mixture of system types. For example, although the United States has a mainly private payment system of health care, some publicly funded programs assist elderly and poor people. Even with these programs, it is estimated that 25 percent of Americans have no health insurance and therefore are limited in their ability to access health care.

Type IV Systems

On the opposite end of the spectrum from type I is type IV. This type of health-care system focuses on keeping the general public healthy so that they can continue to contribute to society and the economy. Health care is considered an essential service or even a right, not necessarily involving compassionate motives, and the goal is to keep the population healthy so that national productivity will remain high. Physicians are considered agents of the state who work to keep others working efficiently.

In Canada, the type IV structure is seen in such organizations as the military, hockey teams, and other sports teams. Physicians are hired by these organizations to ensure the players stay healthy and can do their part to achieve the goals of the group.

Type III Systems

Between the extremes of type I and type IV health-care systems are two less extreme types. The type III system is funded and operated by the government, as was seen in Great Britain some years ago. With this system, the state-operated and state-funded health services were based on an egalitarian value. Public management of each service was considered key to efficient and effective operation.

Type II Systems

The type II system is a hybrid of type I and type III systems. Egalitarian values are given high priority,

Table 18.1 Types of Health-Care Systems in the Western World

Type I	Type II	Type III	Type IV
Private health insurance Primary goal: preserve autonomy Secondary effect: acceptance of social differences	National health insurance Primary goal: egalitarian Secondary effect: preserve autonomy	National health service Primary goal: egalitarian Secondary effect: public management	Socialized health system Primary goal: essential service Secondary effect: physicians as state employees

Source: Najman J, Western J: A comparative analysis of Australian health policy in the 1970s. Social Science and Medicine 18(1):949–958, 1984, with permission.

but so are practitioner and client autonomy. The type II system uses tax dollars to pay for health services through health insurance available from a nonprofit agency (e.g., government).

Each health service is operated more or less autonomously by others, including municipalities, citizen groups, physicians, nurse practitioners, and physiotherapists in private offices, group practices, and other groups. All services rendered to clients are then paid from the central pool of health insurance funds created through taxation. This type of system is used in Canada and embodies the collective sharing of burdens and benefits while allowing a degree of autonomy in delivery.[15]

Third World Alternatives

It is important to note that the four systems described above exclude a group of third world countries that cannot afford the type of health care enjoyed in most developed countries. Yet many third world countries have managed to develop primary care systems that are not as institution dependent as the systems found in Canada and the United States. In their systems, primary care includes preventive health care, first point of contact, and continuing care. However, in some countries, the primary and preventive systems have been undermined by the influence of Western countries promoting high technology and institutionalization.

What Do Taxes Cover?

Even in countries that finance health insurance through tax dollars, there are variations in services provided. For example, some fund home care but others do not; some provide coverage for prescription drugs

and others do not. Regardless of the type of system, it is important to reflect on the influences that have created it and continue to maintain it.

What Do You Think?

What type of health-care system was used the last time you accessed health care? Did you use the health-care system for preventive care or illness care?

ADMINISTRATION AND FUNDING OF HEALTH-CARE SYSTEMS

Health Care in Canada

Financing and administering health-care systems can be an overwhelming responsibility. In Canada, health-care services are provided under the Canada Health Act. The Canadian federal government collects funds through taxes and gives the responsibility of administering health-care services to the provinces. As in the United States, the cost of financing health-care services has risen tremendously since the first Medical Care Act was introduced in 1967–1968. In Canada, medical insurance premiums became an increasing burden for the federal government as a result of the improved services promised to all Canadians.

Federal Transfer Payments

In an attempt to control the costs to be paid to all provinces, the Canadian government proposed a system of block funding. In 1977, the Federal–Provincial Fiscal Arrangements and Established Programs Financing Act was established after lengthy negotiations with all provinces. The formula for federal transfer payments consisted of four components:

1. Per capita payments were made on the basis of previous expenditures and adjusted regularly in relation to the gross national product.
2. Tax points were transferred by the federal government, allowing provinces to reduce their tax contribution to the government and at the same time increase the portion of tax collected at the provincial level.
3. Equalization of tax points was distributed among poorer provinces.
4. Additional per capita payments were indexed to help pay for nursing home, residential, home, and ambulatory care.

This new act changed the funding formulae from a 50-50 cost-sharing arrangement to one that gave taxation points to the provinces in exchange for lower cash transfer payments. The provinces were initially very receptive, as this meant they had more taxation power in an economy that was very healthy. However, with rising costs of health care, owing in part to an aging population and increased technology, some physicians and provinces struggled with health-care coverage. With extra billing or balance billing becoming prevalent, there was a heated public debate, and the new Canada Health Act was passed in 1984.

The Canada Health Act

Although the Canadian federal government has a limited constitutional basis for making health-care decisions, it has considerable economic clout to develop and shape a national health-care plan. To support their positions on health care, the federal government enacted the Canada Health Act (CHA). The purpose of the CHA is to "establish criteria and conditions in respect of insured health services and extended health-care services provided under provincial law that must be met before a full cash contribution may be made."[16]

The insured health services defined by the CHA include all medically necessary hospital services and medically required physician services, as well as medically or dentally required surgical–dental services that needed to be performed in a hospital

for safety. New criteria, conditions, and provisions were formulated to eliminate extra-billing and user charges.

For the provinces to qualify for full cash refunds from the federal government under the Canada Health and Social Transfer (CHST) agreement, they must meet five basic criteria and conditions. These criteria and conditions must be met for each fiscal year and include:

1. *Public Administration:* The health-care insurance plan must be administered and operated on a non-profit basis by a public authority, responsible to the provincial government and subject to audit of its accounts and financial transactions.
2. *Comprehensiveness:* The plan must cover all insured health services provided by hospitals, medical practitioners, and dentists and, where permitted, services rendered by other health-care practitioners.
3. *Universality:* One hundred percent of the insured population of a province must be entitled to the insured health services provided for by the plan on uniform terms and conditions.
4. *Portability:* Residents moving to another province must continue to be covered for insured health services by the home province during any minimum waiting period, not to exceed 3 months, imposed by the new province of residence. For insured persons, insured health services must be made available while they are temporarily absent from their own provinces on the following basis:
   - Insured services received out of province, but still in Canada, are to be paid for by the home province at host province rates unless another arrangement for the payment of costs exists between the provinces. Prior approval may be required for elective services.
   - Out-of-country services received are to be paid, as a minimum, on the basis of the amount that would have been paid by the home province for similar services rendered in the province. Prior approval may be required for elective services.
5. *Accessibility:* The health-care insurance plan of a province must provide for:
   - Insured health services on uniform terms and conditions and reasonable access by insured persons to insured health services not precluded and unimpeded, either directly or indirectly, by charges or other means

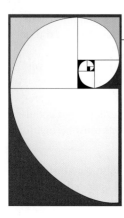

Issues in Practice

National Coalition on Health-Care Findings

A recent survey by the National Coalition on Health-Care Findings developed some interesting information:

- In a survey, the primary reason given by people for being uninsured is the lack of health insurance coverage.
- As health-care costs rise, the number of insured decreases.
- Almost half the American public surveyed indicated that they are very worried about how they will meet the increased premiums for health insurance; and 42 percent are worried that they may not be able to afford health insurance at all.
- Twenty-five percent of Americans identified paying for health insurance as a problem during the past year.
- Medical debt was a leading reason (50%) for people to file for bankruptcy, with the average medical debt being $12,000 per person.
- Elderly couples who retire today will need between $200,000 and $300,000 just to pay for medical coverage.

Sources: Piamjariyakul U, Ross VM, Yadrich DM, Williams AR, Howard L, Smith CE: Complex Home Care: Part I—Utilization and costs to families for health care services each year. Nursing Economics 28(4):255–263, 2010.

Health insurance costs: National Coalition on Health Care. Retrieved November, 2010 from http://www.nchc.org/facts/cost.

- Reasonable compensation to physicians and dentists for all insured health services rendered
- Payments to hospitals in respect to the cost of insured health services

Although discussion and debate continue surrounding the federal and provincial responsibilities for health-care funding and the escalating costs associated with health care, the Canada Health Act of 1984 continues to be the operating model for the Canadian health-care system.

Health-Care Systems in the United States

The United States has a far different method of funding and administering health-care services. According to the World Health Organization, the United States spends more per person on health care than any other country, yet in overall quality its care ranks 37th in the world and last among the seven leading industrialized nations.[17] This disparity is attributed in large part to the cost of health-care services, not the quality of the services available.

In the attempt to contain some of these costs, professional standards review organizations

(PSROs) were introduced to review the quality, quantity, and cost of hospital care through Medicare. The primary goal of PSROs was to review the care provided by physicians to determine whether the best diagnostic and treatment approaches were being used. Another measure was the introduction of utilization review committees, requiring Medicare-qualified facilities to review admission, diagnostic testing, and treatments with the goal of eliminating overuse or misuse of services.

What Do You Think?

Review the bill from your last hospitalization or the bill of a family member. What do you think about the charges listed? Does the bill seem excessive?

Prospective Payment Systems

Although these measures have assisted with cost containment to some degree, one of the most significant factors that have influenced cost control was the prospective payment system (PPS) established by the

U.S. Congress in 1983. This system required facilities providing services to Medicare clients to be reimbursed using a fixed-rate system and included monetary incentives to reduce the length of hospital stays. Medicare clients are classified using a diagnosis-related group (DRG), and the facilities are reimbursed a predetermined amount. Clients may be classified into one of 468 DRGs, and reimbursement occurs regardless of the length of stay.

If the client is discharged sooner than anticipated, the facility keeps the difference. If the client requires a lengthier hospital stay, the hospital pays the extra cost. Under the PPS, the emphasis is on the efficient delivery of services in the most cost-effective manner.

Capitated Payment Systems

Capitation, or a capitated payment system, was introduced to encourage cost effectiveness in a growing health-care system. In a capitated payment system, participants pay a flat rate, usually through their employer, to belong to a managed care organization (MCO) for a specified period of time. The health-care providers who serve the participants receive a fixed amount for each participant in the health-care plan.

Controlled Access

The goal of capitation is to have a payment plan for selected diseases or surgical procedures that provides the highest quality of care, including essential diagnostic and treatment procedures, at the lowest cost possible. Any expenses in excess of the capitated rate are the responsibility of the MCO. If the MCO spends less on the care of a client than it is given for delivery costs, it can keep the excess as profit, providing it with a strong incentive to reduce the cost of services.

Another goal of managed care is to enhance the efficiency and effective use of health-care services. A key underlying concept of managed care is to maintain administrative control over access and provision of primary health-care services for the members of the plan. The MCO controls all aspects of care including delivery, financing, and the purchase of health-care services for clients who are enrolled in the program. Clients are allowed to use only the services of primary care physicians who are approved by the organization. Any referrals to other medical specialists must be approved by the MCO. The MCO contract determines what treatments or procedures will be reimbursed.

A Spending Increase

The effectiveness of the MCO plan rests on the theory that health-care costs can be reduced by decreasing the number of hospitalizations, shortening the length of inpatient stays, providing less expensive home-care services, and keeping people healthy through health promotion and illness prevention services. It is logical to conclude that if people stay healthy, the cost of health-care services should decline.

Although much debate surrounds managed care and its advantages and disadvantages, the reality is that managed care has *not* reduced health-care costs nationally. Increases in spending are attributed to rising health-care wages, legislation that increased Medicare spending, increasing insurance premiums, technology, and consumer demands for less restrictive plans.

QUALITY ASSURANCE

Continuous Quality Improvement

Quality assurance initiatives are essential when efforts are being made to cut costs and, at the same time, maintain high standards of care. To ensure high-quality care, the health-care industry borrowed the philosophy of **continuous quality improvement (CQI)** from the business world. The Joint Commission was so impressed with its potential to improve health-care delivery that in 1994 it began requiring hospitals to implement CQI strategies.

Exceeding Expectations

Continuous quality improvement, also known as **total quality management (TQM),** is based on the belief that the organization with the higher-quality service will capture a greater share of the market than competitors with lower-quality services. Emphasis is placed both on meeting the expectations of the customer (in this case the health-care consumer) and on exceeding those expectations.

According to the CQI philosophy, there are internal customers and external customers. The external customers are clients and their families; internal customers are individuals working within the health-care setting. Delivering high-quality services is valued above all else, and the ideal goal is that every constituent be completely satisfied with the services provided.

A Proactive Approach

Continuous quality improvement requires that the service delivery process receive close and constant scrutiny, and everyone is encouraged to generate ideas for improving quality. Although CQI encourages change on the basis of systematically documented evidence, it also values standardization of the process so that efficiency is maximized. CQI is proactively oriented so that emphasis is placed on anticipating and preventing problems rather than reacting to them after the fact.

Nurses are in an excellent position to implement CQI strategies. On a daily basis, they assess the functioning of the health-care delivery system and the effectiveness of specific treatment approaches. For example, on the basis of evidence that inexpensive saline is as effective as heparin in keeping intermittent intravenous catheters patent, nurses at one hospital implemented a new protocol and saved $70,000 within 1 year.[18]

Case Management Protocols

There is another mechanism for monitoring cost-effective, high-quality care: outcomes-based case management protocols, also known as **clinical pathways.** The development of clinical pathways grew out of a need to assess, implement, and monitor cost-effective, high-quality client care in a systematic manner.

Clinical pathways were an outgrowth of nursing care plans but have the advantages of streamlining the charting process, encouraging documentation across multidisciplinary teams, and systematically monitoring variances from prescribed plans of care. The ability to identify how client care and progress vary from a predetermined plan enables more accurate assessment of client-care costs and maintenance of quality-control measures. Integration of clinical pathways into practical use has been enhanced by computerization of client records and online bedside documentation.

Six Sigma Quality Improvement

The Tail of the Curve

Although **six sigma** was developed and used initially for the manufacturing industry in the early 1980s, it found its way into the health-care system in the mid- to late 1990s. Its origins can be traced back to the 1920s and are based on the statistical model bell-shaped curve. In the perfect bell curve, there is a mean exactly in the center at the highest point of the curve. Away from the mean, the curve slopes down at a predictable rate on both sides and is divided into standard deviations. Each standard deviation is designated sigma and given a number (e.g., plus or minus 1 sigma). Six standard deviations (six sigmas) are so far out in the tails of the bell curve that they are generally considered a total lack of error; in other words, "perfection" (statistically, 3.4 defects per million).

Six sigma technique was initially used by Motorola to improve the quality of their products and was then adopted by such well-known corporations as General Electric and Honeywell. It can be used to reduce the costs of manufacturing items or the steps in manufacturing, making the manufacturing process more "lean." This has led to the use of the term *lean Six Sigma.*[19]

> *The United States ranks last among seven industrialized counties, although it spends more per patient.*

The traditional Six Sigma process comprises five distinct phases that somewhat parallel the steps of the nursing process:

1. *Define:* The problem is identified. Why are the customers dissatisfied? Why are the costs excessive? Why does it take so long to complete the process?
2. *Measure:* Data are collected to pinpoint the exact issue. The whole process is reviewed in detail and time or other types of measurement are given numerical values.
3. *Analyze:* The root causes of the problem are identified, and the relationships of external or environmental influences are analyzed. All factors must be considered, no matter how remote.
4. *Improve:* Strategies, based on the previous three phases, are developed to correct the problems. Any number of techniques may be used to make the process error-proof and more efficient. Pilot projects are then established to demonstrate the success of the efforts to correct the problems. Several attempts may be tested before the best one is identified.
5. *Control:* Systems are put in place to continuously monitor the changes in the process. The goal is to detect errors before they affect the whole system.

A statistical process may be used to determine the level of correction and as an early warning system for new problems. [20]

Six Sigma in Health Care

How does the health care system use Six Sigma to improve the quality of care? Traditionally in health care, finding and defining the specific cause of errors has been extremely difficult. Six Sigma provides a wide-reaching and more pragmatic approach to identifying and measuring the problem. By adapting and modifying the traditional Six Sigma methodology, health-care providers can develop more inclusive objectives to increase reliability and quality. The overriding goal of Six Sigma is to develop a fully reliable process or system of care. Such a system will deliver the same quality of care to all clients all the time regardless of who actually delivers the care. Optimal care is provided when it is evidence based.

As a highly structured approach to identifying fundamental problems, the Six Sigma process guides nurses and others through the five-phase process using statistical tools. Specialized training is required to employ Six Sigma, and individuals can become certified as Six Sigma Consultants through the Institute of Industrial Engineers or the American Society for Quality. Trained individuals can then serve as well-paid consultants for hospitals and other institutions that believe Six Sigma may be the answer to their problems.[19]

When the Six Sigma process is used to analyze a problem, it looks primarily for two types of statistical anomalies or variations. The primary one, usually at the root of most problems, is called "special" or "assigned" variation and shows a pattern of activity outside the patterns expected to produce high-quality care. Once this variation is detected, the five-step statistical process can be applied. The second type of anomaly is called "common" or "chance" variation and is usually attributed to environmental factors that cannot be controlled. However, in some situations, chance variations can become so significant that they affect the process and have to be addressed.

As a newcomer to health care, the Six Sigma process has been used on a limited basis. There is only a relatively small body of publications about the successes and problems of using it in the health-care setting. The Commonwealth Health Corporation in Kentucky was one of the first to use Six Sigma in 2002. It was used to streamline their radiology department and increase its bottom line by reducing costs. Six Sigma has been used successfully in other hospitals to increase nurse satisfaction and retention by eliminating annoying factors in day-to-day operations, to reduce clients' length of stay, and to speed up the process for transferring clients from outpatient areas to inpatient rooms.

There are critics of Six Sigma, and several drawbacks to its use have been identified. Six Sigma is effective in modifying existing processes; however, it tends to stifle creative approaches and "thinking outside the box." Although achieving perfection at the statistical 3.4 errors per million level might be adequate for situations such as client satisfaction and nurse retention, it seems to fall short for such activities as administering medications and operating a ventilator. When Six Sigma is implemented in the health care setting, it is often used as an add-on project not connected with existing quality improvement efforts. Nursing staff tend to resist the strange-sounding jargon and statistical emphasis and may actually attempt to sabotage implementation. Six Sigma has little regard for the interpersonal and institutional culture that is so important in the effectiveness of health-care institutions.

The overall objective of Six Sigma is to increase the reliability of processes by eliminating defects and reducing system variation. Its five-phase structured approach requires high-quality discrete data that are often difficult to obtain in the health-care setting. Its orientation is more industrial than health related: it uses tools such as statistical process control and root cause analysis to identify anomalies in the processes it is examining. Although yet to be

> " *The effectiveness of the MCO plan rests on the theory that health-care costs can be reduced by decreasing the number of hospitalizations, shortening the length of inpatient stays, providing less-expensive home care services, and keeping people healthy through health promotion and illness prevention services.* "

used on a wide scale in the health-care setting, Six Sigma is gradually gaining a following, and its use in health care will probably increase in the future.[20]

Overview of Health-Care Plans

See Boxes 18.1 through 18.5 to compare the principal features of different health-care models.

HEALTH-CARE LEVELS AND SETTINGS

Even though there are many methods for providing and funding health care, high-quality health-care services remain the highest priority. Consumers who

---

Box 18.1

Managed Care Organizations (MCOs)

Definition: Provide comprehensive, preventive, and treatment services to a specific group of voluntarily enrolled persons.

Managed Care Structures
Staff model: Physicians are salaried employees of the MCO.
Group model: MCO contracts with single group practice.
Network model: MCO contracts with multiple group practices and/or integrated organizations.
Independent practice association (IPA): MCO contracts with physicians who usually are not members of groups and whose practices include fee-for-service and capitated clients.
Characteristics: Focus on health maintenance and primary care. All care provided by a primary care physician. Referral needed for access to specialists and hospitalization.

Medicare MCO
Definition: Program same as MCO but designated to cover health-care costs of senior citizens.
Characteristics: Premium generally less than supplemental plans.

Box 18.2

Provider Organizations

Preferred Provider Organization (PPO)
Definition: One that limits an enrollee's choice to a list of "preferred" hospitals, physicians, and providers. An enrollee pays more out-of-pocket expenses for using a provider not on the list.
Characteristics: Contractual agreement exists between a set of providers and one or more purchasers (self-insured employers or insurance plans). Comprehensive health services at a discount for companies under contract.

Exclusive Provider Organization (EPO)
Definition: One that limits an enrollee's choice to providers belonging to one organization. Enrollee may or may not be able to use outside providers at additional expense.
Characteristics: Limited contractual agreement; less access to specialists.

Box 18.3

Medicare

Definition: Federally funded national health insurance program in the United States for people older than 65 years. Part A provides basic protection for medical, surgical, and psychiatric care costs based on diagnosis-related groups (DRGs). Part B is a voluntary medical insurance plan that covers physician and certain outpatient services.
Characteristics: Payment for plan deducted from monthly individual Social Security check; covers services of nurse practitioners (varies by state); does not pay full costs of certain services; supplemental insurance is encouraged.

Box 18.4
Medicaid

Definition: Federally funded, state-operated medical assistance program for people with low incomes. Individual states determine eligibility and benefits.

Characteristics: Finances a large portion of maternal and child care for the poor; reimburses for nurse midwifery and other advanced practice nursing (varies by state); reimburses long-term care facility funding.

Box 18.5
Private Insurance

Traditional Private Insurance

Definition: Traditional fee-for-service plan. Payment, computed after services are provided, based on the number of services used.

Characteristics: Policies typically expensive; most policies have deductibles that clients must meet before insurance pays.

Long-Term Care Insurance

Definition: Supplemental insurance for coverage of long-term care services. Policies provide a set number of dollars for an unlimited time or for as little as 2 years.

Characteristics: Very expensive; good policy has a minimum waiting period for eligibility, payment for skilled nursing, intermediate or custodial care, and home care.

have access to multiple types of health care may not always understand the differences among them.

In the past, health-care services were primarily illness or institution based and focused primarily on treating the ill or injured. The emphasis is now shifting slowly toward prevention and health promotion in the population. It is believed that a focus on

wellness and a population living a healthier lifestyle will reduce the number of people who require expensive illness care services.

Levels of Service
Health-care services are frequently categorized according to the complexity or level of the services provided. This complexity relates to the kinds, or levels, of services: primary, secondary, and tertiary.

Primary Care
In nursing, primary care refers to health promotion and preventive care, including programs such as immunization campaigns. Primary care focuses on health education and on early detection and treatment. Maintaining and improving optimal health is the overriding goal.

Secondary Care
In the secondary level, the focus shifts toward emergency and acute care. Secondary services are frequently provided in hospitals and other acute care settings, with an emphasis on diagnosis and the treatment of complex disorders.

Tertiary Care
The tertiary level emphasizes rehabilitative services, long-term care, and care of the dying. Nursing services are essential in all three levels of health care, including both hospital and community settings.

What Do You Think?

Have you ever received care in a "nontraditional" health-care setting? What was it? What role did nurses play in the delivery of care?

Health-Care Settings
While nursing care is provided in traditional settings such as the hospital and the community, nursing services are also delivered in a growing number of nontraditional locations. One growing trend in care is seen in the outpatient departments attached to some hospitals. Outpatient services are used by clients who require a relatively high level of skilled health care but who do not need to stay in a hospital for an extended period of time. An inpatient is a

person who enters a setting such as a hospital and remains for at least 24 hours. Whether clients are inpatients or outpatients, they often need assistance from the nurse to identify which services best suit their needs.

Public Health

Public health departments are government agencies that are established at the local, provincial or state, and federal levels to provide health services. The goal of early public health departments was to prevent and control communicable diseases that were rampant in the 18th and 19th centuries, producing epidemics that killed millions of people. Today, the scope of public health, while retaining its contagious disease control and prevention mission, has expanded to areas such as child health, obstetric, and pregnancy care, and more recently into the early detection and treatment of terrorist acts, particularly bioterrorism (see Chapter 23).

Home Health Care

Care of the ill and injured in the home is the oldest of all the health-care modalities. If you were to go back far enough, it might even be called "cave health care." The modern hospital and clinic are relatively new entities in the health-care system, having their origins in the industrial revolution. Before that time, the only place a person could receive care was at home, usually from a female relative.

> *It is believed that a focus on wellness and a population living a healthier lifestyle will reduce the number of people who require expensive illness care services.*

Care in the Home Setting

Although the interest in and use of home health care have waxed and waned over time, its benefits have received new attention in the era of an aging population and health-care reform. Currently, the number of clients receiving care in the home exceeds 1.4 million, and some of this care is at a high-acuity level.[21] Gone are the days when home health care consisted of a quick visit by a nurse or aide taking vital signs, changing a dressing, and cleaning the house. Home health care now combines the advantages of health care in a safe and familiar setting with the high-tech treatment modalities found in the most advanced hospitals.

The goal of home health care is to make it possible for clients to remain at home rather than use hospital, residential, or long-term care facilities. Most clients prefer the familiar atmosphere of their own home and neighborhood. Clients experience lower stress levels at home and have a more positive outlook, which studies have shown hastens recovery. They are active participants in their own care, increasing their independence and giving them a sense of control over the outcome. Usually the home contains far fewer invasive pathogens than the hospital, so clients have a lower rate of infection with the medication-resistant bacteria commonly found in hospitals and extended care facilities.[22] When nurses and other health-care professionals do visit the home-care client, the client and his or her health needs are the sole focus of the care provided.

The majority of home health care remains informal and is mostly provided by relatives and friends. When professionals provide care in the home, nurses are the primary group involved. Other providers include physical therapists, home health-care aides, respiratory and occupational therapists, social workers, and mental health professionals. Professional-level home health-care services can include physical and psychological assessment, wound care, medication and illness education, pain management, physical therapy, speech therapy, and occupational therapy. Assistance with activities of daily living and other daily tasks such as meal preparation, medication reminders, laundry, light housekeeping, errands, shopping, transportation, and companionship is sometimes referred to as life assistance services.[21]

The technology long considered the sole domain of the acute care hospital has found its way into the home. Clients who previously could only receive treatment in a hospital can now remain at home and receive the same quality of treatment. A rapidly growing industry of high-tech home care is breaking down the walls between the acute care unit and the bedroom. From the intravenous infusions of antibiotics and total parenteral nutrition to the use of ventilators and hemodialysis machines, the level of high-tech home treatments continues to grow.[23]

Although it might seem logical that hospitals would resist a trend that reduces the number of clients, the opposite is true. Current funding restrictions for clients who return to the hospital too quickly with the same condition, or who have acquired a hospital-source infection, make earlier client discharge very attractive. More continuity of care is guaranteed when clients are observed in the home. Research shows that home care reduces emergency department visits and unnecessary readmissions to the hospital. Overall, clients report an increased level of satisfaction with the care provided and the improvement of their conditions.

A Need for Skilled Care

Not just anybody can be covered to receive home health care. When a client is referred for home health care by a physician or nurse practitioner, the provider must demonstrate that the client requires skilled needs that can only be provided by a professional nurse or other professional, depending on the client's diagnosis. These skilled needs fall into three categories:

- *Management of care* (e.g., injections, intravenous (IV) lines, wound care, diabetes or its complications, urinary catheters, rehabilitation, respiratory therapies)
- *Client evaluation* (e.g., unstable conditions, pain, response to medications, neurological functioning, environment)
- *Client education* (e.g., medications, glucose monitoring, disease management, prevention measures, activities of daily living)[22]

A Rewarding Practice

Not all nurses are attracted to home health care as a career path. Individuals who thrive on the fast pace and perpetual motion of acute care or intensive care units would find the laid-back pace of home health care boring. Additionally, the mountain of paperwork that accompanies home health-care clients might deter even the most dedicated super-nurse. However, many nurses find it a rewarding area of practice. The one-on-one interaction with clients and their families permits a level of care only dreamed of in the acute

care setting. The ability to observe a client over an extended period and to watch his or her condition improving makes all the effort seem worthwhile.

However, the nurse who provides care in the home setting must develop a number of important skill sets. Probably most important of all is **ethical practice.** In the home care setting, the nurse practices with virtually no supervision. It is up to professionals to maintain their competency and provide a high level of skills. Ethical practice is at the heart of establishing trust with the client and his or her family.

Flexibility is another quality that home health-care nursing requires. Things do not always go as planned. Even though appointments are scheduled well ahead of time, clients often have last-minute condition changes or conflicts that require a reschedule. Even during the visit, the nurse may find that the client is not physically or mentally able to do the required skills or learning. Nurses are visitors in the client's home, and the client sets the pace for the care that is provided. It is sometimes difficult for nurses to let go of the control they had over clients in the acute care setting, but it is one of the keys to success.

> *Today, the scope of public health, while retaining its contagious disease and prevention mission, has expanded to areas such as child health, obstetric, and pregnancy care, and more recently into the early detection and treatment of terrorist acts, particularly bioterrorism.*

Nurses must also increase their skills in cultural competency. Each home has its own unique cultural context. To become **culturally competent,** nurses must develop a high level of cultural sensitivity by respecting and believing that all cultures are equally valid and not attempting to impose values from the nurse's culture. Using a cultural assessment such as is found in Chapter 22 can be a great help in providing culturally sensitive care. By learning about a client's beliefs, value systems, attitudes, and customs, the nurse can enrich his or her own life.

Often home health-care nurses find that the home is not a very peaceful environment, but rather, filled with tension and conflict. The ability to apply the principles of **conflict management** is a skill that home health-care nurses must master early in their careers. Illness is an automatic stressor, and often the families of ill clients do not know how to deal with the increased levels of stress. Family members may have widely different views of care, and clients themselves may have a variant understanding of what they can and cannot do. It is not unusual for a nurse to hear from family members: "Tell Mama she's too sick to fix supper anymore!"

The most important skill in conflict management is active listening. It is essential for the nurse to listen to clients' fears, concerns, and even anger about their condition and their families' reaction and actions. The nurse must also be on the lookout for signs of elder abuse and neglect. It is not uncommon for family caregivers, either intentionally or unintentionally, to harm the client through threats, withholding care and medications, or negative communication.

The future of home health care is full of opportunity. As the population ages, home health care will allow them to stay at home while receiving the same treatments and technology as they would receive in the acute care setting. Health-care reform has placed a brighter spotlight on the areas of quality and cost. Home health care allows for increased continuity of care, increasing the quality of care while significantly reducing its cost.

School-Based Services

Nurses provide a variety of services within local school systems. These services include screenings, health promotion and illness prevention programs, and treatment of minor health problems. Emphasis is placed on physical, social, and psychological well-being. Concerns relating to self-esteem, stress, drug abuse, and adolescent pregnancy are frequently addressed by the school nurse. In addition, children and adolescents with long-term health problems often attend school, and it is not uncommon for the nurse to be consulted about such issues as seizure management, colostomy care, or gastric tube feedings.

Students who have health concerns are frequently referred to providers within the community, and an important role of the school nurse is that of community liaison. For this reason, the nurse must be knowledgeable about community resources and adept at getting clients into the system in a timely and efficient manner.

Community Health Centers

Community health centers are being more frequently used in many communities. Most centers use a team approach involving physicians, nurse practitioners, and community nurses working together to provide health services. Most centers have diagnostic and treatment facilities that provide medical, nursing, laboratory, and radiological services. Some centers may also provide outpatient minor surgical procedures that allow clients to remain at home while accessing health services as needed.

Physicians' Offices and General Clinics

The physician's office continues to be the location where most North Americans access primary health care. The majority of physicians in North America continue to work either in their own offices or with other physicians in a group practice. Services range from routine health screening to illness diagnosis and treatment and even some minor surgical procedures.

The responsibilities of nurses who work in physicians' offices or in general clinics include obtaining personal health information and histories of current illness and preparing the client for examination. Nurses also assist with procedures and obtain specimens for laboratory analysis. Teaching clients basic health information and home management of treatments and medications is also a responsibility of the clinic nurse.

Occupational Health Clinics

Maintaining the health of workers in their workplaces to increase productivity has long been recognized as an important role for nurses. In response to rising health insurance costs, today's employers are increasingly supportive of workplace health promotion, illness prevention, and safety programs. Many companies provide wellness programs and encourage or even require their employees to participate. These services range from providing exercise facilities and fitness programs to health screenings and referrals. Illness prevention focuses on topics such as smoking cessation, stress management, and nutrition. Although some companies may hire health educators to manage their clinics, community health nurses often provide these services.

In Canada, occupational health nurses are registered nurses (RNs) holding a minimum of a diploma or a Bachelor of Science degree in nursing. Many may also have occupational health certification, or a degree in occupational health and safety from a community college or university. Nurses who are certified in occupational health nursing must meet eligibility requirements, pass a written examination, and be recognized as having achieved a level of competency in occupational health. The certification is granted by the Canadian Nurses Association.

Hospitals

Hospitals, the traditional provider of health-care services, are still an essential part of the health-care system and still provide the majority of nurses with employment. Hospitals range in size from small, rural facilities with as few as 15 to 20 beds to large urban centers that may exceed a bed capacity of several thousand.

Depending on the services they provide, hospitals will have varying classifications. General hospitals offer a variety of services, such as medical, surgical, obstetric, pediatric, and psychiatric care. Other hospitals may offer specialized services, such as pediatric care. Hospitals can be further classified as acute care or chronic care, depending on the length of stay of the client and the services available. Large hospitals may be designated as specific centers for treatment, such as a trauma or cardiac center, because they can offer specialized services.

Long-Term Care Facilities

The majority of senior citizens in North America continue to live in their own homes. However, a growing group of seniors have health needs that require long-term care or extended care services. Some individuals may require rehabilitation or intermediate care, whereas others require extended, long-term care. These services are provided for both elderly and younger clients who have similar needs, such as clients with spinal cord injuries.

The current trend in extended care facilities is to provide care in a homelike atmosphere and base programs on the needs and abilities of the clients, or residents as they are commonly called, of the facility. Many of these residents require personal services such as bathing and assistance with activities of daily living. Others may require higher-level skilled nursing care such as tube feedings and catheter management or even occasional medical attention. Because of the range of needs of clients, some facilities will

admit clients with specific needs to specific areas of the facility where the appropriate services are provided.

In Canada, admission to long-term care facilities must meet specific guidelines. Assessments of client needs and the nursing services available must be completed before the client is admitted to the facility. Frequently, there are waiting lists for admission to extended care facilities.

In the United States, many long-term care facilities are for-profit institutions that rely heavily on Medicaid and Medicare reimbursements.[24] When Medicare coverage is limited, the resident must use private insurance or personal resources to pay the difference in cost.

Retirement and Assisted Living Centers

As the population continues to age, assisted living centers are increasing in popularity because they allow clients, or residents, to maintain the greatest amount of independence possible in a partially controlled and supervised living environment. These centers consist of separate apartments or condominiums for the residents and provide amenities such as meal preparation and laundry services.

Many centers work closely with home care and other social services to provide the resources required for maintaining a degree of independence. Case coordinators, often nurses, help residents navigate their way through the complex paperwork usually involved in obtaining required services. Some assisted living centers are attached to long-term care facilities. According to the level of care required, residents may be transferred to various facilities as their care needs change.[25]

Rehabilitation Centers

In many acute care facilities, discharge planning and rehabilitative needs are discussed at the time of admission. Rehabilitation centers or units are similar to some extended care facilities where the client goal is to restore health and function to an optimum level. Often clients are admitted to rehabilitation units after recuperating from the acute stage of an injury

> *Hospitals, the traditional provider of health-care services, are still an essential part of the health-care system and still provide the majority of nurses with employment.*

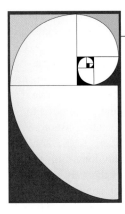

Issues Now

Nursing Home Fall Pays Big

An 82-year-old nursing home resident fell twice within a 6-week period. When she was admitted to the nursing home, the RN assessed that she had an unsteady gait and mild dementia from poor circulation and that she was at high risk for falls. The family also reported that she had fallen several times at home, and the falls were one of the primary reasons for her admission to the nursing home. The care plan recommended the use of seatbelt restraints and a seat alarm.

The first fall occurred in the dining room when the resident pushed her wheelchair away from the table and attempted to stand. The incident report noted that the wheelchair locks were not engaged. The second fall happened in the recreation room. The client was left alone in her wheelchair and again the wheel locks were not engaged. She attempted to stand by herself and fell again. She did not receive serious injuries from either fall.

The client's lawyer argued that the care plan was not followed and that the staff at the facility had neglected the protocols that called for locking of wheelchair wheels when clients were left unattended. The case was settled out of court by the nursing home's insurance company. The client and her family received $150,000 for the falls.

Source: Cebollero vs Hebrew Home, 2009 WL 2989743 (Westchester County Court, New York, March 16, 2009).

---

or illness. The rehabilitation unit then provides services to complete the recovery and restore a high degree of independence.

Some common types of rehabilitation units include geriatric, chemical dependency, stroke, and spinal cord injury units. Nurses who work on these units have the responsibility of coordinating health-care services, providing skilled care when required, supervising less educated personnel, and ensuring client compliance with treatment regimens.

Day-Care Centers

Day-care centers can be used by any age group. Traditionally, "day-care center" has referred to the care of children; however, during the past 12 years or so, adult day-care centers have become relatively common. Adult day-care centers provide services for elderly adults who cannot be left at home alone but do not require institutionalization.

Services provided by adult day-care centers include health maintenance classes, socialization and exercise programs, physical or occupational therapy, rehabilitative services, and organized recreational activities. Nurses who are employed in adult day-care centers may administer medications,

give treatments, provide counseling and teaching, and coordinate services between day care and home care.

Rural Primary Care

A Problem of Distance

Delivering health-care services to the rural areas of North America is a challenge because of the great distances between homes. In many rural towns, it is common to have small hospitals or other health-care facilities available to provide basic health-care services. Most of these facilities have basic laboratory and radiological services available.

In the far north of Canada, aboriginal communities have nursing stations or health centers in the community to provide basic health services. The centers are staffed by nurses. Visiting physicians come in occasionally to provide additional services. The nursing stations also provide emergency services to people who require stabilization before being transferred to a larger facility.

A Problem of Cost

In the United States, paying for health-care services in rural areas is a concern. Many of the residents in rural areas are farmers or employees of small businesses that do not offer health insurance. A type of group insurance called health insurance purchasing cooperatives (HIPCs) is now available to Americans who are self-employed or who do not have health insurance for other reasons. This program allows larger groups of individuals or employers to band together to purchase health insurance at a reduced cost.

Hospice Services

Hospice care originated in Great Britain and has changed the way end-of-life care is delivered. Disillusioned with health-care services that focused on technology and the preservation of life at all costs, the hospice movement gained momentum in the 1970s. Hospice care emphasizes physiological and psychological support for clients who have terminal diseases. Hospice care provides a variety of services in a caring and supportive environment to terminally ill clients, their families, and other support persons. The central concept of hospice care is not saving life, but improving or maintaining the quality of life until death occurs.

Telehealth and E-Health

Telehealth, or telephone health, advice services have experienced major growth in Canada in recent years. These services are generally available 24 hours a day, 7 days a week. Nurses answer the phones, supply answers to health-related questions, and advise callers on how to handle nonurgent health situations.[26]

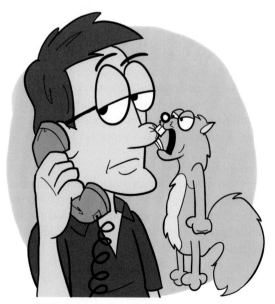

"FOR ANIMAL BITES, PLEASE PRESS 3."

Although telehealth activities have grown significantly in the past 5 to 6 years, their full potential has not yet been reached. The success of telehealth rests on a full and seamless integration of the service as part of the health-care delivery system. Understanding and eliminating barriers to the use of telehealth while capitalizing on the opportunities it presents will eventually improve the acceptance and mainstreaming of telehealth technologies. Telehealth is discussed in detail in Chapter 19.

E-health, electronic health advice, takes the telephone into the computer age. Rather than calling a resource center for information, the client can use a computer to access any number of sites that provide health-care information. Unfortunately, some of the information available online may not be completely accurate. Persons who use these resources need to evaluate their quality and the accuracy of the information they provide.

Parish Nurses

It is estimated that approximately 2000 parish nurses throughout the United States are attempting to meet the needs of individuals who are without adequate primary care or who are experiencing escalating health-care costs. Many of these nurses work part-time or are volunteers, and some work in conjunction with community-based programs. Churches engage parish nurses to:

- Serve as health educators and counselors
- Do health assessments and referrals
- Organize support groups
- Visit parishioners who are sick or elderly
- Serve as client advocates or case managers

Parish nurses are in a unique position to exercise their skills as case managers. As nurses, they possess clinical knowledge and skills, understand the health-care delivery system in their communities, and know many of the key health-care providers. As members of their parish, they are intimately familiar with their communities, understand the cultural climate of their clientele, and are familiar with the services that are available. Moreover, as members of the church community they serve, they are likely to be familiar with the spiritual, psychosocial, and financial needs of their clients. However, direct reimbursement is not yet available for parish nurses.

Voluntary Health Agencies

Since their inception in 1892, voluntary health agencies have experienced steady growth and now number more than 100,000. The first voluntary health agency was the Anti-tuberculosis Society of Philadelphia. Some of the more well-known agencies that exist today include the American Cancer Society, American Heart Association, National Foundation for the March of Dimes, National Easter Seal Society for Persons with Disabilities, and Alliance for the Mentally Ill.

These agencies provide many valuable services, including fundraising in support of cutting-edge research and public education. Some, such as the American Cancer Society, which has a strong emphasis on education and research, also help individuals secure special equipment, such as hospital beds for the home and wigs for chemotherapy clients. The Alliance for the Mentally Ill is politically active and organizes support groups for the mentally ill and their families. These groups are not-for-profit organizations, so all revenue in excess of cost goes toward improving services.

Independent Nurse-Run Health Centers

Similar to community health centers, nurse-run health centers tend to focus on health promotion and disease prevention. Historically, they have been service rather than profit oriented and remain so today. Nurses who are interested in autonomous practice often work in these settings.

Several types of nurse-run health centers have been identified. Among these are community health and institutional outreach centers. These facilities may be freestanding or sponsored by a larger institution, such as a university or public health agency. Primary care services are generally offered to the medically underserved, and these centers are typically funded by public and private sources.

Wellness and health-promotion clinics are another type of nurse-run clinic and offer services at work sites, schools, churches, or homeless shelters. Many of these centers are affiliated with schools of nursing, providing health-care services while offering educational experiences for nursing students.

A final type of nursing center includes faculty practice, independent practice, and nurse entrepreneurship models. These facilities are owned and operated by nurses and may be solo or multidisciplinary

practices. Services are typically reimbursed through fee-for-service plans, grants, and insurance. The ability of nurses in these centers to secure payments through the newly emergent and complex health-care reimbursement network will largely determine the future financial viability of these types of clinics.

HEALTH-CARE COSTS AND THE NURSING SHORTAGE

A Cost-Cutting Measure

The origins of the current nursing shortage can be traced directly back to the implementation of managed care in the 1990s as a method of controlling health-care costs. Managed-care companies required many procedures to be performed outside the hospital, leading to clients being sicker when they do enter the hospitals.

An Expensive Mistake

Health-care facilities trying to cut costs hired fewer expensive RNs in favor of less-expensive personnel. Nursing service at most facilities is the largest single budget item, averaging between 50 and 60 percent of the overall operating budget. At first glance, this seemed like a promising way to control health-care costs, but in the long run it turned out to be a very expensive mistake. RNs who were employed in acute care settings moved in droves to the home health-care and primary care settings. At the same time, the population was aging, resulting in a need for more nurses who could deliver high-quality specialized care in the acute care facilities.

As a result, the health-care industry has seen a trend of closing hospital units because of a lack of RNs. It is estimated that a closed 20-bed general medical-surgical unit will cost a hospital approximately $3 million in lost revenue per year.

Stress on the Nurse

The nurses who remain are finding working conditions to be less than ideal. Mandatory overtime, short staffing, and increased acuity of client conditions all are adding to the stress these nurses experience. As a result, they call in sick more often or leave for other facilities that have fewer demands. Sick time, recruitment, and orientation costs for many facilities have skyrocketed as a result.

Stress on the Facility

The other area in which health-care institutions feel the cost of the RN shortage is in lawsuits and rising insurance costs. During periods when there is a shortage of RNs, the quality of health care decreases, clients become dissatisfied with the care they are receiving, and serious mistakes are made in care, resulting in injury or death of clients. It only takes relatively few of these cases with awards in the tens of millions of dollars to re-emphasize the correlation between RN care and high-quality care.

Staffing Ratio Laws

One proposed solution to the nursing shortage problem is the passage of mandatory staffing ratio laws. Of course, hospital associations see these as increasing operating costs. However, the presumption is that more RNs will equate with higher quality of care and ultimately reduced long-range health-care costs.

Although laws have been passed in California, Florida, and other states, their implementation seems to be inconsistent. Hospital association groups in several states have challenges to the laws that have effectively blocked their implementation for the time being. However, nursing groups generally support these laws and see them as a way to solve staffing shortages by enticing inactive nurses or nurses who have sought employment in other health-care areas to return to the bedside in acute care facilities.

A Lack of Information

Not everyone, including some in the nursing profession, is convinced that enforced staff-to-client ratios will cure an ailing health-care system. One of the key issues is a lack of documented research that demonstrates that more RNs per clients equals higher-quality care. Intuitively, it would seem that putting more RNs back into the hospital would improve client care, yet more than 8 years ago the Institute of Medicine identified a dearth of information about the quality of care being delivered in the nation's acute care facilities.

The documentation and research have been slow to develop, although an increasing body of knowledge is now available. Leaders in the nursing profession hope the new staffing ratio laws will help demonstrate the important and critical part nurses play in providing high-quality care.

This study is one of a series that tracked RN staffing ratios and client outcomes. It validates what the American Nurses Association has been saying since the early 1990s—that there is a direct correlation between the care provided by RNs and positive client outcomes. The American Hospital Association (AHA) has formally acknowledged that RNs are critical to ensuring good client care. The AHA still resists the move toward mandatory staffing ratios, characterizing them as an "oversimplistic" solution to a complex problem. It is evident, however, from this study that in hospitals with low numbers of RNs, clients are more likely to stay longer, suffer more complications, and die from complications that, if they were identified and treated sooner, would be survivable.

Passing staffing ratio laws may be a quick fix to an emotional and dramatic concern, but it does not address a much wider range of problems hospitalized clients face every day. What is needed to ultimately cure the industry is a long-range plan for systemic reform on the basis of client needs, not the needs of a profit-motivated insurance industry.

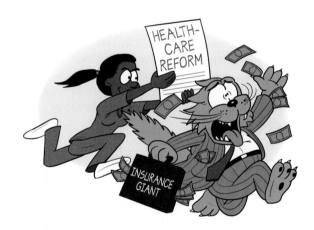

Clients educated to understand what high-quality care is, and how it can best be achieved, will ultimately be the most powerful force for attaining the care they require. When managed care facilities begin to really listen to the clients they are supposed to be serving, nurse staffing ratio laws will no longer be necessary. The facilities will meet the quality expectations by making sure that the needed number of nurses are there to provide the care the client expects.

Although laws may not be the ultimate solution to a much deeper problem, clients in the states with staffing ratio laws will be reassured to know they will have a well-educated, skilled professional nurse nearby who can act as an advocate for their needs and monitor the care they are receiving when they are most vulnerable.

Beyond the Numbers

Some in nursing are concerned that managed care facilities will use the mandated staffing ratio as a ceiling number rather than the minimum number of nurses required to provide safe care. There is also a fear that the facilities will look only at the numbers and not at the educational, skill, and experience levels of the nurses they use to meet their quotas. Without consideration of the acuity of client conditions on a unit and the care needs related to their illnesses, staffing ratios may actually lower the quality of care and threaten the safety of the clients. In addition, some fear that facilities in which the staffing ratio laws are unworkable will close only units where sicker clients are being treated, thus reducing access to care.

A More Acute Problem

Some farsighted nursing leaders see the passage of staffing ratio laws as an important but short-term solution to a much broader problem. Decreasing nurse-to-client ratios are just a symptom of a much more acute systemic problem in the health-care industry. The underlying problem revolves around an overly aggressive policy of cost cutting by managed care, often at the expense of the very clients who support the system with their insurance premiums.

Conclusion

Health-care delivery systems are complex and multifaceted. Nurses continue to provide the majority of health-care services to North Americans and need to understand the important role they play in the system. Changes in the health-care system are neverending. By understanding the various health-care systems and how they are related to each other, nurses put themselves at the forefront of change and advocate changes that benefit the health of all people.

Nursing is as complex as the health-care systems. It occurs in a wide variety of locations, and the role of the nurse will vary just as much as the health-care systems do. How a nurse functions in a hospital is different from how a nurse functions in parish nursing, but the caring and compassion that nurses bring to their roles will not vary. Nurses need to understand and develop their roles, and they will undoubtedly continue to have a significant impact on the further development of the health-care system.

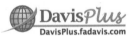
DavisPlus.fadavis.com

Critical Thinking Exercises

- Select three clients you are familiar with who have different health-care needs. Describe these clients' medical histories, current problems, and future health-care needs, then determine which health-care setting and which health-care practitioners would be most appropriate for them. Identify any difficulties that might be encountered during their entry into the health-care system. How can the nurse facilitate the process?
- Skilled nursing facilities, subacute care facilities, and assisted living facilities all are forms of long-term, or extended, health care. Identify five specific problems that nurses working in such facilities encounter. What is the best way to resolve these problems?
- Identify cost-cutting measures used at a health-care facility with which you are familiar. Have these measures affected the quality of client care? What other measures to cut costs can be implemented? How have changes within the health-care delivery system altered nursing practice?
- Identify four health-care priorities that may be initiated by the year 2015. How are these likely to affect the profession of nursing?
- Describe the advantages and disadvantages of various health-care reimbursement plans. Which ones will produce the highest-quality care? Which ones are best for the profession of nursing? Are there any payment plans that do both?
- Identify the most important elements in health-care reform. Should nurses support these changes? Why?

19

Nursing Informatics

Kathleen Mary Young

Learning Objectives

After completing this chapter, the reader will be able to:

- Discuss the impact of the information revolution on society in general and on health care specifically.
- Define nursing informatics.
- Explain the importance of nursing informatics to nursing practice.
- Analyze the availability of resources and references in the practice site.
- Evaluate the importance of human factors engineering on equipment design.
- Compare the electronic health record with the paper record system.

INFORMATION CHANGES EVERYTHING

The information revolution continues to expand exponentially, pushing the systems of modern culture to the breaking point. The information revolution is changing both the way teachers teach and the way learners learn. It is changing the way people work, communicate, and play. Teaching in public schools and even colleges now demands fast-moving, entertaining lessons that capture the students' attention because classroom teachers must compete with television and the computer games with which this generation has been raised.

Schoolchildren and college students no longer read as extensively as they once did. Media technology has accustomed many to 30-second "sound bites" of information. Libraries are evolving from repositories of hardbound volumes and journals to providers of Internet access to online journals and books. Many people spend 8 to 10 hours a day in front of a computer. People who have lost traditional jobs in manufacturing and service industries are finding that, to become marketable in today's workplace, they must have computer skills.

TECHNOLOGY AND COMMUNICATION

The information revolution has changed both the form and the format of communication. Before the advent of the telephone, people communicated through the written word. Letter writing was an art. Before television and the computer were invented, people gathered together in neighborhoods and developed a sense of community.

Today the whole world is the community, and every corner can be reached from a home computer. Senior citizens use their computers not only to chat but also to organize get-togethers and other social activities. Younger people use their cell phones and text-messaging to meet friends and stay connected, even when they are in the bathroom with their pajamas on.

Asymmetrical Information

Not only does technology change the way in which people communicate and work, but it also creates new decision-making processes that affect all aspects of industry and commerce, including health care. Informed decisions produce better outcomes. When people are able to sift through and use the vast amount of information available to them, it gives them a decided advantage in conducting business.

The use of multiple data sources in economics and business is called **asymmetrical information.** Many businesses currently work with asymmetrical information: individuals on one side of the transaction may have much better information than those on the other. Borrowers know more than lenders about their repayment prospects, managers and boards know more than shareholders about the firm's profitability, and prospective clients know more than insurance companies about their accident risk. The fact that the person with more information has an advantage seems like common sense, but a grasp of the impact of asymmetrical information will lead to a better understanding of day-to-day economic activity.

> *Not only does technology change the way in which people communicate and work, but it also creates a new decision-making process that affects all aspects of industry and commerce, including health care.*

Competitive Health Care

One of the key elements of health-care reform is the increased use of informatics to help drive down the cost of health care. The goal is to have every U.S. citizen's medical record in electronic storage. When the Health Care Reform Act was passed, only 8 percent of the more than 5000 U.S. hospitals had completely computerized medical records and charting.[1]

Competition has long been a driving force in the pricing and marketing of health care. Payment methods that promote competition are encouraged by Medicare and Medicaid prospective payment systems (PPSs), health maintenance organizations (HMOs), preferred provider organizations (PPOs), and managed care. For an organization to offer competitive and high-quality services, information must be available for decision making. More information is available to decision makers with information technology.

Technologically driven organizations have a competitive edge through the collection of large amounts of information and its application to decision-making in health care. To stay competitive in national and international health care, the health-care delivery system—specifically nursing—must open itself to new information and ideas.

The health-care information revolution is progressing seemingly at the speed of light. Computers are involved in almost every area of client care today, including assessment of the quality of care, decision-making, management, planning, and medical research.[2]

DEFINING INFORMATICS

Two definitions of informatics are commonly used in health care. The term *medical informatics* was coined in the mid-1970s. Borrowed from the French expression *informatique medicale,* it included all the informational technologies that deal with the medical care of the client, medical resources, and the decision-making process.[3]

Health informatics is a more comprehensive term, defined as the use of information technology with information management concepts and methods to support health-care delivery. Health informatics includes the medical field but also encompasses nursing, dental, and pharmacy informatics as well as all other health-care disciplines. The definition of health informatics focuses attention on the recipient of care rather than on the discipline of the caregiver.

Models for Nursing Informatics

The nursing community has been working toward developing a discipline of informatics that is specific to the delivery of nursing care based on the science of nursing. Nursing has distinct and discrete information needs. The content and application of nursing information are substantively different from those of other disciplines. Data gathered by the nursing profession present unique problems for the use of information in the delivery of nursing care based on critical thinking.

Three Basic Elements

An early model for nursing informatics can be traced back to 1989. Although somewhat simplistic, it primarily combined computer science, information science, and nursing science in a manner that would help the nurse in planning and delivering care. These technologies aid in the collection and analysis of data so that the nurse can make informed and accurate decisions about the type of care clients require.[4]

In this early definition of nursing informatics, computer science was seen primarily as the computer and the institution-wide system to which it was connected. Information science refers to the computer software, including how data or tasks are processed, how problems are solved, and where products are produced. Nursing science is all the research data from nursing and other associated disciplines that relate to and support nursing practice.

More Complex Elements

In newer models of nursing informatics, a fourth element, cognitive science, has been added. Cognitive science combines psychology, linguistics, computer science, philosophy, and neuroscience in a way that enhances the delivery of client care. Cognitive science is also concerned with perception, thinking, understanding, and remembering. This model unites information science, computer science, and cognitive science into a framework of nursing science.

It is also believed that wisdom should be added as a component of nursing informatics along with data, information, and knowledge. With wisdom, the nurse is able to know how and when to use the available information in managing clients' problems and meeting their needs.[5]

Data, Information, and Knowledge

In most theories of nursing informatics, *data* are defined as raw and unstructured facts. For example, the numbers 102 and 104 are raw data: by themselves, these numbers have little meaning because they lack

interpretation. *Information* consists of data that have been given form and have been interpreted. If the number 102 is given additional data so that it becomes a 102°F oral temperature of a 25-year-old man taken at 9 a.m., it becomes information that has meaning to the nurse.

Knowledge takes the process one step further because it is a synthesis of data and information. Knowing that an oral temperature of 102°F is higher than normal for a 25-year-old man, and combining that information with an understanding of human physiology and pharmacology, the nurse is able to decide what treatment should be given.

> **What Do You Think?**
>
> Have you used computerized health-care records? Describe your experience.

> *The nursing community, however, has been working toward developing a discipline of informatics that is specific to the delivery of nursing care based on the science of nursing. Nursing has distinct and discrete information needs.*

This process relies on critical thinking and decision-making and can be used in research to create new knowledge.

The data-to-information-to-knowledge model of informatics is linear, but the process of synthesizing data into information to create knowledge is circular. New knowledge creates new questions and areas of research, which in turn lead to more new knowledge. To answer any research question, new data are required that must be processed into information to create more knowledge. The goal of this process is to provide the most accurate and current information so that nurses can make informed decisions in their daily practice.

Areas of Focus in Informatics

Over the years, the specialty of nursing informatics has evolved through three levels of special interest: technology, concepts of nursing theory, and function.

Technology. The earliest attempts to define nursing informatics focused solely on the use of technology. A commonly used early definition of nursing informatics stated that it existed whenever the nurse used any type of information technology in delivering nursing care or in the process of educating nursing students.[6] Some key points in the use of technology or computer systems to store, process, display, retrieve, and communicate health-care information quickly in the health-care setting include:

* Administering nursing services and resources
* Managing the delivery of client and nursing care
* Linking research resources and findings to nursing practice
* Applying educational resources to nursing education

Nursing Theory. As nursing informatics evolved, it began to combine nursing theory and informatics. Without a well-articulated theoretical basis to guide the gathering of data, nurses soon become overwhelmed with meaningless data and information. Obviously, there is a need for common definitions, a standardized nursing language, and criteria for organization of the data.

Function. An additional step in the evolution of nursing informatics is the inclusion of the concept of function. The function of nursing informatics is to manage and process data to help nurses enter, organize, and retrieve needed information. Technology is then developed to achieve specific purposes related to client-care needs. Although technology forms the foundation of informatics, the nurse's ability to use that technology and make it function to meet clients' needs is the real test of the system's effectiveness.

In reality, nursing informatics includes all three of these areas—technology, nursing theory, and function. However, the field of informatics has become so large that it is difficult for any one person to be an expert in all three areas.

INFORMATICS AS A SPECIALTY

A Broader Definition

A broader definition of nursing informatics is provided by the American Nurses Association (ANA). It defines nursing informatics as

A specialty that integrates nursing science, computer science, and information science in identifying, collecting, processing, and managing data and information to support nursing practice, administration, education and research; and to expand nursing knowledge. The purpose of nursing informatics is to analyze information requirements; design, implement and evaluate information systems and data structures that support nursing; and identify and apply computer technologies for nursing.[7]

Nursing informatics is now recognized as a nursing specialty for which a registered nurse (RN) can receive certification. The catalogue of the American Nurses Credentialing Center (ANCC) states that the nursing informatics practice

. . . encompasses the full range of activities that focus on the methods and technologies of information handling in nursing. It includes the development, support, and evaluation of applications, tools, processes, and structures that assist the practice of nurses with the management of data in direct care of patients/clients. The work of an informatics nurse can involve any and all aspects of information systems, including theory formulation, design, development, marketing, selection, testing, implementation, training, maintenance, evaluation, and enhancement.[8]

Nursing informatics supports all areas of nursing, including practice, education, administration, and research. It facilitates and guides the management of data.

Articulation

Informatics is no longer just an elective subject. In today's competitive and rapidly changing health-care delivery system, mastery of informatics is a basic requirement. The importance of the role of informatics is apparent in the need for the articulation of nursing practice. **Articulation** is an important way for nursing to demonstrate its accountability and credibility so that it can remain an essential element of the health-care system.

> *Informatics is no longer just an elective subject. In today's competitive and rapidly changing health-care delivery system, mastery of informatics is a basic requirement.*

The Need for a Standard

Historically, the nursing profession has had difficulty in locating relevant nursing information quickly because there was no universally accepted nomenclature and taxonomy for either nursing clinical information or management data. In the past, this lack of access to information has presented several seemingly insurmountable challenges for nurse executives, including identifying what the nursing staff actually does, determining the impact nurses have on outcomes, and establishing appropriate reimbursement for nursing activities.

For example, how does a nurse interpret the term *weak grasp* in a client's chart? The meaning of "weak grasp" differs widely depending on the client. If the client is a premature infant, the term has an entirely different meaning than if the client is a 25-year-old professional football player with a head injury or a 60-year-old with a stroke. Imagine the difficulty that a researcher will have when investigating the phenomenon of weak grasp—there is no standardized definition among the nursing community. Because a standardized nursing language is needed to name and communicate what nurses do, nursing classification schemes, taxonomies, and vocabularies have come to the forefront with the evolution of nursing informatics.

What Do You Think?

Think of four terms, not defined actions, carried out by nurses that have multiple meanings. How could these terms be clarified?

Unified Nursing Language System

The ANA Database Steering Committee was formed in 1991 to develop a common nursing language called the Unified Nursing Language System (UNLS). UNLS maps concepts by identifying common terms from different vocabularies and acknowledging them as synonyms of the same concept.

Twelve classification systems are recognized by the ANA as uniquely developed to documenting nursing care. They are designed to record and track the clinical care process for an entire episode of client care in the acute, home, or ambulatory setting or any combination of these. Standards and scoring guidelines for nursing languages can be found in Box 19.1.

Box 19.1

Standards and Scoring Guidelines for Nursing Languages

1. Terms in data dictionaries and tables are appropriate to the domain of nursing.
2. Terms from ANA-recognized languages for nursing are used as a core for the nursing vocabulary.
3. The system allows for the development and addition of new terms as needed, without duplicating existing terms or disrupting the integrity of existing languages.
4. In "local" languages, terms are mapped to appropriate ANA-recognized nursing languages, which may include reference terminologies.
5. The system accommodates the use of reference terminologies to map nursing languages to other existing standardized data sets, classification systems, or nomenclatures.

Nursing Minimum Data Set

Standardization of the data in a client's record is the first step toward unifying information to make it usable to the bedside nurse. The second step is the development of criteria to determine the necessary elements that must be included in every client record or encounter. The Nursing Minimum Data Set (NMDS), developed in 1985 and accepted by the ANA in 1998, is a list of the data elements necessary in any computerized client record system or national database. The NMDS is considered to be the umbrella for other nursing process schemes. The purpose of the NMDS is to

1. Describe the nursing care of clients and their families in various settings, both institutional and noninstitutional.
2. Establish comparability of nursing data across clinical populations, settings, geographical areas, and time.
3. Demonstrate or project trends regarding nursing care provided and allocation of nursing resources to clients according to their health problems or nursing diagnoses.

4. Stimulate **nursing research** through linkages of detailed data existing in nursing information systems and in other health-care information systems.
5. Provide data about nursing care to influence health policy and decision-making.[9]

The NMDS has 16 elements divided into 3 main categories: nursing care (e.g., nursing diagnosis, intervention, outcome, and degree of nursing care), client demographics (e.g., the client's personal identification, date of birth, gender), and service elements (e.g., the unique service agency number, the admission and discharge dates, client's condition, and the expected payer).

Accountability

Intuitively, the nursing profession has long known that the presence of RNs improves the quality of care and client outcomes while decreasing the cost of health care. According to the Congressional Office of Technology Assessment, better use of nurse practitioners could result in savings for clients, employers, and society owing to the cost-effectiveness of both their training and their services. Nurses affect client outcomes positively and contribute measurably to the goals of a competitive health-care delivery system. However, nurses traditionally have not been very good at documenting their worth and effectiveness.[10]

To measure effectiveness with accurate information about client care and outcomes, nurses must use standardized language in both practice and documentation. The ability to measure the resources used and the client outcome achieved will help distinguish one health-care provider from another. This process forms the basis for evidence-based practice (EBP).

As nursing practice becomes more efficient and can demonstrate improved client outcomes, the quality of care will increase, and health-care organizations will become more financially stable.

Credibility

The credibility of the nursing profession rests on its ability to document how nursing care improves clients' health and saves money for health-care institutions. Nurses must be able to measure their effectiveness with accurate information about both the care given and the client outcomes achieved. Having control over the process of care, as well as the information and assessments of the quality of care, is an important element in achieving this goal.

Improvements in quality do not occur in isolation. They result from a continual process of assessing care and measuring outcomes that improves treatments, changes care procedures, and increases the number of support services.

A standardized language will facilitate the nursing profession's ability to distinguish the costs and benefits of nursing care from the costs and benefits of other health-care providers. If the nursing profession cannot articulate and measure the unique contributions that nurses make to the client's health and well-being, the profession will continue to have difficulty justifying its higher costs over less educated and less qualified health-care providers.

Accessing Information
An Information Explosion

Health-care journals and textbooks form a key element in the information explosion. The amount of health-care information contained in scientific journals has grown to a point at which no individual is able to read all of the material. With just a nightly perusal of the latest journals, even the most conscientious practitioners will have difficulty keeping up with all the current research and new developments in their specialty field.

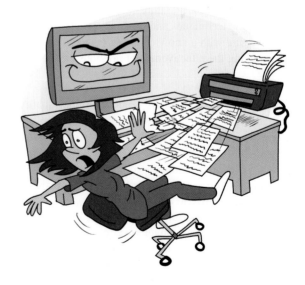

Coping with the volume of biomedical and nursing literature is an enormous task. Since 2005, 34,000 references from 4000 journals were added each month to the National Library of Medicine Medline database from among the more than 100,000

scientific journals published. More than 712,000 references were added in 2009 alone.[11] In the past 20 years, the number of articles indexed annually in the Medline database has nearly doubled, the number of clinical trials in cardiology has increased five times, and the number of clinical trials in health services has increased 10 times. One new article is added to the medical literature every 26 seconds.

Conflicting Paradigms

Although a large amount of new information is available, only a small portion is read by and incorporated into the practice of many health-care professionals. The traditional paradigm that still seems to guide the decision-making process for many nurses is to:

• Refer back to the knowledge learned in school
• Confer with a colleague
• Look up the problem in any textbook or reference book available in the work setting
• Use previous experiences and "gut" instincts

Although this process is useful and has some merit, it is questionable whether it is adequate for the delivery of high-quality care in today's complex health-care system. For the information age, EBP is more appropriate.[12] This process includes:

• Accessing current literature concerning the latest diagnostic techniques and treatment modalities
• Conferring with a knowledgeable colleague
• Evaluating the effectiveness of previous experiences

Research on the Job

Ironically, even though EBP produces higher-quality care, the nursing profession has only recently embraced its use. However, with increasing client-care responsibilities, nurses rarely have time to go to the library to research solutions to client-care problems. Furthermore, nurses still are not being rewarded for taking the initiative to use EBP.

One development encouraging the use of EBP is that nurses no longer have to leave the practice setting to access relevant information. Literature can be searched from the nurses' station or even the client's bedside using available information systems. Nurses find that having access to literature about clinical issues increases their confidence levels in dealing with clients and other health professionals. It also allows them to contribute more fully to the multidisciplinary health-care team.[13]

Nurses must continue to make time for information searches that promote improved client care (Box 19.2). The creation of workplaces in which nurses can easily access client information, including research information, is essential to high-quality nursing practice.

THE HUMAN FACTOR

Is the System Friendly?

When information tools, machines, and systems are developed, they must include recognition of human factors, including knowledge about human capabilities, limitations, and characteristics that may affect the use of the system. The terms *human factors, human engineering, usability engineering,* and *ergonomics* are often used interchangeably.

The study of human factors examines how to make the interaction of people and equipment safe, comfortable, and effective. Cognitive science, one of the components of informatics discussed earlier, forms part of the foundation for the study of human factors. Cognitive science includes the human acts of perception, thinking, understanding, and remembering.

Box 19.2
Principles for Access to Library and Information Services

1. All nurses should have access to a free library service funded by their employer that contains appropriate literature and multimedia resources.
2. Library services should have flexible opening hours and be staffed by qualified librarians.
3. Nurses should have equal rights, similar to those of other health-care professionals, to paid study time to update their practice.
4. Every nurse should have access to training on the Internet and appropriate databases.
5. Every nurse should be educated in electronic systems and services to support evidence-based practice.

Source: Urquhart C, Davis R: The impact of information. Nursing Standard 12(8):23–31, 1997.

In order to manage and process information, especially with an automated system, the individual must be able to understand and remember a great deal of data. The more logically this information is arranged, the easier it is to use the system. "User-friendly" systems are intuitive, self-evident, and logical, even if they are complicated.

Does the System Make Sense?

Every day in their client care, nurses use complex machinery, including many types of monitors, ventilators, intravenous (IV) pumps, feeding pumps, suction devices, electronic beds and scales, lift equipment, and assistive devices. The directions for using many of these machines are not self-evident and may be highly complicated. Although hospital equipment producers are becoming better at incorporating the human factor in the design and use of this complicated equipment, consulting with practicing nurses or "field testing" equipment in the workplace before its mass production would make it more user friendly.

Confusing Technology

New computer systems present many learning challenges for health-care providers. Many computer systems are not as user friendly as they might be. Computer system designers are notorious for supplying computers with numerous advanced but obscure functions. These systems often seem to make relatively simple daily tasks much more complicated. Millions of dollars have been wasted on computer systems that are not used or are underused because the user's needs were not considered before the systems were designed.

Individuals encountering complicated computer systems for the first time commonly feel that they are stupid, incompetent, or too old to learn because they cannot quickly master the new technology. However, the fault often lies not with the individual but with the design of the technology.

Nurses, through their education and philosophical orientation, are generally more in tune with the human factor than computer designers, particularly as it relates to client care. Nurses can use their human factor orientation in the process of evaluating new technology before it is purchased. Also, nurses may

be able to make suggestions to medical equipment producers to help improve the equipment after it has been used for some time.

Is the System Well Designed?

There has been an ongoing concern in the United States about the problem of health-care error and the large number of client deaths attributed to it. Estimates of how many people die annually in the United States as a result of medical error range from 44,000 to almost 100,000. On the basis of these numbers, medical error ranks as the eighth leading cause of death in the United States.[14]

Medical Error

The most common type of health-care error was related to medications, followed by wound infections; technical complications were ranked in third place. The proliferation of new medications and the increasing complexity of medication therapy have dramatically increased the risk for medication errors and adverse drug events both inside and outside hospitals.

Also, the increased use of "fast-tracking" medications through the testing process has led to withdrawal of several medications from the market because of long-term complications not seen in the initial shortened testing phase. Well-designed computerized physician-order entry systems can reduce serious prescribing errors by more than 50 percent.[14]

> *If the nursing profession cannot articulate and measure the unique contributions that nurses make to the client's health and well-being, the profession will continue to have difficulty justifying its higher costs over less educated and less qualified health-care providers.*

Poor Design

Poor user design is responsible for thousands of health-care "accidents" each year. Complex medical devices are often used under extremely stressful conditions in which the user's cognitive abilities are not as focused as they might be in a less stressful situation. Often the users are not considered during the design phase because the designers believe they know what is needed.

Errors Increase

The inevitable result of poor design in all types of equipment, ranging from laboratory forms to life-support devices, is an increased error rate. Cognitive science studies have shown that the average person's memory can retain only six to eight pieces of information at a time. A well-designed system takes these elements into account (Box 19.3) and should reduce the number of errors. However, a poorly designed system can just as easily increase the number of errors as than reduce them.

Training Doesn't Compensate

Employees are commonly trained to use an information system to reduce errors. Although training is important, by itself it may not be adequate. In one study, there was no reduction in the number of errors even with an increase in training time. However, well-designed computer-based reminder systems did help clinicians reduce errors significantly. Even after the clinicians received additional training, errors returned to the previous level when the computerized reminder system was removed.[15]

When automated and computer systems are made user friendly by incorporating engineering techniques based on human needs, they can make a valuable contribution to monitoring and preventing error in clinical practice. Nursing professionals need to understand that human performance is not perfect and that education and training cannot make it so. Professionals must look for well-designed systems that can reduce and even eliminate errors.

B o x   1 9 . 3
Elements of a Good Technology Design

- Intuitive operation with minimal reliance on complicated manuals
- Easy-to-read displays that are logically arranged
- Controls that are easy to use and reach
- Positive, safe electrical and mechanical connections
- Alarms that sound only when there is a real problem so that they are not turned off because of annoyance
- Long-life reliability with few malfunctions
- Easy, quick repair and maintenance

THE ELECTRONIC HEALTH RECORD

A health record serves multiple purposes. It is used primarily to document client care. It also provides communication among health-care team members. It acts as a financial and legal record and is used for research and continuous quality improvement (CQI). Although the health record can take many forms, the most common form is either paper or electronic. Both forms have advantages and disadvantages (Box 19.4).

Advantages

Electronic health records (EHRs) have many advantages. Multiple care providers can access them simultaneously from remote sites. They can provide reminders about completing information or carrying out protocols as well as warning of incompatibilities of medications or variances from normal standards.

B o x   1 9 . 4
Advantages and Disadvantages of the Paper Record

Advantages
- People know how to use it.
- It is fast for current practice.
- It is portable.
- It is unbreakable.
- It accepts multiple data types, such as graphs, photographs, drawings, and text.
- Legal issues and costs are understood.

Disadvantages
- It can be lost.
- It is often illegible and incomplete.
- It has no remote access.
- It can be accessed by only one person at a time.
- It is often disorganized.
- Information is duplicated.
- It is hard to store.
- It is difficult to research, and continuous quality improvement is laborious.
- Same client has separate records at each facility (physician's office, hospital, home care).
- Records are shared only through hard copy.

Redundancy is reduced with the EHR. Rather than every health-care worker asking a client for his or her health history, allergies, and current medications, the information is captured once and then transmitted to every record requiring the information. EHRs require less storage space, are more difficult to lose, and are much easier to research. Improved communication, increased completeness of documentation, and reduction in error are the most important advantages of the EHR.

Disadvantages

Electronic health records have some obvious disadvantages. There is a high front-end cost in buying an electronic system and converting from a paper system. Employees may have problems adapting to the new system because of the steep learning curve involved. EHR systems are becoming more portable with the advent of the wireless network; however, they are also subject to all the glitches of electronic systems.

Decisions must be made about who can enter data into the system and when the entries should be made. The Health Insurance Portability and Accountability Act (HIPAA) regulations currently creating so many headaches for health-care providers were written specifically to address the many legal and ethical issues involving privacy and access to client information (see Chapter 9). Some issues still remain to be resolved.

The Ideal Record

The ideal EHR would be a lifelong continuous record of all the care that the client has received, rather than the episodic, piecemeal data that it now provides. This one record would reflect an individual's current health status and lifetime medical history. It would be unique to the person and not to the institution. This record would reside in multiple data sites and would accept multiple data types (e.g., graphs, pictures, x-rays, text) and be accessible worldwide.

Several Places at Once

The information on the EHR does not physically have to reside in one place, like a paper record.

When viewed from a computer workstation, the EHR only appears to be in one place. In reality, the individual records are retrieved from many information systems, such as laboratory, radiology, document imaging, anatomic pathology, anesthesiology, bedside, and accounting.

With proper authorization, this record could be accessed from anywhere in the world, at any time. Many people around the world could look at the same record simultaneously. If an individual became critically ill on a cruise ship or in a foreign country, the local health-care provider would be able to access the medical record to facilitate the client's diagnosis and treatment.

New Forms of Access

Health-care providers and technology designers are still working to resolve the many barriers to implementation of the ideal EHR. The issues of maintaining confidentiality and security are now closer to resolution. The high cost of starting up the system is still a barrier.

Access to the system would probably require a universal ID code or a unique client identifier.[16] Many organizations may resist a universal ID because they now use either their own client numbering system or Social Security numbers to identify individual records. Neither of these systems is adequate for the global access of the future. Fingerprinting, iris and retinal imaging, face prints, and voiceprints all are identification methods under investigation for use as the universal ID.

Bedside or Point of Care?

Bedside System. Some currently used systems allow nurses to enter information through bedside systems. A bedside system, as the name implies, is a computer terminal installed in each client's room or next to each bed.

Point-of-Care System. A point-of-care system has a broader meaning and includes not only the bedside but also many other points of care in the health-care environment and community, including the laboratory, radiology department, outpatient clinics, and even the client's home for home health-care providers. Many facilities currently have a unit system that can

> *The creation of workplaces in which nurses can easily access client information, including research information, is essential to high-quality nursing practice.*

be accessed at only one terminal in the client-care area (e.g., the nurses' station).

A Process Redesigned

Taking a paper record and typing it into a computer does not, in itself, constitute a modern electronic record. Automating the paper record in its present form only automates inefficient practices based on outdated requirements. Modern systems go beyond merely computerizing paper records. These new systems gain control over the generation of information and develop new techniques for using it creatively.

One of the most important characteristics of a bedside or point-of-care system is that client information can be input directly from the terminal. Then the nurse is freed from having to keep notes or chart from memory at the end of the shift. Documenting at the time of care is an important change in workflow for most health-care workers, who are accustomed to documenting at the end of a shift in a workroom with other professionals.

The re-engineering and streamlining of departmental workflow is accomplished by the automatic and continual routing of electronic documents and medical images from one person or department to another throughout the shift. With this system, traditional manual tasks are now automated, increasing the efficiency of management decisions and improving the distribution and evaluation of complex client records and electronic documents by authorized staff. This redesign of the old manual processes provides the real return on investment for implementing the electronic health record.

> *Estimates of how many people die annually in the United States as a result of medical error range from 44,000 to almost 100,000. On the basis of these numbers, medical error ranks as the eighth leading cause of death in the United States.*

ETHICS, SECURITY, AND CONFIDENTIALITY

Information for Sale

Most people assume that all doctor–client communications are strictly confidential. However, in the new electronic world, confidential information has become a commodity that is bought and sold in the electronic marketplace. Although the HIPAA laws have tried to deal with this issue (see Chapter 9), people who use the Internet or e-mail quickly realize that their personal information is no longer so personal.

Examples of violations of client confidentiality abound. In 1996, a convicted child rapist working as a technician in a Boston hospital rifled through 1000 computerized records looking for potential victims. He was caught when the father of a 9-year-old girl used caller ID to trace a call back to the hospital.

A banker on Maryland's State Health Commission pulled up a list of clients with cancer from the state's records, cross-checked it against the names of his bank's customers, and revoked the loans of those clients. At least one third of all Fortune 500 companies regularly review health information before making hiring decisions. More than 200 subjects in a case study published in *Science and Engineering Ethics* reported that they had been discriminated against as a result of genetic testing.

A Question of Ownership

One of the key ethical questions is, "Who owns the client's health-care data?" Does the individual's health-care information belong exclusively to the individual? Does it belong to the organization (e.g., insurance company, PPO) that paid for the care, or should it belong to the physician who directed and ordered the care? What about the facility in which the care was given—can they claim some ownership to the information, particularly if it is stored there? Do all these groups and individuals own a part of the information?

Should Society Benefit?

Those who argue the "individual rights" end of the ethical spectrum believe that each individual should have total and exclusive control over the information concerning his or her health and the care rendered. Those on the utilitarian, or "social good," end of the ethical spectrum believe that society as a whole benefits from shared information about disease occurrence and treatment. Therefore, the information should be available to all interested parties. As with most ethical dilemmas, a single definitive answer has not been proposed regarding who owns the data.

However, public policy debates have increased concerning the collection of health-care information for use as aggregate databases to underpin health-care planning. Many consumers are concerned about the status of future physician–client relationships. Driving the development of data collection policy is the public's fear about the damage that may result from excessive and uncontrolled disclosures through automated health-care information systems.[17]

The Implications of Consent

When clients enter the health-care system, they are generally asked to sign consent forms so that other organizations can obtain information about their health status and the care that they received (particularly insurance companies so that bills can be paid). They are usually unaware that this information can be supplied to many other organizations or institutions.

For example, reports are made to the trauma registry about injuries resulting from accidents. The tumor registry collects information about benign and malignant tumors, and infectious disease reports are made to the Public Health Department. Currently, health-care information is shared to develop payment systems, examine access to care, identify cost differences in treatment modalities, research disease trends and epidemiological implications, and expand consumer information.

The Evolution of HIPAA

The HIPAA policies covering the collection, development, and use of client data are based on issues of confidentiality and security. In 1996, the federal government started to develop the guidelines that have become HIPAA. The primary objectives of HIPAA include:

- Ensuring health insurance portability
- Reducing health-care fraud and abuse
- Guaranteeing security and privacy of health information
- Enforcing standards for health information

In 2000, rules governing the exchange of electronic administrative health-care information were developed and added to HIPAA. The object of these rules was to simplify and standardize the electronic forms required for claims for services rendered. Every organization must now use the same form.

Rules for Disclosure

In 2001, HIPAA was modified by the addition of rules that address the use and disclosure of individually identifiable health information in any form, electronic or paper. Health-care providers and facilities must obtain client consent before using or disclosing client information for treatment, payment, or health-care operations. The full HIPAA was enacted in 2004.

What Do You Think?

Who do you think owns health-care information? How does your decision affect health-care policy in the future?

Even with HIPAA regulations, confidential client information can be legally used for such purposes as quality assurance, institutional licensing and accreditation, biomedical research, third-party reimbursement, credentialing, litigation, regional and national databases, court-ordered release of information, and managed-care comparisons. Although automated information systems did not cause these information uses, automation does make acquiring this information much easier.

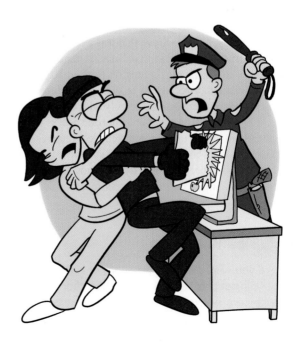

Threats to Security
Unauthorized Access

Unauthorized sharing of health-care information is generally unethical and now is always illegal. The code of ethics for most health-care professionals prohibits unauthorized or unnecessary access to client information. In addition, most health-care institutions have policies prohibiting unauthorized access to confidential information. Individuals can lose their jobs because of unauthorized access or sharing of client information and, under HIPAA laws, may be convicted of a crime.

A new wrinkle has been added to unauthorized access to health-care information. Under the policies of the previous administration's Patriot Act, some national governmental agencies, such as the Federal Bureau of Investigation (FBI) and National Security Administration (NSA), now have the authority to wiretap or access, without court approval, any electronic information they believe may be associated with a terrorist threat. This information includes physicians' and nurses' records, laboratory information such as DNA profiles and blood type, and financial information. Although some believe this unrestricted access is necessary to prevent future attacks against the United States, others believe that it is a major violation of U.S. citizens' right to privacy. It certainly seems to violate the regulations set forth in HIPAA.[18]

Unauthorized access or sharing of information is not a new problem associated only with the electronic age. It is just as easy to gain unauthorized access to a paper record as it is to the automated electronic record. The professional codes of ethics that stress confidentiality have always been the primary protector of client information. Still, access to the paper record is available to anyone who picks up the chart.

> *... most health-care institutions have policies prohibiting unauthorized access to confidential information. Individuals can lose their jobs because of unauthorized access or sharing of client information and, under recently enacted HIPAA laws, may be convicted of a crime.*

What Do You Think?

Have you witnessed any violations of HIPAA in your clinical practice or in your interaction with the health-care system? How could they be prevented?

In some ways, the automated electronic record provides greater privacy. Access to the automated record is generally restricted to employees who have been issued a password. Also, most organizations have periodic **audits** that can track each person who has accessed a record, and some systems can even detect unauthorized access at the time of entry into the system.

Accidents

Threats to information security can be either accidental or intentional and can affect both paper and electronic systems. Accidental threats involve naturally occurring events such as floods, fires, earthquakes, electrical surges, and power outages.

The paper record has little security against natural events. Typically, paper records are secured in a locked file cabinet or medical records room. Although current safety regulations require fire detection and suppression systems in these areas, even a small fire can destroy a large number of paper records very quickly. Little can be done to protect paper records against major flooding. Once the charts are destroyed, they cannot be reproduced.

Facilities with automated systems usually have well-developed natural disaster plans built into the system design. These plans include the automatic production and storage of a backup tape at a protected location some distance from the health-care facility. The frequency of data backup varies with the organization's requirements. Most systems automatically save all the data in the system every 24 hours, although this time interval can be shortened or increased to meet the facility's needs.

Although these measures provide a high degree of protection from major natural events such as floods and fires, power surges and outages create problems for electronic systems but leave paper systems unaffected. Anyone who works with computerized equipment recognizes the major disruptions in service and work that occur when the system goes down. Again, some safeguards can be built into the system so that not all the most recent information is lost when the power goes out. Power surges can be controlled with surge protection devices.

Intentional Acts

Intentional threats to the security of information involve the actions of an individual or individuals who wish to damage, destroy, or alter the records. In most cases, it is difficult to protect paper records from intentional tampering. It is a rather simple task for a determined individual to gain access to paper records and erase, add to, or rewrite sections of the chart. These changes are often very difficult to detect. In addition, a person could simply remove the chart and destroy it so that there would be no record left at all. Although automated electronic records are vulnerable to several kinds of intentional threats, they are, overall, more secure than the paper record. All current automated systems have computer virus–checking programs that protect the automated record from both intentional and accidental introduction of destructive computer viruses into the system.

Once data have been entered into the automated system, they are difficult to alter. Modern automated systems are designed with "write once, read many" (WORM) programs. If a legitimate change in the electronic record needs to be made, it must be an addendum. Any changes made in the electronic record are logged by the time and the person who made them and can always be tracked to the point of origin.

> *Although automated electronic records are vulnerable to several kinds of intentional threats, they are, overall, more secure than the paper record.*

Although a determined and gifted hacker can still obtain access to almost any electronic database, electronic security systems are becoming more and more difficult to breach. However, terrorist acts, ranging from detonation of bombs in key locations to development of "superviruses" to destroy electronic records, are difficult to defend against and present an increasing threat.

USES OF THE INTERNET

For nursing professionals, the Internet has become a valuable resource for communicating with colleagues and professional organizations, researching clinical information, and educating consumers about health resources and information. Because of the lack of standardization and regulation, it is important that the nurse evaluate each site for accuracy of information, authority, objectivity, currency or timeliness, and coverage.

A Resource for Professionals

Most professional organizations maintain a website containing information about the organization. Many include policy statements and lists of publications. **Continuing education units (CEUs)** can be obtained through the Internet to help nurses remain current and retain licensure. The Nurses Network (http://www.nursesnetwork.com), for example, is a site that lists education courses, position vacancies, conferences, and other pertinent information. News groups, such as those listed at http://www.nursingworld.org, provide professional information and access to experts in specific areas of interest.

Disease-specific websites publish clinical information for both the consumer and the professional. OncoLink is an example of a resource for information about cancer. Often the most recent information about a disease is found on the Internet. Publishing is quicker and easier on the Internet than in a peer-reviewed journal. Web-based support groups disseminate information on both technical and consumer levels. Protocols and policies are shared through websites and news groups.

A Guide for Consumers

Today, consumers are more knowledgeable about health care through use of the Internet. Clients are better informed than they were in the past because they now have easy access to a wide range of health-care information. Preventive and wellness services are available electronically through articles, chat groups, and health risk assessment surveys posted on consumer websites. Clients can now purchase medications over the Web, often at a much lower cost than they can get from their local pharmacies.

Healthfinder is a consumer health and human services information website created and maintained by the federal government. The site links the user with online government publications, clearing-houses, databases, websites, and support and self-help groups, as well as the government agencies and not-for-profit organizations that produce reliable information for the public. The goal of this information source is to help consumers make better choices about health and human services needs for both themselves and their families.

TELEHEALTH

Health Care at a Distance

From its fledgling beginnings more than 40 years ago, clinicians, health services researchers, and others have been investigating the use of telecommunications and information technology to improve health care. Physicians examine and treat clients from distant sites with video cameras, thus saving money by exchanging office visits for online appointments.

The terms *telehealth* and *telemedicine* are often used interchangeably.[19] As defined here, telehealth is the use of electronic information and communications technologies to provide and support health care when distance separates the physician and the client. Telehealth includes a wide range of services and technologies, from "plain old telephone service" (POTS) to highly sophisticated digitized cameras, telemetry, voice systems, and even interactive robots. Telemedicine is just one of the services provided by the overall telehealth system that primarily involve consultation with a physician.

Telehealth is being used in emergency departments (EDs) across the United States. The University of Pittsburgh offers neurological consultations to physicians at seven linked hospitals. In Baltimore, providers are using cellular telephone technology to transmit live video and client data back to home base.

Some uses of telehealth, such as emergency calls to 911, are so common that they are often overlooked as part of telehealth systems. Other applications, such as telesurgery, involve advanced technologies and procedures that are being used on a limited basis and are still considered experimental.

Serving Remote Populations

Historically, consumer concerns about access to health care have been the driving force behind the development of many clinical telehealth systems. Early applications focused on remote populations scattered across mountainous areas, islands, open plains, and Arctic regions where medical specialists, and sometimes even primary care practitioners, were not available.

Many telehealth projects from the 1960s through the early 1980s failed because they were expensive, awkward to use, and often not guided by the strategic plans of the facilities using them. However, as the technology has become more common, the costs of many systems have decreased dramatically. With the development of cellular technology, many of the newer systems are tapping into the systems already in place for telephone service.

Renewed interest in telehealth has been spurred by managed-care initiatives seeking to reduce health-care costs while maintaining or increasing quality and access to care. Overall costs have decreased for many of the information and communications technologies used by telehealth systems. In addition, the ever-developing National Information Infrastructure is making these technologies more accessible and user friendly. Medicare reimburses some types of telehealth care, although other third-party payers have been slow to include reimbursement for telehealth services.

Telehealth in an Emergency

Telehealth offers many advantages that will affect the cost of and access to future health care. The telehealth system allows access to centralized specialists who can support primary care providers in outlying areas. Outlying areas can be either rural or urban areas that lack access to the full range of health-care services. Outlying clinics staffed only with nurse practitioners or physician assistants have immediate access to physician referrals through the telehealth system. Many are now using handheld devices for telehealth applications.[20]

University medical centers can offer specialist consulting services to primary care physicians at distant locations, thus reducing unnecessary travel and increased cost to clients. Here is an example of how the telehealth system functions in an emergency situation:

In 1996, a 72-year-old man with a collapsed lung walked into the ED in a small town in North Dakota. The general practitioner, who usually saw routine emergency cases, immediately called the trauma II medical center in Bismarck and arranged a teleconsult with an

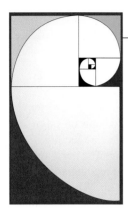

Issues Now

Are the Five Rights Enough?

Nursing students have had the five rights of medication administration drilled into their heads all through nursing school. Recent research indicates that five rights may not be enough. Although the majority of medication errors are caused by failures in the systems of obtaining and administering medications, up to 38 percent of errors can be attributed directly to nurse mistakes. When it comes to medications, the nurse serves as the last line of defense between the system and the client.

Traditionally the five rights are:

1. Right patient
2. Right drug
3. Right route
4. Right time
5. Right dose

However, in today's complex health-care system, many potentially lethal medications are used in all settings. Safe medication administration now seems to demand more than following the basic five rights, a system developed almost a century ago. Research shows that even nurses who meticulously observe the five rights are prone to medication errors. While the nine rights system does not guarantee error-free medication administration, it does increase the safety and quality of client care throughout the process.

The four additional rights are:

6. Right documentation
7. Right action
8. Right form
9. Right response

Right documentation: It is a major legal requirement that after nurses administer a medication, they must sign the medication sheet or make the appropriate entry in the electronic health record. The signature is legal evidence that the client received the medication. Students are taught to never sign the medication chart before administering the medication. Doing so is illegal and endangers the client, who may refuse the medication; in some cases, the nurse may forget to administer it. More dangerous is failing to sign when a medication has been administered. Another nurse may conclude that it has not been administered, and the client will end up with a double dose. For prn medication, it is essential to document the reason for administering the medication and what effect it had on the client.

Right Action: For many years now, the legal defense of, "I was just following the physician's orders" has not been available to nurses. Nurses need to know why the client is receiving a medication and how the medication works. They need to know if the prescribed medication and its dose are appropriate for the client. Administering an antihypergylcemic agent to a client who does not have diabetes but does have an infection is a medication error even if the medication was prescribed. Nurses also need to be aware of laboratory values associated with certain medications. Administering a daily dose of potassium to a client whose

(continued)

Issues in Practice continued

morning laboratory work shows a blood potassium of 7 mEq/mL could lead to cardiac arrest.

Right Form: This one is similar to right route, although it goes one step further. It is possible to administer various medications by different routes. For example, an licensed practical nurse (LPN) in a long-term acute care facility became confused about how to administer a bag of tube feeding. The nurse on the shift before had mistakenly put an IV tubing on the bag of tube feeding and had hung it at the bedside to save the next nurse time in hooking it up. When the LPN on the next shift heard the pump alarm that the bag was empty, he came in and hooked the tube feeding to the IV. The client died about an hour later. In another case, a pharmacist drew up an oral medication in a syringe to obtain a more accurate measurement. The nurse was not familiar with the medication and, because it was in a syringe, gave it by IV.

Right Response: This could also be called "right assessment" or "right observation." After the medication is administered, the nurse must go back to evaluate whether the medication is doing what it is supposed to do. Most nurses know this is mandatory for pain medications and recognize the need to chart whether or not the pain level was reduced. However, it is also important for almost all other medications. If the client was given an antacid for ulcer pain, the nurse needs to note whether or not it helped. Right response is particularly important for dangerous medications such as insulin, anticoagulants, and cardiac medications.

The nurse must respond quickly if a client on anticoagulants begins to have blood in his urine or is oozing blood from the IV site. This may indicate that he is receiving too high a dose of the medication. And of course it is essential to check for allergic reactions to antibiotics and other medications.

The goal, as always, is to make the client's stay as safe and beneficial as possible. Observing the four additional rights can help to achieve this outcome.

Sources: Elliott M, Liu Y: The nine rights of medication administration: An overview. British Journal of Nursing 19(5):300–305, 2010.

Health system sets "zero errors" as its goal for patient safety, quality. Healthcare Benchmarks & Quality Improvement 17(4):37–41, 2010.

ED physician and a thoracic surgeon. The man would have died without a thoracotomy. Following the surgeon's instructions, the physician was able to insert the chest tubes needed to safely transport the client by helicopter to Bismarck.

Telehealth services often save lives and prevent permanent disability, especially when time is a factor in treatment. For example, health-care providers know that if thrombolytic medications are given within 3 hours after the onset of stroke symptoms, the likelihood of death or permanent disability is reduced by 50 percent. Using telehealth technology, neurology specialists can evaluate a client's condition while he or she is still in the ambulance en route to the hospital, thus saving valuable time in deciding about using lifesaving medications. The ED is prepared to administer the medications as soon as the client enters the department, rather than having to wait several hours for all the routine evaluations and consultations to be completed.

Issues for the Future
A Boost for Home Care

In the future, home care may benefit the most from telehealth. By investing in telehealth technologies, home care providers should be able to balance cost reductions with increased quality of care.

Clients can be monitored at home using a combination of telephone calls, home visits, video visits, and in-home monitoring using the telehealth system. In-home monitoring devices for conditions ranging from congestive heart failure and diabetes to cancer and cardiac conditions can send information from the client's home to a central base for assessment by professionals.

Future Challenges

System Design. Many of the older systems are poorly designed and may be totally incompatible with the systems used in modern health-care facilities. The human factor design and user assessments must be carefully considered in developing any new technologies.

> *Nurses who practice in rural and underserved urban areas will have more autonomy and provide higher-quality care when linked electronically with the support services of a large medical center.*

Expense. Although the overall costs of electronic systems continue to decrease gradually, initial expenditures are still a barrier to implementation, especially in smaller facilities. Lack of **third-party payment** for telehealth systems also limits their development and use.

Legal Issues. Several legal issues still need to be resolved, including health-care provider licensure when consultations are given across state lines, and the liability incurred by providers who examine a client by television rather than in a face-to-face, hands-on encounter. Federal and state policies protecting privacy and confidentiality need to be developed with specific provisions for telehealth systems.

Effects on Nursing Practice. The telehealth system also affects nursing practice. Nurses are the primary users of telephone triage systems that rely on computerized decision-making trees to suggest appropriate actions when given a set of client symptoms. Nurses who practice in rural and underserved urban areas will have more autonomy and provide higher-quality care when linked electronically with the support services of a large medical center. The use of remote monitoring devices provides nurses with immediate information about changes in their clients' conditions, improves outcomes, reduces complications, and lowers the number of readmissions to the hospital.

Education and Conferencing. The same types of technology used for telehealth can be used for distance and **nontraditional education** applications. Widespread use of **continuing education** is achieved through distance technology. Courses are video-conferenced with two-way interaction. Continuing education credits can be earned through courses on the Internet. Even college credits can be earned through Internet access. Grand rounds are conducted at multiple sites with video-conferencing equipment, and in-services are beamed to multiple locations.

Conclusion

The demand for nurses trained in informatics will continue to grow at a prodigious rate and presents nurses with exciting opportunities. The federal incentive to develop the industry will make it a highly sought after health-care specialty. The information revolution affects every aspect of health care, not only in the United States but also throughout the world. Advanced communications technology and its increased availability worldwide promote ties between people and nations, bridging the gap between isolated rural communities and major metropolitan areas.

The nursing profession needs to be actively involved in developing clinical information systems and the electronic health record, establishing care standards, safeguarding client privacy, using the Internet, and researching better ways of improving access and the quality of care through technology. The nursing profession is transformed, enhanced, and enriched as nurses become active participants in the information revolution.

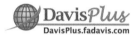

DavisPlus.fadavis.com

Critical Thinking Exercises

- Debate the ethical issues of personal privacy and the greater social good in relation to availability of health-care information.
- Discuss how the design of equipment increases or decreases error rates.
- Discuss uses of telehealth for patient teaching and monitoring of home health clients.
- Write a vision paper describing your view of technology in health care in the year 2030.
- List all the pieces of data you had to give at your last visit to the doctor or hospital. Was all of the information necessary for your care? Who needed the information? How was the information recorded or transmitted?

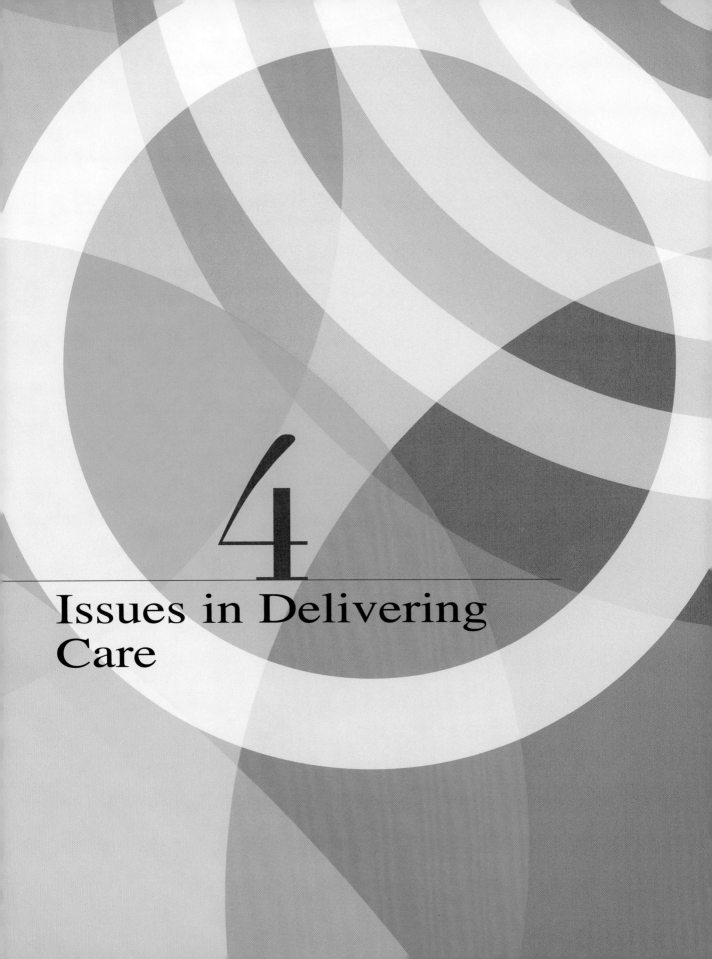

4

Issues in Delivering Care

20

The Politically Active Nurse

Donna Gentile O'Donnel

Learning Objectives

After completing this chapter, the reader will be able to:

- Explain why it is important for nurses to understand and become involved in the political process.
- Discuss how a bill becomes a law.
- Identify the major committees at the federal level that influence health policy.
- Identify four points at which nurses can influence a bill.
- Give examples of how nurses may become politically involved.
- List and describe four methods of lobbying.

A NUTS-AND-BOLTS APPROACH

The word *politics* conjures up various images—some positive and some negative. There are images of great statesmanship and political achievement, like the election of the first African-American president and the passage of landmark health-care legislation. There are also images of ignoble moments, like the Abramoff lobbying scandals and the huge infusion of foreign money to pay for negative TV adds to sway elections. Like it or not, politics touches people's lives at all levels, crossing national boundaries, affecting individual states, and permeating local governments.

This chapter provides a foundation for understanding the political basics by using a nuts-and-bolts approach. The goal is to motivate nurses to become active in the political world. Politics is examined both within the profession of nursing and within society at large. In addition, this chapter discusses the forces that drive politics and the three concepts it comprises: partisanship, self-interest, and ideology.

Almost everyone, ranging from political candidates, academicians, and members of the press to regular citizens, has something to say about politics. People define politics in many ways. One of the most cynical definitions of politics is offered by Ambrose Bierce in *The Devil's Dictionary,* where it is described as "A strife of interests masquerading as a contest of principles. The conduct of public affairs for private advantage." Other, more widely accepted definitions include "the art or science of government," "the art or science concerned with guiding or influencing government policy," and "the total complex of relations between [people] in society."[1]

THE NURSING SHORTAGE

The nursing shortage is a good example of where nurses' concerns intersect with the political process. In many areas of the United States, the nursing shortage has reached crisis levels, and there do not appear to be any permanent cures on the near horizon. Different areas of the country are attempting to deal with the shortage in the short term with quick, stopgap political measures that may have an adverse effect on the nursing profession in the long term.

Foreign Recruitment

One quick and easy solution some hospitals are initiating is recruitment of nurses from outside the country. Hospitals in various parts of the country have started programs to bring nurses from countries such as the Philippines. These foreign nurses generally receive the same pay and benefits as the American registered nurses (RNs). They also often receive permanent resident visas and housing if they desire it. The percentage of foreign-born RNs has seen a steady if gradual increase in the workforce over the past decade.[2] From a facility viewpoint, foreign nurse recruitment plans often do not address obtaining U.S. licensure, an issue that affects the state boards of nursing and nurse practice acts.

Institutional Licensure

In regard to foreign nurses, the issue American nurses should be concerned with is legislative, namely institutional licensure (see Chapters 3 and 12). The practice of institutional licensure has been universally rejected by every major nursing organization; however, health-care facilities continue to attempt "back-door" institutional licensure. When foreign nurses are allowed to practice in specific institutions without taking the American licensure examinations, de facto institutional licensure exists even if it is not called by that name.

What's so bad about institutional licensure? The primary problem is the lack of external standards to determine the level of competency. Obviously,

> *Politics touches people's lives at all levels, crossing national boundaries, affecting individual states, and permeating local governments.*

when the representatives of hospitals planning to hire foreign nurses interview candidates, they are looking for certain characteristics or qualities. What are these qualities? Ability to speak English? Not having a family? Knowledge in critical care, obstetrics, or pediatrics? The hospital establishes the criteria, and no one outside the administration really knows how the finalists are selected.

Without external standards, the designations of RN or LPN/LVN (licensed practical nurse/licensed vocational nurse) become relatively meaningless. In addition, without an American nursing license, these foreign nurses are not under the control of the state board of nursing. What if the foreign nurse was practicing unethically or made grievous negligent errors that caused harm to the client? Who would be responsible? Who would discipline the nurse? Most health-care facilities now require criminal background searches for all employees. How do they obtain these from countries that do not keep records of arrests or convictions for crimes?

Nurses practicing in states where the importation of foreign nurses is being planned or actually practiced need to contact their state board of nursing. It is highly probable that the practice violates a standard in the nurse practice act and the facilities conducting the practice should be investigated.

What Do You Think?

What experiences have you encountered, either as a client or as a health-care worker, related to the nursing shortage? How might the political system help solve the shortage?

Magnet Hospitals

Another, more positive, approach to the nursing shortage is the establishment of "magnet hospital" status for hospitals that retain a high percentage of the nurses they hire. In 1980, the American Academy of Nurses conducted a study to identify the elements present in hospitals that attracted and retained nurses. Several key factors were identified in hospitals that seemed to fulfill the magnet status, including a participative management style, allowing the nurses a relatively high degree of autonomy in practice and decision-making, high-quality leadership at the unit level, a horizontal organizational structure, allowing nurses to practice as full professionals, opportunities for career development, and high-quality client care. Nurses employed at magnet hospitals have a high degree of job satisfaction and a much lower than average turnover rate than nurses in other hospitals of similar size.[3]

The magnet hospital program has grown markedly since the original study. The American Nurses Association (ANA) has established rather rigorous standards for hospitals to meet to obtain the magnet designation. Most hospitals have found achieving magnet status to be very challenging, and only a small percentage are able to achieve it on the first try. However, hospitals that do obtain magnet status have achieved a well-deserved level of prestige among their peers. Nurses working at these hospitals have more control over their practice, and the end result is that higher-quality care is provided to the clients.[4]

> *Nurses employed at magnet hospitals have a high degree of job satisfaction and a much lower than average turnover rate compared with nurses in other hospitals of similar size.*

Late-Entry Nurses

A recent trend being studied indicates that, whereas the number of "traditional" early-20s college students entering nursing has declined, more students in their late 20s and early 30s are seeking admission to nursing schools. These are often students who have gotten an associate degree and come back after several years to complete their baccalaureate degree. Almost as many did not attend any institution of higher education after high school, working at entry level–pay jobs or staying at home to raise families.

One factor that may be attracting this cohort of "20-somethings" into nursing is the well-publicized nursing shortage and the promise of a well-paying career with lots of job security. Older students are

generally looking for a new start, whereas younger students are often looking for jobs in one of the few fields they believe are open to them. So far, the effect of this trend has not reduced the nursing shortage or its projections for the future. Increasing the supply of nurses by any means remains a high priority for heading off the impending nursing shortage.[5]

A Long-Term Solution

None of the previously mentioned measures really addresses the underlying problem of the nursing shortage. The long-term solution is to increase the supply of nurses by encouraging more young men and women to enter schools of nursing and by providing the schools with sufficient funds to educate those who apply.

National trends in nursing school enrollments have shown a gradual increase in enrollment over the past few years, offering some hope for a long-range cure. However, because of an acute shortage of nursing faculty, many nursing schools are turning away qualified students. Data collected by the National Council of State Boards of Nursing (NCSBN) estimates that in 2009, more than 140,000 qualified applicants were turned away from entry into nursing schools because of the shortage of nursing faculty, clinical sites, and classroom facilities.[6] For those who do choose to enter the nursing profession and manage to get into nursing school, the future looks bright. There are many opportunities, and health-care facilities are beginning to appreciate and reward nurses at the level they deserve.

Legislating Nurse-to-Client Ratios

One attempt to legislate a fix to the nursing shortage occurred in California in 1999. The California state legislature made the precedent-setting move to establish minimum nurse-to-client ratios by enacting legislation. The regulations were phased in over several years and took full effect in 2003.

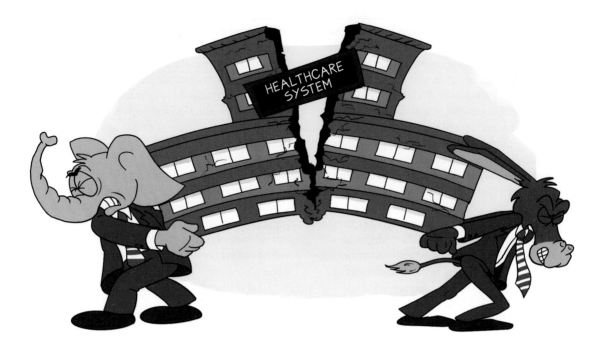

After several years of implementation, the evaluation of the results remains mixed. Nurses' unions and consumer advocacy groups, such as the American Association of Retired Persons (AARP), point to the increase in client safety, the reduction in medical errors, and the increased nurse retention rates as indications that the program has been a success. Groups opposed to this type of legislation, such as state hospital associations and state medical associations, believe that mandated staffing ratios have failed, citing decreases in physician and hospital income and reduction in the total number of clients seen. Several other states implemented similar staffing ratio measures, with results similar to those of California. However, few states currently seem interested in mandating staffing ratios. An unintended result of mandated staffing ratios is that, to avoid legislative action, many health-care facilities have moved to self-regulate their ratios. The increased interest in the magnet program may be an offshoot of legislated staffing ratios.

The nursing shortage and the various attempts to resolve it are health-care issues that have become political. They have the potential to significantly affect the profession of nursing, and nurses need to get out in front of the issues if they want to have a say in what is decided about their future.[7]

GOVERNMENT AND POLITICS

Keep in mind that *government* is a very broad term referring to almost any type of hierarchical structure that organizes and directs an organization. From this context, the governance structure of any health-care facility can be considered a type of government that has its own politics. At this level, nurses potentially have a considerable amount of political influence.

Relevance to Nursing
Historically, most nurses have avoided becoming engaged in government, perhaps because they agree with definitions similar to the one presented by Bierce. However, nurses, both as individual citizens and as a professional group, need to recognize that their personal lives and professional practice are affected by the political world. Some recent trends in health care, particularly the nursing shortage, managed care, and cost containment, have made nurses increasingly susceptible to the "bottom line."

State Level Organization
To increase their effectiveness and power, nurses need to organize at the state level. The ANA has been involved in politics at the federal level for several years and has raised money through telemarketing in

every state in the country. Many nurses do not realize that the ANA Political Action Committee (PAC) is now the second-largest federal PAC in Washington focused on political activities exclusively at the federal level. However, it is important to realize that many of the political battles nurses have to fight are at the state level.

There is an ongoing discussion between the federal and state governments about what constitutes a legitimate course of action for the federal government and what constitutes the same for the state government. The 10th Amendment to the Constitution says essentially that any powers not expressly articulated as part of the federal government mandate go to the states. This amendment underlies the current debate about Medicaid and Medicare and whether or not the states should be responsible for their administration.

The Role of State Nursing Organizations

The concept of unfunded mandates has come to the forefront in the past few years as a result of the states' rights push. There is an ongoing discussion among members of the National Governors' Association demanding that the federal government give governors more latitude in governing their states. They are saying, "Don't give us mandates. Give us the opportunity to set our own standards, our own regulatory actions, and our own legislative and governmental agenda." The nation is moving toward greater state control governmentally. It would be ideal if nurses could organize and just concentrate on issues at the federal level Washington, but because most nursing issues are at the state level, this strategy would probably not work.

For nursing organizations to be effective, there has to be organized political action among nurses and by nurses in every state in this country. In states where nurses are not active and organized politically, there is going to be trouble, and the nurses in them will fare badly. Nurses need to realize that the trend is toward state nursing organizations becoming more active politically and determining their own fate. Consequently, nurses need to organize politically at the state level to increase their political power.

Another thing to keep in mind is that nurses' licensure, as well as the certification and regulation of hospitals, is a function of the state. Again, it does not make sense to concentrate all the resources of

nursing at the national level. Of course, there are some issues and programs, particularly with respect to funding, in which federal action is necessary. However, most of the issues nurses will be dealing with occur at the state level, and that is where attention needs to be focused. The reality is that the states have the capacity to define and regulate objective standards for both nurses and hospitals. The mandate for nursing is to define how those standards are established and then develop an achievable agenda for political action by nurses at the state level.

In addition, because of politics, nurses are confronting major changes in health care on a daily basis. They have experienced the erosion of the profession through their replacement with less-educated personnel and have seen the quality of client care deteriorate. Nurses, if they decide to act, are not powerless against such trends.

The Sleeping Giant

As a large group of voters, nurses have the power, influence, and skill to take an active role in the political process. Because of their large numbers, nurses are sometimes regarded as the sleeping giant in health care. Nurses can gain much by using the tools of political action, and now more than ever their professional survival depends on it.

Individual nurses can take attainable, deliberate actions that can create a powerful political force. However, before nurses can realize their full potential, a basic knowledge and understanding of the political system is necessary. Nurses, who are among the most astute observers of human nature, are in many ways ideally suited to the art and science of politics.

WHY SHOULD NURSES BE INVOLVED?

Every Aspect of Life

A widely accepted definition of politics is the process of influencing *public policy,* including all forms and levels of governmental regulations. The effects of politics are pervasive and related to almost every aspect of life.

On a personal level, politics influences where children go to school, the quality of food, the water that flows from your kitchen tap, what medications are prescribed, and the speed limit on roadways. On a professional level, politics influences where nurses work, what they do and how they do it, the ability to organize professionally, and even the nurse's professional status through licensure and certification. The effects of politics on a person's life seem to have no limits.

Is Acceptance Necessary?

Nurses experience the effects of governmental regulations both directly and indirectly. Examples of directly experienced government regulations include some recent reforms that many states have initiated. Some state legislatures have enacted nurse-to-client ratios. All states now have granted prescriptive privileges to advanced practice nurses, although the regulations governing their implementation vary widely from state to state.

National health-care reform is an excellent example of nurses' involvement in policy making. Because of the large number of Americans who do not have any type of health-care coverage, many hidden costs are added to the health-care system and force the insurance rates up for those who do have insurance. These realities pushed politicians to develop new legislation. Nurses were at the table from the beginning of reform development, helped guide it through the legislative process, and are now playing key roles in its implementation.[8] One of the positive offshoots of health-care reform is the significantly increased amount of money that has become available for nursing students and nursing programs in general.

POLITICS AND POLITICAL ACTION

Politics

As a dynamic process, politics plays a key role in all forms and levels of government, including federal, state, and local government. It can be seen as the complex interaction between public policy and various public and constituent interests.

Politics is directly and indirectly influenced by the self-interest of political officials, both elected and appointed. The mass media also have both a direct and indirect impact on the political process through numerous political commentators, commercials, and investigations into the backgrounds of selected political figures.

Political Action

Political action is a set of activities, methods, tactics, and behaviors that affect or potentially affect governmental and legislative processes and outcomes.[9] Examples of political action include grass-roots efforts to change policies, the activities of lobbyists to change elected officials' opinions or votes, the give and take of political compromise within legislative bodies, and even the power of veto by the chief executive of a governmental structure.

A Series of Processes

Government is often thought of as a series of processes used to maintain society. As both an element of and a result of politics, government is also influenced by the forces that drive politics and the three concepts that constitute it:

- Partisanship
- Self-interest
- Ideology

Partisanship

Partisanship refers to membership in a political party. Because of its limited scope, this chapter focuses on Democrats, Republicans, and to a lesser extent, Independents.

Self-Interest

Self-interest is almost always the most important factor in politics. It dictates the kind of issues that legislators become involved in and present to their constituencies as the key issues. For instance, a congressman who resides in a blue-collar industrialized district that has a majority of constituents who support unionization will most likely be pro-union. The legislative structure in the United States was designed so that elected officials represent the people in their districts rather than having the whole population of the country trying to make policy decisions. If a candidate does not represent the beliefs of the district, it is unlikely that he or she will succeed in that district.

In the larger world of electoral politics, the principle of self-interest often means that an elected official will not make legislative or political decisions that could lead to professional damage, namely loss of an election. Occasionally there are exceptions to this rule. There have been a few cases in which elected officials were so ideologically committed to an issue that they defied conventional wisdom and made decisions that went against their self-interest. Generally, to be effective in politics, a person needs to understand and accept the self-interest of his or her constituents and use it as the driving force in political decision-making.

Ideology

Ideology is a broad concept that embodies the beliefs and principles of an individual or group. Conservatives, liberals, populists, Libertarians, and radicals represent five examples of ideologies.

Conservatives

Traditionally, conservatives support fewer governmental regulations, less involvement in everyday life, lower taxes, and smaller social programs. The general characterization of the conservative belief system is "less government equals better government." Applied to the current range of issues, conservatives tend to be pro-life, pro–gun ownership, anti–stem cell research, anti–universal health care, pro–death penalty, pro–choice on education, and pro–self-regulation of banks and big business. They believe that free enterprise and unrestricted capitalism, not government, will improve wages and the general welfare of U.S. citizens. Conservatives have also wrapped themselves in the mantle of "antiterrorism," suggesting that they are the best qualified to protect the country from terrorist attacks.

However, in recent years, conservative politicians have moved away from some of their core values. During the first decade of the century, under a self-proclaimed conservative president and congress, national spending and debt reached all-time record highs, with huge deficits that will take generations to pay off. The power of the executive branch was greatly expanded. Government inserted itself more and more into citizens' daily lives. Examples include government intervention in the right-to-die case of Terri Schiavo, the use of warrantless wiretapping, and the use of government appropriations to fund religious schools.

Liberals

In recent years, the term "liberal" has taken on a negative connotation falsely associated with the idea that anything goes. More recently, the term "progressive" has been used and seems to have fewer negative connotations. However, traditional liberals believe that government has a moral responsibility to do good for society and that government intervention is necessary for the greater good of the citizens. They believe that

only government can do certain things because of its size and funding ability. This ideology traditionally translates into larger government structures, taxes at a level to maintain programs without deficit, and more spending for a wide range of social programs. Liberals are traditionally pro-environment, pro-choice on abortion, pro-gun control, pro-universal health care, anti-choice on education, and supportive of women and minority groups.

Populists

Populists are probably the most dominant political force in the United States at a grassroots level. Although populists in general do not like paying high taxes, ideologically they may represent a variety of positions on any particular issue. For instance, one group of populists may be anti-abortion, whereas another may be pro-choice.

The common bond among all populists is that they have a sense of being burdened by a large, oppressive government structure. Populists constitute the middle ground between liberals and conservatives and are often considered the group that has the most influence in deciding national elections.

Libertarians

Libertarianism is both a political party and an ideology. As a political partisan group, Libertarians represent an electoral fringe element. Ideologically, they differ from populists because they do not have the underlying middle-class anger that often drives the populists to take political action. Although they do believe in fiscal conservatism and dislike paying high taxes, Libertarians tend to be "laid back" in their approach to politics. Typically, they avoid ideological battles and choices on gun control, health care, schools, or abortion.

Radicals

Radicals exist at both ends of the ideological spectrum in both of the major parties. It is important to recognize that, although most voters tend toward the middle of the political spectrum between conservatism and liberalism, radicals attempt to force their parties to the extreme ends of the spectrum.

For instance, Republicans are challenged by the radical right, which consists of the anti–big government and pro-life forces that make conspicuous demands on the party. To counteract the rhetoric of the radicals, the Republican party tries to find candidates who are ideologically near the middle of the spectrum because they know that most Republican voters have similar opinions.

UNDERSTANDING THE PLAYING FIELD

Structure

The three branches of the United States government are the executive, judicial, and legislative branches. These branches exist simultaneously at the federal, state, and local government levels.

The Executive Branch

At the federal level, the executive branch consists of the president, vice president, cabinet, and various executive administrative bodies. The executive of a state is the governor. Boards and commissions can also be construed as part of the executive branch because they are appointees of the chief executive. In county government, one or more county commissioners function as executives. Larger cities usually have a mayor. Smaller cities and townships sometimes also elect mayors (Fig. 20.1; Box 20.1).

The Judicial Branch

The judicial branch is the court system. It is important to note the distinction between state court and federal court; appeals and supreme courts are found at both levels. At the state level, there are supreme courts, appeals courts, and the lower courts. At the federal level, there are the Supreme Court, federal courts of appeal, and district or circuit courts. Additionally, many cities and counties have a local court system.

The judicial branch of government should not be discounted as unimportant to nurses. Over the years, courts have decided several important issues that have an effect on the practice of nursing. These include the Supreme Court's decision regarding the right of nurses to organize into collective bargaining units (see Chapter 17), the requirement of health-care providers to report potentially violent clients to the police, the obligation of nurses to refuse to carry out physician orders they deem dangerous, and criteria permitting nurses to withdraw life support measures. New test cases that are continually being brought before the Supreme Court have the potential to dramatically change the way nurses are perceived and what they are permitted to do in the workplace.

The Legislative Branch

At the federal level, the legislative branch of government consists of the House of Representatives and the Senate. Each state also has a legislative branch of government, and, except for Nebraska, all states have a bicameral legislature with both a house of representatives and a senate. The primary function of the legislative branch of government is the formation of policy by the making of laws.

Key Players in the Legislative Process

Members of the legislative branch of government have a wide range of ability and influence. It is important to remember that legislators are human and respond to the same forces that all people respond to, including interpersonal dynamics, peer pressure, and both internal and external factors.

The Majority Leader

The majority leader in the House of Representatives is the person who generally supervises and directs the activities on the House floor. Some consider this to be the most powerful job in politics. The majority leader has control over the legislative calendar, which ultimately determines when many of the House session activities take place and even when bills are introduced for consideration. The majority leader is also the central figure in crafting the budget, which is the most important activity the legislature performs on an annual basis.

The Majority Whip

The majority whip is responsible for collecting votes when legislators may be leaning toward voting against their party. At the same time the majority leader is supporting a bill, the whip is negotiating on the House floor for the votes necessary to pass the bill. The whip is responsible for collecting support and votes for various issues both during the legislative session and when it is in recess.

The Minority Leader

The minority leader represents the party that does not have a numerical majority in the House and helps organize support against bills introduced by the majority leader. The minority leader presents an alternative point of view. There is an expression in the legislature: "The majority will have their way, and the minority will have their say."

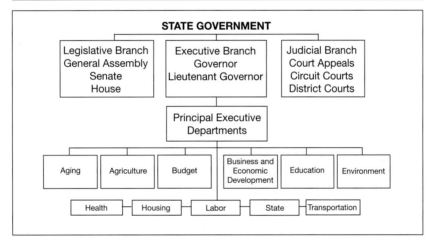

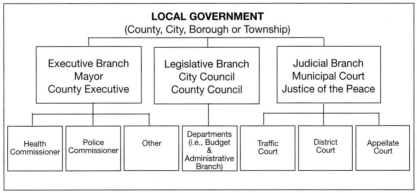

Figure 20.1 The organizational structure of the U.S. government.

Box 20.1
Know the Structure to Play the Game

One of the keys to creating power is understanding the organizational structure of the government. The Constitution of the United States establishes three separate branches of the federal government: legislative, judicial, and executive. The Constitution also ascribes certain auxiliary powers to the individual states. It is the role of the state governments to serve their citizens within these parameters and to delegate discrete areas of activity to local governments.

Beneath the federal and state level of government in the United States, there exist five layers of local government identified by the U.S. Census Bureau: county, municipal, township, school district, and special district governments (which include various utility, construction, and facility authorities). The qualifications for the classification of these local government structures are generally determined by the parent state governments. State governments are defined by their individual state constitutions and in turn delineate responsibility for the local governments.

Nurses must understand that there are three levels in each governmental sector: federal, state, and local. These distinctions are important and are the most common source of confusion for nurses.

In most cases, the majority party has the capacity to pass almost any bill they support over the objections of the minority. The minority leader usually only has the capacity to speak against it. However, there are some issues that legislators will almost never vote against: "mom," "pop," and "the little guy." When these issues are included in a bill, most legislators will support it even if they must vote against their party.

The Conference Committee
The conference committee attempts to reconcile differences in bills from the House and the Senate. The rules governing the structure, composition, and function of the conference committee vary from state to state. Generally, they consist of an equal number of appointed members from both the House and the Senate. Often a specified combination of votes, such as two votes from the House and two votes from the Senate, is necessary to approve a compromise bill and move it out of committee.

What Do You Think?

Who do you know in the legislature of your state government? Who is your representative or congressperson? Make a list of the things you would want that person to do for health care.

Caucuses
Caucuses are formed when the legislature divides into groups consisting of people with mutual interests. These groups operate as a unit, trading on their capacity to bring a block of votes for or against an issue or bill, rather than an individual vote. Examples are the Black Caucus, the Women's Caucus, the Hispanic Caucus, and the Business Community Caucus.

Although caucuses may be bipartisan, many are partisan. For example, the largest caucus groups are the Democratic Caucus and the Republican Caucus. Each caucus develops its own internal governance structure and leadership, including a speaker who leads the caucus and speaks for the group. After a group member achieves a leadership role, he or she must try to balance the wishes of the group against his or her own political survival in the caucus and the political pressures exerted by the larger world.

THE POWER OF THE MEDIA

When Is It News?
The media and the voters are external forces that influence policy makers. The media have become a tangible power in government, often driving and shaping public opinion that eventually evolves into a legislative agenda. The public often perceives media personalities as the people who know, write, and

speak about important public issues and matters of substance.

Although they claim to be objective, the major news organizations decide what is and what is not news. For many years, conservatives have accused the major news media outlets of a "liberal bias." To act as a counterbalance to this perceived bias, other networks have purposely taken a conservative spin. In the 2010 election, one news network became openly partisan when it donated $2 million to only one party for election of its candidates and hired several candidates as "commentators" for their various opinion programs.

In recent years, the Internet has become a force with which politicians must reckon. Politicians well versed in electronic media have learned to use them as a tool to get their message out. Younger voters no longer rely on the national networks' nightly newscasts to get their information about politics and most all other issues, but use the Internet and the short "sound bites" through which it conveys ideas. Some politicians have learned that the Internet is a practically free and unrestricted way to publicize their positions and slant their information.

However, politicians are now dealing with new issues related to the Internet. Often, fringe radical groups put rather sophisticated and professional-looking political advertisements on the Internet attacking the other candidate in a personal way or falsely attributing a radical viewpoint to their own candidate. These ads are picked up by the mainstream media, and then candidates have to spend time and money letting the voting public know that the ads were not from them and that they do not support the position.

Election by Media

Before media campaigns became the norm, with millions of dollars being spent on television and radio advertising, the printed news media used to publish what the candidate said and often printed whole speeches. This approach allowed the public to read the speeches and make up their minds about which issues the candidate supported. Today, the trend is to give a 30-second sound bite of a speech,

then have 10 minutes of political analysis by a well-known commentator who tells the public what the candidate is saying.

Some of the printed media have adopted a similar approach to political issues. In newspapers, it is not unusual to see a lengthy editorial comment positioned next to a statement made by a candidate. Elected officials have a great respect for the power of the media to influence public opinion. Those who learn to use the media to their advantage get elected.

Unfortunately, in recent elections, huge sums of money from foreign countries with business interests in the United States has been funneled through recognized U.S. political entities. The result has been a blizzard of negative political attack ads that influenced the outcomes of several elections.

Legislator Beware

Legislators, while recognizing and using the power of the media, have also become wary of it. They know that although they can use the media to proclaim their message, the media also pose a risk to their political survival, depending on the vulnerability of their position. Some legislators have a false sense of invulnerability because of the nature of their constituency.

> *The media have become a tangible power in government, often driving and shaping public opinion that eventually evolves into a legislative agenda.*

A Story With Legs

For example, a legislator may have a large population of senior citizens in his district who have supported him for many years. The legislator publicly supports senior citizen issues and believes that the senior citizen support will always be there. However, during an election campaign, a political opponent's investigation uncovers information that the legislator voted against several bills that would have increased senior citizens' benefits. In addition, the opponent discovers that the legislator is having an affair with his married secretary.

In recent years, stories involving sexual misconduct have overshadowed all other issues, even those as serious as violations of the U.S. Constitution, such as the erosion of separation of powers and misuse of executive power. It would seem that everyone understands sex but that many people have difficulty understanding the more serious and complicated issues that will have long-term effects on their lives.

The legislator's opponent leaks this information to the media, which immediately put it on television and report it in the newspapers. If the story develops "legs," meaning it takes on a life of its own and continues to grow without further information from the opponent, it will be on television news programs and in the newspapers every day. The major networks will do investigative reporting on the issues. Eventually the talk show and television tabloid programs will become interested and begin interviewing people who know or have heard more "dirty little secrets" about the legislator.

The Internet has contributed to the "legs" phenomenon. Today, almost everything a person in a public position has ever said or done is recorded on tape somewhere, and political websites show these recorded clips. If they are entertaining enough, they are often picked up by the mainstream media and shown over and over again, giving the information a much wider audience than it might otherwise have had. Internet-savvy people are proficient at "data mining" and can obtain private records and information on individuals running for office. This information can become a potent tool in the hands of a political rival.

At this point, the legislator who is the subject of that story is in political jeopardy. There is little that a politician fears more than being the subject of this type of negative story.

THE POLITICAL PROCESS

Who Introduces Legislation?
Where Laws Begin
Laws maintain order in a complicated society and regulate the interactions of its citizens. As society becomes more complex, more laws are needed to ensure the survival and smooth functioning of the population.

For example, although computers and electronic communications have increased the quantity of information individuals can process and the speed at which it is transmitted, they have also added to the complexity of the world. Just a few years ago, there were no laws that dealt with hacking, computer fraud, computer theft of bank funds, or online pornography. Today, there is an ever-growing body of law that deals with computers, and whole sections of police agencies, such as the Federal Bureau of Investigation's Computer Crime Unit, are dedicated to enforcing these laws. Where do ideas for laws and policies come from, and how do these ideas become laws?

Elected Officials
Any elected official, including governors, mayors, county commissioners, and city council members, can propose a program or initiative that requires passage by the legislature. This initiative is called a *bill.* The elected official goes to the legislative leadership in the parties and asks them either to submit the bill or to help move the bill through the legislative process.

Lobbyists, constituency groups, and advocates are a major source of proposed legislation. They represent various interests ranging from public interest groups to corporate lobbyists. Lobbyists frequently craft legislation and then pass it on to a friendly legislator. Consumer groups are often visible at the legislature through demonstrations and lobbying.

Constituency groups can best be described by example, such as the AARP. These groups are made up of individuals interested in advancing an agenda that promotes a range of issues based on self-interest. Advocates, in contrast, are groups that have a single issue or point of view that they are trying to advance, such as housing or abortion rights.

Government Agencies
Legislation is also generated from government agencies. When agencies are seeking fee increases or another type of policy reform, they can introduce legislation. For example, policy reforms in the Internal Revenue Service are a type of agency-initiated legislation. Frequently the employees of the agency draft the legislation and then direct it toward a supportive legislator.

What Drives Legislation?

Funding. Because almost all government agencies depend on legislative funding to sustain their operations, they become actively engaged, overtly or covertly, in seeking the passage of a budget that will sustain their survival.

Public Demand. Legislators are very careful to listen to the demand of their voters and avoid voting against an issue to which the public is emotionally attached. A classic example of this process was seen in New Jersey, where a child was sexually molested and murdered by a known convicted sex offender who moved into the child's neighborhood. The tragedy prompted a public outcry: How could this happen? Something needs to be done! Ultimately, the outcry produced the now famous Megan's Law, which requires public disclosure of a known sex offender's residence.

Program Issues. These issues recur periodically and require legislative attention. Requests for increases in television cable rates constitute an example of a programmatic issue. The cable industry will be very interested in the outcome of legislation that may affect what they can charge for their services. Both cable and consumer group lobbyists actively seek the ear of key legislators at these times.

Constituent-Specific Issues. Groups of voters may have specific interests that can lead to introduction of a bill. For example, in legislative districts where a large population of senior citizens resides, the escalating cost of prescriptions may be an important issue. Legislation specific to that constituency will be introduced at a greater rate than in areas with fewer senior citizens.

How Bills Become Law
The Tracking Number
Any legislator can introduce a bill from any source. Additional legislators can sign on as the bill's cosponsors. A bill is considered to be strong if it has strong sponsorship, including a number of powerful cosponsors, a high degree of bipartisanship, and the interest of powerful individuals, both political and nonpolitical. After the bill is introduced, it is taken to the chief clerk, who assigns it a number that permits it to be tracked throughout the process.

What Do You Think?

Contact your state legislature's website and identify two bills that deal with health care. How do you feel about these bills? How should your representative vote on this issue?

The Committee
After the bill is assigned a number, it is referred to a **committee.** The house and senate leaders decide which committee considers the bill. This decision, greatly influenced by politics, is critical to the survival and ultimate passage of a bill.

It is no coincidence that most bills die in committee. Invariably, the leadership discusses their expectation for the bill with the committee chairs. If the leadership wants a bill to fail, it is referred to a committee that will never vote on it or will pass it on to the House.

Full Committee Hearing
At the federal level, bills are referred to a full committee and generally, because of the enormous number of bills being introduced, to a subcommittee. Most of the work of Congress takes place within the committee structures. Committee action is perhaps the most important phase of the congressional process; this is where the most intensive consideration is given to proposed measures and where people are provided with an opportunity to be heard.

Subcommittee Hearing
The subcommittee studies the issue carefully, holds hearings, and reports the bill back to the full committee with recommendations. There are numerous standing committees in the House and Senate. In addition, there are several select committees and several standing joint committees. Each committee has jurisdiction over certain subjects and often has two or more subcommittees.

In the U.S. Congress, the committees with greatest jurisdiction over health matters and their subcommittees are:

- *House Ways and Means Committee:* Social Security and Medicare (health-care subcommittees)
- *House Commerce Committee:* Health legislation including Medicaid (Subcommittee on Health and the Environment)
- *Senate Finance Committee:* Medicare and Medicaid (health subcommittees)
- *Senate Labor and Human Resources Committee:* Health legislation in general; also works cooperatively with the Senate Finance Committee in considering issues involving Medicare and Medicaid
- *House and Senate Appropriations Committee:* Authorizes all money necessary to implement

action proposed in a bill (subcommittees for labor, education, and health and human services)

The Next Step

As a result of full committee hearings, several things may happen to a bill. It may be:

• Reported out of committee favorably and be scheduled for debate by the full House or Senate
• Reported out favorably, but with amendments
• Reported out unfavorably
• Killed outright

For example, a bill reforming the way judges are elected ideally would go to the judiciary committee. However, there is no legal requirement that the speaker or the Senate pro tem president send the bill to any particular committee. For political reasons, the speaker may refer the bill to the committee on intergovernmental affairs, where it will languish and die.

Can the Bill Survive?

For a bill to survive, its sponsor must have the knowledge and the political standing to move the bill out of committee. If sponsors are truly committed, they will trade on their political capital. *Political capital* generally refers to some type of favor or action that a politician can exchange for something he or she wants. It is an extremely important element in the legislative process and consists of, but is not limited to, votes, amendments to bills, appointments, and support from constituency groups. Political capital often consists of an "If you vote for my bill, I'll vote for your bill" type of exchange.

A Scheduled Debate

After a bill has been reported out of a House committee (with the exception of the Ways and Means and appropriations committees), it goes to the Rules Committee, which schedules bills and determines how much time will be spent on debate and whether or not amendments will be allowed. In the Senate, bills go on the Senate calendar, after which the majority leadership determines when a bill will be debated.

After a bill is debated, possibly amended, and passed by one chamber, it is sent to the other chamber, where it goes through the same procedure. If the bill passes both the House and the Senate without any changes, it is sent to the president for signature.

Opposing Versions

If the House and Senate pass different versions of a bill, however, the two bills are sent to a conference committee, which consists of members appointed by both the House and the Senate. This committee seeks to resolve the differences between the two bills; if the differences cannot be resolved, the bill dies in committee. When the conference committee reaches agreement on a bill, it goes back to the House and Senate for passage. At this juncture, the bill must be voted up or down, because no further amendments are accepted.

Passage or Veto?

If the bill is approved in both houses, it then goes to the chief executive—at the federal level, the president, or at the state level, the governor—who makes determinations about the bill. Governors can do one of two things: sign the bill into law or actively **veto** it. At the federal level, the president has the same options, with the addition of the pocket veto. Pocket vetoes, found only at the federal level, occur when the president, rather than actively vetoing a bill, simply does not sign it so that it does not become law. If vetoed, it is sent back to the House and Senate. To override the veto, a two-thirds vote by both chambers is required.

The Fiscal Note

Clearly, the passage of a law can be a long and difficult process. This is often quite frustrating for action-oriented nurses who are used to seeing immediate outcomes—forming plans and making things happen quickly.

All bills that are passed need a fiscal note attached to them. Therefore, the appropriations committee is operationally very powerful. A piece of legislation that is passed without a fiscal note attached will never become a law. Over the years, many pieces of legislation have been passed by the legislature but have been starved to death financially. These are called unfunded mandates.

Housekeeping Bills

Major regulatory change occurs in laws in the form of housekeeping bills. Legislators can use this tactic to move a piece of legislation through the process, especially when the bill is more significant than the leadership acknowledges it to be. Although regulatory reform and change may seem tedious, they are important to the legislative process and have the capacity to do enormous public good or harm.

Executive Orders

Executive orders provide the chief executive, the governor or the president, with a means for moving an agenda item forward. Executive orders are in many cases a convenient way to formulate policy with minimal involvement of the legislature. They also allow the executive to make a statement about an issue that can be entered on the public record.

The legislature can leave executive orders uncontested or challenge them by characterizing them as beyond the scope of the executive branch. This may involve turning to the third branch of government, the judiciary.

Regulatory Agencies

Regulatory agencies are also arenas where policies are made and amended. For instance, the role of the Intergovernmental Regulatory Reform Commission is to examine regulatory issues across the state.

HOW TO BE POLITICALLY ACTIVE

Why Be Active?

The first step in becoming politically active is to identify the specific goals that nurses, as a group, want to accomplish. Nurses recognize many important issues in today's health-care system, including:

- Increasingly acute conditions of hospitalized clients, who require higher levels of care and more complex levels of support than ever before
- Increasing responsibilities for nurses in supervision of rising numbers of unlicensed health-care personnel
- Loss of control of the work environment caused by managed care organizations
- Ever-shortening hospitalizations resulting in clients being sent home "quicker and sicker"

Any one of these issues can become a focal point at which nurses aim their considerable political power.

For example, most nurses are concerned that RNs, who have traditionally been at clients' bedsides, are being replaced by individuals who are less prepared and less able to deal with high-acuity clients. Nurses believe that when they are replaced in large numbers by unlicensed assistive personnel, including nursing assistants, as well as with personnel who provide specific services, such as technicians who sit in front of cardiac monitors, the quality of client care decreases. Nurses know that these technicians often take on responsibilities for which they have had little training. Rarely are there established national standards that require these assistive personnel to demonstrate their ability to provide a specific level of care, or even standards that protect the public safety.

Feeling Powerless

Nurses are usually employees at will and can be fired for any reason. Although some efforts have been made in this direction, whistle-blower protection is generally not available to protect nurses who wish to speak out against unsafe staffing levels or employment practices. Nurses are, at times, torn between their obligations to maintain high standards of safe, ethical care and their obligations to their families.

Although nurses often feel powerless against a monolithic health-care bureaucracy, in reality they have the potential to be a potent political force. Nationally, with almost 3 million nurses licensed to practice, the nursing profession constitutes the largest single body of health-care providers in the country.

Finding a Voice

Nurses in all health-care settings are saying, "Somebody's got to do something about this situation." The reality of the situation is that the "somebody" is nurses themselves. Once nurses identify exactly what it is that needs to be accomplished and understand what is possible within the political framework, they can use their considerable political power to make changes that will benefit both the clients and the profession.

Three Groups of Constituents
Group 1: Have a Little

One problem nurses in this group encounter is the ongoing conflict between the status quo and progress. They want to obtain more power and control, gain more benefits, earn more money, and have more respect as professionals. However, the strong desire to advance is counterbalanced by fear of jeopardizing their current jobs and their professional standing. Their motivation to be something more, to do something new, or to believe in something bigger is held back and pulled in another direction by their fear of change. The result of this internal tug-of-war is an attitude of inertia and ambivalence that has prevented nurses from organizing politically and effectively using their numerical power.

Group 2: Want More

Despite the inertia and ambivalence problems of individuals in the "have a little and want more" category, some of the most notable revolutionaries in history have come from this group, including Thomas Jefferson, Napoleon Bonaparte, Martin Luther King, Jr., and Vladimir Lenin. Each of these individuals came from the working middle class with a belief that it could be made better. Nurses can use their actions as examples of what individuals can accomplish to raise their own motivation levels to a point at which they overwhelm the inertia of the status quo.

Group 3: Sit Back and Watch

A third group of people, who share the inertia found among the "have a little, want more" group, are the "do-nothings." These individuals can be heard saying things like, "I agree with what you are saying, I just don't agree with your means," "I'm not going to get involved in this," or "I'm too busy to belong to the organization." The do-nothings tend to watch the activities of others, and if their efforts are successful, then they will join in as beneficiaries because they feel they have supported the effort from an ideological standpoint. However, they avoid any active involvement in politics. The 18th-century British politician Edmund Burke recognized the danger of the do-nothings. He said, "The only thing necessary for the triumph of evil, is for good men [and women] to do nothing."

What Can One Nurse Do?

It is important to remember that politics is a free-market enterprise open to anyone who is willing to become involved and play the game. Success in the political arena is contingent on three elements:

1. Knowledge and understanding of the process
2. The ability to offer something of value to the political figure
3. The capacity to identify what will be necessary to accomplish the objective

Anyone who is interested in becoming politically active must recognize that all candidates and elected officials need three things: resources to run their political operation (money and volunteers), votes, and a means to shape public opinion.

Resources
Money

Sufficient resources are essential to running a political campaign. The first and most necessary resource is always money. Would-be candidates soon discover that a lack of money to fund a campaign will inevitably lead to political failure. An unfunded candidate cannot travel, send mailings, produce radio and television commercials, post signs, or organize a telephone bank.

Voters often fail to realize that political candidates are only as available as finances permit. Frequently, good candidates lose because they fail to garner the financial resources necessary to run an effective campaign. Nurses can gain a candidate's support for issues by donating to his or her campaign chest.

Volunteers

A second important resource in an election campaign is volunteers. Volunteers work in campaigns by manning telephone banks, making literature drops, placing signs, and conducting voter registration drives. Usually political candidates are very glad to have free help for their campaigns.

Although nurses may not be able to make large monetary contributions to a candidate's campaign, they can always volunteer some time. Working closely with a candidate on a volunteer basis allows individuals to discuss important issues and helps candidates who support issues important to nurses. Most candidates need a considerable amount of education about health-related issues because of their lack of knowledge about medical and nursing concerns.

Votes

Obviously, votes are essential to any candidate. If a candidate does not have votes, he or she will not be elected. One of the most significant activities nurses can become involved in is to join and support a political party. The chosen party should reflect the nurse's value system and fundamental beliefs.

Keep in mind that there is never a perfect fit with any political party. Almost everyone who belongs to a political party will disagree at some point with some element of the party, usually with the extremist views. However, differing opinions and beliefs should not be a barrier to membership in a political party. The only way to change a view or opinion is by active participation from within the party.

The ultimate political power is the vote. Nurses must be registered to vote and must go to the polls on election day. They can make the difference for a candidate who supports legislation that empowers nurses and who recognizes what is needed for beneficial health-care reform.

Shaping Public Opinion
Public Trust in Nurses

Candidates need endorsements from their constituents so they can build their support base. They generally consider endorsements from nurses as one of the most valuable assets to their campaign. By careful selection of candidates who support legislation favorable to nursing and health care, endorsements can give nurses the capacity to shape public opinion. Periodic polls conducted by national news magazines, asking readers to rank various professions by how much they are trusted, have consistently shown that the public views nurses very highly, in the same category as police officers, firefighters, and teachers.

Why the Governor Matters

Nurses should use endorsements by choosing candidates in campaigns that have an impact on important issues. Often the campaign for governor falls into this category because governors, as chief executives, have a great deal of political power and can appoint people to a number of boards, committees, and other positions. Nurses need to recognize that the members of the board of nursing in their state, as well as other important appointed positions in health departments and other regulatory agencies, may be appointed by the governor and that this board has the final decision on the way that nurses practice.

When nurses establish a working political relationship with the governor, the governor is more likely to look favorably on them as those who have sustained him or her, provided financial support, and given endorsements during the political campaign. They will be the people the governor appoints to a board position.

Targeting endorsements will prevent nurses from making blind political decisions. Candidates

should be assessed first on their willingness to support issues that nurses are interested in and then on their capacity to win the election.

Grassroots Effort

A model for individual political development encourages grassroots involvement in local issues. This model is based on the belief that grassroots efforts may be more fulfilling than involvement in partisan politics.[10] This model is an activity-oriented ladder, including activities at four distinct levels:

- *Rung 1: Civic involvement.* Children's sports, parent–teacher association (PTA), neighborhood improvement group.
- *Rung 2: Advocacy.* Writing letters to public officials and newspapers and making organized visits to officials to discuss local issues.
- *Rung 3: Organizing.* Independent organizing on local issues, incorporation of single-issue citizens' groups, and networking with similarly situated citizens' groups.
- *Rung 4: Long-term power wielding.* Campaigning for oneself or another, local government planning, and agenda setting.

Sometimes grass root movements are not so grass roots. An organization, developed for the 2010 election and advertised as grass roots, actually was organized and funded by a large corporation with conservative leanings. It tapped into a radical wing of the party that had high levels of anger and resentment over the recent election of an African American president. The group effectively rebranded the party, moved the focus away from its previous president, and got several candidates elected. Unfortunately it also produced the "arrow shot in the air" effect: no one knows where the arrow will land when it comes down. Unleashing a group of radical ideologues produced considerable backlash and actually cost the party several elections.

Nurses in Office

Nurses usually shudder at the thought of running for political office. They tend to perceive political campaigns as something underhanded and tawdry and do not want to be involved. However, it is not impossible for nurses to achieve high status in public office.

One way that nurses can direct their political activities is to develop a political relationship with a legislator or a political operative who can mentor and guide the nurse in finding a route through the political maze. As discussed earlier, the principle of self-interest is one of the most critical elements in politics, and to establish a relationship with a political figure, nurses must demonstrate that the issues they support have value to both themselves and to the politician.

Making Alliances

There are several ways that a nurse can decide whom to support when becoming involved in the political process. A first step is to begin identifying the issues particular legislators are interested in and will vote for. Editorial opinion pieces in newspapers can give legislators a sense of the issues of concern.

It is a good idea to begin with local legislators and candidates, such as the state representative, state senator, or councilperson serving the neighborhood. Call their offices and find out when and where they are scheduled to speak, then go and listen to the speech to get a sense of who they are and what issues they support. Their speeches and the way they answer questions will reveal their ideology and partisanship. Also, during question-and-answer periods, ask elected officials what they think about issues important to you.

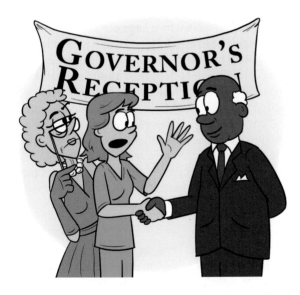

Another way to become familiar with prominent political figures is by attending some of the many partisan events that occur during an election season. A good way to visualize the local political landscape is by observing who is talking to whom at the event. Nurses can make their own assessments of political candidates by observing the candidates in action, calling their offices for information, reading published literature, and talking to people who know the candidates.

Beginning the process may seem difficult, but once you decide to become politically active, you'll become more confident.

Know the Issues

For nurses to be successful in the political process, they must know and understand the issues. At times an issue may be readily apparent in a nurse's community, for example, an increased number of homeless people. Other issues are easily identified by reading newspapers. Issues are generally presented in the editorial section; most newspapers also have a political watch section, which reports the results of any significant votes at the state and federal levels.

The American Nurses Association (ANA) newspaper, *American Nurse,* is an excellent source of information on issues of concern to the profession. In addition, the *American Journal of Nursing* Newsline feature and *Nursing and Health Care's* Washington Focus are excellent, easily readable sources of information in journals. *Capitol Update,* the ANA legislative newsletter for nurses, reports on the activities of its nurse lobbyists and on significant issues in Congress and regulatory agencies. This publication requires a subscription but is available in most nursing school and hospital libraries.

State nurses' associations and many specialty nursing groups also publish newsletters or legislative bulletins. Many of these are free to members but may be sent only when requested. Action alerts may also be sent to inform members of vital issues and the action needed by nurses. Most state legislatures now have online access to their proceedings so that bills of interest to nurses can be tracked as they progress through the legislative process.

Tactics

Tactics, essential tools for those who desire to be politically active, are the conscious and deliberate acts that people use to live and deal with each other and the world around them. In a political sense, "tactics" usually means the use of whatever resources are available to achieve a desired goal.

Nurses, with their long history of accomplishing much with few resources, are natural tacticians. As nurses learn how to organize themselves for political purposes, they can use their well-developed tactical skills to achieve important political goals. Listed below are some easy-to-use tactics for political action.

Engage in Bipartisan Tactics

Both Republican and Democratic nurses need to be politically active to achieve unified goals. Political action across the spectrum of issues and across partisan lines is necessary to achieve the goal of bipartisanship. Nurses should understand that only by supporting candidates who favor nursing and its agenda, whether Democrat or Republican, can the profession make changes that will advance its agenda. The most important thing, always, is the issue being addressed, not the personality or party of the candidate.

Lobbying

Sometimes communication with legislators takes the form of lobbying. Lobbying may be defined as attempting to persuade someone (usually a legislator or legislative aide) of the significance of one's cause or as an attempt to influence legislation. Lobbying methods include letter writing; face-to-face communication or telephone calls; mailgrams, telegrams, or e-mail; letters to the editor; and providing testimony (verbal or written).

To lobby effectively, one should be both persuasive and able to negotiate. Lobbying is truly an art of communication, an area in which nurses can become skilled. Before beginning any lobbying effort, it is vital to gather all pertinent facts. If the legislator asks you a question you do not know the answer to, be honest and reply that you will get that information. Then get back to the legislator as soon as you can.

In politics, getting the facts and laying the groundwork are analogous to developing a nursing care plan. Before visiting or writing a legislator, gather facts, delineate a problem or concern you wish to discuss, and develop a plan to articulate your concerns. Determine a method for evaluating your effectiveness.

Nurses need to recognize that the communication skills they use on a daily basis, as when explaining complicated medical jargon to clients, are the same skills they can use in translating health-care issues into language that the public and elected officials can understand.

If the plan is to visit the legislator's office, an appointment should be set up in advance. Usually, the meeting will actually be with the legislative aide, particularly at the federal level. This should not be discouraging because this individual is often responsible for assisting in the development of position statements and offering committee amendments for the legislator.

To ensure that legislators listen to your concerns, it is important not only to be well prepared but also to show that others support your position. When one person speaks, legislators may listen, but when many people voice the same concern, legislators are much more likely to pay attention. Always leave a business card, contact sheet, or both with your personal information so that the legislator can contact you. Send a thank-you note expressing your gratitude for the meeting.

Collaborate with Constituency Groups

Nurses can increase their political power by making alliances with other powerful constituency groups that support similar issues, such as the AARP. The AARP is very interested in health-care issues, particularly managed care, national health insurance, and the decreased quality of care from the increased use of unlicensed personnel. Nurses who are organized into collective bargaining units can use an alliance with powerful unions. Unions are traditionally concerned with issues such as working conditions, including staffing patterns in hospitals, wages, job security, and benefits. Nurses are concerned about the same issues.

How to Organize

"Know thine enemy" is one of the most fundamental rules that tacticians must follow, whether in war or politics. Napoleon was successful as a tactician and general because, before he fought any battle, he walked the battlefield. He knew what the terrain was like and where the rocks and crevices were. He knew what to anticipate when he arrived on the battlefield. Nurses who want to be successful in a political battle must first learn the hills, valleys, rocks, and crevices of the primary political battlefield, their own state demographics.

Comparing numbers helps define the political landscape of a state. Important demographics for organizing nurses at the state level include:

- Total population of the state. This provides a demographic overview of the political arena.
- Total number of registered voters
- Total number of registered voters by political party
- Total number of likely voters in any given election cycle. To determine this number, the difference between an on-year and an off-year election cycle should be understood. An on-year election cycle occurs when there is a major race in the state, usually during a presidential or gubernatorial race. An off-year cycle occurs when a major race is not being run. Lower levels of political activity are seen in an off-year election cycle.
- Total number of registered nurses. This information can be obtained from the state board of nursing. Comparing the number of actual voters with the number of RNs in a state provides an indication of the potential power of an RN voting block. For example, if there are 800,000 people who regularly vote in a state and there are 100,000 nurses in the state who are organized into a voting block about a particular issue, that group of nurses represents a significant percentage of voters, and candidates running for statewide office will be interested in having nurses' support. Nurses must be encouraged to register and vote to increase the power of the block.

Important Characteristics of an Organizer

Many of the characteristics of an organizer listed in Box 20.2 are the same characteristics that are required of nurses on a daily basis in the practice of their profession. Although these characteristics may have varying degrees of value for the organizer, the one critical element a political organizer has to have is the capacity to communicate. Although nurses usually have a well-developed ability to communicate at the bedside, they may lack the confidence to communicate in the larger public and political arenas. Nurses need to recognize that the communication skills they use on a daily basis, as when explaining complicated medical jargon to clients, are the same skills they can use in translating health-care issues into language that the public and elected officials can understand.

Box 20.2

Characteristics of an Organizer

- Curiosity
- Motivation
- Reverence
- Realism
- Flair for the dramatic
- Sense of humor
- Charisma
- Self-confidence
- Communication skills
- Clear vision of the future
- Capacity to change
- Persistence
- Ability to organize
- Imagination

One way to gain the public's interest and elected officials' support is to personalize health-care issues by stressing the fact that nurses are the professionals who provide the bulk of direct care for their mothers, fathers, siblings, and children. Communication of issues that touch people personally is usually the most effective method.

WHAT FOLLOWS ORGANIZATION?

Drafting Legislation and Creating Change

Certain critical questions must be asked. The first question always must be, "Who is the decision maker?" For example, if an issue needs to be resolved in the state board of nursing, the first step is to identify who makes the decisions at the board. Although the board members make decisions, it is important to remember that the people who sit on the board are appointed. Who appoints them and what is the basis of those appointments? If they are political appointees, they usually have some sort of political benefactor or a political relationship with someone in power.

Understanding these types of relationships makes it easier to determine the appointees' ideological and partisan positions on many issues. For example, if a nursing board is newly appointed by a recently elected Republican governor, it is probably safe to assume that most of the board members are Republicans who agree with the governor on many key issues.

The second question to address is, "How accessible is the appointee's benefactor?" Sometimes board members are appointed by the legislative leadership, not the governor. It is important to discover who appointed the board and whether or not individual voters have access to them. Generally, access by individual voters to the power figures who make these types of appointments is very limited. Organized groups, such as the ANA, provide the best avenue of access at the federal level.

Questions About Health Care

Other questions that need to be answered include:

- How successful have nurses been in the past in achieving specific goals?
- What positions do nurses hold in government?
- What does the state board look like politically?
- Which legislators have supported nursing issues in the past?
- Which legislators traditionally oppose nursing and health-care issues?

Because of the failure to ask and answer these questions, numerous pieces of pro-nursing legislation have died in committee or lacked sponsors to move the bill through the process. In states where nurses are in tune with the political issues and powers, they have more success moving bills through the legislative process so that they become law than in states where nurses are apathetic about the political process.

If a Bill Doesn't Pass

Even if a bill favorable for nurses or health care does not pass the first time, the fact that it was brought to a vote is important for several reasons. First, it has brought an issue to the attention of the whole legislature that they might otherwise have dismissed as unimportant.

Second, the legislative process brings to light the proponents and opponents of the issue and allows nurses to specifically target legislators who voted against the bill. One of two approaches can be used at this point. Nurses can either communicate with the legislators to explain why the bill is important in hopes of changing their minds, or they can organize as a voting block and attempt to vote the opposing legislators out of office.

Third, after a bill has gone through the process the first time, it becomes much easier to identify the obstacles and sticking points in the language of the bill. Before the bill is reintroduced in a later session of the legislature, it can be modified and amended to eliminate those parts that may have caused ideological problems for specific legislators.

The Nurse as Political Ally

Very few nurses have sought or been elected to governmental positions. However, it is important to realize that not all nurses who hold elected positions are allies for nursing. Currently there are approximately 80 nurses in state legislative positions or high administrative positions across the nation. There are no nurses in the U.S. House of Representatives or the Senate. Unless elected nurses identify themselves as nurses and support the profession, they may not be willing to support nursing issues politically.

Conclusion

There is nothing magical about nurses becoming involved in politics. It is simply a matter of hard work and use of the critical thinking skills nurses already possess. It is clear, however, that nurses can and do make a difference in the political arena. Nurses must ask how and where they can make a difference and how they can become involved in the process. Not every nurse will choose to run for political office, but each nurse can and should make a contribution. The willingness of nurses to become involved in politics is the key to developing legislative respect for the profession and improving health care.

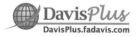

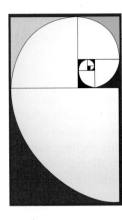

Issues in Practice

How Do Politics Affect You and Your Family?

Why should nurses be involved in politics? Does it really make a difference who is elected and who makes the laws? Take a minute to go through the questions below and check the items you think may be affected by politics.

Between the time you wake up and the time you leave the house, several things usually happen to you. Do you think any of the following subjects are affected by politics?

- The water with which you wash your face and brush your teeth
- The electricity that lights the room
- The price and quality of food you have for breakfast
- The safety of the products you buy

As the average person's life span grows longer and the retirement age is lowered, these later years become more meaningful. Are any of the following decisions affected by our political systems?

- The age at which you can retire
- The income that you get during retirement
- The quality and cost of health care
- Our life expectancy

We value our leisure time and the chance to get away from it all. Are any of the following areas affected by politics?

- The parks and lakes where vacationers fish and swim
- The air you breathe
- The radio and television programs that entertain you

Take some time to think about these questions. The answers will make you think some more.

21

Spirituality and Health Care

Roberta Mowdy

Learning Objectives

After completing this chapter, the reader will be able to:

- Develop a working definition of spirituality.
- Distinguish spirituality from religion.
- Describe what is meant by the nursing diagnosis "spiritual distress."
- Describe research that supports the health benefit of spiritual practices.
- Describe the relationship between spirituality and one alternative healing modality used within nursing.

ROUGH SPOTS ON THE TRAIL

The road of life often is filled with twists and turns, ups and downs, and precipitous waysides. People who are facing potentially long-term or debilitating illnesses, confronting acute health crises, or suffering from loss and grief may find themselves reexamining the foundational beliefs they have held since childhood. Usually, at no other time in a person's life is he or she so focused on evaluating the spiritual self than during such crises. Yet the times when clients are most vulnerable also can be opportunities for personal and spiritual growth.

Nurses have the unique task of working with clients at various points throughout their life journeys. Often nurses encounter clients during the "rough parts of the trail." The holistic nursing perspective requires nurses to view each person as a biopsychosocial being with a spiritual core. Each component of the self (physical, mental, social, and spiritual) is integral to and influences the others (Fig. 21.1). Nurses spend more time with their clients than do other health-care workers. Therefore, the spiritual needs of clients must be recognized as a domain of nursing care. Holism cannot exist without consideration of the spiritual aspects that create individuality and give meaning to people's lives.[1] Thus, nurses must be sure to address the spirit along with the other dimensions to provide holistic care.

NURSING AT LIFE'S JUNCTURES

It is universally true that the human life cycle is marked by a rhythm of transitions: birth, the entry of a child into society, puberty, sexual awakening, entry into adulthood, marriage, parenthood, illness, loss, old age,

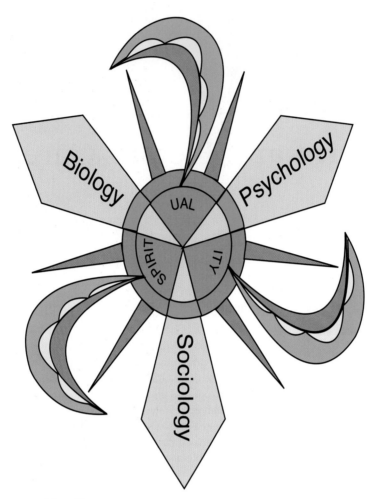

Figure 21.1 Components of the self.

and death. In all cultures there are other rhythms that people honor, such as the solar and lunar cycles, the agricultural cycle, and the reproductive cycles. These cycles constitute the rhythm of human life.

Developmental Crisis

All people recognize the importance of transitions and in some way have ritualized them through their religions or through custom. People learn from their own cultural groups how to behave during each transition, and each cultural group has conceptualized an understanding of these human experiences. Their importance is universally recognized.

Nurses primarily have contact with clients in the health-care setting within the context of these transitions. Developmental crisis theory holds that transitions are times of anxiety and vulnerability for families. Therefore, nurses are required to treat people who are going through transitions with great tenderness and care. It is a sacred trust for nurses to be allowed into a family system in transition. Clients and families may seek spiritual support or may feel spiritual abandonment. Ideally, nurses can help people identify and find the spiritual support they require.

Science as Magic

Over a long period of time, from the enlightenment of the 17th century to the dawn of the 21st century, political leaders and educated people in Western cultures came to believe that all the answers to human suffering could be found in science and technology.

For example, early in the 20th century, antibiotics were thought of as "magic bullets" that cured diseases and reduced suffering. People were eager to take part in research studies to solve their health-care problems.

It was in this context that the nursing profession embraced the Western scientific method as the measure for defining itself. Nurses believed, and some still do believe, that rigorous research involving testing of hypotheses would provide the theoretical base for the practice of professional nursing.

SOCIAL AND SCIENTIFIC EFFECTS ON SPIRITUALITY

To Be Fully Human

More recently, the horrors of terrorism, the harnessing of nuclear power, space exploration, and the mapping of the human genome are among the new capabilities that have given urgency to reconsideration of the question, "What does it mean to be fully human in the universe as it is now understood?" It is evident that science and technology cannot offer the solutions to all human problems; in fact, they have contributed to many of them.

> *Spirituality may be regarded as the driving force that pervades all aspects of and gives meaning to an individual's life.*

What Do You Think?

Make two lists: a list of the problems that science and technology have caused during the last 20 years and a list of the problems that have been solved by technology and science. Which list is longer? Why?

Science, electronic communications, and the great social experiments of the past two centuries are among the influences directing humans to a consciousness that individuals are connected to the whole of creation and to all peoples. One of the ways in which both health-care consumers and professionals are responding to this realization is by reintegrating spirituality and spiritual modes of healing into health and illness practices. Another response is the growing inclination to examine and adopt the spiritual wisdom of traditions other than one's own.

Phenomenology

A feature of postmodernism is the realization that the concept of truth as relative, allowing for an appreciation of diverse perspectives on what is true. Science, including nursing science since the mid-1980s, has expanded its ways of discerning truth, leaving behind traditional hypothetico-deductive, quantitative research. The emergence of **phenomenology** within the discipline of philosophy is one major influence that has led nursing to appreciate qualitative methods of discovery. As a philosophical approach to understanding truth, phenomenology parallels and is closely related to existentialism, advocating the view that consciousness determines reality and truth in space and time.

In the health-care setting, a phenomenological approach recognizes the belief that the client's observations may be more objective than those of the nurse: they are attached to the client's past experiences and knowledge, which include rich descriptions of the person's life transitions. In nursing, intuition has emerged as a phenomenon worthy of further investigation. This change in viewpoint coincides with increased interest in complementary and alternative therapies and with the importance of spirituality in healing and wellness.

THE NATURE OF SPIRITUALITY

What Is Spirituality?

Spirituality is a broad and somewhat nebulous concept that has to do with people's search for answers to certain questions and issues (Box 21.1). Similar concerns have been identified among children of various cultural backgrounds in research on the development of spirituality.

A Diverse Heritage

A rich heritage of spiritual practices, including systematic reflection for growth toward wholeness, is

Box 21.1
Spiritual Questions

Why are we here?

How do we fit into the cosmos?

What power or intelligence created and orders the universe?

What is the nature and meaning of divine or mystical experiences?

How are we to make meaning of suffering?

How are we to behave toward other people?

How are we to deal with our own shortcomings and failures?

What happens to us when we die, and where were we before we were born?

found in all the major religions of the world. The roots of the great traditions, including each religion's prayer practices, can be traced to the shift in human consciousness that occurred around 500 B.C. During this period, many great teachers and spiritual leaders emerged, including Confucius; Lao-tzu; Siddhartha Gautama, who became the Buddha; Zoroaster; the Greek philosophers Socrates, Plato, and Aristotle; and the Hebrew prophets Amos, Hosea, and Isaiah.

St. Augustine, a Roman Catholic bishop who lived in North Africa during the 5th century, is credited with first identifying the relationships among contemplation, action, and wisdom within the Christian tradition. For Augustine, the contemplative life was properly focused on the discernment of truth and was open to all people. Augustine equated truth, ultimately, with God.

Hope Through Compassion

Spirituality is often defined as integrative energy, capable of producing internal human harmony, or holism. Other definitions refer to spirituality as a sense of coherence. Spirituality also entails a sense of transcendent reality, which draws strength from inner resources, living fully for the present, and having a sense of inner knowing. Solitude, compassion, and empathy are important components of spirituality for many individuals.

The concept of hope is central to spirituality. Spirituality may be regarded as the driving force that pervades all aspects of and gives meaning to an individual's life. It creates a set of beliefs and values that influence the way that people conduct their lives. Spiritual activity involves introspection, reflection, and a sense of connectedness to others or to the universe. For many people, this connectedness focuses ultimately on a supreme being who is sometimes called God.

When providing spiritual care to their clients, nurses must base their actions on compassion, or sensitivity to the suffering of others. Compassion is a way of living born out of an awareness of one's relationship to all living creatures, a sensitivity to the pain and brokenness of others. The Greek word for compassion literally means "to feel in one's innards." Given this definition, one can easily see how compassion is part of spirituality and the life journey.

A Sense of Meaning

Traditionally, the term *spirituality* has been defined as a sense of meaning in life associated with a sense of an inner spirit. However, it is difficult to identify what such a spirit is like and how it can be observed. Spirituality can be defined from both religious and secular perspectives. A person with spiritual needs does not necessarily need to participate in religious rituals and practices.

Despite the lack of consensus regarding the definition of spirituality, several themes emerge from an interdisciplinary review of the literature:

- All human beings have the potential for spirituality and spiritual growth.
- Spirituality is relational.
- There is a necessary link among religion, moral norms, and spirituality.
- Spirituality involves lived experience; it is a way of life.

In some ways spirituality is a mystery. Although human beings can experience spirituality, appreciate it, and grow in it, there is much about spirituality that cannot be explained or reduced to human language.

On the basis of these themes, spirituality is defined as a way of life, usually informed by the moral norms of one or more religious traditions, through which a person relates to other persons, the universe, and the transcendent in ways that promote human fulfillment (of self and others) and universal harmony.

The Religious Perspective

From the religious perspective, spirituality can be defined as encompassing the ideology of the *imago dei* (image of God), or soul, that exists in everyone. The soul makes the person a thinking, feeling, moral, creative being, able to relate meaningfully to a supreme being and to others. This being or force may be called God, Allah, the divine creator and sustainer of the universe, the divine mystery, or other names that convey a profound sense of transcendence and awe. A religious perspective often entails a set of beliefs that help explain the meaning of life, suffering, health, and illness. These beliefs can be crucial to a believer's well-being.

Beyond Religious Practice

Spirituality is often mistakenly understood to mean just religious practice; however, it should be considered in the broader sense of the term. Religion can be an approach to or expression of spirituality, and spirituality is a component of religion, but the two concepts are different.

It is quite possible for the members of a specific religion to be limited in their spirituality. Most people have known individuals who dutifully follow the rules of their religious tradition. They strongly believe that if they have adhered to the rules correctly, God will reward them with blessings such as health, success, affluence, social status, and power. For these individuals, adverse events like disease, death of a loved one, or loss of investments can be devastating because they are perceived as a failure in religious practice or punishments from God. On the other hand, there are many deeply spiritual persons who do not belong to any organized religion but who may be profoundly reflective about the meaning of their life and experiences.

Specific Values and Beliefs

Current religious leaders attempt to help a diverse population appreciate religious traditions other than their own. They point out that all the world's major religions seek to answer the same questions: "Why are we here?" "What does it all mean?" and "What,

if anything, are we supposed to be doing with our lives?" All religions taken together can be perceived like a stained-glass window that refracts the light in different colors and offers reflections of different shapes. Each of the world's religions is different because it has evolved to respond to unique histories and different cultural developments.

Definitions of religion usually identify a specific system of values and beliefs and a framework for ethical behavior that the members must follow. Religion can be thought of as a social construct that reflects its cultural context and specific philosophical influences. A religion evolves within a specific cultural group, situated in history, and attempts to discern what the group beliefs are and how the group has come to understand God's commandments.

Religion, as an institutionally based, organized system of beliefs, represents only one specific means of spiritual expression. Participation in a religion generally entails formal education for membership, an initiation ceremony, participation in worship gatherings, adherence to set rules of behavior, participation in prescribed rituals, a particular mode of prayer, and the study of that group's sacred texts. Religious groups vary widely in their tolerance of intragroup diversity of beliefs and behaviors as well as their respect for the belief systems of others. In addition, a specific religious group may encompass a wide range of understanding of what its practices represent.

Occasionally, health-care professionals may encounter individuals whose spiritual practices are highly questionable or discomforting to witness (e.g., worshippers of Satan or those who seek to invoke harm to others through their prayers and rituals).

The Secular Perspective

From a secular perspective, spirituality is seen as a set of positive values, such as love, honesty, or truth, chosen by the individual to ultimately become that person's supreme focus of life and organizing framework. These values have the capacity to motivate the individual toward fulfillment of personal

> *Occasionally, health-care professionals may encounter individuals whose spiritual practices are highly questionable or discomforting to witness (e.g., worshippers of Satan or those who seek to invoke harm to others through their prayers and rituals).*

needs, goals, and aspirations, leading ultimately to self-actualization.

Manifestation of Spirituality

The religious and secular perspectives can exist together in the totality of a person's life. A person's spirituality may be nourished by the ability to give and receive touch, caring, love, and trust. Spirituality may also entail an appreciation of physical experiences such as listening to music, enjoying art or literature, eating delicious food, laughing, venting emotional tension, or participating in sexual expression. A series of four developmental stages have been proposed for human spirituality:

- Stage 1: The chaotic (antisocial) stage, with its superficial belief system
- Stage 2: The formal (institutional) stage, with its adherence to the law
- Stage 3: The skeptic (individual) stage, with its emphasis on rationality, materialism, and humaneness
- Stage 4: The mystical (communal) stage, with its "unseen order of things"[2]

A SPIRITUAL TRADITION IN NURSING

Modern nursing has a rich legacy of the appreciation of spirituality in health and illness. Florence Nightingale's views of nursing practice were based on a spiritual philosophy that she set forth in *Suggestions for Thought.* She was the daughter of Unitarian and Anglican parents, and among her ancestors were famous dissenters against the Church of England. The skepticism fostered by her Unitarian upbringing may have influenced her to question and critique established religious doctrine. Her search for religious truth caused her to become familiar with the writings of Christian mystics (e.g., St. Francis of Assisi, St. John of the Cross) and also with various Eastern mystical writings, including the *Bhagavad-Gita.*

What Do You Think?

How would you define your spirituality—religious or secular?

The Lady of the Lamp

Most modern nurses consider Florence Nightingale (1820–1910) to be the mother of the nursing profession (see Chapter 2). Most know her as "the lady of the lamp," who almost single-handedly brought about sweeping changes in British medicine, care delivered on battlefields, and public health. Nightingale realized a call to care early in her life. She was a sickly child, and as the recipient of care from family members, she began to reciprocate in kind by nursing other sick relatives.

A Modern Prophet?

Nightingale sought places where she could learn to care for the sick and dying in a way that distinguished what she did from the work of common chambermaids. She attended the Institution of Deaconesses at Kaiserwerth in Dusseldorf, Germany. This was a Protestant training hospital that taught something akin to nursing as a call from God and a diaconal function. Through her time at Kaiserwerth and her contacts there, she came to believe that all persons on a mission or quest to become Christlike are given certain gifts and talents. Some say Nightingale was a modern prophet of God and saw herself as a liberated human being.

For Nightingale, spirituality involved a sense of a divine intelligence who creates and sustains the cosmos, as well as an awareness of her own inner connection with this higher reality. The universe, for Nightingale, was the embodiment of a transcendent God. She came to believe that all aspects of creation are interconnected and share the same inner divinity. She believed that all humans have the capacity to realize and perceive this divinity. Nightingale's God can be described as perfection or as the "essence of benevolence."[3]

The Thoughts of God

Nightingale saw no conflict between science and mysticism. To her, the laws of nature and science were merely "the thoughts of God." Spirituality for Nightingale entailed the development of courage, compassion, inner peace, creative insight, and other "God-like" qualities. Based on this belief, Nightingale's convictions commanded her to lifelong service in the care of the sick and helpless.

Nightingale endorsed the tradition of contemplative prayer, or attunement to the inner presence of God. All phenomena, Nightingale believed, are manifestations of God. A spiritual life entails wise stewardship of all the earth's resources, including human beings. She saw physical healing as a natural process regulated by natural laws, and as she stated in her *Notes on Nursing,* "What nursing has to do ... is to put the client in the best condition for nature to act upon him."[3]

Spirituality and Religion in Nursing Theory

As nursing sought to establish itself as a profession with a legitimate knowledge base, the concern with human spirituality was downplayed and even consciously ignored until the early 1980s. Typically, the spiritual domain is assigned to the art rather than to the science of nursing because its seemingly subjective nature is mistakenly equated with esthetics and intuition. Paying attention to the spiritual domain in providing holistic care depends on the beliefs and values of both the nurse and the client.

> *Nightingale saw no conflict between science and mysticism. To her, the laws of nature and science were merely 'the thoughts of God.'*

There are 26 major nursing theories and conceptual frameworks that have been developed since the 1960s. Although 14 of them recognized the spiritual domain of health somewhere in their assumptions, only 2 theories mention it by name.

Energy Fields

Martha Rogers' Science of Unitary Human Beings is an example of a profoundly spiritual view of humanity that does not directly name the concept of spirituality. Rogers' framework suggests that there are unbounded human energy fields in interaction with the environmental energy field. Rogers' spiritual definitions can apply as well to the concept of the soul (discussed later). Rogers, who grew up in Tennessee amidst fundamentalist Christians, was loath to be interpreted in that light; moreover, she had to establish her credibility at New York University during the 1950s, before nursing was accepted as a scientific discipline.

An Aspect of Holistic Health

Betty Neuman, in the later development of her theory, and Jean Watson are the only theorists who clearly acknowledged the impact of spirituality in the development of their theories (see Chapter 4). Watson alone defined and explained the spiritual terminology she used to discuss the spiritual aspect of holistic health.

Watson specifically identifies the awareness of the clients' and families' spiritual and religious beliefs as a responsibility of a nurse.[4] She advocates that nurses should appreciate and respect the spiritual meaning in a person's life, no matter how unusual that person's belief system may be. Watson states that nurses have an obligation to identify religious and spiritual influences in their clients' lives at home and to help clients meet their religious requirements in inpatient settings. For example, nurses can facilitate clients' use of measures, such as the lighting of candles (real or electric), put flowers and personal objects in the room, ensure privacy, and play music to promote increased comfort and to relieve anguish.

Spiritual Distress

Since 1978, the North American Nursing Diagnosis Association (NANDA) has recognized the nursing diagnosis of spiritual distress.[5] It has most recently been defined as "disruption in the life principle that pervades a person's entire being and integrates and transcends one's biological and psychosocial nature."

Defining characteristics of spiritual distress include concerns with and questions about the meaning of life and death, anger toward God, concerns about the meaning of suffering, concerns about the person's relationship to God, the inability to participate in preferred religious practices, seeking spiritual help, concerns about the ethics of prescribed medical regimens, black humor, expressing displaced anger toward clergy, sleep disturbances, and altered mood or behavior. Spiritual distress may occur in relation to separation from religious or cultural supports, challenges to beliefs and values, or intense suffering.

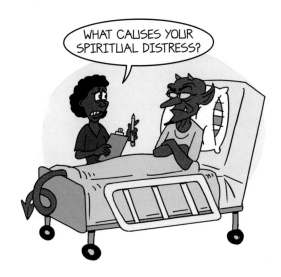

WHAT CAUSES YOUR SPIRITUAL DISTRESS?

Illness as Punishment

Nurses should be aware that some individuals have been seriously harmed by their religious communities. Examples of harm might include being shunned or excommunicated, being told that they are evil, being forced into a rigidly controlled lifestyle by a cult, or being physically or sexually assaulted by members of the religious community. For these people, illness may be seen as punishment for some sinful action, and they may perceive any offer of spiritual support from the religious community as profoundly threatening. They may believe that God has abandoned them or that the idea of God is foolish or even destructive.

Given the rapid turnover of clients in most health systems, there may be little that the nurse can do other than to acknowledge their spiritual pain and accept them, with the assurance that "I am here for you now." If there is more time for contact, the nurse may be able to refer a client or family to appropriate support groups or clergy.

Going Against Tradition

At times clients make health-care decisions that conflict with the beliefs of their religious communities. These often produce high levels of spiritual distress that may affect both the mental and physical well-being of the client. Consider the following case study:

When I was a nursing student in the early 1970s, I cared for a woman who was undergoing a

therapeutic abortion because of several medical complications of her pregnancy. She had her first child before RhoGAM was available, and she, an Rh-negative mother, had borne an Rh-positive baby. She had only one kidney, and her physicians were concerned that the immunological complication of carrying a second Rh-positive baby would jeopardize that kidney's function. The decision was difficult for the woman and her husband to make, but they believed the first priority was to care for and raise their 7-year-old son. She needed to protect her kidney so that she could live and participate fully in the child's upbringing.

The night before I cared for this woman, her clergyman came to the hospital and told her that she would go to hell for her decision. Being a devout church member, the woman was extremely distressed the next day. The primary nurse assigned to this woman recognized the spiritual distress caused by the clergyman and requested that a hospital chaplain spend time with her. The chaplain talked and prayed with the woman for several hours. These actions brought great comfort to the woman, who proceeded with the abortion.

Clients often make choices that are difficult for nurses to accept. For instance, because of religious beliefs, clients may refuse commonplace treatments, such as blood transfusions, medications, and even minor surgeries. End-of-life decisions are often based on family members' spiritual beliefs and can be controversial among the health-care personnel who are involved in the decision. In some acute care settings, chaplains and psychiatrists conduct regular group sessions with staff nurses to assist them in understanding and accepting controversial client decisions. The Schiavo case in Florida demonstrates how well-meaning people with strong religious beliefs can be diametrically opposed when it comes to end-of-life decisions.

The Human Energy System and the Soul

Most religious traditions include a concept called "the soul." Religious traditions usually offer explanations of what the soul is, how and when human beings acquire a soul, and what happens to the soul after death, but "soul" need not be a religious concept.

Images of the Soul

Thomas Moore, a psychotherapist who has written extensively about spiritual development, describes the soul "not as a thing, but a quality or a dimension of experiencing life and ourselves. It has to do with depth, value, relatedness, heart, and personal substance ... [not necessarily] an object of religious belief or ... something to do with immortality."[6] Yet Moore observes that the soul must be nurtured, and religious practices can provide that nurturance. For Moore, spirituality is the effort a person makes to identify the soul's world view, values, and sense of relatedness to the whole of the person and of creation. The work of the soul is the quest for understanding or insight about major life questions.

Some people may depict the soul as an image of the person that extends several feet beyond the physical self, or characterize it by color and energetic movement. Many people believe that the soul enters the body at some point during gestation and leaves the body at approximately the moment of death. Reincarnation, or the return of a soul for many earthly lifetimes, is a concept encountered in many religious frameworks, including certain mystical traditions within Judaism and Christianity, although not all denominations subscribe to it. The reason for the soul's return to earthly life is to learn, to develop, and to be purified. Some traditions express this process in terms of earning an improved position in the spiritual world to become closer to God after the final judgment.

The soul would seem to be an exquisitely precise and vast center for communication. Souls have the capacity to communicate with one another, with all living things, and with the divine source of all energy. Their capacity is not limited by the laws of physical matter. Some alternative modalities of healing rely on energy movement through the soul.

Examples of therapies that capitalize on knowledge of the soul and the movement of a divinely generated energy, life force, or grace (*chi* in Chinese, *ki* in Japanese, *prana* in Indian traditions) include therapeutic touch, Reiki, and shiatsu. Energy can move in many directions. When a person needs it, energy can be drawn from its divine source into the person. Excess energy can be moved from one person to another, and the flow of energy throughout the person's energy field can be balanced to achieve a state of health.

> *At times clients make health-care decisions that conflict with the beliefs of their religious communities. These often produce high levels of spiritual distress that may affect the client's mental and physical well-being.*

Human Energy Centers

Some alternative healing practices that use colors, herbs, aromas, and crystals can be regarded as consistent with a paradigm of repatterning the human energy field or altering the flow of energy throughout the person's body. The circulation of divine energy may be thought of as coming from God and circulating through all living things, the earth, and all the celestial bodies, thus interconnecting all creation.

Religious traditions of India and other Eastern cultures teach that the human energy system contains seven energy centers, or chakras. These can be considered the primary openings in the human energy system through which energy flows. Each center has or controls a unique type of energy and spirituality that it allows to enter or leave the body. The root chakra is located at the base of the torso or the perineum, and its energy has to do with the material world. The crown chakra, the highest level of energy at the top of the head, relates to spirituality.

Examining the religious art of many cultures, over many centuries, artists depict these areas of their subjects' bodies in similar ways. For instance, holy people are depicted with vivid, large, or colorful hearts, and their heads are surrounded by halos. At the very least, the chakras represent a paradigm for ordering the archetypal issues of human life.

What Do You Think?

What sources of religious energy do you have? When and how do you use them?

Communication Between Worlds

Some individuals seem to be more aware of the non-physical or spiritual realms than others. Many people have had a precognition or déjà vu experience during their lives. However, nurses may have more opportunities to glimpse a different reality than laypeople. Nurses have been involved in research on the near-death experience for more than 20 years.

The Near-Death Experience

Across religious and cultural traditions and throughout history, a common near-death experience has been documented, but only since the early 1980s has it gained credence among Western health professionals.

Many clients describe the experience of near death as a sensation of floating in the air while visualizing their body lying below on a hospital bed, at the scene of an accident, or where the near death occurred. They often watch health-care personnel who are working to resuscitate the body. The person then experiences being drawn into a tunnel, perhaps accompanied by other forms or spiritual beings, and moving toward a bright light that exudes great energy or love. They also describe a communication with the light being, generally identified as God, about whether they are to remain there or return to the earthly body.

Obviously, in cases of near death, the decision is made to return. Individuals who have experienced near death often report that they have developed a great inner peace, that they no longer fear death, and that their lives have been transformed by what they experienced.

Nurses who spend much of their time working with clients who are near death, such as hospice nurses, are most likely to have witnessed the experience of deathbed visions and gained a glimpse of a different realm of reality. Dying clients who are having a deathbed vision are often aware of multiple realities: the tangible here and now that family members and caretakers can observe, and "the other side," where they see loved ones who have died and are waiting for their arrival.

Some medical researchers attribute near-death and deathbed experiences to progressive hypoxia in specific brain centers. However, others give the experiences a spiritual interpretation. Could a husband, for example, really come to meet his wife of many years past? A vast amount of literature on angels and spiritual guides emphasizes that people need not feel alone or frightened by future situations or crises. Angels and other spiritual guides are available to comfort them just for the asking.

Spirituality in Children

Some authorities believe that children are more open to communication from the spiritual world than adults because they have not yet been contaminated by the laws of natural science that are generally accepted by Western society. Nurses can watch for and nurture spirituality in children. When a nurse is open to such an occasion and acts on it, an opportunity for transcendent and reciprocal spiritual growth is available to both the child and the nurse.[7]

Mysticism

Mystics are people believed to have a different relationship to time, space, matter, and energy than most of the population. It seems that they are able to understand the real nature and full capability of their souls and can apply that knowledge and ability to the physical world, producing changes that science has difficulty explaining and that some call miracles. For example, a current-day Hindu holy man in India, Sai Baba, generates ash that has brought miraculous healing to some people who have touched it. Also, many healing miracles were documented by physicians and

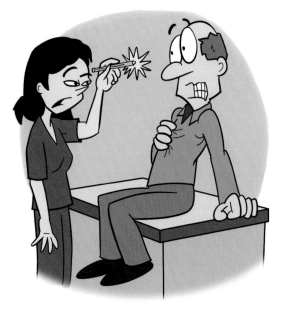

"SIR, THE BRIGHT LIGHT YOU SEE
IS MY PENLIGHT, NOT THE AFTERLIFE."

scientists during the lifetime of the Italian Franciscan priest Padre Pio before his death in 1968.

The common message of mystics from around the world is that people are to live lives of love and compassion for all. The extraordinary love and compassion that most mark the early life of the Dalai Lama, a Buddhist holy man, is depicted in the historical films "Seven Years in Tibet" and "Kundun."

SPIRITUAL PRACTICES IN HEALTH AND ILLNESS

Nurturing the Spirit

The way that nurses care for and nurture themselves influences their ability to function effectively in a healing role with another person. The spiritual path is a life path. Attentiveness to one's own spirit is a key component of living in a healing way and is fundamental to integrating spirituality into clinical practice. Care of their spirit or soul requires nurses to pause, reflect, and take in what is happening within and around them; to take time for themselves, for relationships, and for other things that animate them; and to be mindful about nourishing their spirits. The many ways to nurture their spirits and respond to their spiritual concerns are the same as those that they suggest to their clients.

Spiritual Assessment Questions

Nurses may have some difficulty assessing the spiritual status of a client. Some questions that facilitate gathering this information include:

- What is strength for you?
- Where can you get your strength?
- Who gives you strength?
- How can you increase your inner strength?
- What does peace mean to you?
- Where do you feel at peace?
- Who makes you feel more peaceful?
- What situations will increase your sense of peace?
- When do you feel most secure?
- Where do you get your security from?
- Who makes you feel secure?
- How can you increase your security?[1]

A Professional Responsibility

Care of the spirit is a professional nursing responsibility and an intrinsic part of holistic nursing. Nurses must become confident and competent with spiritual caregiving, expanding their skills in assessing the spiritual domain and in developing and implementing appropriate interventions. A caring relationship with a client is necessary to show the person that he or she is significant. Effective spiritual care requires self-awareness, communication, trust building, and giving hope.[8]

The nursing profession must understand and support holistic care. Therefore, spirituality and the delivery of spiritual care become fundamental content areas for nursing students. Guidelines and policies must be developed to fully support nurse educators in their endeavors.

A persistent barrier to the incorporation of spirituality into clinical practice is the fear of imposing particular religious beliefs and values on others. Nurses who integrate spirituality into their care of others need to recognize that, although each person acts out of and is informed by her or his own spiritual perspective, acting from this foundation is not the same as imposing these beliefs and values on another. In fact, many practitioners believe that the more grounded they are in their own spiritual understandings, the less likely they are to impose their values and beliefs on others.

A number of organizations and agencies encourage the incorporation of spiritual practices into health care (Boxes 21.2 to 21.4).

Prayer and Meditation

Prayer and meditation are spiritual disciplines practiced in many traditions, both cultural and religious. Appreciating the personal nature of these disciplines, the nurse, with respect and sensitivity, can help clients remember or explore ways in which they reach out to and listen for God or the absolute.

> *Some authorities believe that children are more open to communication from the spiritual world than adults because they have not yet been contaminated by the laws of natural science that are generally accepted by Western society.*

B o x   2 1 . 2

American Holistic Nurses' Association

The American Holistic Nurses' Association (AHNA) was founded in 1980 by a group of nurses dedicated to bringing the concepts of holism to every arena of nursing practice. They define holism as wellness, that state of harmony between body, mind, emotions, and spirit in an ever-changing environment.

The AHNA offers certification in holistic nursing and has endorsed programs in aromatherapy, interactive imagery, and healing touch.

Source: Visit the AHNA website at http://www.ahna.org.

B o x   2 1 . 3

Parish (Congregational) Nursing

Parish (congregational) nursing is a movement of the past two decades in which churches, synagogues, mosques, and other faith communities designate nurses to serve their membership. Parish nursing is viewed as a healing ministry, and parish nurses are attuned to spiritual issues raised by health transitions, as well as the healing nature of spiritual practice. They may assist people to remain in their own homes, connect them with other health services for which they are eligible, or provide needed health teaching and support. At times their role is simply to be present with them.

The International Parish Nurse Resource Center is located in St. Louis, Missouri. They can be contacted at 314-918-2559, 314-918-2527, or on the Internet at http://www.parishnurses.org.

B o x   2 1 . 4

International Center for the Integration of Health and Spirituality

The International Center for the Integration of Health and Spirituality (ICIHS) in Rockville, Maryland, disseminates research on the benefits of spiritual practices to health professionals through their publication, conferences, and speakers.

For further information about this resource, contact ICIHS at their website at www.encognitive.com.

In the clinical setting, both the nurse's and the client's understanding of prayer will determine its role. Clarifying the client's understanding of and need for prayer is part of holistic nursing. Some clients want others to pray with or for them, whereas others do not believe in prayer. Nurses should support each client's request and needs for prayer, which may mean inviting others to take part in various forms of prayer with and for the client, or simply praying with the client themselves. Facilitating the appreciation and practice of prayer in a client's life is an important aspect of caring for the spirit.

Relief Through Imagery. When a person is physically confined to a hospital room, the practice of imagery may enable him or her to experience another space. Imagery can take a person to a temple, an ocean, a place of religious worship, a breakfast nook, or any "sacred space," that is, a life-giving and healing place for the client. In this other space, the client may feel more comfortable in spirit and more able to engage in prayer. Family and friends, as well as other clients and other staff, may be resources in this practice of imagery.

Exploring as many aspects of the prayer experience as possible enriches both the nurse's and the client's understanding of the nature and place of prayer. Sacred or inspirational readings, music, drumming, movement, light or darkness, aromas, and time of day are among the many factors that may be important considerations in one's prayer life.

Recalling the place and meaning of prayer and the ways in which they experience the presence of and communion with God or the absolute provides clients with a rich resource.

The client's prayer life, in all of its fullness and meaning, nurtures the spirit, and the nurse may be able to support the client's prayer needs by facilitating changes in the environment or schedule. It is wise to remember that merely the process of listening to and appreciating the prayer life of another nurtures the spirit and acknowledges the spiritual dimension of that person.

Relaxation Response
Remembered Wellness
The relaxation response and prayer have been demonstrated to affect illnesses. The ability of people to participate in their own healing through prayer or meditation may use a source of healing power called "remembered wellness," sometimes also called "the placebo effect." It is based on the belief that all people have the capacity to "remember" the calm and confidence associated with emotional and physical health and happiness. As a source of energy that can be tapped into, remembered wellness should not be regarded suspiciously but instead used for healing. However, its effectiveness depends on the individual's belief system.

Remembered wellness depends on three components: belief and expectation of the client, belief and expectation of the caregiver, and belief and expectation generated by a caring relationship between the client and the caregiver. A warm and trusting relationship seems to enhance the effectiveness of the care provided.

Everyone involved in providing health care is in a position to use remembered wellness as an energy source to enhance the healing process. One thing health-care providers can do to promote healing is to speak positively of treatments and medications being used. For example, positive reinforcement occurs when the nurse refers to the clients' medication as the "drug your doctor prescribed to help your heart" or the food tray as "nutrition to help your body fight your infection."

The Nocebo Effect
In contrast to the placebo effect, the "nocebo" (negative placebo) effect is the fulfillment of an expectation of harm. It is also an effect that health professionals can cause. Examples of the nocebo effect include advising clients that a medicine will probably make them sick, telling them that chemotherapy will drain their energy and cause their hair to fall out, or informing them that a certain percentage of people die from a given procedure. Such warnings can actually bring about the complications.

A Quiet Focus
The relaxation response entails 20 minutes, twice each day, of quiet meditation on a word or image that is spiritually meaningful to the person. When an intrusive thought enters the person's consciousness, the person should lightly dismiss it, as if gently blowing a feather away, and return to the meditation word or image. Over time, individuals who use this method have lowered blood pressure, decreased incidents of dysmenorrhea, reduced chronic pain, and brought about improvement in a number of illnesses.

Peace Through Awareness
Relaxation, meditation, visualization, and hypnosis can help seriously ill clients, including many with cancer. Meditation is a technique of listening. However, listening is not a passive process. Rather, it is a way of focusing the mind in a state of relaxed awareness to pay attention to deeper thoughts and feelings, to the products of the unconscious mind, to the peace of pure consciousness, and to deeper spiritual awareness.

Some teachers of meditation suggest that the person select a spiritually symbolic word (e.g., God, love, beauty, peace, Mary, Jesus) on which to focus, whereas others suggest watching a candle flame. Still others teach practitioners to focus on their breathing. All these methods are intended to bring the person to a deeply restful state that frees the mind from its usual chatter. This is the experience of being centered. People may experience spiritual insights, but more often they experience a gradual enhancement of well-being.

Visualizing an Outcome
Visualization is the practice of meditating with an image of a desired outcome or the process of attaining it. It is preferable that the image be selected by the person using it rather than someone else. For

> *Care of the spirit is a professional nursing responsibility and an intrinsic part of holistic nursing.*

example, a person with a tumor might visualize miniature miners mining the unhealthy tissue and carting it away. Hypnosis is a process of suggesting an image of a desired reality to someone. Both these techniques have been demonstrated to stimulate the immune system.

Researchers have also observed that some seriously ill people believe that they deserve their illness as a punishment for something they did in the past. Helping them forgive themselves often brings about dramatic improvements in their conditions. Releasing fear and hate has a similar effect. This process reflects back to Nightingale's belief that nurses need to help clients get out of the way of their own healing.

It might seem logical to conclude that clients who do not recover from illness, or who die, have failed to help themselves or did not adequately use their spiritual powers. That is not the case. Spiritual modes of healing do not always lead to cure. Spiritual healing takes a much broader view and includes enhanced comfort and an inner peace with disability or death.

Therapeutic Touch

Therapeutic touch (TT) is an active alternative healing modality that involves redirecting the human energy system. In recent years, TT has been retrieved from ancient traditions, studied, and refined.

Altered Wave Patterns

As a healing practice, TT is consistent with the Science of Unitary Human Beings developed by Martha Rogers. The Science of Unitary Human Beings defines people as energy fields interacting with the larger environmental energy field. The energy fields are characterized by patterns of waves. One way of altering the wave patterns of the human energy field is to use TT to move energy into and through it in deliberate ways.

The practitioner of TT acts with the intent of relaxing the recipient, reducing pain and discomfort, and accelerating healing when appropriate. Early controlled studies showed that the hemoglobin levels of a group of clients who received TT increased significantly more than the levels in a control group who did not receive TT.

The TT practitioner should approach the client with compassion and the intent to heal, and the recipient of care ideally approaches the healing encounter with receptivity and openness to change. The practitioner of TT first centers and then assesses the state of the recipient's energy field, noting energy levels and movement around the chakras. Cues may be determined through physical sensations in the practitioner's hands, direct visualization, inner awareness, or other intuitive modes of insight.

After assessing the recipient, the TT practitioner, working from the center of the client's energy field to the periphery, directs energy from the environment into the client's field as needed, stimulates energy flow through the client's field, clears congested areas in the energy field, dampens excess energetic activity, and synchronizes the rhythmic waves of the energy flow depending on the client's needs. The practitioner is not diverting his or her own energy into the client because it would be detrimental to the practitioner. Rather, the TT practitioner redirects the client's energy field or directs energy from the environment outside the client.

> *Therapeutic touch (TT) is an active alternative healing modality that involves redirecting the human energy system.*

An Expression of Care

Families and friends may need encouragement to share physical expressions of care and concern in the sometimes intimidating hospital environment. Nurses may encourage them with statements such as, "It's OK to hold her hand; you won't interfere with the tubes." "He mentioned that you give a wonderful back rub; would you like to give him one today?" "She seems to know when you are in here holding her hand." "I can show you how to massage her feet." "Would you like to brush her hair?"

Persons vary in their degree of comfort with touch and the conditions in which they may want to share touch. The nurse's own personal feelings about and comfort with touch help in assessing the place and potential use of touch in the client's situation. At times when words cannot be found, or in circumstances in which people are more

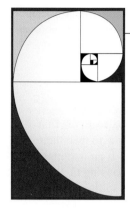

Issues in Practice

Religious Issues Versus Care Issues

Angie and Edward are a young couple with two teenage children. They are a close and loving family who have a large network of family and friends. The entire family is active in their church, school, and other community groups.

Alan, 15 years old, has just been severely injured in a high school soccer game. Angie and Edward are summoned to the hospital where they are told that Alan has multiple fractured bones and possible internal injuries. While they are waiting for the surgical team to arrive, the couple keeps vigil at their son's bedside in the pediatric intensive care unit (PICU). The surgeon informs the distressed parents that there is evidence that Alan's injuries are more serious than previously diagnosed. Alan has active internal bleeding and will need a blood transfusion to survive. Although genuinely devastated, the parents adamantly refuse to sign for the lifesaving blood transfusion, stating that they are Jehovah's Witnesses and that receipt of blood is against their religion. The surgeon asks you, Alan's nurse, to get the parents to change their minds. You talk with the couple, but they continue to refuse to sign the surgical consent form.

- What are the primary underlying spiritual principles involved in this dilemma?
- Do Alan's parents have the right to refuse their consent for a blood transfusion on the basis of religious beliefs?
- Do you think that the fact that Alan is a minor (under 18 years old) may make a difference in this situation?
- What actions do you think the charge nurse should take?
- How would you resolve this dilemma?

comfortable with physical expression than with words, touch is a powerful expression of spirit and instrument of healing.

NURSING PRACTICE AND SPIRITUAL WELLNESS

Profession or Vocation?
Although the nursing profession is deeply rooted in religious traditions, modern nursing has spent considerable energy attempting to distance itself from this aspect of its history. Nursing as vocation has given way to nursing as profession (see Chapter 1). The current health-care system has required nurses to shift their identity from vocation to profession in order to achieve appropriate value in a system that is increasingly economically oriented.

Nursing as Spiritual Calling
Nursing is much more than the mere secular enterprise the modern world perceives it to be. Perhaps it is time that nurses re-evaluate the work they do and consider it a vocation, that is, a life calling in the spiritual sense of that word. The world's religions consistently allude to the symbolic and deep meaning of the work that nurses do. Nursing practice has the capacity to be richly imaginative and to speak to the soul on many levels. Nursing practice can be carried out mindfully and artistically, or it can be done routinely and unconsciously, like any other job. When nursing is practiced with deep consciousness and purpose, it nurtures the nurse as well as the client.[9]

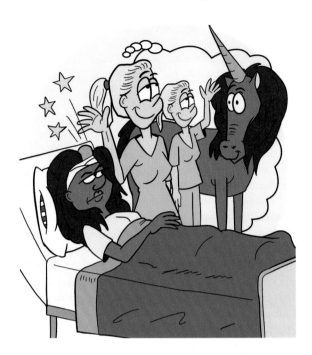

Some experts perceive that nursing is directly connected to the nurse's fantasy life, family myths, ideals, and traditions. The profession of nursing may be one way nurses sort out their major life issues. Although the choice of nursing as a career may often seem to have been serendipitous, in the spiritual context it is reasonable to question whether anything really happens by accident. As nurses practice nursing, they craft themselves, undertaking the soul's lifetime work of self-definition and self-identification.

When the Well Runs Dry

As with most professions, at times it may become difficult, even impossible perhaps, to feel good about the work that one is doing. Negative attitudes about work are detrimental to a person's self-development and often cause people to become overly invested in the surface trappings of work, such as money, power, and success. The phenomenon of burnout among nurses has been identified and studied for many years (see Chapter 12). Burnout can be viewed from a spiritual perspective, in which the well runs dry, energy fields become unbalanced, or the person experiences a prolonged "dark night of the soul," or even feels that the nurse's life work is devoid of meaning.[10]

People working in the helping professions, whose work is rooted in compassion and concern for others, are prone to depression and burnout. A concerted effort at spiritual development, or the nourishment of the soul, is essential to nurses' overall mental and physical well-being.

Maintaining Balance
Self-Restoration

To maintain an internal state of balance, the first thing nurses need to do is take time to feed their spirit. Daily prayer or meditation is an important source of insight and energy. Belonging to a group or community that actively pursues spiritual growth is also a powerful source of spiritual nourishment. Many individuals find that their spirits are nourished within the setting of a formal religion, although not necessarily the one in which they were reared. It is not uncommon for people to seek a faith community in midlife or later life, perhaps after being away from one for many years. The experience of trying various religions and modes of worship is by itself a broadening, nurturing experience.

A Sense of Sacredness

Periodic retreat from the hustle and bustle of modern living can be highly restorative to the spirit. A retreat may be for a few hours, a half-day, a weekend, a week, or longer. For some people, keeping a journal is a retreat-like experience. For others, it may be a stroll through a beautiful park, a few hours watching waves on a beach, or a trip to the woods. Retreat is most effective when time is consistently set aside for introspection and reflection rather than for tasks.

A sense of sacredness can infuse everyday life with meaning and zest if nurses open themselves to it. It is a part of normal human activity to celebrate seasonal and family holidays with specific rituals, music, decorations, group gatherings, and foods. These types of activities honor life cycles that are greater than the individual and nurture important relationships that serve as a **support system.**

Enjoy Special Moments

Many people have routines for their weekends or days off that allow time for self-restoration. These special activities may include a large country breakfast while listening to favorite music; baking cookies, bread, or a pie; sitting for an extended period of time in a favorite easy chair; or even playing a physically demanding sport like basketball. Many people have favorite coffee mugs or dishes or special objects in their homes that are not only beautiful but may remind them of loved ones, wonderful trips, religious experiences, or other events that nourish them each time they view the object.

One of the most spiritual aspects of a person's life is the enjoyment of beauty. It costs little or nothing to plant or cut flowers or to listen to music. It is in these moments that a person's creativity and insight are most evident.

Regaining the Center

The hectic modern world continually urges people to enhance their capacity for dealing with multiple concerns at the same time. Some people even define success by looking at how many tasks they can juggle simultaneously. *Multitasking* is the new buzzword for the health-care environment of the 21st century. Nurses must be able to talk on the

> " *People working in the helping professions, whose work is rooted in compassion and concern for others, are prone to depression and burnout.* "

telephone, send faxes and e-mail, surf the net, and use a word processor for entering client data at the same time that they are developing care plans, evaluating clients, answering call lights, supervising unlicensed assistive personnel, and providing physicians with information.

Although this is highly productive, the more nurses multitask, the more disconnected they become from themselves. Multitasking can be thought of as the antithesis of spiritual nurturance. Spirituality is about personal wholeness, whereas multitasking is about fragmentation.[10] Only when nurses begin to slow down and start centering their energy fields will they have the capacity to be fully present and be able to attend with complete consciousness to their loved ones, colleagues, and clients and focus completely on the present moment.

Conclusion

Spirituality within the nursing context needs to be seen as a broad concept encompassing religion but not equated with it. Fundamental to this concept is a search for meaning within life and its particular events, such as ill health. Nursing students need to be made aware of the many forms that spiritual distress may take.

Nurses are in an ideal position to provide spiritual care that positively affects the mental and physical health of their clients. To be able to focus clearly on clients' spiritual needs, nurses must first consider their own spirituality as a starting point for self-knowledge. The means of supporting clients with spiritual problems must be explored. Teaching methods should be participatory and student centered; the means of assessing and meeting spiritual needs hinges on effective communication skills and determines whether the nurse is "being with" the client as opposed to merely "being there."

The meaning of the holistic moment emerges through the synergistic interaction among its elements (Fig. 21.2). Just as a person is greater than the sum of her or his parts, so is the holistic moment greater than the sum of its parts, namely spirituality, presence, and relationship to others.[11]

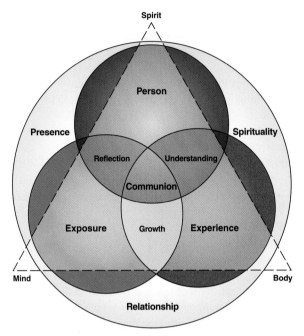

Figure 21.2 Elements involved in experiencing spirituality and presence in the nurse–client relationship. (Adapted from Rankin EA: Finding spirituality and nursing presence. Journal of Holistic Nursing 24[4]: 286, 2006.)

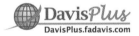
DavisPlus.fadavis.com

Critical Thinking Exercises

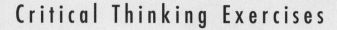

rs. Jan Steiner, 73 years old, has outlived two husbands. Ted, her second husband, died 20 years ago. Reared in the Roman Catholic faith, Mrs. Steiner converted to Judaism when she married Ted. Her two daughters by her first husband were also reared in the Roman Catholic tradition. One of them, Kathy, continues to practice her religion. The other daughter, Judith, is Unitarian.

Mrs. Steiner experienced a stroke 2 years ago that left her moderately disabled. At that time she moved into a long-term care facility. She was still able to read and to enjoy visits with friends and family, but a second stroke 3 months ago left her incontinent and aphasic.

Mrs. Steiner has just had a major heart attack. Although bypass surgery could extend her life, she has never articulated any end-of-life desires. Her daughters are in conflict over how Mrs. Steiner's medical management should proceed. Kathy strongly believes that as long as Mrs. Steiner is alive, life should be actively supported. It would be morally wrong to do less than that. Judith, on the other hand, believes that what had been the "life" of Mrs. Steiner is essentially over and it is a waste of resources to merely delay the inevitable. The nursing staff, as they attempt to facilitate communication between the family and the medical staff, feel caught in the middle.

- What are your own spiritual beliefs about the proper approach to Mrs. Steiner's medical management?
- Analyze the positions of Kathy and Judith from both their ethical and spiritual contexts.
- What resources are likely to be available in the hospital or the community to help the daughters come to a decision?

Bypass surgery is not performed, and Mrs. Steiner returns to her long-term care facility. Her overall condition continues to deteriorate, and within 3 months she is very near death. She seems to have little awareness of her surroundings and does not consistently recognize or respond to her daughters.

- Knowing the religious divergence within Mrs. Steiner's family, how might the nursing staff facilitate their preparation for the death of their mother and her funeral?
- What would happen within Mrs. Steiner's circle of family and friends if any "side"—Catholic, Jewish, or Unitarian—"won" in planning her end-of-life care?
- Have you seen blending of religious traditions in rituals of marriage or burial? What are the advantages and disadvantages of such an approach?
- What might be the outcomes of handling their mother's death in a strictly secular or nonsectarian way and allowing all relatives and friends to mourn privately in accordance with their own spiritual traditions?

22

Cultural Diversity

Joseph T. Catalano

Learning Objectives
After completing this chapter, the reader will be able to:

- Define culture and identify its expression.
- Compare and contrast the "melting pot" and "salad bowl" theories of acculturation.
- Identify the components of an accurate cultural assessment.
- Distinguish between primary and secondary cultural characteristics.
- List and define the key aspects of effective intercultural communication.
- Name two sources of information about transcultural nursing.

TRANSCULTURAL NURSING

Culture is a powerful influence on how nurses and clients interpret and respond to health care. Both nurses and clients expect to be treated with respect and understanding for their individuality no matter what their cultural origins. Nurses who understand essential characteristics of transcultural nursing will be able to provide competent and culturally sensitive care for clients from all cultural backgrounds.

WHAT IS CULTURE?

Culture is defined and understood in several ways. Culture may be seen as a group's acceptance of a set of attitudes, ideologies, values, beliefs, and behaviors that influence the way the members of the group express themselves. For example, members of a political party, although diverse in other ways, may be viewed as a culture because of their beliefs and ideologies. Cultural expression assumes many forms, including language; spirituality; works of art; group customs and traditions; food preferences; response to illness, stress, pain, **bereavement,** anger, and sorrow; decision making; and even world philosophy.

A Powerful Influence
An individual's cultural orientation is the result of a learning process that literally starts at birth and continues throughout the life span. Behaviors, beliefs, and attitudes are transmitted from one generation to the next. Although expressions of culture are primarily unconscious, they have a profound effect on an individual's interactions and response to the health-care system.

Mrs. Su Sung, who is 74 years old, is brought into the emergency department (ED) by her family because of "very bad indigestion that won't go away." Three family members (a middle-aged man and woman and a younger woman) accompany the elderly lady. They are discussing her condition in a mixture of English and another language the nurse does not recognize. Because the client does not seem to understand any English, the nurse attempts to address the family. The younger woman speaks only broken English but manages to explain that the client is her grandmother and that she is accompanied by her mother and father, who speak even less English than she does. By default, the granddaughter serves as the translator. After much prompting, she explains that her grandmother arrived in the United States for a visit only 2 days ago from a small mountain village in Korea where she has lived all her life. She had been having periodic episodes of "indigestion" for several weeks before the visit and used traditional herbal teas prescribed by the local healer to treat her condition. On the basis of further assessment and a diagnostic test, it is determined that Mrs. Sung had an extensive myocardial infarction at least 1 week before her trip and is currently in a mild state of congestive heart failure (CHF).

She is given medications for the chest pain and CHF and is started on anticoagulant medications in the ED. She is then transferred to the coronary care unit (CCU), where she is scheduled to have coronary angiography the next day. The angiogram shows multiple blockages in her coronary arteries and extensive myocardial damage. Because of her age and the extensive damage to her heart, the physician thinks it would be too risky to attempt bypass surgery and decides to monitor her closely and treat her medically until she is stable enough to have a balloon angioplasty.

When the CCU nurse assigned to Mrs. Sung enters the room at the beginning of her shift the day after the angiogram, she finds the client covered with four heavy blankets and a bedspread and sweating profusely. When the nurse attempts to remove the excessive bed covers, the client's daughter protests vehemently in Korean and puts the blankets back on as soon as the nurse leaves the room. The daughter seems to think that her mother is sick because she is too cold and gives the elderly woman hot herbal drinks from a thermos bottle she has brought from home.

When the granddaughter arrives, the nurse explains to her why excessive heat is harmful to the client's cardiac status and why she needs to follow the diet restrictions prescribed by the physician. The ingredients of the herbal drinks are unknown, and there may be some serious interactions with the numerous medications the client is receiving. The granddaughter translates this information to her mother, who seems to become even angrier with the nurse.

Although she outwardly seems to comply with the restrictions, she continues the traditional folk treatments in secret, believing the Western hospital food is bad for her mother's health.

Culture is not a monolithic concept. Any individual probably belongs to several subcultures within his or her major culture.

Mrs. Sung is very quiet and hardly ever asks for help. When she does talk to her family, the conversation is usually about the airplane flight to the United States and the belief that high altitude probably caused all Mrs. Sung's problems.

Her condition gradually deteriorates during her hospitalization, despite all the medical treatment. The nurse and physician tell the family about the client's worsening condition and the likelihood that she will not survive the hospitalization, but they refuse to relay the information to the client.

Although this situation is fictitious, it demonstrates some of the potential problems that nurses may encounter when interacting with clients who come from a strong traditional cultural background. Culture is, among other things, a belief system that has been developed over a person's lifetime and, like all strongly held belief systems, is difficult to change. In the case of Mrs. Sung, it is easy to see the futility of attempting to change her belief system in a short period of time with a limited number of interactions. Another important aspect of the situation is the effect of the family. Rather than being helpful to the care of this client or attempting to alter her belief systems to follow care recommendations, the family reinforced the client's beliefs.

Concepts of Culture

Culture is not a monolithic concept. Any individual probably belongs to several subcultures within his or her major culture. Subcultures develop when members of the group accept outside values in addition to those of their dominant culture. Even within a given culture, many variations may exist. For example, it is logical to conclude that people who live in the United States all belong to the American culture and are very similar in most ways. However, teenagers living in the rural areas of Oklahoma may find it difficult to relate to teenagers raised in the inner city of Philadelphia. Even though they speak the same language and share some similar interests, they have so many different past experiences that change their perspectives on life that it may be difficult for them to relate to each other.

> *Many individuals who migrate to the United States from other countries now cling tenaciously to their traditional cultural practices and languages, resulting in a phenomenon called multiculturalism.*

Culture can be considered a type of flawed photocopy machine that makes duplicates of the original document with minor differences. As a society attempts to preserve itself by passing down its values, beliefs, and customs to the next generation, slight variations in the practices inevitably occur. The key parts of the culture remain similar, but other parts change greatly owing to effects from both within and outside the group.

Diversity

Diversity is a term used to explain the differences between cultures. The characteristics that define diversity can be divided into two groups: primary and secondary.

1. Primary characteristics tend to be more obvious, including nationality, race, color, gender, age, and religious beliefs.

2. Secondary characteristics include socioeconomic status, education, occupation, length of time away from the country of origin, gender issues, residential status, and sexual orientation. These may be more difficult to identify, although they may have an even more profound effect on the person's cultural identity than the primary characteristics.

When individuals make generalizations about others based on the obvious primary characteristics and do not take the time to consider the secondary characteristics, they are stereotyping the other person. Stereotyping is an oversimplified belief, conception, or opinion about another person (or group) based on a limited amount of information.

MELTING POT VERSUS SALAD BOWL

The United States has traditionally been considered a melting pot of world cultures. Early in the history of the United States, most people who came from distant lands were eager to be assimilated into American culture. Many people Americanized their names, shed their traditional dress, learned American manners and customs as quickly as possible, and made heroic attempts to learn English without the benefit of formal schooling—all so they could "fit in" with their new homeland. Until recently, most people who immigrated to this country were very willing to acculturate (i.e., to alter their own cultural practices in an attempt to become more like members of the new culture). The end result was a blending, or melting pot, of cultures.

Multiculturalism

Since the early 1970s, the practice of intentional acculturation by immigrating cultures seems to have fallen by the wayside. Many individuals who migrate to the United States from other countries now cling tenaciously to their traditional cultural practices and languages, resulting in a phenomenon called multiculturalism. Rather than blending smoothly into the bigger pot as former immigrants have done, the modern immigrants maintain their own unique flavors and textures, much like the ingredients in a large tossed salad. As an ever-growing phenomenon, multiculturalism is something that health-care providers need to be aware of; they must learn ways of adapting their health practices to allow for these differences.

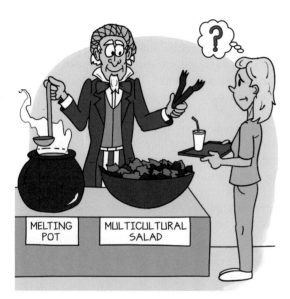

Drawbacks and Benefits. There are drawbacks and benefits to both approaches. In the era of the melting pot, individuals who attempted to retain their native beliefs, customs, and languages were often ridiculed, scorned, and generally made to feel they were outsiders to the mainstream culture. When they did become homogenized into the American culture, learned the language of the dominant society, and made an effort to be seen as belonging, they were more likely to be accepted as equals and quickly advanced up the socioeconomic ladder.

Cultural Relativism

The current salad bowl trend has the advantage of allowing individuals in the dominant culture to gain an appreciation of other cultures for their unique contributions to society. The drawback of the salad bowl is that it tends to create pockets of culturally different individuals who live in, but only have minimal interaction with, mainstream American society. Because they do not speak the language or refuse to accept the customs of the dominant culture, it may

be more difficult for them to advance their socioeconomic status.

The salad bowl process has also given rise to cultural relativism among some groups. Cultural relativism occurs when members of a strong cultural group understand their culture and group members only from their own viewpoint rather than from that of the larger culture. They do not try to understand the larger culture's unique characteristics, values, and beliefs.

Heritage Consistency

Some cultural groups manage to blend the melting pot and the salad bowl together through a rather complex process sometimes called heritage consistency. Outwardly, they may become acculturated to the point where they wear business suits, speak passable English, eat fast food, and go to movies. However, when they are at home, or with groups from their traditional culture, they speak their native language, wear their traditional clothes, eat ethnically correct meals, and generally follow their native customs.

> ### What Do You Think?
>
> Identify and rank by priority at least five of your own health-care values (e.g., exercise, immunizations). Identify five health-care values of a culture with which you are familiar. How do these values compare with your own?

This approach to acculturation has the advantages of allowing them to fit in and advance in the larger culture while retaining many of the elements of their traditional culture that provide a sense of stability to their lives. It does, however, create in some individuals a type of cultural confusion that may lead to increased tension and anxiety.

U.S. ETHNIC POPULATION TRENDS

A Population Shift

Rapid population growth in ethnic groups has been the trend in the United States for many years. According to U.S. Census Bureau statistics, in the year 2006 (the last year data were available) approximately 100 million, or 33 percent, of the entire U.S. population was composed of minority groups, up from 30 percent in the year 2000. If current trends continue, it is projected that by the year 2080, the Caucasian population will be a minority group constituting 48.9 percent of the total population of the United States. In states such as California, the white population may be a minority as early as 2030.

Contributing to the rapid growth in minority populations is the increasing number of immigrants coming to the United States. Between 1920 and 2000, the number of legal immigrants each year increased from 500,000 to more than 6 million. Currently the largest numbers of immigrants are from Asia, Mexico, and Central and South America. Fewer immigrants have come from Africa and Europe than in previous years.

The Need for Transcultural Nursing
Culturally Competent Care

The percentage of minority nurses does not reflect the national population trends. Despite efforts on the part of the National League for Nursing (NLN), American Association of Colleges of Nursing (AACN), and other organizations concerned with nursing education, minority nurses have remained constant at approximately 10.7 percent of the registered nurses (RNs) practicing in the United States. The percentage of men who are RNs is 5.8 percent, up slightly over the past decade. The latest reported statistics from the NLN in 2009 demonstrate a marked increase in the number of minority students enrolled in basic nursing programs, from 15 percent in 2000 to 29 percent in 2009. In a perfect world, the percentage of RNs from various minority groups should be approximately 33 percent and would mirror the percentage from each minority group.

Despite the relatively low number of minority nurses, it is expected that nurses from one culture should be able to give culturally competent care to individuals from any other culture. Being on the front lines of health care, nursing is the one profession that is continually confronted with cultural changes that result from ethnic shifts in the population. Nurses now recognize they can no longer use traditional ethnocentric models to guide their practice

Despite the relatively low number of minority nurses, it is expected that nurses from one culture should be able to give culturally competent care to individuals from any other culture.

and protocols. Nurses are beginning to promote an understanding of individuals from other cultures and improve the overall quality of health care.

Coverage for Minorities

The Medicare and Medicaid laws that evolved out of the social programs of the 1960s have increased the number of culturally diverse clients with whom nurses come in contact. Historically, many minority groups tend to be among the poorest segments of the population. Before the Medicare and Medicaid legislation that expanded government-funded health care to cover all welfare recipients, some ethnic minorities were unable to afford health care and were seen in the health-care setting only when severely ill. Ethnic minorities are now covered by these laws and, by their increasing numbers in all levels and areas of health care, have prompted nurses to become more sensitive to the transcultural aspects of their work.

Since the 1970s, transcultural nursing has become an important subject in most nursing programs. However, nursing education has taken only the first unsteady steps on the path to seeking a true integration of cultural competence into daily practice. As technological and transportation advances bring more and more people from different cultures closer together, there will be an increased demand for nurses who can practice effectively in a culturally diverse society. Many challenges still lie ahead.

DEVELOPING CULTURAL AWARENESS

Developing cultural awareness is the first step in becoming a culturally competent nurse. One of the main challenges for nurses who practice in a culturally diverse environment is to understand the client's perspective of what is happening in the health-care setting. From a cultural viewpoint, it may be very different from what the nurse believes is occurring.

Awareness Begins at Home

A nurse develops cultural awareness only when he or she is able to recognize and value all aspects of a client's culture, including beliefs, customs, responses, methods of expression, language, and social structure. However, merely learning about another person's culture does not guarantee that the nurse will have cultural awareness. Nurses must first understand their own cultural background and explore the origins of their own prejudiced and biased views of others. Several tools have been developed to measure a person's cultural awareness.

Cultural awareness begins with an understanding of one's own cultural values and health-care beliefs. To those unfamiliar with a particular culture's health-care beliefs, many of the health-care practices may appear meaningless, strange, or even dangerous.

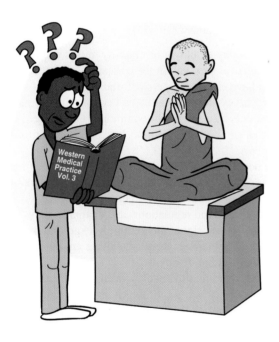

Beliefs about health care are based in part on knowledge and are often related to religious beliefs. For example, if a particular society has no knowledge of bacteria as a cause of infection, antibiotics may seem useless in achieving a cure for the disease. On the other hand, if a society believes that illness is caused by evil spirits entering the body as the result of curses by witches or medicine men, practices such as incantations; use of ritualistic objects like bones, feathers, or incense; and even blood-letting and purgatives to release the spirit from the body are logical approaches to achieving a cure.

Cultural Belief Systems
The Purpose of Tradition

Cultural belief systems are highly complex. For example, some Native American groups attributed twin births to witchcraft and believed that one of the twin infants had to die so that the other might live. These beliefs and practices are usually kept as closely guarded secrets among the group's members, and there may even be some type of sanction or punishment for members who reveal the belief.

Many cultural beliefs develop over time from a trial-and-error process that has both benefits and drawbacks. For instance, several Native American tribes that live in the Western desert have developed the practice of keeping infants in cradle boards until they begin walking. This practice, from a safety viewpoint, protects the crawling infant from injury and bites from creatures that are commonly found in the desert, such as scorpions, rattlesnakes, and poisonous insects or lizards. However, the practice tends to delay the leg muscle development of the child and increases the incidence of hip dysplasia because of the child's position in the cradle board.

Some cultural beliefs have a primary purpose of explaining unusual or unpredictable events. For example, many traditional Vietnamese Americans believe that mental illness results from some action that offended one or more of the gods. They also believe that a family member who is mentally ill brings disgrace on the family, and thus knowledge of the illness must be kept secret, especially from strangers. As a result, traditional shamans, or priest-doctors, are sought to attempt to appease the offended deity through rituals and prayers. Only with great reluctance will a traditional Vietnamese American family seek therapy or medication for a mental illness.

Cultural Values

The several sources of the development of cultural values include religious beliefs, world view and philosophy, and group customs. The values that underlie any particular culture are powerful forces that affect all aspects of a person's life, ranging from individual actions and decision-making to health-care behaviors and life-goal setting. Values, which are discussed in Chapter 7, are the ideals or concepts that give meaning to an individual's life. They are deeply ingrained, and most individuals will strongly resist any attempt to change their value structure.

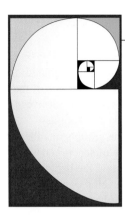

Issues Now

Minority Nurses Needed for the Future of Nursing

Recruiting, retaining, and reshaping the role of minority nurses has been a primary concern of the health-care industry for almost a decade. Initiatives have been implemented by both the private sector and governmental agencies to increase the numbers of minority nurses and meet the needs of the ever-shifting client demographics.

Recent studies have shown that there has been only a slight increase in the number of minority nurses. Based on the estimated number of 2.9 million licensed RNs in the United States, the following percentages are found in each minority group:

- African American, 4.2 percent (122,495)
- Asian, 3.1 percent (89,976)
- Hispanic, 0.3 percent (48,009)
- American Indian or Alaska Native, 1.4 percent (19,473)

Hospitals have been the primary employer of minority nurses and recognize that their employment is a matter of survival. In the competition to attract clients, hospitals cannot afford to have clients feel uncomfortable because of cultural diversity issues. A recent survey showed that 88 percent of minority nurses are employed in nursing, whereas only 82 percent of nonminority nurses are. Also, 85 percent of minority nurses are working full-time, but that number drops to 65 percent for nonminority nurses.

Although hospitals and health care in general acknowledge the need for more minority nurses, some nurses are experiencing barriers to their career mobility. Although the core issues are not unlike those that all nurses experience—understaffing, frustration with paperwork and regulations, and unappreciative administration and physicians—they also feel that their ethnic background may be hindering their chance for promotion. Sometimes their capabilities are questioned because of their differences, and that is a big deterrent.

The role of minority nurses continues to develop as an issue for the future of health care. Not only are they necessary because of the changing demographics of the population, but many in the health-care system believe that it is a sound economic policy to have more minority nurses. To help recruit nurses and retain those who are already practicing, several organizations have been established that nurses can contact. The National Coalition of Ethnic Minority Nurse Associations and the Tennessee Hospital Association's Council on Diversity are available for assistance.

Sources: Nursing Statistics 2009. Retrieved December, 2010 from http://www.minoritynurse.com.
Percentage of Students Enrolled in Basic Nursing Programs 2008–2009. Retrieved December, 2010 from http://www.nln.org/research/slides.

Cultural values are neither right nor wrong; they exist in a culture as the result of a long-term process of development that can often be traced back to a need for group survival. However, when judged from the perspective of other cultures, they may seem strange or perhaps harmful. Because it makes nurses feel secure and even superior, there is a tendency to transfer to clients health-care expectations based on the nurse's own cultural framework. This approach often leads the nurse to fail when trying to change health-care behaviors.

Recognizing Health-Care Practices
Changing the Client's Values

It is important to recognize that one of the primary functions of nurses is to change clients' values, particularly values about health care. It is not an easy task. The first step, always, is to recognize that the nurse comes from a particular culture that has its own set of health-care values. Like all values, these have developed over time and are dependent on the nurse's education, upbringing, religious beliefs, and cultural background.

The next step is to identify the culture of the client and recognize specific health-care practices that are both similar to and different from those of the nurse. The nurse must then make a decision about whether it is desirable or possible to change the client's values and if the end result would be worth the effort.

When Is Persuasion Appropriate?

For example, many cultures have strong values concerning pregnancy and the birth of children. In traditional Middle Eastern families, the birth process is valued as an event strictly involving women, and the father is usually not present to either witness or assist in the delivery. However, midwives and obstetric nurses from the current American culture place a high value on the father's participation in the birth event as a way of promoting stronger family ties and starting the bonding process as soon as possible. The nurse who takes care of a Middle Eastern family must decide whether to try to convince the father to stay in the delivery room during the delivery. In any event, the ultimate outcome remains relatively unchanged. Even without the father in the delivery room, the child is delivered safely, and only the bonding process with the father is delayed.

Some African cultures have discovered over time that a woman who delivers a small infant will have a much easier time during labor and delivery. Small infants usually have fewer traumatic birth defects, and there are fewer stillbirths and a higher maternal survival rate. In some traditional central African homeland settings where there is little skilled health care available, the value of having small infants helps in the survival of the group. The custom of feeding pregnant women only a corn-mush cereal throughout their pregnancies ensures small babies at birth.

In the United States, where good prenatal nutrition is highly valued, this traditional practice is seen as dangerous to both the mother and the infant. Poor prenatal nutrition has been related to developmental delays, mental retardation, and skeletal deformities in infants as well as maternal malnutrition that can lead to infectious diseases and inability to breast-feed. In this situation, changing such practices of traditional African American women would be rewarded by healthier babies and mothers.

Assessing Culture

Obtaining accurate cultural assessments can be time consuming and difficult. However, the only way nurses can avoid imposing their cultural values and practices on others, and develop plans of care based on their knowledge about others' beliefs and customs, is to make a concerted effort to obtain this information. Several cultural assessment tools for clients have been developed—some short and directed, others lengthy and complicated. One of the most thorough cultural assessments developed to date is based on Purnell's Model for Cultural Competence (Box 22.1). Although this tool is lengthy, it can provide a good overview of the client's culture. Nurses should not neglect completing an assessment of their own culture as well.

Beginning the Assessment

Most busy nurses do not have the time to complete this assessment on every client from a different culture. However, the following key questions can serve as a starting point for a cultural assessment:

- Why do you think you are ill? What was the cause of the illness?
- What was going on at the time the illness started?
- How does the illness affect your body and health?
- Do you consider this to be a serious illness?
- If you were at home, what type of treatments or medications would you use? How would these treatments help?

B o x 2 2 . 1

The 12 Domains of Cultural Assessment: Purnell's Model for Cultural Competence

I. Overview, inhabited localities, and topography overview
  A. Heritage and residence
  B. Reasons for migration and associated economic factors
  C. Educational status and occupation
II. Communications
  A. Dominant language and dialects
  B. Cultural communication patterns
  C. Temporal relationships
  D. Format for names
III. Family roles and organization
  A. Head of household and gender roles
  B. Prescriptive, restrictive, and taboo behaviors
  C. Family roles and priorities
  D. Alternative lifestyles
IV. Workforce issues
  A. Culture in the workplace
  B. Issues related to autonomy
V. Biocultural ecology
  A. Skin color and biological variations
  B. Diseases and health conditions
  C. Variations in drug metabolism
VI. High-risk behaviors
  A. High-risk behaviors
  B. Health-care practices

VII. Nutrition
  A. Meaning of food
  B. Dietary practices for health promotion
VIII. Pregnancy and childbearing practices
  A. Fertility practices and views toward pregnancy
IX. Death rituals
  A. Death rituals and expectations
  B. Responses to death and grief
X. Spirituality
  A. Religious practices and use of prayer
  B. Meaning of life and individual sources of strength
  C. Spiritual beliefs and health-care practices
XI. Health-care practices
  A. Health-seeking beliefs and behaviors
  B. Responsibility for health care
  C. Folklore practices
  D. Barriers to health care
  E. Cultural responses to health and illness
  F. Blood transfusions and organ donation
XII. Health-care practitioners
  A. Traditional versus biomedical care
  B. Status of health-care providers

Source: Purnell LD, Paulanka BJ: Transcultural health care. Philadelphia, F. A. Davis, 1998, with permission.

- What type of treatment do you expect from the health-care system?
- How has your illness affected your ability to live normally?
- If you do not get better, what do you think will happen?

Because clients from different cultures may feel uncomfortable revealing information about cultural beliefs, values, and practices to strangers, it is a good idea to begin your assessment by asking some general questions. A client is more likely to trust a nurse who demonstrates interest in that person as an individual. Only after a warm and trusting environment has been established will a client be willing to reveal the more hidden aspects of his or her culture to the nurse.

Understanding Physical Variations

Physical assessments made on individuals from other cultures require a certain level of cultural awareness and competence. Although the assessment techniques used for different individuals may be identical, the nurse needs to know the basic biological and physical variations among ethnic groups. The interpretation of assessment findings may be affected by ethnic variations in anatomical structure or characteristics (e.g., children from some Asian cultures may fall below the normal growth level on a standardized American growth chart because of their genetically smaller stature).

Changes in skin color may also affect the interpretation of assessment findings (e.g., cyanosis

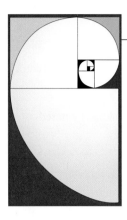

Issues in Practice

Cultural Aspects of Organ Donation

"Sarah, are you going to ask them?" The tall, haggard third-year trauma resident stood across the desk from me and eyed me with apprehension.

"Well," I sighed, "he's medically suitable and has been declared brain dead. So, yes. I'm going to ask them." I had been Coordinator of the New Mexico Organ Procurement Organization for more than 2 years and had asked families for permission to obtain organs for transplantation literally hundreds of times.

"But they're Navajo," he said.

"Organ donation is an option for them," I replied. "They deserve to be offered the option at the very least."

"Can I come in with you?" he asked. "There's a lot of them in there."

"Sure," I said. When a traditional Navajo came to the hospital for treatment with "white man's" medicine, often the whole family came too.

So, after reviewing the client's case file to identify the legal next-of-kin and doing a few laps around the intensive care unit (ICU) to work out my adrenaline, the resident and I went into the ICU conference room to approach a traditional Navajo family for consent for organ donation.

As I entered the room, 13 pairs of dark eyes looked up at me. I ran through in my head all the things I had learned regarding the American Indian culture in my training. Keep it low-key. Don't make prolonged eye contact. American Indians are stoic in their grief. I took a deep breath, let the resident introduce me, and we began our conversation.

The family was young, and the patient had never married, so the oldest daughter was making the decisions. She had a lot of good questions for me, as did the rest of the family, and I sat on the floor in front of them with my knees drawn up to my chest and talked with them for a long time.

"You know we're Navajo?" one of her brothers asked me. "Organ donation is against our beliefs."

"I realize that," I said. "But you have the option to save a life, possibly as many as three lives, and I wanted to let you know."

"Our uncle got a kidney transplant last year," the oldest daughter said while looking at her brother. "I think we owe something back. Can we have some time to talk about this?"

I thanked them for their time, expressed my condolences again, and left the room with the resident.

Once we were back on the unit, the resident got excited.

"Oh, man. I think they're going to say yes," he said, shifting from one foot to another. "That would be so awesome to have the first Navajo donor here."

I could see the story starting to form in his head and smiled at him when I saw the anticipation and hopefulness in his eyes. I helped with that American Indian donor. It was so cool.

Just then, the doors to the ICU swung open and a pair of elderly, withered-looking American Indian women walked into the unit and right up to the desk where I was sitting. They inquired as to which room my client was in and went into the room after I told them. They hovered at the client's bedside for several

(continued)

Issues in Practice continued

minutes, regarding the beeping medication pumps, the monitors and the ventilator with disdain.

"Don't get your hopes up," I said to him under my breath.

Silently, the pair left the unit through the doors they had just entered, making eye contact with no one, and showing no emotion.

"Who are they?" the resident asked.

"I believe those were the tribal elders," I said.

He looked at me with disbelief. "What do we do now?"

"Now we wait," I said.

I kept myself busy shuffling papers and returned a couple of phone calls. I was playing Free Cell on the computer when the oldest daughter appeared around the corner. I could tell she had been crying.

"Can we see the doctor in our room?" she asked.

"Sure, wait here and I'll go get him," I said.

I went around the corner where he was lounging with his feet propped up on the desk. He was chatting with the unit clerk. "I really think they're going to do it," he said.

"The family wants to see you," I interrupted.

When he looked at me, I saw a question mark on his face. I returned the look with one of my own. Having been in this situation a couple of times before, I had a feeling I knew what the outcome would be.

We walked around the corner, and he went into the conference room with the family, and I returned to my desk to wait.

Two minutes later he was back. He slumped into the chair beside me. "They declined," he sighed disappointedly. "What do I do now?"

"You," I said, "are done. Thank you very much for all your time and hard work. I've got to do some paperwork and call in the decline, and then I'm going home."

He sighed again and then patted my leg. "Well, good effort."

QUESTIONS FOR THOUGHT

1. Was it ethical to ask the family about organ donation when American Indian beliefs generally prohibit it? Do you know of any American Indian organ donors?

2. Was there another possible approach to seeking permission from the family?

3. Why are American Indians opposed to organ donation when they routinely accept organs for transplantation?

Source: Sarah T. Catalano, Coordinator, New Mexico Organ Procurement Organization.

in people with a light versus a dark complexion). To determine whether the client's skin color is normal or abnormal, the nurse must know what constitutes the normal color for a particular ethnic group. In assessing for cyanosis, the nurse may need to examine the client's oral mucosa and may also need to measure capillary refill times to determine whether the client has cyanosis.

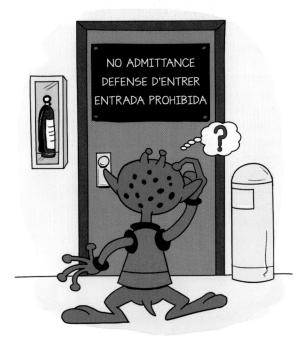

The ultimate goal of cultural assessment, as with all assessments, is to provide the best care possible for the client. A fundamental belief that nurses hold to strongly is that all clients have a right to self-determination, including the customs, practices, and values that emanate from their culture. By considering both the cultural and ethnic variables of each client, nurses will avoid practice that is ethnocentric and conducted strictly from the nurse's cultural viewpoint.

PROVIDING CULTURALLY COMPETENT CARE

Transcultural Understanding
Cultural competence has become a buzzword in the health-care system. The term has several divergent definitions, with little consensus among cultural experts. However, cultural competence as it relates to

nursing can be regarded as the provision of effective care for clients who belong to diverse cultures, based on the nurse's knowledge and understanding of the values, customs, beliefs, and practices of the culture.

What Do You Think?
Using Purnell's cultural assessment tool, assess your own cultural background. In what areas of your own culture are you lacking knowledge?

Provision of culturally competent care requires the development of certain interpersonal skills that allow nurses to work with individuals and groups in the community. The primary skills required for cultural competence include communication, understanding, and sensitivity. Although the basic types of cultural skills are similar, their application within and between cultural groups may differ greatly. The development of cultural competence is not a one-time skill to check off on a skills checklist; rather, it is an ongoing process that continues throughout the nurse's career.

Transcultural Communication
The ability to communicate is the foundation on which culturally competent care is built. The most obvious barrier to culturally competent care for the non–English-speaking client is the lack of a common language (Box 22.2). Communication is a highly complex process that requires both verbal and nonverbal exchanges. Nonverbal communication includes (but is not limited to) body language, facial expressions, eye contact, personal space, touch and body contact, formality of names, and time awareness. Other factors that affect communication are volume of voice, tone, and acceptable greetings. Often clients communicate differently with family and friends than they do with health-care personnel. Nurses should be aware that in some cultures (e.g., those with a strong caste system, which involves a class structure) communication between those in the upper and lower classes may be affected by tradition. For example, some cultures hold the role of women in health care in high esteem, whereas other cultures may consider women in health care as the bottom rung on the ladder.

Nonverbal Responses
Nurses who work with non–English-speaking clients need to develop alternative ways to measure a client's

Box 22.2

Guidelines for Communicating with Non–English-Speaking Clients

1. Use interpreters rather than translators. Translators just restate the words from one language to another. An interpreter decodes the words and provides the meaning behind the message.
2. Use dialect-specific interpreters whenever possible.
3. Use interpreters trained in the health-care field.
4. Give the interpreter time alone with the client.
5. Provide time for translation and interpretation.
6. Be aware that interpreters may affect the reporting of symptoms, insert their own ideas, or omit information.
7. Avoid the use of relatives who may distort information or not be objective.
8. Avoid using children as interpreters, especially with sensitive topics.
9. Use same-age and same-gender interpreters whenever possible. However, clients from cultures who have a high regard for elders may prefer an older interpreter.
10. Maintain eye contact with both the client and the interpreter to elicit feedback and read nonverbal clues.
11. Remember that clients can usually understand more than they express; thus, they need time to think in their own language. They are alert to the health-care provider's body language and may forget some or all of their English in times of stress.
12. Speak slowly without exaggerating mouthing, allow time for translation, use active rather than passive tense, wait for feedback, and restate the message. Do not rush; do not speak loudly. Use a reference book with common phrases, such as *Roget's International Thesaurus* or *Taber's Cyclopedic Medical Dictionary.*
13. Use as many words as possible in the client's language and use nonverbal communication when unable to understand the language.
14. If an interpreter is unavailable, the use of a translator may be acceptable. The difficulty with translation is omission of parts of the message; distortion of the message, including transmission of information not given by the speaker; and messages not being fully understood.
15. Note that social class differences between the interpreter and the client may result in the interpreter's not reporting information that he or she perceives as superstitious or unimportant.

Source: Purnell LD, Paulanka BJ: Transcultural health care: A culturally competent approach (3rd ed). Philadelphia, F. A. Davis, 2008, with permission.

understanding rather than depending only on a verbal response. Nurses must be cautious when interpreting the nonverbal responses from some cultural groups. Some cultures respond to all questions with the reply "yes," a nod, or a smile. This response, in the American culture, usually indicates understanding and **compliance.** However, particularly in Asian cultures, nodding and smiling can be signs of respect for the nurse's position or an attempt to avoid confrontation. The following is a classic example:

An English-speaking nurse gave a non–English-speaking Asian client preoperative instructions about how to prepare an abdominal surgical site. She thought that she had shown the client how the bottle of povidone-iodine, a powerful skin disinfectant, was to be used in scrubbing the area. The client smiled and nodded throughout the instruction. When asked whether he had any questions, he did not respond. The nurse took the silence to mean that he had no questions. When the nurse left the room, the client promptly drank the whole bottle of povidone-iodine. Fortunately, the error was discovered immediately, and no long-term complications occurred from the accident.

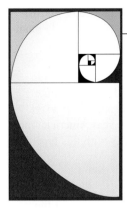

Issues Now

Informed Consent Requires Understanding

Sinwan Ho is an elderly woman from an Asian culture who speaks very little English. She was admitted to the Gastromed Health Care center for a routine colonoscopy and polypectomy which was performed on May 20, 2003, by Lawrence Kluger, MD. During the procedure the bowel was perforated. The next day Ms. Ho underwent a laparotomy with removal of the damaged part of the colon and the formation of a colostomy.

Ms. Ho was readmitted on September 2, 2003 to have the colostomy closed and the colon reconnected. She recovered well, but several years later she began experiencing abdominal pain and gastrointestinal symptoms. It was determined that lesions had formed in the reconnected bowel and were closing the bowel. On April 20, 2006, Ms. Ho was readmitted and another colostomy was performed. Later that year on September 6, 2006, the colostomy was again closed with reconnection of the bowel. The client had a total of five surgeries related to the first routine procedure.

Initially sued for malpractice, the court could not find conclusive evidence that Dr. Kluger had committed any medical errors, and the case was dismissed as a "bad outcome."

Later a suit was filed on behalf of Ms. Ho. According to her testimony and that of a friend, Kenneth Lee, she had not been properly informed of the possible complications of the procedure in language that she could understand. She did sign the informed consent form when it was handed to her. The court determined that lack of clear communication of the possible complications was a deviation in the standard of care.

In further testimony, Dr. Kluger admitted that he knew the client did not speak much English and that he had made no attempt to find an interpreter to help explain the procedure and the possible complications such as bowel perforation and colostomy. However, his lawyer argued that because the possibility of an intestinal perforation with a resulting colostomy is so low, revealing that information did not meet the state's requirement as a "reasonable degree of medical probability."

The court ruled that Dr. Kluger's failure to communicate the complications of the procedure adequately did not meet the requirement for malpractice. However, it did rule that there was a case for medical negligence based on the premise that failure to disclose what a reasonable and prudent client would want to know is a deviation from a standard of care.

The case is still under appeal.

Source: Ho v. Kluger, A.2d, 2009 WL2431591 (N.J. App., August 11, 2009). Retrieved November, 2010 from http://findacase.com/wfrmdocviewer.aspx/xq/fac

Speech Patterns

The use of silence by some cultural groups has led to misunderstandings in the health-care setting. For example, Asian Americans consider silence to be a sign of respect, particularly for elders, whereas Arab Americans and the English use silence to gain privacy. Among many people in Europe (e.g., the French, Russians, and Spanish), silence often indicates agreement.

Variations in communication style also account for misunderstandings and miscommunications. Factors such as loudness, intonation, rhythm, and speed of speech all are important in communication. Among certain cultural groups, American nurses have a reputation for speaking at a rapid rate and for using medical jargon. Some nurses also have a reputation for their tendency to increase the volume of their voices when communicating with clients who do not speak English, as if talking more loudly will increase understanding.

On the other hand, groups such as American Indians and Asian Americans speak more softly and may be difficult to hear even when the nurse is standing at the bedside. These groups may misinterpret the louder, more forceful tone of the American nurse as an indication of anger. Arab American groups are often noted for their dramatic communication styles. Nurses may misinterpret this behavior as hostility, when in reality the client is merely trying to demonstrate a point using an emotional communication style. Nurses need to analyze their own speech patterns and consciously modify their tone and pace when working with different cultural groups to prevent misunderstandings.

Personal Matters

Nurses also need to recognize that certain groups are much less willing to disclose private matters or personal feelings than others. In general, clients from American or European origins tend to be less secretive about almost all issues because the practice of sharing has been encouraged from an early age. However, many Asian cultures, particularly the Japanese, are highly reluctant to discuss personal topics with either family or health-care providers.

Other groups, such as Mexican Americans, discuss personal issues openly with friends and family members but are reluctant to do so with health-care providers whom they do not know well.

Even within these groups there are wide variations. American women probably constitute one of the most open groups when it comes to expressing personal feelings, whereas American men tend to have much more difficulty with this type of communication.

Open-Ended Language

Nurses presume that all clients should trust them instantaneously just because they are nurses and should answer even the most personal questions immediately. As discussed earlier, it may be much more productive to start the communication process with small talk and general, nonthreatening questions to establish an atmosphere of trust.

> *Nurses who work with non–English-speaking clients need to develop alternative ways to measure a client's understanding rather than depending only on a verbal response.*

Often the use of open-ended questions and statements allows the client to express beliefs and opinions that would be difficult to discover through closed-ended questions that the client can answer with a simple "yes" or "no."

As the level of trust increases, the client will be more likely to reveal important information in the more sensitive areas of the assessment. In addition, sensitivity to the nonverbal aspects of the communication process allows nurses to use behaviors that increase trust and to avoid gestures, facial expressions, or eye contact that may relay a message of superiority, hostility, anger, or disapproval.

Touch Misinterpreted

The touching of clients from different cultures in ways that they consider inappropriate is a leading cause of miscommunication. American nurses are taught early in their first nursing classes, usually physical assessment or basic skill courses, that it is necessary to "lay on hands" in order to provide good care. Students who are reluctant to palpate the femoral pulses of their laboratory partner or remove a client's shirt to auscultate anterior heart and breath sounds may receive a failing grade for the course.

However, touching in other cultures conveys a number of alternative meanings, ranging from power, anger, and sexual arousal to affirmation, empathy, and cordiality. For example, it is generally not acceptable for men and women to touch in many Arab cultures, except in the privacy of the home and in the context of marriage. American women nurses who palpate pulses, listen to breath sounds, or palpate for tactile fremitus when assessing men from an Arab culture may be communicating a message that they never intended.

Some groups, such as Mexican Americans and Italian Americans, who frequently touch and hug family members and friends, are much less receptive to touching by strangers during health-care examinations, particularly if the health-care provider is of the opposite gender. In these situations it is extremely important for the nurse to explain, before the particular physical contact occurs, what he or she is going to do and why it should be done. The nurse should also avoid any unnecessary contact, such as palpation of femoral pulses when the client has pneumonia.

Personal Space

Closely related to the issue of touch is the concept of personal space. Personal space is a zone that individuals maintain around themselves in most casual social situations. When a person's personal space is violated, it often creates a generalized feeling of discomfort or threat, which causes the person to move away from the offending individual. Nurses routinely violate clients' personal space when performing physical assessments or providing basic care.

The distance required to maintain a comfortable personal space varies widely from one culture to another. People who belong to the European, Canadian, or American cultures usually require between 18 and 22 inches of distance for a comfortable personal space when communicating with strangers or casual acquaintances. In contrast, individuals from the Jewish, Arab, Turkish, and Middle Eastern cultures may require as little as 3 to 5 inches of personal space when talking with another person and often interpret physical closeness as a sign of acceptance. In addition, they prefer to stand face to face and maintain eye contact when they are talking.

> " *. . . touching in other cultures conveys a number of alternative meanings, ranging from power, anger, and sexual arousal to affirmation, empathy, and cordiality.* "

It is easy to understand why misinterpretations in communication might arise. A client from a Middle Eastern culture might judge an American nurse to be cold and aloof, although she is merely maintaining a comfortable personal space from the client. Likewise, an American nurse may feel physically threatened by the close communication style of a Turkish-American client and continually back away from the client in an attempt to re-establish his or her personal space.

Eye Contact

Similarly, eye contact communicates different messages to different cultures. Among American and many European cultures, making periodic eye contact during conversations indicates attentiveness to the communication and is a means of measuring the person's sincerity. Common sayings such as, "Look me in the eye and say that," and admonitions for public speakers to make eye contact with the audience emphasize the underlying positive value these cultures place on eye contact. Lack of eye contact may be interpreted as inattention, insincerity, or disregard.

In contrast, some American Indian cultures believe that the eyes are the windows of the soul and that direct eye contact by another may be interpreted as an attempt to "steal the soul" from the body. Between American Indian men, direct eye contact is a sign of challenge and aggression and may precipitate a violent, physical confrontation. Among some South American cultures, sustained eye contact is a sign of disrespect, whereas in other cultural groups, particularly Mexican Americans, eye contact with a child is believed to convey the *mal de ojo,* or "evil eye." Many childhood and adult illnesses among these cultures are attributed to the effects of the evil eye, and practices such as tying red cloths or strings around children's wrists are used to ward off illnesses. Eye contact, a routine part of American culture, has diverse and powerful meanings to clients from other cultures.

The complexity and importance of communication should never be underestimated when working with clients from diverse cultures. Merely speaking a language does not encompass the entirety of communication. Awareness of the meanings of gestures, body positions, facial expressions, and eye movements is essential in culturally competent communication.

LOOKING DEEPER

Several other elements must be considered for effective transcultural nursing, including passive obedience, cultural synergy, building on similarities, and conflict resolution. The term *passive obedience* refers to a type of behavior that develops when clients from a different culture believe that the nurse is an authority figure or expert in health-care matters. Although many cultures may display this type of behavior to some extent, it is most commonly seen among Asian American groups. These cultures try to cope with the uncertainty of their health status and the threat of an authority figure by becoming passively obedient. Rather than asking questions they think will reveal their lack of knowledge or confusion about some health-care issue or that they believe may challenge the authority of the nurse, they become passively obedient and compliant.

Cultural Conflicts
It is inevitable that conflicts will arise from time to time when a nurse cares for clients of different cultures. It is important to recognize that the origins of many conflicts reside within the individual. Nurses may label clients from other cultures as noncompliant, when in reality the nurse has an incomplete understanding of the client's culture or unrealistic expectations for behavior.

> **What Do You Think?**
>
> Think of the last client for whom you provided care. What were the cultural differences that affected the care you gave? What measures did you use to overcome these? What might you have done differently to improve care?

Other common reasons for noncompliance among culturally diverse clients include the lack of external symptoms of disease, inconvenient or painful treatments, and lack of external support from family members or close friends.

Respect for Healing Traditions
The nurse first needs to ask the client what traditional treatments are used in dealing with this disease. In some cases, in which the traditional treatments are similar to the ones used by the health-care facility, the nurse may be able to demonstrate this similarity to the client.

In other cases, the treatments may be very different. However, if culturally based alternative treatments do not interfere with the prescribed treatment plan or threaten the client's health, they can be used simultaneously with the standard medical treatments. For example, nurses who work in the American Indian health-care system and hospitals have become accustomed to finding bone fragments, feathers, and leather medicine pouches in the beds of their clients.

Cultural Synergy
Nurses who work actively to develop cultural synergy tend to be more successful in the delivery of competent transcultural care. *Cultural synergy* is a term that implies that health-care providers make a commitment not only to learn about other cultures but also to immerse themselves in those cultures. Nurses achieve cultural synergy when they begin to selectively include values, customs, and beliefs of other cultures in their own world views. The first step in cultural synergy is the desire to know everything about another culture and to purposely establish relationships with individuals from other cultures.

More Alike Than Different
Closely related to cultural synergy is the recognition that cultures are much alike in many aspects. It seems that most books and publications written about cultural diversity present only the diversity of cultures and not the similarities. Although recognition of cultural differences is important, it should be just one step toward the ultimate realization that there are more similarities than differences among diverse cultures.

Many colleges offer courses in comparative religions identifying the many similarities of the fundamental beliefs that underlie the major religions. However, many college courses on cultural diversity have not evolved past the point of identifying cultural differences. Perhaps this is due in part to the salad bowl approach to cultural communication that exists in current society. Perhaps a new approach to acculturation, based on the similarities between cultures rather than on the differences, needs to be developed.

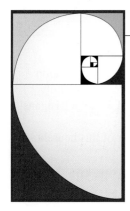

Issues in Practice

Case Study: Cultural Conflict Within a Family

In 1990, Jose Bisigan, aged 87 years, and his wife Carmen, aged 85, sold their small restaurant and immigrated to Los Angeles from a small town in the Visayan region of the Philippines. They came to join their firstborn daughter, nurse Felicia, aged 54, her husband, and their three children, aged 10 to 18. Mr. Bisigan speaks limited English and is in a poststroke rehabilitation unit. Since the stroke, he has had mild aphasia, mild confusion, and bladder and bowel continence problems. His hypertension and long-standing diabetes are controlled with medication and diet. His wife, daughter, and grandchildren have been supportive of him during this first hospitalization experience. Mr. Bisigan's family has cooperated with the health team, often agreeing with minimal resistance to the prescribed treatment management. The rehabilitation team recommended subacute rehabilitation treatment as part of the discharge plan.

As a businessman and the elder in the family household, Mr. Bisigan is looked to for counsel by the immediate and extended family. Mr. Bisigan's status, however, has caused friction between Felicia and her husband, Nestor, an American-born Filipino who works as a machinist. Nestor has accused Felicia of giving excessive attention to her mother and father. Felicia's worries about her parents' health have made Nestor very resentful. He has increased his already daily "outings with the boys." Felicia maintains a full-time position in acute care and a part-time night shift position in a nursing home.

Mr. Bisigan's discharge is pending, and a decision must be made before Medicare coverage runs out. Felicia has to consider the possible choices available to her father and the family's circumstances and expectations. Mrs. Bisigan, who is being treated for hypertension, has always deferred decisions to her husband and is looking to Felicia to make the decisions. Because of her work schedule, the absence of a responsible person at home, her mother's health problems, and inter-generational friction, Felicia considers nursing home placement. She is, however, reluctant to broach the subject with her father, who expects to be cared for at home. Mrs. Bisigan disagrees with putting her husband in a nursing home and is adamant that she will care for her husband at home.

Felicia delayed talking to her father until the rehabilitation team requested a meeting. At the meeting, Felicia indicated that she could not bring herself to present her plan to put her father in a nursing home because of her mother's objection and her own fear that her father will feel rejected. Feeling very much alone in resolving the issue about nursing home placement, she requested the team to act as intermediary for her and her family.

- Identify cultural family values that contribute to the conflicts experienced by each family member.
- Identify a culturally competent approach the team can use when discussing nursing home placement with the Bisigans.
- How might the rehabilitation program be presented to Mrs. Bisigan and still allow her to maintain her spousal role?
- Discuss at least three communication issues in the family that are culture-bound and suggest possible interventions.

(continued)

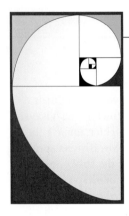

Issues in Practice   <small>continued</small>

- Identify psychocultural assessments that should be done by the rehabilitation team to have a greater understanding of the dynamics specific to this family.
- Identify health promotion counseling that might be discussed with the Bisigans' grandchildren.
- Identify and explain major sources of stress for each member of this household.

Source: Purnell LD, Paulanka BJ: Transcultural health care: A culturally competent approach (3rd ed). Philadelphia, F. A. Davis, 2008, with permission.

INFORMATION SOURCES FOR TRANSCULTURAL NURSING

From a Conference . . .

The recent explosion of interest in cultural diversity and transcultural nursing has led to a proliferation of literature on the topic. The origins of the current transcultural movement can be traced back to 1974, when a transcultural conference on communication and culture was held at the University of Hawaii School of Nursing. Following the success of this conference, a series of transcultural conferences were planned over the next year to bring together nurses, sociologists, anthropologists, and other social scientists to discuss issues that would eventually form the basis for transcultural nursing.

Not long after the Hawaii conference, the Transcultural Nursing Society was organized. It was incorporated in 1981 and began publishing its semiannual official journal, *Journal of Transcultural Nursing,* in 1989. It is now being published four times a year. In 1976, the American Nurses Association (ANA) recommended that multicultural content be included in nursing curricula. Since then, the ANA has organized the Council on Intercultural Nursing, which publishes the *Intercultural Nursing Newsletter.*

. . . to a Specialty

Since the 1980s, more and more universities and colleges have started offering graduate degrees in transcultural, cross-cultural, and international nursing. Graduates are now able to become certified transcultural nurses (CTNs) by completing oral and written examinations offered by the Transcultural Nursing Society. Nurses do not need to be from minority groups to obtain the CTN qualification.

Society has not remained stagnant during this period of development and organization. Growing numbers of immigrants, changing governmental regulations, and grassroots movements all have contributed to the pressure placed on nursing to recognize and effectively care for clients from different cultures.

Conclusion

The major changes in U.S. demographics that began in the 1980s—and have been accelerating ever since—require nurses to provide culturally sensitive care. A fundamental belief of professional nursing holds that all individuals are to be cared for with respect and dignity regardless of culture, beliefs, or disease process. Therefore, nurses must actively seek multicultural education.

However, nurses need to keep in mind that cultural assessments and decisions about care are relative to the nurse's personal experiences, beliefs, and culture. There is a natural tendency to unconsciously stereotype individuals from other cultures on the basis of one's internal value system. There is also a tendency to batch all individuals from one culture into a single group, when in reality there may be wide variations within the group.

It is a well-accepted belief that nurses who value cultural diversity will deliver higher-quality care. Nurses who have a high level of cultural knowledge and sensitivity maximize their nursing interventions when they become coparticipants and client advocates for individuals who might otherwise be lost in an impersonal health-care system. Only when nurses can understand the client's perspective, develop an open style of communication, become receptive to learning from clients of other cultures, and accept and work with the ambiguities inherent in the care of multicultural clients will they become truly culturally competent health-care providers.

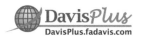

DavisPlus.fadavis.com

23

Developments in Current Nursing Practice

Barbara Bellfield
Joseph T. Catalano

Learning Objectives

After completing this chapter, the reader will be able to:

- Discuss the nurse's role in forensics, bioterrorism, disasters, entrepreneurship, legal consulting, and case management.
- Discuss ways in which to develop a nurse-run business.
- Identify factors that indicate the need for case management.
- Discuss the importance of the nurse's early recognition of a bioterrorist attack.
- Give examples of organizations that nurses can become involved in to provide assistance in the event of a disaster.

NEW ROLES FOR THE NURSE

The profession of nursing is dynamic and ever-changing. Nursing roles evolve and develop in response to societal needs. The recently passed Health Care Reform Act will open even more doors for professional nurses and provide opportunities for expanded practice. This chapter discusses the new and exciting practice roles in nursing. Included are discussions of forensic nursing, bioterrorism and disaster nursing, nurse entrepreneurs, nurse case managers, and legal nurse consultants.

FORENSIC NURSING

Forensic nursing is an emerging field that forms an alliance among nursing, law enforcement, and the forensic sciences. The term *forensic* means anything belonging to, or pertaining to, the law.

An Emerging Discipline

Forensic nursing, as defined by the International Association of Forensic Nurses (IAFN), is "the application of nursing science to public or legal proceedings; the application of the forensic aspects of health care combined with the bio-psycho-social education of the registered nurse (RN) in the scientific investigation and treatment of trauma and/or death of victims and perpetrators of abuse, violence, criminal activity and traumatic accidents." Forensic nurses provide a continuum of care to victims and their families, beginning in the emergency room or crime scene and leading to participation in the criminal investigation and the courts of law.[1]

Nurses, particularly emergency department (ED) nurses, have long provided care to victims of domestic violence, rape, and other injuries resulting from criminal acts. They have collected, preserved, and documented legal evidence, often without formal training. It was not until 1992 that the term *forensic nursing* was coined.

What Do You Think?

Do you know any nurses who are involved in forensic nursing? Is this a role that you might be interested in pursuing after graduation?

The IAFN was founded in the summer of 1992. Seventy-four nurses, primarily sexual assault nurse examiners, came together in Minneapolis, Minnesota, to develop an organization of nurses who practice within the arena of the law. This very diverse group includes, but is not limited to, legal nurse consultants, forensic nurse death investigators, forensic psychiatric nurses, and forensic correctional nurses.

The organization's membership tripled within its first year. By 1999, the IAFN had more than 1800 members. The American Nurses Association (ANA) recognized forensic nursing as a subspecialty in 1995, and the Scope and Standards of Forensic Practice was established in 1997. Because this is a new field, the definition of the forensic nurse role is continuing to evolve. With the formation of the IAFN and the designation of the forensic specialty, nurses were given an identity and recognition for a role they have long been performing.

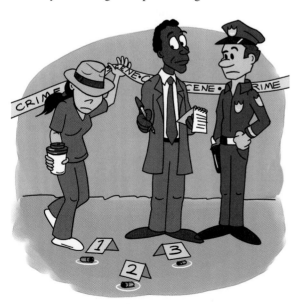

Forensic nurses specialize in several diverse roles and are beginning to find employment in a variety of settings. These roles include the sexual assault nurse examiner (SANE), the forensic nurse death investigator, the forensic psychiatric nurse, the forensic correctional nurse, and the legal nurse consultant.

Sexual Assault Nurse Examiner

A SANE is an RN trained in the forensic examination of sexual assault victims. A SANE has an advanced education and clinical preparation specialized in this area.

Clients who have been sexually assaulted have unique medical, legal, and psychological needs. As crime victims, they require a competent collection of evidence that assists in both investigation and prosecution of the incident. Their bodies and clothing become a key part of the crime scene and are essential for collection of evidence. The SANE offers the type of compassionate care that is often lacking among law enforcement personnel. The care provided by SANEs has been designed to preserve the victim's dignity and reduce psychological trauma. Research data collected in recent years indicate that the SANE's comprehensive forensic evidence collection leads to more effective investigations and more successful prosecutions.[2]

Usually SANEs work in a hospital or ED with other members of a sexual assault response team (SART). The other team members may include physicians, law enforcement personnel, social workers, child and adult protective service workers, and therapists.

In their training, SANEs learn all aspects of the care of sexually assaulted clients. Their responsibilities include interviewing the victim, completing the physical examination, collecting specimens for forensic evidence, and documenting the findings. They also provide emotional support for victims and family members. When the case goes to court, the SANE testifies as an expert legal witness about how evidence was collected and the physical and psychological condition of the client. The SANE may offer an opinion as to whether a crime occurred.

To become a SANE, an RN must complete an adult/adolescent SANE education program. These programs are available through a traditional university setting and online. The training includes either a minimum of 40 contact hours of instruction or three semester units of classroom instruction by an accredited school of nursing. Trainees also must have clinical supervision until they demonstrate competency in SANE practice. After successful completion of the program, the candidate is able to take the certification examination.

Legal Nurse Consultant

The legal nurse consultant is a licensed RN who critically evaluates and analyzes health-care issues in medically related lawsuits. Because the legal system is involved, nurses acting as consultants are considered to be practicing forensics. Nurses uniquely combine their medical expertise with legal knowledge to assess compliance with accepted standards of health-care practice.

Legal nurse consultants work in collaboration with attorneys and other legal and health-care professionals. They may have independent practices, work in the hospital setting in risk management, or be employed by law firms or health insurance companies.

The following is a list of activities performed by legal nurse consultants that distinguishes their specialty practice:

1. Drafting legal documents under the supervision of an attorney
2. Interviewing witnesses
3. Educating attorneys and other involved parties on health-care issues and standards
4. Researching nursing literature, standards, and guidelines as they relate to issues within a particular case
5. Reviewing, analyzing, and summarizing medical records
6. Identifying and conferring with expert witnesses
7. Assessing causation and issues of damages as they relate to the case
8. Developing a case strategy in collaboration with other members of the legal team
9. Providing support during the legal proceedings
10. Educating and mentoring other RNs in the practice of legal nurse consulting[3]

Forensic Nurse Death Investigator

The role of the nurse death investigator is to advocate for the deceased. In general, a death investigator is a professional with experiential and scientific knowledge who can accurately determine the cause of death. The forensic nurse death investigator is an RN with specialized education who is functioning in the death investigator's role.

The forensic nurse death investigator may assume several different titles such as forensic nurse investigator, death investigator, or deputy coroner. In some areas of the country, nurses actually practice as coroners. In the United States, there are currently no standard definitions of "nurse death investigator" or any national credentialing or education requirements. Each region of the country specifies the requirements in its own jurisdictions.

The basic knowledge and skills in which all nurses are educated, such as physical assessment, pharmacology, anatomy, physiology, growth, and development, are minimum requirements for the death investigation role. This nursing knowledge allows the investigator to sort out factors involved in a death. Nurses also learn advanced communication skills and knowledge of the grief process during their education. These skills are required for notifying next of kin and interviewing witnesses.[4]

Forensic nurse death investigators have a number of responsibilities. They respond to scenes of deaths or accidents and work in collaboration with law enforcement. At the scene, they examine the body, pronounce death, and take tissue and blood samples. They take pictures of the body and evidence at the scene. Nurse death investigators must be able to recognize and integrate other evidence collected during the investigation, such as patterns of injury, types of wounds, and estimated time of death. They are responsible for record keeping and arranging for the transport of the body to the morgue or to the coroner's office to undergo autopsy for further examination. Nurse death investigators work with the forensic pathologist to collect additional evidence in the lab during the autopsy.

What Do You Think?

Have you ever been involved in a court case or lawsuit? What was your role? How would being a nurse trained in legal issues have changed what you did or said?

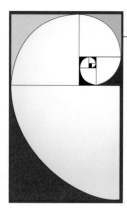

Issues in Practice

If You Were the Nurse on Duty, What Would You Do?

Below are scenarios that exemplify typical situations for the nurse in general practice. Identify your probable response. Critically analyze each situation in terms of what you know and do not know. What types of facts or skills are not part of your current knowledge base?

You are working on a maternity unit when a woman who is an inmate from a correctional institution is admitted in an advanced stage of labor. A correctional officer is in attendance; the woman is shackled at the feet and hands. As she is wheeled to the labor room, you note that the client has had 10 previous pregnancies and four live births.

- What factors make the care of this woman different from that of other pregnant women?
- Is she dangerous?
- How do you maintain confidentiality with this client?
- As an offender in custody, does she surrender any rights?

You work in a hospital setting that is experiencing an increase in workplace violence. Perpetrators of street, child, and domestic violence often follow their victims to the hospital and continue to pose a significant threat to the whole hospital community. It is important to assess the potential for violence.

- How will you contribute to the reduction of risk in the workplace?
- Identify risk factors and cues for violence.
- How would you implement strategies to assist violence management in the acute care setting?

A halfway house for paroled offenders is due to be constructed in your community. Residents are angry and afraid to have ex-convicts living in their neighborhood. A town meeting is scheduled in which the issue will be discussed. Does nursing have anything to contribute to the discussion?

- What do we know about mentally ill offenders, sex offenders, perpetrators of domestic violence, and others?
- What is the therapeutic outcome for those mentally ill offenders who have completed rehabilitation programs?
- What is the risk to the community?
- What stress management strategies are helpful to a community?

You work at a junior high school, providing sex education and health promotion programs for young teenagers. You notice that more and more young people are wearing gang colors and using gang-related language and hand signals.

- How does this affect your work?
- Does this change your priorities?
- Are there referrals or strategies that should be initiated because of the gang affiliations of your students?

Forensic Psychiatric Nurse

Forensic psychiatric nurses work with individuals who have mental health needs and who have entered the legal system. These nurses generally practice in state psychiatric institutions, jails, and prisons.

Nurses in this role perform physical and psychiatric assessments and develop care plans for the clients entrusted to their care. At the most basic level, forensic psychiatric nurses assist clients with self-care, administer medical care and treatment, and monitor the effectiveness of the treatment. Psychiatric interventions are developed to promote coping skills and improve mental health in a therapeutic environment.[5]

Forensic psychiatric nurses may also have advanced practice certification. RNs who have master's degrees in psychiatric–mental health nursing practice work as clinical nurse specialists or nurse practitioners. Nurses in this role are able to diagnose and treat individuals with psychiatric disorders and often are allowed to prescribe medications. They may function as primary care medical and mental health providers, psychotherapists, and consultants. Advanced practice forensic psychiatric nurses may practice independently or in mental health centers, state facilities, and health maintenance organizations (HMOs).

> *Legal nurse consultants work in collaboration with attorneys and other legal and health-care professionals. They may have independent practices, work in the hospital setting in risk management, or be employed by law firms or health insurance companies.*

Forensic Correctional Nurse

Correctional facilities reflect the demographics of the general population, with an increasingly aging incarcerated population who have age-related health-care problems. Forensic correctional nurses provide health care for inmates in correctional facilities such as juvenile centers, jails, and prisons. They manage acute and chronic illness, develop health-care plans, dispense medications, and perform health screenings and health education. Forensic correctional nurses conduct psychiatric assessments and respond to emergency situations. The role of the forensic correctional nurse offers a high level of autonomy compared with other nursing roles.

Evolving Requirements

There is no official certification as a forensic nurse in the United States except for the SANE certification. Many nurses working in forensic roles believe certification requirements will develop as the specialty of forensic nursing continues to evolve and becomes better defined. In the near future, nursing education will be required to develop classes that teach forensic nursing as a part of their curriculum.

NURSE ENTREPRENEUR

Should You Be Your Own Boss?

An entrepreneur is someone who establishes and runs his or her own business. A nurse entrepreneur starts a business by combining nursing experience and knowledge with business knowledge. Starting a business can be risky financially and certainly is far different from the nurse's traditional role as an employee in an institution.

However, nurses are educated to think independently and are sometimes willing to take risks for the benefit of their clients. As professionals who can translate their expertise and confidence into new arenas, nurses are capable of achieving personal and financial success running their own businesses.[6]

Historically, nurse-run businesses have usually focused on temporary staffing agencies, nursing education, or consultant roles. Nurse entrepreneurs can also include nurse attorneys, nurse case managers, nurse educators, nurse death investigators, nurse midwives, nurse paralegals, psychiatric nurses, legal nurse consultants, and sexual assault nurses. Nurse practitioners in rural areas set up their own primary care clinics and provide care for populations who do not have access to any other type of primary care.

Assess Your Nursing Skills

In making the decision to start a business, nurses need to first assess their nursing experience to determine what type of business would be appropriate for their skill and knowledge levels. For example, a SANE may contract services to EDs or law enforcement agencies. A critical care nurse may start a home care agency offering high-tech services. Nurses may develop self-defense courses they can market to high-risk professions, such as forensic psychiatric and forensic correctional nurses.

After nurses determine what skills and knowledge they possess, they need to develop a plan on how to establish the business. A basic level of knowledge about finances and the business start-up process is essential for success. The hopeful entrepreneur needs to consider the customer who will be seeking his or her services, what customers need and desire, what start-up costs will be, and who the competition may be. Answering these questions will allow the nurse to assess the potential success of the business.[7]

Any nurse can start a business. Generally, no advanced degrees are required unless the business involves diagnosis and treatment. Key qualities needed for success are a high degree of self-motivation and a passion for the business to succeed. Nurse entrepreneurs are limited only by their creativity and desire to succeed.

CASE MANAGEMENT

The Case Management Society of America (CMSA) defines case management as ". . . a collaborative process of assessment, planning, facilitation and advocacy for options and services to meet an individual's health needs through communication and available resources to promote quality, cost-effective outcomes."[7] Effective collaboration among all members of the health-care team is essential to meet the needs of clients in today's complex heath-care system.

A Care Coordinator

Nurse case managers act as advocates for clients and their families by coordinating care and linking the client with the physician, other members of the health-care team, resources, and the payer. The goal of the nurse case manager is to help the client obtain high-quality, cost-effective care while decreasing the duplication and fragmentation of care. Research data indicate that active participation by a nurse case manager in the care of a client positively affects the outcomes experienced by the client.

What Do You Think?

Do you know any nurses with the title of "case manager"? Interview them and note what duties they perform as part of their roles.

Nurses are uniquely prepared by their education and professional experiences to fulfill the role of case manager. The holistic health-care approach has been an underlying principle of nursing care since the time of Florence Nightingale. Nurses have experience in arranging referrals, providing client education, and acting as a liaison between physicians and specialty care.

Any client who may face challenges regarding care and recovery can benefit from case management. Included are hospitalized clients, those with complex medical conditions, those requiring specialty care, and those who have personal or psychological circumstances that may interfere with recovery.

Factors that indicate the need for a nurse case manager include:

> " *The role of the forensic correctional nurse offers a high level of autonomy compared with other nursing roles.* "

1. A complex treatment plan that requires coordination or a plan that is unclear
2. An injury or illness that may permanently prevent the client from returning to a previous level of health
3. A preexisting medical condition that may complicate or prolong recovery
4. A need for assistance in accessing health-care resources
5. Environmental stressors that may interfere with recovery

Physicians Catch Up

The CMSA Standards of Practice for Case Management cite the physician and case manager collaboration as essential for successful case management. Although recent research shows that clients benefit from case management, it has been underused by physicians. Case managers and physicians met in 2003 to identify barriers to the use of case management and to explore ways to increase the use of case managers. One result of this meeting was the development of the "Consensus Paper of 2003 Physician and Case Management Summit:

Exploring Best Practices in Physician and Case Management Collaboration to Improve Patient Care." This paper identified both barriers and ways to promote effective, collaborative use of case management by physicians (Box 23.1).

The research that attributes improved client outcomes directly to case management is compelling. It appears that nurse case managers will continue to expand their role in the health-care system of the future.

Box 23.1
Collaboration of Case Managers and Physicians

Barriers to the Use of Case Managers by Physicians
1. Lack of resources and financial incentives in medical practice to integrate case management
2. Resistance to change by, and time pressures imposed on, physicians
3. Insufficient awareness of the role of the case manager among physicians and consumers
4. Insufficient promotion of their value by case managers
5. Lack of evidence of the value of case management

Facilitators of the Use of Case Managers by Physicians
1. Recognition, understanding, and use of case management
2. Standardization of the education and definition of case managers
3. Education for physicians and consumers about case management
4. Compensation for physicians who use case manager services
5. Education of clients in accessing case management
6. Validated research on the effectiveness of case management
7. Recognition of the CMSA Standards of Practice for legitimacy and credibility of the nurse case manager role.

Healthy People 2020

The Healthy People 2020 initiative, begun by the U.S. Department of Health and Human Services, is formulating objectives for the coming decade. Its purpose is to improve the health and longevity of Americans using governmental agencies to strengthen the policies that lead to better health. Key to this initiative is the provision of information to the public on strategies for living long, healthy lives. Healthy People 2020 is discussed in detail in Chapter 24.

BIOTERRORISM

An Acute Health Issue

Bioterrorism is the use of microorganisms with the deliberate intent of causing infection to achieve military or political goals. Biological weapons are relatively easy and inexpensive to produce. The use of microorganisms is a particularly effective means of killing large numbers of people. Biological agents can be spread through the air, through water, or in food. It is also possible to use robotic delivery of agents by remote-control devises such as model airplanes. Most frightening of all, biological agents can be spread by "suicide coughers" who have the disease and spread it from person to person in a crowded space such as a subway or an airport. After being released, microorganisms can go undetected for an extended period because their effects are not immediate and the initial symptoms are often nonspecific or "flu-like." Person-to-person transmission may continue for days or even weeks before the source is detected.

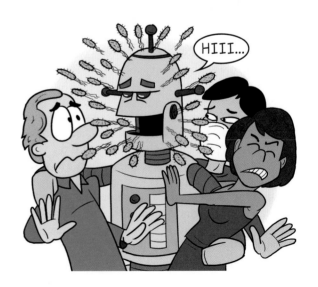

The vulnerability of the United States to a biological attack became painfully apparent with the delivery of anthrax spores through the postal system as an infective agent after the 9/11 attacks. The need to protect a vulnerable American population from further terrorist attacks became an acute public health issue.[8] Also, the offensive biological weapons programs of the former Soviet Union produced some weaponized biological agents that cannot be located; this knowledge has increased the national anxiety level concerning bioterrorism in the United States. Since 1998 the ANA has worked in conjunction with the American College of Emergency Physicians (ACEP) to develop strategies for health-care providers to use in responding to nuclear, biological, and chemical incidents.

Early Recognition

For nurses and other clinicians, the key to an effective response is training in the early recognition of a bioterrorist attack. Studies conducted over the past decade provide data indicating that nurses are still poorly prepared to respond to biological warfare agents.[9] Nurses have been and will remain the frontline first responders to all emergency situations, including biological attack. Nurse preparedness can only increase through improved education and training in the early recognition, detection, and treatment of infected persons. To help achieve this goal, several computerized education programs have been developed to raise the knowledge level of nurses and other first responders.

To educate nurses about bioterrorism, the Centers for Disease Control and Prevention (CDC) have produced online teaching and learning modules. A more comprehensive education program has been developed by the University of California, Los Angeles, in conjunction with content experts. It consists of six interactive case studies that require participants to use their knowledge to identify each biological agent. Pretest and post-test results indicate a marked increase in participant knowledge and ability to detect and distinguish among various biological agents.[9]

Recognizing and treating outbreaks as early as possible is critical for rapid implementation of measures to prevent the spread of disease. Response to bioterrorist attacks is similar to the traditional public health response when communicable disease outbreaks occur naturally, but the focus must be on early detection. However, early recognition is challenging because terrorists may use weaponized biological agents that cause highly variable initial symptoms.

Clinical Presentation

Nurses and other clinicians must be familiar with the specific symptoms and clinical syndromes caused by bioterrorism agents (Box 23.2). One of the first indications of a biological attack will be an increase in the number of individuals seeking care from public health agencies, primary care providers, and EDs. Hospitals, doctors, nurses, and public health professionals will be on the front lines of any attack. A heightened level of suspicion, plus knowledge of the relevant epidemiological clues, should help in the recognition of changes in illness patterns.[10]

Biological Agents

The CDC has developed a list of biological agents that are considered the most likely to be used in a bioterrorist attack (Table 23.1). Infective agents were included for their ability to produce widely disseminated infections, high mortality rates, potential for major public health impact, and ability to cause panic and social disruption. Those that require special action for public health preparedness were also included. Category A agents possess the highest immediate risk for use as biological weapons; category B agents pose the next highest risk. Category C agents have a potential for use, but are not considered an immediate risk as biological weapons.

Box 23.2

Epidemiological Clues to a Biological Attack

Presence of a large epidemic
Unusually severe disease or unusual routes of exposure
Unusual geographic area, unusual season, or absence of normal vector
Multiple simultaneous epidemics of different diseases
Outbreak of zoonotic disease
Unusual strains of organisms or antimicrobial-resistant patterns
Higher attack rates in persons exposed
Credible threat, as determined by authorities, of biological attack
Direct evidence of biological attack

T a b l e 2 3 . 1   Critical Biological Agent Categories for Public Health Preparedness

Category	Biological Agent	Disease
A: Highest immediate risk	Variola major	Smallpox
	Bacillus anthracis	Anthrax
	Yersinia pestis	Plague
	Clostridium botulinum (botulinum toxins)	Botulism
	Francisella tularensis	Tularemia
	Filoviruses and arenaviruses (Ebola and Lassa viruses)	Viral hemorrhagic fevers
B: Next-highest risk	Coxiella burnetii	Q fever
	Brucella species	Brucellosis
	Burkholderia mallei	Glanders
	Burkholderia pseudomallei	Melioidosis
	Alphaviruses	Encephalitis (VEE, EEE, WEE)
	Rickettsia prowazekii	Typhus fever
	Toxins (e.g., ricin, staphylococcal enterotoxin B)	Toxic syndromes
	Chlamydia psittaci	Psittacosis
	Food-safety threats (e.g., Salmonella species, Escherichia coli 0157:H7)	Salmonellosis Diarrheal illness, sepsis, hemolytic uremic syndrome
	Water-safety threats (e.g., Vibrio cholerae, Cryptosporidium parvum)	Cholera Cryptosporidiosis
C: Potential, but not an immediate risk	Emerging-threat agents (e.g., Nipah virus, hantavirus)	

EEE = eastern equine encephalitis; VEE = Venezuelan equine encephalitis; WEE = western equine encephalitis.

Effective Response
Identification and Management

In the event of a widespread bioterrorism attack, nurses in all levels and types of health-care settings have the potential to become involved. To develop a prompt and effective response, nurses and other health-care providers must know the modes of transmission, incubation periods, symptoms, and communicable periods of these diseases as outlined by the CDC.

Once a potential outbreak is detected, it must be brought to the attention of the appropriate health-care agencies or specialist in infective diseases. All nurses should have accurate around-the-clock information on the resources available for their geographic area. Once appropriate notifications have been made, nurses will use their skills of clinical evaluation and history taking to identify the infective organism, mode of transmission, and source of exposure. In addition, nurses play a critical role in managing postexposure prophylaxis and its complications, as well as psychological and mental health problems brought on by the event.

What Do You Think?

Have you received any specialized training in disaster or bioterrorism preparedness? If you have, how does it make you better able to care for victims of disaster or bioterrorism? If you have not, why? Do you feel prepared to care for these victims?

Response Training

The ACEP, in alliance with the ANA, submitted a list of recommendations to the Health and Human Services Office of Emergency Preparedness in April 2001. Included was the recommendation that all basic nurse education programs include information on how to respond to mass casualty events. The task force also recommended that self-study modules and other types of specialty programs be developed for ED nurses that would contain more in-depth information on the detection and management of bioterrorism.

The ANA is actively involved in developing ways to better prepare nurses to respond to bioterrorist events. In collaboration with the Department of Health and Human Services, they established the National Nurses Response Teams (NNRT). This joint effort was unveiled at the ANA's 2002 biennial convention.

New technology may also play a part in the future early detection of biological agents. The latest research is focused on developing tiny electronic chips containing living nerve cells that could be worn like a radiation detection badge. It would warn of the presence of a wide range of bacterial and viral organisms. Another experimental devise that would help identify specific pathogens such as botulism and smallpox consists of fiberoptic tubes coated with antibodies. Light-emitting molecules would shine through the antibodies, and the different colors produced would indicate which organism is present.

> *Since 9/11 the need to protect a vulnerable American population from further terrorist attacks has become an acute public health issue.*

Activation and Deployment

In the event that the president declares a bioterrorism state of disaster, the NNRT will be activated to respond by providing mass immunization or chemoprophylaxis to a population at risk. The NNRT, under the auspices of the Department of Health and Human Services, will be quickly deployed in response to a major national event.

The goal of the ANA and federal officials is to recruit 10 regional teams of 200 nurses. The ANA is working to recruit these nurse teams and will provide ongoing education to the NNRT in disaster response. The Department of Health and Human Services is responsible for the screening and processing of potential nurse team members after they have been recruited by the ANA.

When the NNRT teams are deployed, the members become "federalized," and the federal government will pay their salaries, reimbursement for travel, and housing costs during the duty period. In case of a terrorism disaster, the deployment will be limited to 2 weeks to minimize the impact on the nurses' employers.

The nursing profession faces serious challenges in the response to threats of bioterrorism. The nation is counting on nurses to play a vital role in bioterrorism preparedness and response. The public depends on nurses to be the frontline responders and to protect them from the effects of bioterrorism. Nurses must be able to communicate medical information and educate the public quickly after a crisis. It is imperative that the nursing profession train nurses in appropriate, effective responses to ensure the best outcome in a frightening, unfamiliar event.

DISASTER NURSING

The United States has witnessed an increase in terrorism-related disasters during the past decade. However, the vast majority of disasters are still considered natural. These range from the catastrophic failure of manmade structures, such as bridge collapses, to weather-related catastrophes, such as hurricanes and floods. Simply defined, a disaster is a catastrophic event that leads to a large number of injuries, displaced individuals, or major loss of life. The American Red Cross defines a disaster as ". . . an occurrence such as a hurricane, tornado, storm, flood, high water, wind-driven water, tidal wave, earthquake, drought, blizzard, pestilence, famine, fire, explosion, building collapse, commercial transportation wreck, or other situations that cause human suffering or create human needs that the victims cannot alleviate without substantial assistance."[11]

Many Roles for the Nurse

Every disaster poses its own unique challenges. The role of the nurse in a specific disaster depends on its nature and on the type and numbers of injuries. Although most nurses are familiar with the type of disaster aid provided by the Red Cross, they may assume many other roles when a disaster strikes. Often in disaster situations, nurses function outside their usual practice setting and may assume a variety of roles in meeting the needs of the disaster victims. Nurses must be able to perform under stressful and sometimes physically dangerous conditions.

After the hurricanes in Florida in 2005, large numbers of disabled and elderly clients who had been living in nursing homes and extended care facilities were displaced to schools and shelters. Nurses assumed the primary responsibility for caring for these individuals who, because they could not care for themselves and lacked essential medications, needed care at a level above what rescue workers could provide.

When the number of injured is very large, more than 1000, the incident is classified as a mass casualty, and multiple agencies, from the local to federal, become involved. Many times a nurse functions as a triage practitioner, assessing victims and prioritizing care for the best use of resources. However, in mass casualty situations, the traditional classification of clients into low risk, intermediate care, and immediate care is reordered. To provide care for the greatest numbers of victims, often workers give only palliative care to those with critical injuries, allowing more resources to be used for those with a better chance of surviving the disaster.

Nurses also provide direct treatment, which may be brief, or may be involved in more complex roles, such as mobile surgical units (Box 23.3).

Box 23.3
Responsibilities of the Disaster Nurse

Short Term
1. Provides emergency medical assistance. Special attention is given to vulnerable groups, such as handicapped people, children, and elderly people.
2. Provides assistance in the mobilization of necessary resources such as food, shelter, medication, and water.
3. Works in collaboration with existing organizational structures and resources.

Long Term
1. Provides assistance with resettlement programs and psychological, economic, and legal needs.
2. Partners with independent, objective media; local and national branches of government; international agencies; and nongovernmental organizations.

However, in the early stages of many disasters, nurses may find a lack of essential resources. Nurses have a long history of being able to improvise and get by with what is available, and a disaster will certainly challenge their creativity.

Disaster Phases
Preparing for Impact
Certain types of natural disasters are preceded by a warning period. For a tornado, this may range from a few minutes to as much as an hour; for hurricanes, it may be as long as several days. During the warning stage, also called the preimpact phase, the focus is on preparation for the aftereffects of the event. This preparation is primarily at the local level.

Even before a catastrophic event is predicted, communities in disaster-prone regions practice with disaster drills. These drills provide valuable training in a low-stress environment and identify the types of resources that may be needed during a disaster. This type of training helps identify unique risk situations for the community and builds the skill and knowledge disaster responders must have to meet the needs of the population. When the disaster becomes imminent and a warning is issued, preparations such as evacuations are put into operation.

Communication is Critical
One key element, brought to the forefront by recent disasters, is the ability of the various agencies involved to communicate with each other. Fire and rescue, first responders, law enforcement, public health, and health-care services must be able to exchange essential information to provide the highest-level care possible. Good communication leads to a well-coordinated response. All agencies must have agreements in place and understand the role that each one is to play in the disaster. This preparation will eliminate the turf arguments sometimes seen among agencies. In rural areas, agreements with nearby communities also become important.

Planning for the news media and the flow of information is often overlooked in disaster preparations. Nurses are likely to hear about a disaster from breaking news reports before they learn about it through official channels. One fear that can become real is group panic. Generally, all information released from a health-care facility should go through the public relations representative or the designated spokesperson for the facility. Before any information is released, it should be determined how the news will affect particular populations. Families of victims often cling to every word and may misinterpret what is being said.

Persons designated to speak for the health-care facility should have experience with public speaking and be able to convey the information clearly and in terms that the general public can understand. They should also be able to "think on their feet" when responding to questions. However, question-and-answer sessions should be severely limited, especially when national media are involved. When people are under stress or have high levels of anxiety, communication must be direct, honest, and to the point. Long technical explanations will only confuse the facts. The public should also be calmed by reassurances that everything possible is being done. Regular updates every 30 to 60 minutes, even if there is little new information, are helpful in reducing anxiety levels.

The following agencies can help with planning during the preimpact phase:

- *Disaster Medical Assistance Team (DMAT):* A group of frontline medical personnel, including nurses, who provide health care after a disaster. These may include terrorist, natural, or environmental disasters.
- *Medical Reserve Corps:* Part of the USA Freedom Corps, which was developed in 2002 in response to Americans' desire to volunteer and serve their communities in the wake of the 9/11 terrorist attacks.
- *American Red Cross:* RNs can join their local Red Cross and receive specialized training in disaster and bioterrorism preparedness.
- Commission Corps Readiness Force: Deploys teams to respond to public health emergencies.12
- *National Disaster Medical System (NDMS):* Mobilizes comprehensive disaster relief and works closely with local fire, police, and emergency medical services. NDMS also uses volunteer disaster response teams called International Medical/Surgical Response Teams (IMSURTs), of which nurses are an essential component. The IMSURTs provide emergency medical services at any place in the world where there is a lack of resources.

> " *Often in disaster situations, nurses function outside their usual practice setting and may assume a variety of roles in meeting the needs of the disaster victims. Nurses must be able to perform under stressful and sometimes physically dangerous conditions.* "

The Impact Phase

When the actual disaster strikes, the impact phase begins. The goal during the impact phase is to respond to the disaster, activate the emergency response, and reduce the long-term effects of the disaster as much as possible. Activation of the emergency response plans developed during the preimpact phase mobilizes all agencies involved. Because fire, rescue, and police are usually the first on the scene, they provide and establish the command post from which all other efforts will be coordinated. Their goal is to identify and remove victims from dangerous situations, deal with unstable structures, and provide first aid to those who have been injured.

Because of the recent heightened concern over acts of terrorism, law enforcement may initially take control of the disaster until it can be determined that the cause was not a criminal act. Nurses working in the early stages of disasters sometimes feel frustrated by law enforcement officers, who may limit their ability to provide care. It is important to remember that law enforcement is concerned with identifying a crime and preserving evidence that may be used later in criminal prosecutions. The whole disaster area is considered a crime scene until released by law enforcement.

The Incident Management System (IMS) is an effective tool in bringing some order to the confusion that always surrounds any disaster event. Based on a military model, IMS is a hierarchy with a well-defined chain of command. At the top is the incident commander or manager, who is responsible for coordinating all rescue efforts. A "job sheet," really a vertical organizational chart, lists all the key people from all the key agencies involved. It also outlines the responsibilities of each person and agency and must be followed throughout the disaster event for the best coordination of emergency services. Most IMS plans now include hospitals within the service area. Information flows freely from the commander down to paramedics and from the street level back to the top.

Medical assistance is provided in hospitals, local clinics, or the field. Deployable Rapid Assembly Shelter Hospitals (DRASHs) are mobile shelters

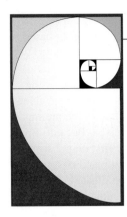

Issues in Practice

The 10 Commandments of Disaster Preparedness

Nurses and the general public should take the following preparation steps well before a disaster strikes:

1. Discuss the type of hazards that could affect your family. Know your home's vulnerability to storm surge, flooding, and high wind.
2. Locate a safe room or the safest areas in your home for high wind hazard. In certain circumstances, the safest areas may not be your home but within your community.
3. Determine escape routes from your home and places to meet.
4. Designate an out-of-state friend as a single point of contact for all your family members.
5. Make a plan now for what to do with your pets if you need to evacuate.
6. Post emergency telephone numbers by your phones and make sure your children know how and when to call 911.
7. Check your insurance coverage—flood damage is not usually covered by homeowners' insurance.
8. Stock nonperishable emergency supplies and a disaster supply kit.
9. Purchase and know how to use a National Oceanic and Atmospheric Administration (NOAA) weather radio. Remember to replace its battery every 6 months, as you do with your smoke detectors.
10. Take first aid, cardiopulmonary resuscitation (CPR), and disaster preparedness classes.

Sources: Goodhue CJ, Burke RV, Chambers S, Ferrer RR, Upperman JS: Disaster Olympix: A unique nursing emergency preparedness exercise. Journal of Trauma Nursing 17(1):5–10, 2010.

James JJ, Benjamin GC, Burkle FM, Gebbie KM, Kelen G Subbarao I: Disaster medicine and public health preparedness: A discipline for all health professionals. Disaster Medicine & Public Health Preparedness 4(2):102–107, 2010.

McCabe OL, Barnett DJ, Taylor HG, Links JM: Ready, willing, and able: A framework for improving the public health emergency preparedness system. Disaster Medicine & Public Health Preparedness 4(2):161–168, 2010.

that can be used by the IMSURT team as a small independent hospital. The DRASH is designed with triage emergency care, intensive care units, and surgical rooms.

Protection for First Responders

Nurses and other first responders must always be aware of the potential dangers of any disaster. If the health-care providers become injured during rescue attempts, they can no longer provide care to the victims. As a result, protecting the lives and health of the first responders takes priority over rescue efforts. Because of the wide range of potential hazards, including chemicals such as nerve gas or toxins, biological substances, radioactive agents, and explosive devices, care providers must wear appropriate protective equipment. Images of rescue personnel wearing bulky white biohazard suits have become ingrained in the public consciousness. The biohazard suits, otherwise known as personal protective equipment, actually have a range of protective abilities against many types of substances (Box 23.4).

Most nurses have not received training in donning, wearing, or performing procedures in biohazard suits. If nurses find themselves in situations in which they may be required to wear such protection, it is important to recognize some of the limitations. The heavy gloves reduce manual dexterity significantly, and even routine procedures, such as starting intravenous (IV) lines or dressing wounds, become extremely difficult if not impossible. The hood restricts peripheral vision and the plastic view plate may distort the visual field. Even cursory physical examination, including the ability to use a stethoscope, becomes more difficult. Nurses may also find that the suit itself causes claustrophobia. The unusual taste and smell of the self-contained breathing equipment have been known to cause nausea.

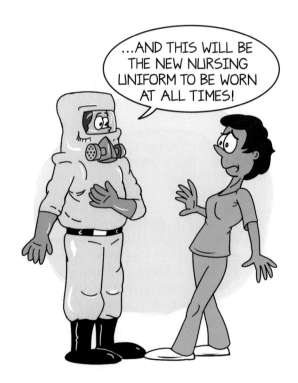

Box 23.4

Protective Levels of Biohazard Suits

Level A: Resistant to all types of chemicals and biological and radioactive substances and is used in situations in which splashing or exposure to unknown agents is possible. Totally encapsulates personnel and has its own internal air supply.

Level B: Has a hood but does not totally encapsulate personnel. Is splash resistant to most chemicals. Has its own internal air supply.

Level C: Has a hood but does not totally encapsulate personnel. Is less resistant to chemical penetration than previous levels. Equipped with a respirator that can filter out most chemical contaminants and biological and radioactive substances.

Level D: Used when there are no chemicals or agents that can affect the respiratory system or penetrate through the skin. Generally consists of a jump suit or scrub suit.

Source: http://www.Firstrespondernetwork.com.

After exposure to any type of chemical, biological, or radioactive agent, personnel must go through a decontamination procedure. These procedures vary widely depending on the type of agent. They range from simply removing clothes and showering with water to extensive treatment with various neutralizing agents. Most emergency response teams have a decontamination tent that provides some privacy and contains the equipment necessary for thorough decontamination.

After the Disaster

The postimpact phase may begin as little as 72 hours after the incident and in some cases may last considerably longer. It may continue for years, as in the aftermath of hurricane Katrina in New Orleans. The activities focus on recovery, rehabilitation, and rebuilding. One of the key activities during the postimpact phase is the evaluation of the disaster preparations and of how rescue and recovery efforts could be improved.

Conclusion

Florence Nightingale wrote in 1859 that "no man, not even a doctor, ever gives any other definition of what a nurse should be than this 'devoted and obedient.' This definition would do just as well for a porter. It might even do for a horse!"[13] The profession of nursing has come a long way since Nightingale made the first efforts to move it out of its position of servitude to physicians.

Nursing is constantly evolving and defining itself as it strives to include expanded roles of practice. Of the many new and exciting roles for nurses, forensic, bioterrorism, disaster, entrepreneur, case management, and legal consultant have developed in response to the needs of society.

The tragic events of September 11, 2001, in New York City, Washington, DC, and Pennsylvania revealed how poorly prepared the United States was to deal with disasters. In response, legislation was enacted on federal and state levels that began to address the many issues associated with terrorist acts. Large sums of money were expended to purchase equipment and train health-care workers to be better able to deal with a variety of potential disasters. Collaboration between groups that often had little to do with each other in the past became an essential component of these plans. The Department of Health and Human Services and the ANA have been working closely to educate nurses in disaster and bioterrorism responses. However, the country still remains woefully unprepared for major disasters, as was seen in the events following Hurricane Katrina in 2005.

Although nurses have practiced in these areas for many years, they are only now beginning to be recognized for the unique skills and qualities they bring to these roles. For example, the job description of an emergency department nurse has long included interviews with and assessments of crime victims, collection and proper handling of evidence, and accurate and complete documentation of injuries and information provided by crime victims. In the role of client advocate, nurses have always been case managers through assessment of client needs, coordination of referrals for specialized or long-term care, and coordination of non-nursing services such as diet teaching and social services.

All nurses have the knowledge of anatomy, physiology, growth, and development that is required for the death examiner position. As more nurses seek the specialized training now available for many of these roles and obtain nationally recognized certification as a demonstration of their knowledge, they will gain acceptance as highly qualified and valuable members of these specialized health-care teams.

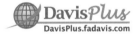
DavisPlus.fadavis.com

ASSOCIATIONS AND WEBSITES

American Academy of Forensic Sciences: http://www.aafs.org

American Association of Legal Nurse Consultants: http://www.aalnc.org

American College of Forensic Examiners International: http://www.acfei.com

American Forensic Nurses: http://www.amrn.com

American Psychiatric Nurses Association: http://www.apna.org

Forensic Nurse Magazine: http://www.forensic-nursemag.com

International Association of Forensic Nurses: http://www.forensicnurse.org; http://www.iafn.org

Legal Nurse Consultant Certificate Program: http://www.continuing-legal@udel.edu

National Alliance of Sexual Assault Coalitions: http://www.taasa.org

National Association of Correctional Nursing: http://www.correctionalnursing.org

National Association of Independent Nurses: http://www.independentrn.com

National Commission on Correctional Healthcare: http://www.ncchc.org

National Nurses in Business Association: http://www.nnba.net

Nurse Entrepreneur Network: http://www.Nurse-Entrepreneur-Network.com

Nursing Entrepreneur: http://www.nursingentrepreneurs.com

Office for Victims of Crime: http://www.ojp.usdoj.gov/ovc

Office for Victims of Crime Resource Center: http://www.ncjrs.org

Public Health Functions Projects: http://www.health.gov/phfunctions/public.htm

Rape, Abuse and Incest National Network (RAINN): http://www.rainn.org

Sexual Assault Resource Service (SARS): http://www.sane-sart.com

Violence Against Women Office: http://www.ovw.usdoj.gov

Critical Thinking Exercises

Application of Human Rights

What information do you need to make a decision? Explore applications of human rights from the point of view of the victim and the perpetrator of the crime. Think about how the issue of human rights would be defined and protected in the following examples. What is the nurse's role?

- A married father of two, an upstanding member of the community, is accused of child molestation and is admitted to the unit for psychiatric evaluation and submission of tissue samples.
- A female inmate becomes pregnant in prison and does not want anyone to know who the father is.
- A young man has a history of substance abuse and mental illness. He refuses medication to control psychotic behavior and is confined in a forensic psychiatric facility because of the claim that he is incompetent to stand trial for car theft.
- A mother of an infant is being interviewed in a suspected child abuse case. She admits that she was sexually and physically abused as a child and throughout her marriage. The priority is to establish her role in the current charges involving injury of her 3-month-old infant.

24

Client Education: A Moral Imperative

Mary Abadie
Sharon M. Bator
Cynthia Bienemy
Sandra Brown
Doris Brown
Joan Anny Ellis

Anita H. Hansberry
Sharon W. Hutchinson
Esperanza Villanueva-Joyce
Karen Mills
Janet S. Rami
Betty L. Fomby-White

Jacqueline J. Hill
Anyadie Onu
Enrica K. Singleton
Wanda Spurlock
Melissa Stewart
Cheryl Taylor

Learning Objectives

After completing this chapter, the reader will be able to:

- Explain the philosophical reason for using the term "client" rather than "patient."
- Describe the quality requirements for computer-based client health teaching.
- Discuss ways to enhance communication with different cultures.
- Discuss the basic literacy requirements for self-management of health care.
- Use the three domains in learning and the six domains in level of understanding to develop a client teaching plan.
- Discuss commonly used teaching strategies and methods appropriate for clients of all ages.
- Describe the nursing skills needed to provide appropriate client teaching.
- Compare the nursing process and teaching process for client teaching.

INTRODUCTION

Some indicators of the considerable growth of nursing as a profession include the expectations of nurses to provide client education, the increased emphasis on ethics, and the legal accountability for safe and high-quality nursing care (see Chapters 7 and 9.) For example, 50 years ago, nurses were prohibited from teaching clients in the U.S. hospital system without direct orders from physicians. Many physicians believed that client teaching in general was not relevant or effective, nor were there third-party payments available for client teaching.[1]

In the current health-care system, client teaching is not only an expectation but an ethical and legal requirement. The enactment of the 2010 healthcare reform act (Patient Protection and Affordable Care Act [PPACA]) provides nurses new opportunities, including preventive teaching.[2] Whether the nurse is providing health promotion, health maintenance, or health rehabilitation, bringing a client to a level of personal understanding is morally and ethically the right thing to do.[3] In recent years, several lawsuits have resulted from the failure of nurses to provide adequate client teaching (Box 24.1).

Physician authors advise clients to be "smart" and learn as much as possible about their health-care needs.[4] Expert nurses have modeled ways to incorporate client education as a priority in care,[5] and nurse theorists such as Stewart and Fomby-White provide world views and theories imbued with the primacy of client education. The nation's

Box 24.1

Documenting What You Teach

Always document what you teach clients and their families and include their understanding of what you taught. The court in *Kyslinger vs. United States* (1975) addressed the nurse's liability for client teaching. In this case, a Veterans Administration (VA) hospital sent a hemodialysis client home with an artificial kidney. The client eventually died (apparently while connected to the hemodialysis machine), and his wife sued, alleging that the hospital and its staff failed to teach her or her husband how to properly use and maintain a home hemodialysis unit.

After examining the evidence, the court ruled against the client's wife as follows: "During those 10 months that plaintiff's decedent underwent biweekly hemodialysis treatment on the units (at the VA hospital), both plaintiff and decedent were instructed as to the operation, maintenance, and supervision of said treatment. The Court can find no basis to conclude that the plaintiff or plaintiff's decedent were not properly informed on the use of the hemodialysis unit."

clients and consumers of health-care services need their most trusted professionals—nurses—to drive substantial initiatives to address health literacy concerns.[3] Toward this end, the American Nurses Association's (ANA's) 2010 House of Delegates approved a literacy resolution. It sets the stage for the ANA to implement the following[3]:

- Promote collaborative nursing initiatives to address health literacy problems
- Use existing research findings to strengthen health literacy knowledge and skills in nursing school curricula and in RNs' workplaces
- Advance nursing research to identify evidence-based practices that promote optimum health literacy

For more information on health literacy, go to http://www.health.gov/communication/literacy/quickguide/resources.htm and http://www.health.gov/communication/HLAction Plan/.

ETHICAL CONSIDERATIONS OF HEALTH SELF-MANAGEMENT

In the United States there has been a lack of adequate preparation for educating clients with self-management concerns, particularly clients with chronic illnesses. This lack of education is a serious violation of ethical responsibilities by health-care providers at all levels. It has the potential to produce harm, such as increased pain, disability, and premature

death. For people in poverty conditions, the negative outcomes can be far worse. The unhealthy outcomes produced by lack of adequate education also cause greater monetary loss and greater loss of productivity.[6]

Since at least 50 percent of deaths occur secondarily to unhealthy lifestyles, Pender's work (Health Promotion Model) is instrumental in helping to change negative spirals of health promotion.[7]

ETHICAL CONSIDERATIONS OF "NURSE, HEAL THYSELF"

In a time of increasing health-care costs and increased incidence of chronic disease, providing high-quality preventive care through health promotion is critical.[8] By assessing their own lifestyle behaviors, nurses and nursing students can invest in their future health and that of their present and future clients.

As obesity has reached epidemic proportions locally, nationally, and internationally, there is increased question of whether overweight health-care workers will be asked to reduce their weight.[9] A survey for nurses, advanced practice nurses, and educators showed that 54 percent were obese or overweight. Some authors believe in the importance of role-modeling diet and lifestyles to positively motivate clients. Put more simply, if experienced health-care providers, knowing the health risks of obesity and informed about intervention techniques, do not follow expert advice, is it realistic to expect nursing students or the public to do so?[10] One study, in which 93 percent of practicing nurses admitted to being overweight or obese, showed that 76 percent did not even pursue the topic with clients they saw as obese. Studies indicate that limited exercise counseling by nurse practitioners does not match the strong values placed on health promotion.[11] Do nurse educators, who are among those surveyed, mirror the same behavior by not pursuing the topic with their nursing students. If so, what are the health implications for the nursing students now and in the future?

MANAGED CARE

Managed care, with its focus on clients' taking greater responsibility for their own health and self-care, has contributed to the increased need for client education.[12] The Institute of Medicine (IOM) has harshly criticized the chasm in quality of health care and strongly recommends placing clients at the center of control, with clients' choices based on the best information and knowledge available to them. The IOM established 10 rules, 4 of which relate to client teaching (Table 24.1).[13] For many years, the rules for redesigning health care to empower consumers and advocate for their specific health needs have been backed by many nursing theorists and by nursing research.[4,10]

The Joint Commission has taken steps to regulate client teaching because it is essential to high-quality care. Not only do The Joint Commission representatives make unannounced visits, they also look for evidence that education standards are being met.[2] The Joint Commission Standards PC.6.1 requires nursing staff to serve as critical resources by acting as skilled client educators. Additionally, The Joint Commission determines whether learning activities relate to assessment of the client's learning needs and any areas in which the client would like more information. The standard requires all providers to communicate whether the client's teaching needs are being met (Box 24.2).[5]

IMPLICATIONS OF TECHNOLOGY

Electronic Records
Electronic charting systems currently help track the teaching standards recommended by The Joint Commission and IOM. As is shown in Table 24.1, the IOM suggests that care should be continuous, customized to each client, and keep the client in control, with freely shared information. Electronic records and charting systems assist in tracking required information. (See Chapter 19 for more detailed information of electronic charting.)

Other technologies include telehealth, biodefense systems, and universal access to the Internet, all of which can serve as teaching tools for

Table 24.1   Building Responsiveness Into Health-Care Systems

Rule	Description
1. Care is based on continuous healing relationships.	Clients should receive care whenever they need it and in many forms, not just face-to-face visits. The health-care system must be responsive at all times, and access to care should be provided over the Internet, by telephone, and by other means in addition to in-person visits.
2. Care is customized according to client needs and values.	The system should be designed to meet the most common types of needs, but should have the capability to respond to individual client choices and preferences.
3. The client is the source of control.	Clients should be given the necessary information and opportunity to exercise their chosen degree of control over health-care decisions that affect them. The system should be able to accommodate differences in client preferences and encourage shared decision-making.
4. Knowledge is shared, and information flows freely.	Clients should have unfettered access to their own medical information and to clinical knowledge. Clinicians and clients should communicate effectively and share information.

Box 24.2

The Joint Commission Focus on Standard PC.6.1

Standard
- Client receives appropriate education and training specific to needs.

Rationale
- Client is given sufficient information to make decisions and to take responsibility for self-management. Family is educated to improve outcomes.

Elements of Performance
- Education is appropriate to client's needs.
- Cultural and religious beliefs, emotional barriers, motivation, and physical or cognitive barriers to communication are assessed.

Educational Content
- Plan for care, treatment, services
- Basic health practices and safety
- Safe and effective medication use
- Nutrition and diet, oral health
- Use of equipment or supplies
- Pain assessment and management
- Habilitation or rehabilitation toward maximal independence

Source: Adapted from The Joint Commission on Accreditation of Healthcare Organizations, 2005, pp. C-26, C-27.

improving client care.[14] Clients at some hospitals, such as the University of Minnesota Health Care Services, can now log onto the website and access their own electronic hospital records. Such advances are also good marketing tools for medical facilities: Well-educated learners can use them successfully in programs such as weight reduction, stress abatement, parenting, and women's health issues.[5]

Working With the Internet

The Internet is the fastest-growing source of health information. Access to the latest information in virtually any subject is just a click away. Electronic networking has created a worldwide learning community that clients and health-care providers can tap into. This technology better enables clients to increase their own level of responsibility for their health care. This factor in itself will change nursing practice profoundly. According to O'Neil and colleagues, "the original purpose of the Web was to communicate and share information, and its development has . . . changed the practice of nursing."[15] Websites such as WebMD, with 16 million users

each month; online "Ask-a-Nurse" sites; and "Tele-Medicine," to name a few, strongly enhance nursing practice. Note that only a few health information websites follow privacy policies; it is common for them to share personal health information without the client's permission or even personal knowledge.[4]

In this growing, complex society, demands from the client for sophisticated and better health care have increased, and online Web-based classes can impart information as never before. Nursing must keep abreast of these trends and devise more Web-based learning opportunities to improve the quality and outcomes of client care.

Using Technology in Teaching

Widespread access to the Internet, and its huge volume of available information, makes it a useful and widely sought tool for both clients and caregivers. The Internet can provide contact with medical publications, caregivers, prescription and nonprescription drug information, other clients or family members, and an almost limitless variety of related sources.

Searching for Information

More than half of Americans who have gone online have searched for health or medical information. On a daily basis, far more people seek such information online than actually visit health professionals. They can also enhance their own knowledge through proper use of the Internet.

Some medical professionals have expressed concern about the poor quality control of Internet information and about the possibility that clients seeking health-care information will be misinformed. The JCAHO has a website, http://www.jointcommission.org, with an icon labeled "Health on the Net Foundation." This icon, used with the Search button, connects the user to any Internet site. If the site meets the rigorous JCAHO criteria, additional information about the website will appear. If nothing appears, the site does not meet the criteria and should be viewed as unreliable.

Table 24.2 lists some helpful online health and medical directories. This list is not comprehensive.

Evaluating Results

Evaluation of the search results is important, and a partnership between caregiver and client is the best way to undertake it. Both the client and caregiver should ask: Does the site or information have credibility? Is it published by a marketing firm or drug manufacturer with a primary focus on sales rather than education? Is the content accurate and aligned with the answer being sought? Can it be checked for accuracy elsewhere? Is it scientifically based or anecdotal? Are disclaimers present, and if so, do they state appropriately that the information is for general use and not diagnostic?

To provide the best of care, nurses will need a thorough understanding of all these Internet learning tools.[5] Of course, nurses must also recognize that some clients, such as economically disadvantaged ones, do not have Internet access. In such cases, the nurse will need to substitute more traditional methods of obtaining information.

To provide appropriate-level reading materials, the nurse must know the client's literacy level.[16] The Joint Commission Public Policy Initiative has a website that helps nurses evaluate literacy for client education quality. The link is http://www.jointcommission.org/PublicPolicy/health_literacy.htm.

Table 24.2 Online Health and Medical Directories

Name	URL Address	Description
Harden Meta Directory	www.lib.uiowa.edu/hardin/md	Health sites listing, selected for connectivity
Health A–Z	www.healthAtoZ.com	Consumer health site maintained by health-care professionals
HealthFinder	www.healthfinder.gov	U.S. government–maintained site; uses colloquial language
Medhunt	www.hon.ch	Sponsored by Health on the Net Foundation, for professionals and clients
MedicineNet	www.medicinenet.com	Doctor-produced information
Mayo Clinic	www.mayoclinic.com	General health information
National Library of Medicine	www.Medline.gov	Current health care information including videotapes
Government	www.nutrition.gov	General nutrition information
Agency for Healthcare Research and Quality	www.ahrq.gov/consumer	Primarily aimed at health-care professionals; informative for some clients
CDC Health Topics A to Z	www.cdc.gov/ncidod/diseases	Information about infectious diseases studied by the Centers for Disease Control and Prevention (CDC)
Safe Medication (American Society of Health System Pharmacists)	www.safemedication.com	Information to help clients use medications safely and correctly

HEALTH PROMOTION FOR OUR TIME

The need for enhanced communication has created a new emphasis on health promotion. One example is the Healthy People 2020 objectives, created by the U.S. Department of Health and Human Services. Healthy People 2020 focuses on 28 areas that center on access to preventive care and developing healthy lifestyle habits.[17] Implied throughout this document is the need for high-quality client education, particularly from nurses.

However, the document does not discuss how best to educate clients to make healthy choices. This educational gap is also reflected by the unacceptable health-care disparities among minority groups. Also, the goal for reducing smoking has not been accomplished since Healthy People 2010 was published in 2000. The number of teenagers who smoke has even increased significantly.

Some people find it difficult to make choices because they have not learned to think critically. A new theory of choices is emerging in the nursing literature, led by the work of Dr. Betty Fomby-White, with the purpose of helping clients make informed choices for equitable care.[18] Chapter 6 discusses critical thinking in greater depth.

CARING RELATIONSHIPS MATTER

If clients feel loved by themselves and others, they will want to learn more and will have more faith in their own ability to learn.[7] Abundant information demonstrates that drug abuse and other destructive habits are linked to lower self-worth. Helping clients develop healthy lifestyles and choices is "one of the most important responsibilities of contemporary nurses."[19]

In the midst of health reform, sustaining a caring orientation is critical for both the health-care provider and the client: ". . . the quality of the relationship is what facilitates health and makes it possible for nurse and client to connect in a way that is transforming."[20] A non-nurturing interpersonal relationship is profoundly negative to body, mind, and spirit for the health-care provider as well as the client. Tables 24.3 and 24.4 reflect the dramatically different consequences of caring and noncaring relationships between nurses and clients. See Chapter 4 for caring theory and models and their impact on care; see Chapter 14 for ways to improve communication.

Research studies show that competent, appropriate interweaving of spirituality and prayer enhances healing. Spirituality can provide support in conditions that include hypertension, stress, cancer, and depression.[21] See Chapter 21, "Spirituality and Health Care," and Chapter 26, "Alternative and Complementary Healing Practices."

CLIENT TEACHING IMPLICATIONS FOR NURSING EDUCATION

Shared power is essential for building a constructive sense of community. Therefore, educators should emphasize the importance of sharing power with clients. Nursing education is essential for mentoring collaboration, increasing cultural competence, and decreasing prejudice and stereotyping.

Table 24.3　Empirical Outcomes of Caring: Clients

Effects of Caring Relationships on Clients (Summary of Findings)	Effects of Noncaring Relationships on Clients (Summary of Findings)
Emotional and spiritual well-being (dignity, self-control, personhood)	Humiliation, fear, despair, perceived lack of control and helplessness, alienation, vulnerability, lingering bad memories
Enhanced healing, more lives saved, increased safety, more energy, fewer costs, more comfort, less sense of loss	Decreased healing
Trusting relationship, decrease in alienation, closer family relations	

Source: Adapted from Swanson, HL. Meta-analysis of 130 empirical studies. In Watson J (ed): Assessing and measuring caring in nursing and health science. New York, Springer, 2002.

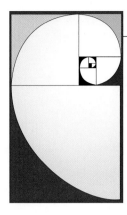

Issues Now

Healthy People 2020

It seems that the Healthy People 2010 campaign was just starting, and now the 10-year revision is already here. The Healthy People initiative is based on the belief that setting objectives and providing benchmarks promotes tracking and monitoring of progress; these in turn can motivate, guide, and focus actions to increase the quality of health on the United States. The initiative, begun by the U.S. Department of Health and Human Services (HHS), has been renewed each decade since its beginnings in 1980. Starting in 2009, HHS began formulating objectives for the next decade. One of the major changes is that the report produced will be available online, as well as on paper, to better deliver the information tailored to the needs of its users. HHS will also be producing a user-friendly disk that will be distributed on request.

Healthy People 2020 envisions the United States becoming a society in which all people live long, healthy lives. The mission of the project is to work though federal and state governmental agencies to strengthen the policies and practices to make people healthier. Some of the strategies include identifying nationwide health improvement priorities, increasing public awareness and understanding of what produces health and causes disease and disability, developing measurable goals and objectives for all levels of government, and using evidence-based practices to guide actions and focus research to collect data in key areas.

Healthy People 2020 rests on four key goals:

- Eliminating preventable disease and death
- Achieving health equity by eliminating disparities and improving the health of all groups
- Creating social and physical environments that promote good health for all citizens
- Promoting healthy habits and behaviors for all ages of the population

The 2020 campaign has increased the number of priority, or focus, areas from 22 in 2000 to 28 in 2020.

Healthy People 2020 is important because it forms a national health agenda that, combined with health-care reform, can be used as a vision and a strategy for the whole nation. Its national-level goals are a road map for where the nation needs to go and how it will get there. Healthy People 2020 will be action oriented and will provide leadership, guidance, and direction for individuals and governmental agencies alike.

For more information about the ongoing developments and plans for implementation, go to http://www.healthypeople.gov/hp2020.

Source: Retrieved December, 2010 from http://www.healthypeople.gov/hp2020.

Table 24.4   Empirical Outcomes of Caring: Nurses

Effects of Caring Relationships on Nurses (Summary of Findings)	Effects of Noncaring Relationships on Nurses (Summary of Findings)
Sense of accomplishment, satisfaction, purpose, gratitude	Hardened affect and feeling of failure
Preserved integrity, fulfillment, wholeness, self-esteem	Obliviousness and apathy
Satisfaction in living own philosophy	Depression
Respect for life and death	Fear of death
Opportunities for reflection	Worn-down feeling
Love of nursing and increased knowledge	Burnout and indifference

Source: Adapted from Swanson, HL. Meta-analysis of 130 empirical studies. In Watson J (ed): Assessing and measuring caring in nursing and health science. New York, Springer, 2002.

Mentoring is a highly effective way of becoming an expert nurse.[22] Through mentoring partnerships and increasing their own cultural competence, health-care providers expand and update their own educational process.

The Nurse's Evolving Role

The National Institute for Nursing Research (NINR) has requested $160 million from a Congressional committee to investigate selected health issues. Among these issues is the need to eliminate disparities in access to health care and quality of health care being provided. In its mandate, the Committee states that, "reducing, and ultimately eliminating, health disparities is a critical priority for all areas of health-care research." To stimulate research on health-care disparities, NINR is encouraging the development of new nurse scientists from underserved populations.[23]

Collaborative Client Teaching for Healthy Communities
Sensitivity and Empowerment

The Pew Commission Final Report stressed that relationship-centered interactions must become central to the education of health professionals.[24] The report emphasized that constructive interpersonal encounters—culturally sensitive, caring, collaborative, and relationship centered—are critical to the promotion of preventive health care. See Chapter 4 for a fuller discussion of the Pew Commission Final Report, including "Twenty-one Competencies for the 21st Century."

For effective partnership and interaction with other health-care professionals, a picture of the health team can show how different professions view their focus on client care (Fig. 24.1).

Health professionals also can use population approaches in client teaching (Fig. 24.2). Effective decision-making and problem-solving are critical and

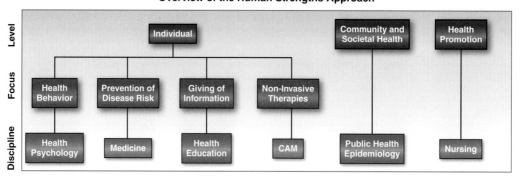

Figure 24.1 The interaction of different health professions with the community. CAM, complementary and alternative medicine. (From Leddy S: Health promotion. Philadelphia, F. A. Davis, 2006, with permission.)

Population Perspective of Health Promotion

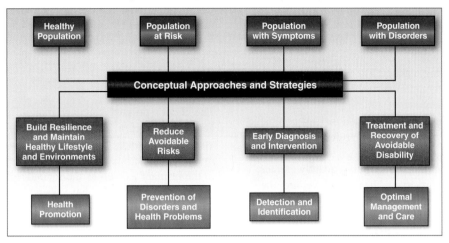

Figure 24.2 Health care for different populations. (From Rankin SH, Stallings KD, London F: Patient education in health and illness (5th ed). New York, Lippincott Williams & Wilkins, 2005, with permission.)

occur when a community is empowered. Such empowerment improves the health of all community members.

An Evidence-Based Example of Collaboration and Partnership

Few social programs can boast scientifically demonstrated outcomes through randomized controlled trials. Even fewer have demonstrated multigenerational outcomes that benefit society economically and reduce long-term social service expenditures.

Box 24.3 summarizes the results of a teaching partnership involving nurses, other health professionals, and first-time parents.[25]

For more than 33 years, Dr. David Olds conducted a model for a Nurse–Family Partnership (NFP) in collaboration with schools and with the fields of medicine, psychology, and public health. This teaching study tracked the effectiveness of home visiting by nurses in improving maternal and child health. First-time parents volunteered to take part in the study.

Box 24.3
Nurse–Family Partnership: Helping First-Time Parents Succeed

At an average savings of $17,500 per client being returned to the government, the following consistent outcomes occurred:
- Improved prenatal health
- Fewer childhood injuries
- Fewer subsequent pregnancies
- Increased intervals between births
- Increased maternal employment
- Improved school readiness

Source: Adapted from Olds DL, Henderson CR, Hanks C, Cole R, Tatelbaum R, et al.: Home visiting by paraprofessionals and by nurses: A randomized, controlled trial. Pediatrics 110(3):486, 2002.

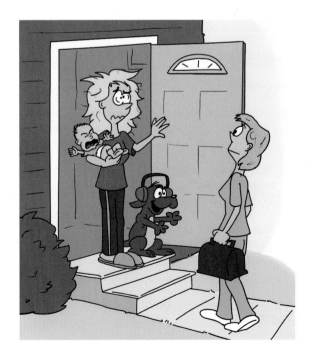

The NFP is committed to enduring improvements in the health and well-being of low-income, first-time parents and their children. Nurses were chosen for this program because of the high public trust of nurses and because nurses can relate to clients in a caring manner. The NFP has evolved to serving 270 counties across 22 states within the United States.[26]

A Denver trial conducted in 1994 compared home visits by nurses with paraprofessionals (workers with no formal education in caregiving professions). The visits by nurses produced significantly greater benefits to the participants' health and welfare; the paraprofessionals' visits produced small effects that rarely achieved statistical or clinical significance. The study concluded that caution should be used in allowing health-care providers other than registered nurses to make home visits, at least until consistent new evidence indicates that other helping paraprofessionals can become effective home visitors.[26]

Cultural Aspects of Teaching

Given the cultural diversity of the United States, nurses and other health-care providers must accommodate to different cultural behaviors. A client's cultural background strongly influences attitudes and beliefs about health. The nurse's knowledge of diverse cultural groups can facilitate a therapeutic approach to the client.

Communication Style

Communication and a caring relationship are profoundly affected by culture. Table 24.5 outlines differences in, and nuances of, some communication styles.

Language

The client's primary language may influence his or her ability to learn, especially if the nurse does not know the language. In conducting a language assessment, the nurse must determine the client's fluency in the primary as well as the secondary language.

Brochures that have been translated directly from English may not convey the intended message, or the words used may not be familiar to the client. In that case, an interpreter may be needed. It is important to ascertain that the interpreter speaks a dialect familiar to that particular client. The following provides an example of the fine discrimination needed in client teaching:

> In the Hispanic groups there are variations to the Spanish language. One example is the word *careta,* which for Mexicans means a cart used by farmers and pulled by oxen. For many Central Americans, *careta* means a taxicab. Using the wrong word can adversely affect a Hispanic individual trying to leave the emergency room to go home.[27]

Table 24.5   Cultural Differences in Communication Styles

Native Americans	Hispanics, Asian Americans	Whites	African Americans
1. Speak softly, more slowly	1. Speak softly	1. Speak loudly and fast to control listener	1. Speak with affect
2. Indirect gaze when listening or speaking	2. Avoid eye contact when listening or speaking to high-status persons	2. Head nods, nonverbal markers	2. Direct eye contact (prolonged) when speaking, but less when listening
3. Interject less, seldom offer encouraging communication	3. Similar rules	3. Head nods, nonverbal markers	3. Interrupt (in turn, when convenient)
4. Delayed auditory response (silence)	4. Mild delay	4. Prompt response	4. Prompt response
5. Low-keyed, indirect manner	5. Low-keyed, indirect manner	5. Objective, task-oriented manner	5. Affective, emotional, interpersonal manner

Source: Adapted from Sue DW, Sue D: Counseling the culturally different: Theory and practice (2nd ed). New York, John Wiley, 1990.

A person may understand elementary English and yet be unable to translate a lengthy or rapidly spoken explanation. When the nurse and client are from different cultures with language variations, more sensitivity and understanding than usual are required. Although television has contributed to wide recognition of terms such as "malignancy" and "cholesterol," the nurse should not take for granted that a client understands such terms and their implications in the same way a nurse does. Nor should the nurse expect the client receiving an explanation to be brave enough to speak up and ask for clarification, particularly if the client has been hiding a literacy problem for years. The following passage illustrates the frustration and fear that can occur in a chaotic cultural misunderstanding:

> A nursing acquaintance tells of a client who became hysterical when an explanation about the presence of a hydatidiform mole aroused fears of a brown, furry animal growing inside her. The client was too fearful and ashamed to tell her husband. She did not follow through on treatment for a long period of time, until a translator determined what the misapprehension was. Then a priest as well as the health-care providers were needed to help the client overcome her emotional turmoil and stress that could have been avoided with a more sensitive communication.[28]

The Office of Minority Health (2011) supports standards needed for cultural competence, language access, and organizational support and recommends the adoption of the National Standards for Culturally and Linguistically Appropriate Standards.[29]

Educational Level and Motivation

The higher a person's educational level, the more likely that person is to have received some formal health education. Research also shows that the higher a person's educational level, the higher the motivation to learn. Physicians often speak of well-educated clients who surf the Internet and learn new information about a disease or diseases. The researcher Goetz has developed data that provide new insight into a collaborative relationship with the client. He uses a decision tree to facilitate clients' decision-making process and motivate them to change their health strategies.[30]

The nurse should ask the following questions before teaching a client: What is the client's level of motivation to learn? What factors will motivate the client to learn healthy behaviors? Outstanding motivational success occurred in the NFP when Olds' five principles were followed (Box 24.4).[26]

These simply stated five principles concur with Peplau's notion of the importance of interpersonal relationships to the practice of nursing.[28] Authoritarian, oppressive, negative communications produce a lack of healing. Simple, sincere, positive exchanges create and reinforce a new health-care communication style and healing. Healing is the most important contribution of health-care providers. They should care for a client as if they were caring for themselves or their loved ones because, at some fundamental level, they actually are. Nurses, being human, are energic beings. As such, they are designed to perceive and translate energy into neural code, which will help them become more aware of their energy and dynamic intuition.[27]

As nurses care for clients and provide education, it is critical to use a positive wavelength to connect with and heal the client (see Table 24.3).

THE NUTS AND BOLTS OF CLIENT TEACHING

Collaborative Skills

Imagine the best-case scenario: caring communication, cultural and environmental sensitivity, attention

---

Box 24.4

Olds' Principles of the Nurse–Family Partnership

1. The client is an expert on his or her own life.
2. Follow the client's heart's desire.
3. Focus on strengths.
4. Focus on solutions.
5. Only a small change is necessary.

Source: Adapted from Olds DL, Henderson CR, Hanks C, Cole R, Tatelbaum R, et al.: Home visiting by paraprofessionals and by nurses: A randomized, controlled trial. Pediatrics 110(3):486, 2002.

to educational and economic considerations, and advanced technology. In these circumstances, nurses can rely on the teaching–learning process just as they do on the nursing process. In fact, the two processes are very similar.

The need for certain collaborative skills is implicit in the teaching–learning process. Health-care providers need these skills to empower their clients and help them achieve the best possible quality of life. Haber[6] recommends the following collaborative skills:

1. Consider yourself a consultant and help clients remain in control of their own health choices.
2. Counsel all clients, and especially reach out to those who differ from you in age, educational level, gender, and ethnicity.
3. Make sure your clients understand the relationship between behavior and health. Understand that, although knowledge is necessary, it is not sufficient to change clients' behaviors.
4. Assess clients' barriers to change, including their lack of skills, motivation, resources, and social support.
5. Encourage clients to commit themselves to change, involving them in the selection of risk factors to eliminate.
6. Use a combination of strategies, including behavioral and cognitive techniques, the identification and encouragement of social support, and appropriate referrals.
7. Monitor progress through follow-up telephone calls and appointments, and activate your health-care team, including the receptionist and other office staff.
8. Be a role model.

Nurses need to not only remember client literacy but also to be "client literate." Every time a client leaves an encounter with a health-care professional, the client should have more knowledge than when he or she entered the system. If clients do not understand the information nurses and other providers are offering or are not given a rationale for lifestyle-change recommendations, they are unlikely to remember the information and may continue making poor decisions that can ultimately cost them their lives.[31] As health-care reform leads the nation toward a client-centered, proactive, and preventive model, consumers must understand their health status and provider's instruction.[3]

Medagogy

Medagogy is one of the first theories focused on client–provider information exchange or client education in the health-care delivery system. Developed by Stewart,[31] the Medagogy model identifies the client and health-care provider as both learner and educator. The model identifies the provider as the *expert of health,* whereas the client serves as the *expert of self.* Both provider and client, through knowledge acquired from each other, are able to make informed decisions about health-care choices.

The goal of Medagogy is to move client education away from the traditional disease-oriented or provider-oriented information toward a more client-oriented focus. The Certified Patient Educator (CPE) is a licensed health-care professional trained in the Medagogy model. CPEs work to ensure that clients succeed in understanding their health status and actions or behaviors that can help improve their health. In their daily practice, CPEs incorporate various Medagogy tools, such as report card teaching plans and evaluation of client understanding. CPEs transition clients by empowering them with knowledge so they can assume a more active role in their personal health care.[31]

Steps in a Process

Table 24.6 outlines the five steps of the teaching–learning process and compares them with the four steps of the nursing process. The following discussion of the teaching–learning process examines each step in detail.

I. Assessment
  A. Learner Characteristics
    In assessing learning needs and learning readiness, nurses should focus on cultural and literacy issues and on the client's age and gender. People with learning disabilities also require special attention.

    The term **health literacy** refers not only to reading comprehension level but also to the ability to act on instructions. Problems with health literacy are associated more commonly with ethnic minorities, who have worse outcomes than the majority of the U.S. population.[32] However, even the most educated may have difficulty understanding health-care instructions. One well-educated

Table 24.6   Comparison of the Teaching-Learning Process with the Nursing Process

Teaching-Learning Process	Nursing Process

I. Assessment
  A. Learner characteristics
  B. Learner needs
	I. Assessment

II. Development of expected learning outcomes through objectives	II. Diagnosis and planning

III. Development of a teaching plan
  A. Content
  B. Teaching strategies and learning activities	

IV. Implementation of the teaching plan
V. Evaluation of expected outcomes
  A. Achievement of learning outcomes
  B. Effectiveness of the teaching process
	III. Implementation of the nursing plan
	IV. Evaluation

Source: Adapted from Edelman C, Mandel C: Health promotion throughout the life span. Philadelphia, Mosby Elsevier, 2006, p 225.

elementary school teacher thought the instruction to take pills with food meant wrapping her pills in cheese and then taking them.[33]

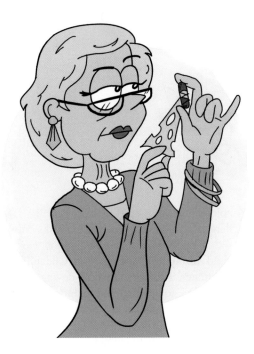

B. Learner Needs
The most effective learning occurs when the client is involved in the process. **Passive learning** does not change behaviors or attitudes and therefore does not change the outcome.[34] Although passive learning is useful when new knowledge must be gained, it becomes unbalanced and lost for lack of application. In either case, the nurse must determine the performance level of any tasks or skills the client may need to learn.[32]

II. Development of Expected Learning Outcomes Through Objectives
Without learning objectives, measurement of learning outcomes is compromised and ineffective. By developing behavioral objectives, the nurse clarifies what behaviors or actions are expected. The best objectives are created by the client in collaboration with first, the health-care team, and second, the family or community to which the client returns. Clients are energized by accomplishing simple behaviors conceived collaboratively.[35]

Objectives fall within three domains, or categories: affective, cognitive, and psychomotor. The **affective domain objectives** concern the feelings, values, and attitudes necessary for a positive effect on the client's life. Affective skills include positive attitudes, constructive feelings, and values (ethics) that underlie the rapport with the client.

Cognitive domain objectives outline the knowledge the client will need, accounting for intellectual ability and age. Cognitive skills include evidence-based knowledge, logical thought processes, and sufficient clarity of vision to understand the client's perception of his or her self-management care needs. The last point is important for promotion of the greatest possible independence.

The cognitive area also involves understanding of both acute and chronic illnesses. Many websites offer suggestions for teaching clients about managing illness. The cognitive domain is divided into levels of understanding, from simple to complex. Box 24.5 shows the different levels of learning.

The **psychomotor domain objectives** comprise expected behaviors, such as a change in diet or weight. For behavioral change to occur, memory from the cognitive domain must be present. Psychomotor skills include modeling the skills clients will need for self-care. For example, an obese 92-year-old white diabetic female, suffering from retinal damage and renal failure caused by untreated hypertension, will need to give injections, take her own blood pressure, check her urine for protein and glucose, and increase possible exercise options, along with trying to improve her deteriorating vision and following a renal diet. A nurse could model these behaviors or involve her with a support group of individuals needing to learn the same skills.[36]

Box 24.5

The Cognitive Domain: Levels of Understanding

- Knowledge: recall of facts and concepts
- Comprehension: understanding of what concepts mean
- Application: use of a concept
- Analysis: ability to examine or explain a concept
- Synthesis: integration of a concept with other learning
- Evaluation: judging or comparison of concepts

Source: Adapted from Bastable SB: Behavioral objectives. In Bastable SB (ed): Nurse as educator: Principles of teaching and learning for nursing practice (p 226). Sudbury, MA, Jones & Bartlett, 2003.

III. Development of a Teaching Plan
   A. Content
   Nurses can gather the content they need from many resources. Some underused but critical sources are nursing organizations and disease-oriented websites, such as that of the American Cancer Society. Good content also helps clients get answers about medical decisions; self-care information; and more complete understanding of their condition, their care, or any area of wellness that needs improvement.[33]
   B. Teaching Strategies and Learning Activities
   Tables 24.7 and 24.8 summarize this part of the outline.

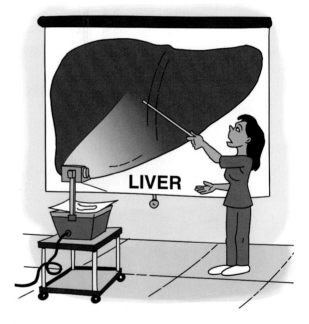

IV. Implementation of the Teaching Plan
   Client education is difficult when tasks outweigh the time needed to do an effective job. Hospitals should introduce a new position: Client Teacher Practitioner. This person would devote the needed time to creating and maintaining the required environments at a primary, secondary, or tertiary setting.

   A study at Georgetown University found that, on an average, $3 to $4 was saved for every dollar invested in client education. A Danish hospital study of clients with chronic obstructive pulmonary disease (COPD) found a savings of $2583 per client. Centers that

Table 24.7 Commonly Used Teaching Strategies and Methods

Strategy/Method	Description
Case study	An actual or hypothetical account of a situation to help the learner apply principles.
	Useful for critical thinking exercises in the classroom. Useful in the clinical setting for comparison with actual situations.
	Helpful in problem solving. The learner moves from a simple formulation of a problem to a complex understanding of it.
Computer instruction (PowerPoint™, Internet) (also called *e-learning*)	Use of computers in the classroom or clinical setting.
	Adds color to presentations. Key words are important in PowerPoint presentations. Includes blogs, iPods, and video games for younger learners.
Demonstration	A skill performed by the teacher and repeated by the learner.
	Useful for developing motor skills in both the classroom and clinical settings.
Discussion	Verbal communication of ideas; information with participation by both teacher and learner.
	Useful in classrooms with fewer than 20 students.
	Useful in clinical settings with an audience of 1 or more.
	Allows for assessment of values and knowledge of the topic.
	Elicits decision-making regarding a situation or a piece of information.
Lecture	Formal oral presentation by the teacher.
	Useful for a group of more than 30.
	Best if oral presentation is accompanied by a handout (e.g., outline, notes, with space to write more notes). Handouts help the learner stay focused.
Media	Use of audiotapes, videotapes, or filmstrips; may be auditory or visual.
	Useful for testing motor-skill development, discussing a particular topic, or assessing comprehension of content.
Modeling	Teaching by example; learners observe the teacher's behavior.
Trial and error	Learning by experience; used sometimes when the learner has little knowledge of content or of a situation.
	Sporadically useful during practice with a computer, engine, or other machine.
	Trial-and-error learning is time consuming and frustrating to learners (especially adults) and should be minimized.
Visual aids	Use of overhead transparencies, slides, pictures, paintings, posters, handouts, brochures.
	Useful for determining knowledge about, for example, objects and organs.
	Useful as adjunct to verbal explanation of concepts.
Role-playing	Acting the part of another person; usually followed by discussion of perceptions or feelings.
	Provides a change in perspective.
	Useful in both classroom and clinical settings.

specialize in asthma care (The Community Asthma Care Centers) save $1.07 million in health-care costs when clients are able to carry out self-care measures properly.

V. Evaluation of Expected Outcomes
A client's ability to meet co-created objectives can be easily monitored if follow-up and communication are embedded in the teaching–learning process. Technology- and computer-based learning programs need further study. That, and time, will determine their contribution to saving lives and improving quality of life for clients, families, and communities.

Evaluating Teaching Effectiveness in Client Education

Health-care providers must educate clients with the intent increasing their knowledge. To ensure

Table 24.8 Matching Teaching Strategies to Learners

Strategy/Method	Learner
Case study	Adolescents, young adults, adults
Computer	All ages; especially appropriate for young learners (born after 1982)
Demonstration	All ages
Discussion	Preadolescents, adolescents, young adults, adults, older adults
Lecture	Adults, older adults
Media (e-learning)	All ages; especially appropriate for young learners (born after 1982)
Modeling	All ages
Trial and error	Adolescents, young adults
Visual aids	All ages
Role-playing	Children, adolescents, young adults

that the context of the intended information is received, the provider must evaluate the client's understanding. An assessment of understanding offers a glimpse into the receiver's comprehension of the information received.

Content evaluation is easily accomplished through testing. True/false, multiple choice, and even essay questions are all viable methods for testing health-care knowledge. Unfortunately, test anxiety is a real phenomenon that can stress a client already challenged by a health problem. Return demonstration is an effective method of evaluating a person's ability to perform a skill. The challenge lies in consistency of behavior as a person transitions from care setting to home.[31]

The Understanding-Personal Perception (UPP) tool offers a new perspective to quantifying client understanding. UPP uses a five-point Likert scale with visual graphics to evaluate how much clients believe they have learned. The UPP tool removes anxiety about wrong answers because it provides a self-reflection of personal knowledge positioning.[37]

Conclusion

With its emphasis on prevention and health maintenance, health-care reform not only has left the door wide open for client education but also demands it as an essential part of high-quality health care. This should not be a surprise to nurses. Since its earliest steps toward a profession, leaders in nursing realized that client education was a moral imperative for nurses. Recent research shows that a large number of unnecessary readmissions to hospitals could have been prevented if clients had received the health-care education they needed before discharge. However, nursing students receive very little education on how to teach clients. As a result, they often feel uncomfortable in the educator role and often will avoid teaching because of feelings of inadequacy. It is imperative that nursing schools increase their content on client education so that graduates will have the skills and confidence to fulfill this important role of the profession. Everyone in society benefits if client education is successfully planned and instituted.

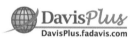

DavisPlus
DavisPlus.fadavis.com

Critical Thinking Exercises

- Take the computer-based learning sites in Table 24.2 and plug them into The Joint Commission icon to determine which ones are approved.
- Look back at your own client teaching and critique what you did well and what could have been improved. Refer to The Joint Commission requirements in Box 24.2.
- Review Chapter 7, "Ethics in Nursing," and apply the concepts to the moral imperative for client teaching.
- Review the legal caveat in charting for client teaching. Reflect on your own client teaching charting and describe your strengths and weaknesses in this area.

25

Nursing Research and Evidence-Based Practice

Mary Ann Remshardt

Learning Objectives

After completing this chapter, the reader will be able to:

- Discuss the necessity of nursing research as an essential component of comprehensive client care.
- Describe ways in which nursing research can be used to enhance communication and understanding between cultures.
- Demonstrate the ability to identify the basic similarities and differences related to qualitative and quantitative research designs.
- Identify at least four strategies that may help promote implementation of valid research findings in clinical settings.
- Define and describe the concept and utility of evidence-based practice.
- Discuss the research–practice gap as this relates to nursing research and identify some ideas for promoting change.

A UNIQUE BODY OF KNOWLEDGE

One characteristic that defines a profession is the creation of a unique body of knowledge and related skills to guide its practitioners. There are many ways of obtaining knowledge. In the nursing profession, the development of a distinct body of nursing knowledge is an ongoing process. Nursing has a long and dignified history as a service and caring profession. In contrast, nursing as a scientific discipline is just now taking its first unsteady steps. As with every profession, nursing continues to evolve to meet the needs of a changing society and the rapid development of new health-care technology.

TRIAL AND ERROR

In the past, much of what constituted the practice of the nursing profession was based on the edicts of those in authority. Founded on experiential learning, nursing focused on doing exactly what was prescribed by a person in charge, usually the physician. Before we built our own body of knowledge, it made sense to rely on the judgment of those who were considered by society to be authorities on issues such as health and illness and with whom nurses worked closely.

In the past, when skills used in the promotion of health and healing were developed, often through trial and error, they were then passed on by tradition. The trial-and-error method (supported by early science) historically served as a primary source of health-care knowledge.

Today the *search* for knowledge within what is *known* is being systematically replaced by *research* that reveals what is *best* in nursing practice. Research is the approach through which nursing knowledge, although not infallible, may be judged much more reliable and transferable than that afforded by authority, tradition, or past experience. Nursing as a science depends on valid research evidence to support best practice. Research provides the crucial link between theory and practice.

This chapter presents an overview of pertinent issues regarding the critical nature of research as scientific support for the profession of nursing.

NURSING RESEARCH DEFINED

Nursing research defines nursing as a profession and therefore must be embraced by nursing professionals. As one of a number of professions involved in providing health care, nursing accepts responsibility for defining its own uniqueness. Scientific inquiry is the tool of choice for tasks related to professional clarification, justification, extension, and collaboration.

The Goals of Inquiry

Nurses are held accountable for their actions and must equip themselves to defend the interventions they initiate through strong empirical evidence. At the very minimum, nursing care must be safe. With contemporary cost-containment issues, nursing interventions are expected to demonstrate practicality as well as cost effectiveness. Research can show which approaches to nursing care are most effective and which do not work. The profession of nursing will not experience a true renaissance until scientific inquiry becomes as much a part of daily practice as caring interventions.

More than a method of inquiry, nursing research is a systematic process for answering questions through the discovery of new information with the ultimate goal of improving client care.[1] The purpose of nursing research is "to test, refine and advance the knowledge on which improved education, clinical judgment, and cost-effective, safe, ethical nursing care rests."[2]

Beyond Clinical Practice

Some authors would limit the scope of nursing research to the clinical practice of nursing. In its fullest meaning, however, nursing research involves a systematic quest for knowledge designed to address questions and solve problems relevant to the profession, including issues related to nursing practice, nursing education, and nursing administration.[3] Nursing research is conducted to expand and clarify the body of knowledge unique to the discipline of nursing.

Redefining the Client. Nurses know that clients are more than just individuals receiving nursing care within selected clinical settings. Nursing clients are family units, communities, organizations, institutions, corporations, local and state agencies, and citizens of a country and of the global community. To accurately measure how effectively it meets the needs of an expanding and diverse consumer base, the nursing profession must integrate an expanding and diverse body of scientific knowledge into its daily practice. Nurses must focus on promoting better understanding of the research process and encouraging their colleagues to seek the evidence needed to explain, modify, and improve nursing practice.

Setting Priorities and Directions. Clinical decisions and the resulting nursing interventions are justified by scientifically documented findings. Using nursing research, nurse investigators not only address issues related to cost, safety, quality, and accessibility of health care but also look ahead to establish priorities and to define the future direction of the nursing profession. Recently, the Institute of Medicine (IOM) has established a list of 100 research topics that are based on comparative effectiveness research (CER). Many of these are community oriented and fit well with nursing's holistic approach to health care.

Crossing Cultural Boundaries. One critical requirement for a dynamic profession is to understand and address cultural issues involved in nursing care and to understand the various cultures within the communities where nurses practice. We must also learn to look beyond perceptual and geographic boundaries to promote dialogue, investigation, and collaboration with our many international nursing colleagues in the interest of culturally sensitive and global concerns. Culturally related issues provide numerous opportunities for nursing research (see Chapter 22).

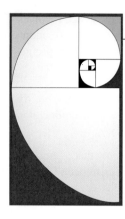

Issues Now

Big Bucks for Nursing Research in Health Care Reform Act

If you had $1.1 billion, what type of research would you conduct? That's the amount that was made available for health-care research with the passage of the American Recovery and Reinvestment Act of 2009 and further clarified in the Patient Protection Affordable Care Act of 2010. If health-care reform is not repealed as promised by the opposition party in the legislature over the next few years, the sum may be increased to as much as $10 billion by the end of the decade. Of course, not all of it is just for nursing research, but nursing will certainly get its share of the pie. Originally the money was to be spent in 18 months, but cooler heads recognized that was not realistic, so now it will be given out at the rate of several hundred million per year until it is gone.

How do you get the money? You must submit a research proposal similar to the ones that have been used for many years for all federal grants. Nursing will be up against stiff competition from the pharmaceutical and biomedical industries, which have well-developed research writing abilities. However, the distribution of the money will not rely totally on the federal government. The health-care reform bill contains provisions that change the oversight of funding from the Federal Coordinating Council of Comparative Effectiveness Research to a new organization called the Patient-Centered Outcomes Research Institute. This is a public–private partnership organization that will base funds distribution on the IOM's list of 100 initial priorities.

Projects to be funded must come under the designation of CER. Best practices development is a key in receiving funding. In addition to the usual ethical compliance and regulatory documentation, researchers will also have to demonstrate that they are pursuing Good Clinical Practice (GCP). GCP guidelines are much more specific about the elements of research protocol. In addition to documenting research methodologies, all researchers will be required to spell out in detail each aspect of the trial. The Research Institute will provide the tools required for the project. Required information includes personnel qualifications, curriculum vitae, Institutional Review Board (IRB) submission and approval documentation, tracking logs, and participant enrollment, just to start with. These documents must all be in a regulatory binder that can be used by others at the research site when the principal investigator is unable to conduct the research.

The IOM's 100 priorities are not individually ranked in any particular order. They are divided up into groups of 25, or "quartile" groups, according to the primary focus of the research. Many of the categories are community based because most health issues occur away from the hospital and outside the physician's office or clinic. Following are listed 10 areas that may interest nurses who wish to apply for some of the research money.

Nursing's Top 10 IOM Priorities for Research (with apologies to David Letterman)

10. Preventing and treating overweight and obesity in children and adolescents through school-related interventions such as healthy meal programs, vending machines that sell healthy snacks, and physical activity.

Issues Now continued

9. Developing more effective treatment strategies for atrial fibrillation by comparing treatments such as surgery, catheter ablation, lifestyle changes, and medications.

8. Identifying risk factors and preventing falls in older adults through primary prevention methods such as exercise, balance training, and various clinical treatments.

7. Evaluating the effectiveness of comprehensive home-care programs for children and adults with severe chronic disease, particularly in minority and ethnic populations that have been identified has having ongoing health disparities.

6. Comparing the effectiveness of hearing loss treatments for children and adults in minority groups and ethnic populations: evaluating various methods including, but not limited to, assistive listening devices, cochlear implants, electric-acoustic devices, rehabilitation methods, sign language, and total communication techniques.

5. Preventing obesity, hypertension, diabetes, and heart disease in at-risk groups such as the urban poor, Hispanic, and American Indian populations: comparing the effectiveness of strategies including, but not limited to, pharmacological interventions, improved community environment, making healthy foods available, or a combination of interventions.

4. Reducing or eliminating health-care associated infection (HAI) in adults and children by testing various techniques, particularly where invasive devices such as central lines, ventilators, and surgical procedures are used.

3. Determining the best methods for early detection, prevention, treatment, and elimination of antibiotic-resistant organisms (e.g., methicillin-resistant *Staphylococcus aureus* [MRSA]) in both community and institutional settings.

2. Determining the best treatments for early detection and management of dementia to be used by caregivers in the community setting.

1. Publishing and distributing the findings of CER so that clients, physicians, nurses, and others can use the data to establish best practices.

Sources: Doherty RB: The certitudes and uncertainties of health care reform. Annals of Internal Medicine 152(10):679–682, 2010.

Elwood TW: Health reform and its aftermath. Journal of Allied Health 39(2):65–71, 2010.

Eastman P: IOM workshop: US clinical research needs major transformation. Institute of Medicine. Oncology Times 31(22):39–41, 2009.

Health care reform and clinical research: Gold rush or drug bust? Millions available, but long-term impact questioned. Clinical Trials Administrator 8(5):49–53, 2010.

Initial National Priorities for Comparative Effectiveness Research. Committee on Comparative Effectiveness Research Prioritization, Institute of Medicine. Washington, DC, The National Academies Press, 2009. Retrieved November, 2010 from http://www.nap.edu.

DEVELOPMENT AND PROGRESSION OF RESEARCH IN NURSING

The Origin of Nursing Research

Florence Nightingale is viewed as the person who first elevated nursing to the status of a profession, as presented in her first book, *Notes on Nursing* (1859).[4] She is also credited with introducing research to the profession. Nightingale believed in the importance of "naming nursing" through the collection and use of objective data to support the need for health-care reforms, including those related to nursing education. Nightingale recognized the impact of combining strong logical thinking and empirical research in developing a sound scientific base on which to build the practices of the nursing profession.

Methodical Observation

As the first recognized nurse epidemiologist, Florence Nightingale systematically collected objective data and in 1855 described environmental factors that affected health and illness. During the Crimean War, appalled by what she observed of the care of soldiers, Nightingale was forward-thinking enough to implement and then demand scientific inquiry in the practice setting. She methodically gathered facts, eventually supporting her claims that lack of cleanliness, fresh air, proper rest, and nutrition contributed to high levels of disease and death seen in the frontline "hospital" during the war.

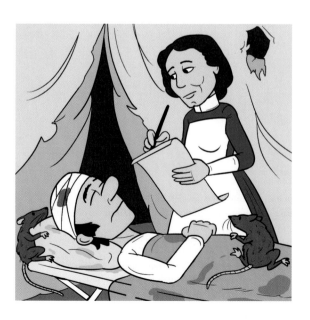

As a result of her research, she petitioned forcefully for more supplies, better food, and cleaner conditions. Her advocacy lowered the mortality rate among wounded soldiers from 42 to 2 percent. Her work during the 1800s was not fully appreciated until more than a century later.[4]

The Development of Research

Even today, the full importance of this one woman's work to the profession of nursing is still being evaluated. Nightingale had few professional role models, relatively little education, a military organization that doubted her value, and meager financial support. Her accomplishments, in view of the challenge, were phenomenal. It is interesting to speculate about how much more progress would have been made in building the unique body of nursing knowledge if other nurses had heeded Nightingale's earliest call for research.

A Look at Nursing Education

During the 1940s, many studies concerning nursing education came to the forefront because of the tremendous demand for educated nurses during World War II. Nursing education practices were evaluated in a study commissioned by the National Nursing Council for War Service. Findings from this study and others at the time uncovered weaknesses in nursing education. This relatively new wave of research spawned several other studies that looked at nurses' functions, roles, attitudes, acceptance, and interactions with clients.

A Center for Nursing Research

Several events that occurred during the 1950s prompted those conducting nursing research to carve out an ever-expanding path for the profession of nursing that continues to widen today. Nurses with advanced degrees were increasing in numbers. A center for nursing research was formed at the Walter Reed Army Institute of Research.

Creation of the American Nurses' Foundation and the journal *Nursing Research* allowed publication of nursing research findings that gave both a face and a voice to the studies. Many of these studies became both the mirror and the microscope through which nurses studied themselves. This self-appraisal was an unprecedented research approach for any profession.

A New Definition of Nursing

In the 1960s, phrases such as *conceptual framework, conceptual model,* and *nursing process* made their first appearances in textbooks and other nursing literature (see Chapter 4). Nursing leaders, now becoming more focused on theoretical support for nursing, continued to lament the relative lack of research.

Many professional nursing organizations set priorities for research during this time. It was also during this time that another visionary nurse heeded the call to logical reasoning and empirical research. Virginia Henderson, one of the early nursing theorists, defined the role of nursing as, "to assist individuals (sick or well) with those activities contributing to health, or its recovery or to a peaceful death, that they perform unaided, when they have the necessary strength, will, or knowledge; to help individuals carry out prescribed therapy and to be independent of assistance as soon as possible."[4]

This definition was so conceptually clear that it was accepted by the International Council of Nurses (ICN) in 1960, and Henderson's work went on to identify many relevant research questions for the practice of professional nursing.

> *Nightingale recognized the impact of combining strong logical thinking and empirical research in developing a sound scientific base on which to build the practices of the nursing profession.*

A Growth in Research Programs

In the 1970s, the number of graduate nursing programs experienced tremendous growth, and so did the number of nurses conducting research. Increases in the number of ongoing research studies pointed out the need for an improved way to publicize those studies. Three more research journals were developed: *Advances in Nursing Science, Research in Nursing and Health,* and the *Western Journal of Nursing Research.* During this time the research focus began to change from the study of nurses to the study of client-care needs. Clinical challenges were identified as having the highest priority for nursing research.

A Source of National Data

The 1980s witnessed another information explosion with the continued growth rate of research-trained, graduate school–educated nurses and the introduction of computers. Research and writing were both enhanced by electronic databases and the expanding World Wide Web. In 1983, the American Nurses'

Association created the Center for Research for Nursing.

The mission of this center is to serve as a source of national data for the profession. In 1986, the National Center for Nursing Research (NCNR) at the National Institutes of Health was established by congressional mandate. The mission of this organization is to support clinical (applied) and basic research to create a scientific foundation for the care of individuals across the life span. During the 1980s, a journal with the specific intention of providing research directed toward the practicing clinical nurse took form in *Applied Nursing Research.*

A New Focus on Practice

In 1993, the NCNR was awarded full institute status, and the National Institute of Nursing Research (NINR; http://www.nih.gov/ninr.org) came into being. In 1996, NINR had a reported $55 million budget, and it was poised to promote and support research priorities established during that decade. Since the late 1990s, studies have become more focused on the practice of nursing, the outcomes of nursing and other health-care services, and the building of a stronger knowledge base by replicating previous research using a variety of settings and situations.

THE NEXT STEP IN NURSING PRACTICE

Evidence-Based Practice

Today, the movement to achieve cost-effective, high-quality care based on scientific inquiry generates the drive for evidence-based practice (EBP). Evidence-based practice is today's nursing issue of priority. Because of the volume of literature being published by all health-care professions, including nursing, it is important to develop critical discernment skills. Critical discernment requires the nurse to understand the research process and to sift through and carefully assess all available and credible research findings. Once the research has been analyzed and judged, recommendations for using the best practice techniques can be made on the basis of best evidence.[5]

Although nurses have been using evidence-based nursing practice in some form since the early days of nursing, it is only recently that the process has become formalized and widespread as a methodology. The current use of EBP in nursing requires a transition from nursing care that is based on opinions, past practices, and precedent to decisions that are based on scientific research and proven evidence. The goal of nurses using EBP is to obtain the best information available and to integrate it into nursing practice. Such practice includes the client's values and self-determination in providing care, as well as those of the client's family. The ultimate outcome sought is improved quality of care.

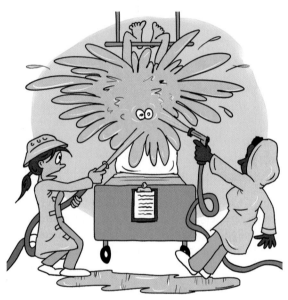

"ARE YOU SURE THIS NEW BATH TECHNIQUE WAS ON THE EVIDENCE-BASED PRACTICE LIST?"

Evidence Reports

Nurses can use numerous sources when incorporating EBP into their care provision. Research reported in the literature is a primary source of high-quality information, but not the only one. Other sources include expert opinion, collaborative consensus, published standards, historical data, local quality assurance studies, and institutional reports including cost effectiveness and client and family preferences and input. The key to using these various sources of information is the ability to grade or rank them so that nursing practice is based on the *best* information available. An excellent way to sort out the quality of information is to visit the website http://www.guideline.gov for evidence reports.

The evidence reports contained at this site provide a scientific basis for a disease or a nursing practice and then integrate the data into actions used in practice. The reports synthesize previous and current knowledge related to the topic, review the information for quality and documentation, explain how EBP is currently being used, and discuss how useful the EBP is to the clinical practice. The reviews in evidence reports are more detailed than a typical literature review and include broad-based information translated into specific approaches to client care. Currently there is a substantial database, and new data are constantly being added to the site.[6]

Nurses should look for several key elements in evidence reports when attempting to integrate EBP into their care. The first part of the report should include a structured summary statement of the problem, practice, or disease that describes what is in the evidence report. The second part should comprise a lengthy and detailed analysis of the published and unpublished data, including reviews of articles and reports, the populations included in the studies, and the nature of the nursing actions investigated. One of the most important elements in the second part of the evidence report is the ranking or grading of the quality of the evidence.

The level of quality of the evidence is sometimes referred to as the "level of recommendation for use" and answers the nurse's question, "Should I value this information and use it in my practice?" Integrative reviews in evidence reports should provide both the type of evidence included and the strengths and consistencies of the information.

Types of Evidence Used

Five types of evidence can be present in an evidence report, ranked from I (strongest) to V (weakest). They are:

I. Meta-analysis of multiple well-designed, controlled studies that examines and synthesizes many studies to find similar results
II. At least one well-designed experimental study with a random sample, control group, and intervention
III. Well-designed, quasi-experimental studies, such as nonrandomized controlled, single-group pretest or post-test, cohort studies, or time series studies

IV. Well-designed nonexperimental studies, such as comparative and correlational descriptive studies and controlled case studies

V. Case reports and clinical examples

The strength and consistency of evidence are also ranked on a five-point scale ranging from A (best) to E (poorest). In general, a "B" or higher should be present before a nurse integrates the data into EBP. The rankings are:

A. There is type I evidence or consistent findings from multiple studies of types II, III, or IV.

B. There is type II, III, or IV evidence, and the findings are generally consistent.

C. There is type II, III, or IV evidence, but the findings are inconsistent.

D. There is little or no evidence, or there is type V evidence only.

E. *Panel consensus:* Practice recommendations are based on the opinions of experts in the field.

One potential problem in using these ranking systems is that they may not be the best method of analyzing the strength of the evidence. In nursing, much of the research is qualitative or descriptive, or even narrative, because of the difficulty in performing controlled studies with large groups of clients. The nurse needs to check the consistency of the results, even though there may not be any type I, II, or III studies in the evidence report.[5]

> " *Understanding research is more than merely learning simple methods of inquiry.* "

The next section of the evidence report focuses on clinical practice and should include practice-focused guidelines or recommendations for specific clinical interventions. Often this section begins with a statement such as, "There is very good evidence that . . ." or "There is no evidence that. . . ." The practices outlined should be specific and relevant to the care being given.

The last section of the evidence report is the report source. Reports should be specific and current and should come from high-quality, refereed professional journals.

Evaluating an Evidence Report

The nurse can evaluate the evidence report by asking three questions. Only after answering these questions will the nurse be able to decide what to do with the information.

1. *Is this the best available evidence?* Best sources include peer-reviewed journals and reports no more than 3 to 5 years old.

2. *Will the recommendations work for my practice given the client population and problems?* If the study population is of young adult white men and the nurse's primary work population is elderly women, the data generated may not apply.

3. *Do the recommendations fit well with the preferences and values of the clients I commonly work with?* If the values of the nurse's primary group vary greatly from those of the study group, it is likely the recommendations may not work well.

Nurses can locate evidence reports from numerous sources:

Clinical Journals
Evidence-Based Nursing
Online Journal of Clinical Innovations
Reformatted STTI
Online Journal for Knowledge Synthesis in Nursing

Other Sources
National Guideline Clearinghouse (U.S. Agency for Healthcare Research and Quality): a repository for clinical practice guidelines
The Cochrane Collaboration (international): develops and maintains systematic reviews
State University of New York (SUNY) website: lists the best sites for information

When nurses begin to take the next step and integrate EBP into the care they provide, they will make a major leap toward raising the level of professionalism in nursing practice. Through the use of EBP in nursing, the quality of client care will improve when that care is based on validated evidence that focuses on what works best.

Currently, nurses have been given the responsibility not only to conduct research but also to evaluate, critique, and apply the research findings of other nurses and health-care professionals in their own practice. Understanding research is more than merely learning simple methods of inquiry.

THE RESEARCH PROCESS

Nursing students, long before graduation, often notice something in the clinical setting that grabs their attention. They may simply wonder if a different approach would work better in a particular situation or if the best technique is currently being used, and what evidence exists to support a particular technique or intervention as "best."

As neophytes, students may question interventions or solutions that seasoned nurses may take for granted. Students may see the experienced nurse's familiar world differently, and their minds may be open to possibilities that others may not see. Questioning the status quo is a key first step in the research process. Employing critical thinking often leads to visualization of a research project, the development of a plan, the implementation of that plan, and finally, sharing of the findings with others. This process follows a logical progression from abstract ideas to concrete actions.

Research Designs

The word *design* implies both creativity and structure. The design for a research study can be seen as a road map or a recipe. It serves as a fairly flexible set of guidelines that will provide the researcher with answers to the questions of inquiry.

To choose a research design, the nurse must first develop a vision of the overall plan for a study, including a general idea of the type of data needed to answer the research question. The design is a critical link that connects the researcher's framework with appropriate types of data. The level of preexisting knowledge in the area of inquiry also helps determine the research design. If little is known about a specific subject, an exploratory study may be the best method for uncovering new information. In exploratory research, there is usually more interest in the qualitative characteristics of data. Hypotheses are usually not required for these studies.

If the researcher is looking at variables that are independent or objective, or that demonstrate cause and effect, a quantitative design is best. If the question invites discovery of meanings, perceptions, and the collection of subjective data, a qualitative design should be used.

Quantitative Versus Qualitative Research

Historically and in the tradition of scientific inquiry, quantitative experimental research designs were the most highly respected. These designs are guided by a somewhat rigid set of rules that gives the most importance to the *process* of inquiry. However, the past 15 years have seen a growing interest in, and respect for, qualitative approaches in research, especially in the social sciences. Social researchers see human interactions as complex, highly contextual, and too intricate to be studied using a rigid framework or standard instrument. Also, attempting to conduct quantitative research on human subjects often produces serious ethical dilemmas.

Qualitative Designs

The purpose of qualitative inquiry is to gain an understanding of how individuals construct meaning in their world, visualize a situation, and make sense of that situation. For example, to nurses, the concept of "caring" is very important, yet the nurse will probably perceive caring differently than the client. The nurse researcher wishing to measure "caring interventions" might find this concept very difficult to quantify, but a qualitative method could yield much usable information.

Because of the nature of nursing and the usual subject matter (human beings), qualitative designs are best suited to answer questions that interest nurses. The most commonly used of these designs are shown in Box 25.1.

Semistructured interviews using open-ended questions and observations are the most commonly used data collection methods in qualitative studies. Knowledge generated by qualitative research answers questions related to the meaning and understanding of human experiences.

Quantitative Designs

Quantitative designs are approaches that seek to verify data through prescriptive testing, correlation, and

---

B o x   2 5 . 1

Qualitative Research Designs

Phenomenology
Ethnography
Grounded Theory
Historical Studies
Case Studies

sometimes description. These designs imply varying degrees of control over the research material or subjects. Control of the research design can range from very tight to somewhat loose.

The design in quantitative research becomes the means used for hypothesis testing. The design also optimizes control over the variables to be tested and provides the structure and strategy for answering the research question. More highly controlled quantitative designs try to demonstrate causal relationships, and more flexible designs address relationships between and among variables. Box 25.2 summarizes and classifies quantitative research designs.

In quantitative experimental design, a comparison of two or more groups is required. The groups under study must be as similar as possible so that results can be credited to the treatment of the variables and not to differences between the groups. The independent variable is the one managed or manipulated by the researcher. The dependent variable *depends on,* or is altered as a direct result of, the researcher's manipulation.

In research, it is good to remember that neither the quantitative nor the qualitative research school is better. Each research approach is useful in different ways, and both expand understanding of health care and the nursing profession. What *is* important is to choose the methodology that best addresses the questions the researcher is asking and collects whatever data are most useful.

NARROWING THE RESEARCH–PRACTICE GAP

Two Different Cultures

More and more, nurses are becoming academically astute in the area of research. Unfortunately, education alone does not ensure transfer of what is learned into the daily practice of nursing. Like the basic but critical skill of sterile asepsis, research will become a part of each nurse's practice only when it becomes a part of each nurse's ideology.

Academic and practice arenas are often, in reality, two entirely different cultures. The critical and creative thinking so valued and promoted in the academic environment may fall victim to time and budget constraints within the clinical setting. To support what is best for clients, clinical practice areas such as hospitals must find ways to ensure that research finds safe harbor in the culture of practice. The implementation of research in practice will depend on inquisitiveness, development of cognitive skills, the ability to question one's own practice, and professional discipline. Nurses must also understand that sometimes research findings may conflict with practices rooted in tradition.[7]

Barriers to Research in Practice

Experts are now asking, "Why generate more research when the research already generated has not been adapted to practice?" The research–practice gap remains a bewildering challenge to the nursing profession.

Box 25.2

Quantitative Research Designs

Experimental Designs
Pretest/post-test control group
Post-test only control group
Solomon four group

Quasi-experimental Designs
Nonequivalent control group
Time series

Pre-experimental Designs
One group pretest/post-test

Nonexperimental Designs
Comparative studies
Correlational studies
Developmental studies
Evaluation studies

Meta-analysis Studies
Methodological studies
Needs-assessment studies
Secondary analysis studies

Survey studies
One-shot case study

An Isolated Skill

A challenge to the use of research in practice is that research skills are often taught to nursing students in isolation from other nursing subjects. This type of teaching may broaden the division between research and practice by separating the two elements early in the nurse's development and education. Unless ways are found to focus inquiry and link research findings to clinical practice early in the education process, the research–practice gap will likely remain.

As the situation currently stands, even though there has been an emphasis on nursing research for more than 2 decades, there are few indications that nurses on the front lines of clinical practice actively use research as a way to inform their practice.

Lack of Understanding

There are several barriers to the implementation of research in the health-care setting. Often, nurses skilled in clinical nursing may not be skilled in conducting research. Nurses who attempt to use research studies to answer practice questions may feel that the research does not provide the practical solutions for which they are looking. This concern may be valid because some researchers do not understand practice issues from the bedside nurse's viewpoint.

Conversely, practicing clinical nurses may lack the knowledge to understand or interpret the language of research. Published research often appears so esoteric and complicated that the message cannot be found in the bottle. The information should be easily accessible to those who provide direct care to clients. Researchers must find ways of packaging the conclusions so that practicing nurses may easily understand and implement clinical solutions to the care issues they are facing.

Unquestioned Practices

Entrenched nursing practices present another challenge. In the not-too-distant past, traditional nursing practices appear to have had a half-life longer than uranium. A few nursing traditions remain so widely accepted as fact that they are never questioned and therefore evade the scrutiny of testing. Best practice may never become evident without testing approaches to practices that have been accepted as necessary, preeminent, and sacrosanct.

Lack of Incentive

With the real challenges of time and budget limitations, very few hospitals or other agencies offer encouragement or rewards to nurses who *are* willing to seek out and use research findings in an effort to improve practice. One survey, conducted to identify barriers to implementation of research from clinicians' perspectives, revealed "insufficient authority and insufficient time" as the two obstacles most often cited.[1]

Resistance From Managers

Some researchers suggest that unit managers may view an environment of updates and change as unfavorable to maintaining a committed and cohesive staff. Some describe change as a threat to the constancy necessary for safe and expeditious client care.[8] Nurses willing to incorporate best practice evidence into clinical protocols must have confidence in their own professional judgment and the courage to stand against nurses who find comfort in unchanging traditional practices.

> *Unfortunately, education alone does not ensure transfer of what is learned into the daily practice of nursing.*

Incorporating Best Practice

Several strategies can help nurses conduct and use research for the improvement of nursing care, such as attending conferences in which clinical research findings and ideas for practice are presented. Other strategies proposed include but are not limited to:

1. Incorporating research findings in textbooks, basic and continuing nursing education programs, and clinical policy and procedure manuals
2. Explicitly connecting research use to institutional goals and objectives
3. Developing joint committees between colleges of nursing and hospital nursing departments
4. Inviting staff nurses to find and present summaries and abstracts, during unit meetings and clinical case conferences, in an effort to increase the interest of colleagues working on their units.[9]

Almost all of the most widely read, clinically focused nursing journals have added research or EBP sections or routinely include research articles. These increase the ease of access to research, ensure a wider distribution of current clinical research findings, and promote the incorporation into clinical settings of best practices based on credible evidence. This mission serves the profession by simplifying some of the language of research and by giving voice to the importance and practical nature of clinical research.

COMPARATIVE EFFECTIVENESS RESEARCH

Improvement of client care is the primary reason for conducting nursing research. It is important to continually update research priorities based on client outcomes in both the hospital and the community setting. Past research often compared two treatments to determine which was more effective, but never took the next step in translating the findings into the practice setting. CER emphasizes the need to use research to establish best practice standards and to sustain research that has proved effective.

Systematic Reviews

Systematic reviews present reliable summaries of past research. The role of such reviews has become more important as the volume of health-care literature has expanded. Other factors favoring reviews include the inconsistent quality of some research produced, the increased number of treatment approaches resulting from the availability of the numerous pharmaceuticals and health-care products on the market today, and the exponential growth of health-related technology.

Consideration of these factors has prompted the proposal that systematic reviews of existing literature replace primary research as a main source of evidence for clinical decision-making. One review of this type could replace many individual studies and free those making clinical decisions from finding, interpreting, and evaluating a collection of published primary research reports and articles.

Some believe that systematic reviews should represent the "gold standard" in research summaries. However, those eager to jump on the review-only bandwagon need to keep in mind that methods currently used for literature review may not most accurately reflect some of the nursing research being reviewed. The challenge exists in the "narrowly defined concept of what constitutes good evidence."[10]

Primary Research

What about only using nursing research studies as a source of information? One recurring criticism of primary nursing research is that much of it is accomplished as single studies. Some nursing researchers believe that many excellent qualitative studies are not followed by rigorous quantification. Other nursing leaders continue to urge nurse researchers to make replication studies a high research priority, particularly for research addressing clinical nursing issues. A single study is rarely adequate for making decisions regarding clinical practice.[11]

A Practical Angle

Evidence-based practice is believed to constitute the best of practice and has garnered the attention of health-care administrators because of its potential to decrease the cost of health-care delivery. Standards of nursing practice, clinical guidelines, and routine performance audits promote the use of research findings to some degree. The availability of electronic databases and emphasis on the teaching of research in nursing curricula, along with such support organizations as the Cochrane Collaboration (http://www.cochrane.org), Best Evidence (http://www.acpinteractiveonline.com), and the Centre for Health Evidence (http://www.cche.net), all endorse the expectation that nurses must be able and willing to use evidence to inform their practice.

How Useful Is It?

Successful implementation of EBP also depends on how practical and useful the information is to the practicing nurse. The usefulness of information requires the nurse to evaluate several factors, including potential benefits versus possible harm, cost effectiveness, availability of ongoing support resources, and willingness of the health-care staff and clients to accept change.

With the emphasis on the urgency for implementing EBP, critical and creative thinking

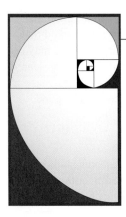

Issues in Practice

Short Staffing in an Emergency

Halley had been working on the medical-surgical unit since her graduation from an Associate Degree in Nursing (ADN) program 2 months ago. She had also had clinical rotations while in nursing school and felt comfortable and confident with the unit's procedures and her own skills. One Sunday evening the house supervisor stopped her just before the beginning of her shift and explained that the registered nurse (RN) on the eight-bed maternity unit had called to say that she was going to be late because of a family emergency. Because of the overall short staffing on weekends at this hospital, Halley would need to be pulled to the maternity unit for no more than 2 hours to cover the RN position and pass medications until the regular nurse could arrive for her shift. That would leave the medical-surgical unit short staffed, but it was relatively quiet and only about three-quarters full.

Halley hurried to the maternity unit and received an abbreviated report from the staff who were waiting to go home. All the clients were stable, and the only potential problem was a client in the emergency department (ED) who was 36 weeks pregnant and might be in the early stages of labor. Although they hadn't received report on the client in the ED, the departing staff joked that it would probably be the next morning before "anything happened."

After conducting an abbreviated initial assessment of the clients on the maternity unit, Halley called the ED to receive report on their client. The client was a 36-year-old woman who had three children, aged 12, 9, and 2 years. The ED nurse also reported that the client's old charts revealed a history of "precipitous labor" (a very rapid labor with the sudden birth of the baby). Given the client's history and the relatively short time of her last delivery, Halley recognized that she did not have the skills or experience to provide safe care for this client.

Halley called the nursing supervisor and explained that she would need a nurse more experienced in obstetrics to help admit and care for this new client. The supervisor responded that the whole hospital was short of nurses and she had no one she could send. Halley would just have to do her best until the regular maternity unit nurse arrived.

A few minutes later, the ED nurses brought the client to the maternity unit. After she was transferred to a unit bed, Halley did an initial admission assessment with the following results: blood pressure 166/123; pulse 134; contractions 2 to 3 minutes apart, regular and strong; fetal heart rate 166, faint but regular; amniotic fluid leaking from the vagina. After making her assessment, Halley again called the supervisor and demanded that she come to the maternity unit immediately to help with this client, who Halley felt was going to deliver her baby very soon. The supervisor responded that she was in the middle of a code blue in the intensive care unit and that Halley would just have to hang on for the half hour or so until the maternity nurse was due to arrive.

- What are the primary underlying ethical principles involved in this dilemma?
- How do an individual nurse's ethical obligations differ from those of a hospital's administration?
- What type of research data would help resolve this issue?
- Do you think this case study reflects a realistic situation?

have become even more important for the following reasons:

- Nurses must access, understand, evaluate, and disseminate a rapidly expanding body of nursing and other health-related information.
- Nurses must be able to recognize commonalities and uncover inconsistencies regarding the values of the profession, the values of the organization that employs them, the needs of clients for whom they advocate, and even the popular culture that exerts pressure on the public's ability to make safe choices.
- Nurses recognize that it takes critical and creative thought to support research into complex health-care issues and to promote successful implementation of changes in professional practice.

Essential Features

The goals of EBP include cost-effective practice based on the data produced by research, the dissemination of data, and the implementation of best practice interventions into the nurse's practice. The following have been identified as essential features of EBP:

- EBP is problem based and within the scope of the practitioner's experience.
- EBP narrows the research–practice gap by combining research with existing knowledge.
- EBP facilitates application of research into practice by including both primary and secondary research findings.
- EBP is concerned with quality of service and is therefore a quality assurance activity.
- EBP projects are team projects and therefore require team support and collaborative action.
- EBP supports research projects and outcomes that are cost effective.[12]

In summary, evidence-based researchers conduct systematic reviews of existing literature. These reviews are necessary because of the large quantity of health-care literature already in existence that has not been assimilated into practice. The mission of EBP researchers is to evaluate and present the available evidence on a specific topic in a clear and unbiased way. Clinical recommendations evolving from this process present nurses with sound decisions based on best evidence. Consequently, researchers not only will know what questions have been satisfactorily answered, but also will be better able to identify where gaps in the knowledge still exist.

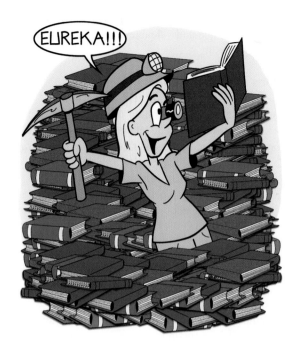

Networking: Where to Begin

As more evidence becomes available to guide practice, agencies and organizations are developing EBP guidelines. The Agency for Healthcare Research and Quality funds several EBP centers that are accessible through its website (http://www.ahrq.gov) and sponsors a National Guideline Clearinghouse where abstracts for EBP are available, at http://www.guideline.gov. The American Pain Society (http://www.ampainsoc.org), the Oncology Nursing Society (http://www.ons.org), and the Gerontological Nursing Interventions Research Center (http://www.nursing.uiowa.edu/centers/gnirc) also provide material. The Best Practices Network presents information from several organizations and is available at http://www.best4health.org.

RESEARCH ROLES BY EDUCATIONAL LEVEL

Leaders and educators within the profession of nursing agree that there is a role for every nurse in research, regardless of level of education. A minimal requirement for all 21st-century nurses is the ability to develop *and use* basic research skills. Nurses striving to improve their individual practice are increasingly committed to building a body of knowledge specific to nursing. Findings from scientific inquiry define the unique and valuable roles and the challenges of nursing.

Areas of Competency

One of the hallmarks of success in the field of research is the identification of research competencies for nurses at each educational level of preparation. In its classic document, *Commission on Nursing Research: Education for Preparation in Nursing Research,* the American Nurses Association (ANA) identified research competencies for each classification of the nursing education program. It is presumed that professional nurses committed to lifelong learning will cultivate their research expertise throughout their careers. Following are the expected research roles by educational level:

Associate Degree Nursing Graduate

1. Demonstrates awareness of the value or relevance of research in nursing
2. Assists in identifying problem areas in nursing practice
3. Assists in collection of data within an established structured format

Associate degree nurses are expected to demonstrate an awareness of the value of research in nursing by becoming knowledgeable consumers of research information and by helping identify problems within their scope of nursing practice that may warrant exploration.

Baccalaureate Degree Nursing Graduate

1. Reads, interprets, and evaluates research for applicability to nursing practice
2. Identifies nursing problems that need to be investigated and participates in the implementation of scientific studies
3. Uses nursing practice as a means of gathering data for refining and extending practice
4. Applies established findings of nursing and other health-related research to practice
5. Shares research findings with colleagues

Nurses with a baccalaureate education are expected to be intelligent consumers of research by understanding each step of the research process to interpret, evaluate, and determine the credibility of research findings. The baccalaureate nurse is able to distinguish between findings that are merely interesting and findings supported by enough data to be included in the nurse's practice. Baccalaureate-prepared nurses also participate in one or more phases of research projects. These nurses must be alert to and uphold the ethical principles of any research involving human participants and oversee the protection of individual rights as specified in the ANA Code of Ethics.[13]

Master's Degree in Nursing

1. Analyzes and reformulates nursing practice problems so that scientific knowledge and scientific methods can be used to find solutions
2. Enhances quality and clinical relevance of nursing research by providing expertise in clinical problems and by providing knowledge about the way in which these clinical services are delivered
3. Facilitates investigation of problems in clinical settings by contributing to a climate supportive of investigative activities, collaborating with others in investigations, and enhancing nurses' access to clients and data
4. Investigates for the purpose of monitoring the quality of nursing practice in a clinical setting
5. Assists others in applying scientific knowledge in nursing practice

Doctorate Degree in Nursing or a Related Discipline

1. Provides leadership for the integration of scientific knowledge with other types of knowledge for the advancement of practice
2. Conducts investigations to evaluate the contributions of nursing activities to the well-being of clients
3. Develops methods to monitor the quality of nursing practice in a clinical setting and to evaluate contributions of nursing activities to the well-being of clients

Graduate of a Research-Oriented Doctoral Program

1. Develops theoretical explanation of phenomena relevant to nursing by empirical research and analytic processes

> *Leaders and educators within the profession of nursing agree that there is a role for every nurse in research, regardless of level of education.*

2. Uses analytic and empirical methods to discover ways to modify or extend existing scientific knowledge so that it is relevant to nursing
3. Develops methods for scientific inquiry of phenomena relevant to nursing[12]

ETHICAL ISSUES IN RESEARCH

The Nuremberg Code

Although guidelines that govern human behavior have always been a part of recorded history, the need for ethical standards in research came to the public's attention in a dramatic way following World War II when evidence of the Nazis' experimentation and torture of selected groups of victims was revealed.

During the trials of Nazi war criminals, the U.S. Secretary of State and the Secretary of War discovered that the defense was trying to justify the atrocities committed by Nazi physicians as merely "medical research." As a result, the American Medical Association was asked to develop a code of ethics for research that would serve as a standard for judging the Nazi war crimes. This standard remains valid to this day and is known as the Nuremberg Code (Box 25.3).

National Research Act

Ethical issues are critical to all research, and researchers from all disciplines are bound by ethical principles that protect the rights of the public. One set of principles addressing the conduct of research came from the 1974 National Research Act. This act established the National Commission for Protection of Human Subjects in Biomedical and Behavioral Research.

Part of that act mandated the establishment of IRBs, whose primary responsibility is to safeguard, in every way, the rights of any individual participating in a research study. IRBs are panels that review research proposals in detail to ensure that ethical standards are met in the protection of human rights. The mission of the IRB is to ensure that researchers do not engage in unethical behavior or conduct poorly designed research studies.

Box 25.3

Articles Adapted from The Nuremberg Code

1. The voluntary consent of human subjects is absolutely necessary.
2. The experiment should yield fruitful results for the good of society.
3. The experiment should be so designed and based on results of animal experimentation and knowledge of ... the disease or problem under study that the anticipated results will justify performance of the experiment.
4. The experiment should be conducted so as to avoid all unnecessary physical and mental suffering and harm.
5. No experiment should be conducted where there is an a priori reason to believe that death or ... injury will occur.
6. The degree of risk ... should never exceed that determined ... by the importance of the problem to be solved by the experiment.
7. Proper preparations should be made ... to protect the experimental subject against even remote possibilities of injury, disability, or death.
8. Only scientifically qualified people must conduct the experiment. The highest degree of skill and care should be required through all stages of the experiment.
9. During the course of the experiment, the subject should be at liberty to bring the experiment to an end....
10. During the course of the experiment, the scientist ... must be prepared to terminate the experiment at any stage....

Source: Adapted from Trials of War Criminals before the Nuremberg Military Tribunals under Control Council Law No. 10, Vol. 2, pp 181–182. Washington, DC, U.S. Government Printing Office, 1949.

Every university, hospital, and agency that receives federal monies must submit assurances that they have established an IRB composed of at least five members. These members should reflect a variety of professional backgrounds, occupations, ethnic groups, and cultures in an effort to uphold complete and unbiased project reviews.[14]

Code of Ethics for Nurses

The profession of nursing also has its own code of ethics to which all nurses are legally and ethically bound. The development of this code was initiated by the ANA Board of Directors and the Congress on Nursing Practice in 1995. In June 2001 the ANA House of Delegates voted to accept a revised Code of Ethics, and in July 2001 the Congress of Nursing Practice and Economics voted to accept the new language, resulting in a fully approved Code of Ethics for Nurses with Interpretive Statements. A read-only version of this document is available at http://nursingworld.org/MainMenuCategories/EthicsStandards/CodeofEthicsforNurses/Code-of-Ethics.aspx. Specific ANA position statements on selected ethics and human rights issues may be viewed at http://www.nursingworld.org/readroom/position/ethics (see Chapter 7).

Nurses must use the moral authority given them by their license and position in the health-care structure to guard against anyone who tries to minimize the importance of that responsibility or, for any reason, attempts to convince nurses to set aside their responsibilities. Nursing research most often addresses the needs and behaviors of human beings. Embedded in nurses' professional code of ethics is the charge to protect every person from harm. This responsibility extends beyond nursing *research* to include any client-related issue, any type of behavioral or biomedical research, and any questionable procedure.

In nurses' position of trust with clients, nurses possess a great deal of influence over a population that is especially vulnerable because of health issues and needs. This unique position of trust gives nurses a higher responsibility to protect and defend those in their care.

Informed Consent

Protection of human subjects underpins the conduct of research and implies that individuals have the information they need to make informed decisions (Box 25.4). They have the right to be fully informed, not only about the care they receive, but also about

Box 25.4

Key Elements of Informed Consent

1. Researcher is identified and credentials presented.
2. Subject selection process is explained.
3. Purpose of the research is described.
4. Study procedures are discussed.
5. Potential risks are identified.
6. Potential benefits are described.
7. Compensation, if any, is discussed.
8. Alternative procedures, if any, are disclosed.
9. Assurances regarding anonymity or confidentiality are explained.
10. The right to refuse participation or withdraw from the study at any time is assured.
11. An offer to answer all questions honestly is made.
12. The means of obtaining the study results is described.

Source: Nieswiadomy RM: Foundations of Nursing Research (5th ed). Upper Saddle River, NJ, Pearson/Prentice Hall, 2008. Adapted by permission of Pearson Education, Inc.

any research in which they participate. Informed consent is both an ethical and a legal requirement in the research process. The ethical principle of self-determination is central to the process.

Besides those with special health considerations, certain groups of individuals are considered particularly vulnerable owing, in part, to their lack of ability to give informed consent or their potential susceptibility to coercion. These groups include children, mentally retarded people, elderly people, those with terminal diseases, homeless people, and those who may have altered levels of consciousness as the result of a condition, medication, or sedation.

Nurses are well aware of the need for informed consent and the provision of information before procedures. This knowledge can serve nurses well in their obligation to obtain informed consent before conducting research. The key elements of informed consent for research can be found in Box 25.4.

The language of the consent form must be clear and understandable, written in the primary language of the client, and designed for those with no more than an eighth-grade reading level. Technical language should never be used. The Code of Federal Regulations states that subjects must never be asked to waive their rights or to release the investigation from liability or negligence. It is important to note that various institutions and researchers, in an extended effort to protect research participants, include more than the 12 elements listed in Box 25.4.

Process Consent

In qualitative research, an important concept is process consent, which requires that the researcher renegotiate the consent if any unanticipated events occur.[15] An example of this might be a situation in which two parents with a small child in the hospital have given consent for the taping and study of "a day in the life of a hospitalized toddler."

During taping of the event, the parents are informed by the physician that a diagnosis is being questioned and their child must subsequently undergo an unexpected lumbar puncture. The parents may become visibly upset by this turn of events. In such a case the researcher should find a way of reconfirming the couple's ongoing interest in being part of the research study. When this family is given the opportunity to renegotiate the original agreement, the nurse researcher is confirming his or her role of advocate and proceeding in the best interest of all participants.

Detecting the Ethical Components of Written Research

It may be difficult to critique the ethical features of written research reports, but if there is evidence that permission to conduct the study was granted by an IRB, it is highly likely that the participants' rights were protected. Nurses have the responsibility of protecting the privacy and dignity of every individual, and the integrity of the nursing profession depends on doing what is right even when no one is watching.

Box 25.5 provides the guidelines for critiquing ethics in research.

IMPLEMENTING RESEARCH IN THE PRACTICE SETTING

Knowledge that is generated by research and then translated into policy and procedure becomes the ultimate guide to the scientific practice of nursing.

Box 25.5

Guidelines for Critiquing the Ethical Features of Research

1. Was the study approved by an IRB?
2. Was informed consent obtained from every subject?
3. Is there information regarding anonymity or confidentiality?
4. Were vulnerable subjects used?
5. Does it appear that any coercion may have been used?
6. Is it evident that potential benefits of participation outweigh the possible risks?
7. Were participants invited to ask questions about the study and told how to contact the researcher, should the need arise?
8. Were participants informed how to obtain results of the study?

Source: Nieswiadomy RM: Foundations of Nursing Research (5th ed). Upper Saddle River, NJ, Pearson/Prentice Hall, 2008. Adapted by permission of Pearson Education, Inc.

A primary responsibility of every nurse conducting research is the distribution of the findings (evidence) that have application in the client-care setting. Conversely, the professional responsibility of every nurse caring for clients requires that all nursing interventions be planned on the basis of reliable research findings.

Nursing research is of no value to the profession, or to the client, if the practice supported by the research is not used in the clinical setting. Unlimited opportunities for the generation and the dissemination of new knowledge exist in nursing, but the truly daunting task addresses the challenge of transforming that knowledge into practice.

The Call for Implementing Research

Research is critical to the professional practice of nursing. The Joint Commission's accreditation guidelines specify that client-care intervention must be based on information from scientifically valid and timely sources.

The mandate of the modern health-care system is that nurses make practice decisions based on the best scientific information available. Standard VII of the ANA Standards of Clinical Nursing Practice states that "the nurse uses research findings in practice." Nurses may participate in research activities in a number of ways. They can conduct reviews of literature, critique research studies for the possibility of application to practice, or "[use] research findings in the development of policies, procedures and guidelines for client care."[16]

Approaches to Using Research

Nursing is not the only profession experiencing reluctance in transforming research into practice. Even though new knowledge is expanding at an exponential rate, every discipline seems to have some type of research–practice gap. Nurses are often hesitant to change current traditional practice to EBP. They often identify significant difficulties involved in the changeover. Currently there are several models to help nurses apply research findings that support EBP. One model that appears both practical and relatively uncomplicated is found in Box 25.6.[17]

Promoting Change

It is often difficult for nurses to promote an environment conducive to change. In many hospitals, maintaining the status quo often appears to carry incentives that may intimidate even the most intuitive and confident change agent. The professional nurse committed to using "best evidence" to provide the best client care can be most effective by finding simple approaches that create an environment receptive to new research findings. Some helpful tactics include:

- Reading clinical journals regularly but also critically. Nursing professionals are well informed and believe in the concept of lifelong learning.
- Attending clinically focused nursing conferences where the latest client-care interventions are presented and discussed.
- Learning to look for evidence that clearly supports the effectiveness and the feasibility of updating nursing interventions.
- Seeking work environments that promote the use of research findings and evidence-based care.
- Collaborating with a nurse researcher. Apprenticeship to one who masters a skill is an old but venerated means of learning that skill.
- Learning to critically scrutinize the status quo. Many worthwhile ideas for change come from those students and nurses "in the trenches" and at the bedside.

Box 25.6

Rosswurm and Larrabee Model for Application of Nursing Research

Assess the need for practice changes:
(a) Involve all nurses that have a stake in the intervention or change.
(b) Identify problems associated with the current practice.
(c) Compare available information.

Link the problem intervention and outcomes:
(a) Identify possible interventions.
(b) Develop outcome indicators.

Produce best evidence for consideration:
(a) Conduct a review of existing literature.
(b) Compare and contrast the evidence found.
(c) Determine feasibility (including cost in dollars and time).
(d) Consider benefits and risks.

Design a proposed practice change:
(a) Define the anticipated change.
(b) Identify necessary resources.
(c) Develop a plan based on desired outcomes.

Implement and evaluate the proposed change:
(a) Conduct a pilot study.
(b) Assess the process and the outcomes.
(c) Make a decision to alter, accept, or reject the proposed change.

Support the change with ongoing evaluations of the outcomes:
(a) Communicate the desired change to those involved.
(b) Conduct in-service education sessions.
(c) Revise standards of practice (policy/procedures) reflecting the change.
(d) Monitor the ongoing process and results.

Source: Rosswurm M, Larrabee J: A model for change to evidence-based practice. Journal of Nursing Scholarship 31(4):317–322, 1999, with permission.

- Pursuing the possibility of proposing and implementing a project. If the nurse finds a research-based idea for clinical care interesting, then taking the steps to research it can be productive.

Conclusion

Modern health care has become so complex and demanding that simple trial-and-error approaches do not provide the high-quality information required for the safe, effective, and economical care demanded by well-informed consumers. The nursing profession is quickly moving away from the "I do it because it's always been done this way" method of care to scientifically rooted care practices based on research. As a result, nurses are gaining increased recognition as key members of the health-care team.

Also, nurses are now required to be able to analyze and evaluate research findings to determine which studies are of high quality and which can be used as a guide for nursing practice. Similarly, nurses are required to contribute to the body of nursing knowledge by participating in nursing research studies conducted at their facilities. It is presumed that nurses with advanced degrees will initiate and conduct high-quality research.

The ability of nurses to make thoughtful use of research is an important first step in the development of EBP. Society's call for cost containment, high-quality care, and documented outcomes of health-care services will continue to fuel the engine of positive health-care developments. As nursing looks to its future, research and EBP will increase in importance as factors that guide and inform the day-to-day practice of nurses.

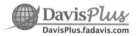
DavisPlus.fadavis.com

GLOSSARY OF TERMS USED IN RESEARCH

Bias An influence that produces a distortion in the results of a research study.

Case study An in-depth qualitative study of a selected phenomenon involving a person, a group of people, or an institution.

Causal relationship A relationship between variables in which the presence or absence of one variable (known as the "cause") will determine the presence or absence of the other variable (known as the "effect").

Collaboration A cooperative venture among those with a common goal.

Comparative Effectiveness Research (CER) A method to determine the priority of research topics developed by the IOM, based on client outcomes both in and outside the institutional setting.

Conceptual framework A framework of concepts that demonstrate their relationships in a logical manner. Although less well developed than a theoretical framework, this framework may be used as a guide for a study.

Conceptual model A set of abstract constructs that explains phenomena of interest.

Correlation The degree of association between two variables.

Empirical evidence Objective data gathered through use of the human senses.

Epidemiologist One who studies the distribution and determinants of health and illness and the application of findings as a means of promoting health and preventing illness.

Ethical standards Standards determined by principles of moral values and moral conduct.

Ethnography A qualitative research approach involving the study of cultural groups.

Evidence-based practice (EBP) The selective and practical use of the best evidence, as demonstrated by research, to guide health-care implementation and decisions.

Experimental research design A quantitative research design that meets all of the following criteria: an experimental variable that is manipulated, at least one experimental and one comparison group, and random assignments of participants to either the experimental or the comparison group.

Exploratory study The descriptive examination of available data to become as familiar as possible with the information.

Grounded theory An inductive approach to research using a systematic set of procedures to develop a theory that is then supported by, or "grounded in," the data.

Historical study Qualitative research involving the systematic collection and synthesis of data regarding people and events of the past.

Hypothesis A formal statement of the expected relationship between variables in a selected population.

Informed consent Consent to participate in a study given by one who has full understanding of the study before the study begins. Informed consent is based on the principle of the right of each individual to self-determination.

Institutional Review Board (IRB) A panel established at an agency, such as a hospital or university, to review all proposed research studies and to set standards for research involving human subjects.

Nonprobability sampling A sampling process in which a sample is selected from elements of a population through methods that are not random. Convenience, quota, and purposive sampling are examples.

Nuremberg code A code of conduct that serves as one of the recognized guides in the ethical conduct of research.

Nursing research A process that permits nurses to ask questions directed at gaining new knowledge to improve the profession, including elements of client care.

Phenomenology Qualitative research studies that examine lived experiences through descriptions of the meanings of such experiences by the individuals involved.

Primary research source A report or account of a research study written by the researcher(s) conducting the study. In historical research a primary source might be an original letter, diary, or other authenticated document.

Process consent A version of informed consent that supports renegotiation when a situation originally consented to undergoes change.

Qualitative research design A systematic but subjective research approach implemented to describe life experiences and give them meaning.

Quantitative research design A systematic and objective process used to describe and test relationships and evaluate causal interactions among variables.

Quasi-experimental design A type of experimental design in which there is either no comparison group or no random assignment of participants.

Random sample A selection process that ensures that each member of a population has an equal probability of being selected.

Reliability The dependability or degree of consistency with which an instrument measures what it is intended to measure.

Replication study A research study designed to repeat or duplicate earlier research. A different sample or setting may be used while the essential elements of the original study are kept intact.

Research design A blueprint for conducting a research study.

Research process A process that requires the comprehension of a unique language and involves the ability to apply a variety of research processes.

Review of literature An exploration of available information to determine what is known and what remains unknown about a subject.

Sample A subset of a population selected to participate in a study as representative of that population.

Scientific inquiry A logical, orderly means of collecting data for the generation and testing of ideas.

Theoretical framework A framework based on propositional statements derived from one theory or interrelated theories.

Validity The ability of an instrument to measure the variables that it is intended to measure.

Variable Any trait of an individual, object, or situation that is susceptible to change and that may be manipulated or measured in quantitative research.

26

Alternative and Complementary Healing Practices

Lydia DeSantis

Learning Objectives

After completing this chapter, the reader will be able to:

- Compare the philosophy and objectives of alternative and complementary healing modalities with those of conventional Western medicine.
- List major reasons why a growing number of people use alternative and complementary healing modalities.
- Describe major types of alternative and complementary healing modalities.
- Summarize methods by which nurses and clients can obtain information about alternative and complementary healing modalities.
- Evaluate a client for use of alternative and complementary healing modalities.
- Identify the strengths and weaknesses of alternative and complementary healing modalities.

A DIFFERENT KIND OF HEALING

Complementary and alternative health-care practices are widely used by a large percentage of the population. Their popularity continues to increase dramatically with clients of all ages and backgrounds. It is important for nurses to have a good understanding of this type of health care to ensure their clients' safety and well-being and to be supportive of their practices.

According to the World Health Organization (WHO), 80 percent of the world's population uses what Americans call "alternative" practices as their primary source of health care. Because of the widely accepted use of these practices, WHO has officially sanctioned the incorporation of "safe and effective [alternative] remedies and practices for use in public and private health services." Currently, between 34 and 42 percent of Americans (60 to 83 million people) use alternative and complementary healing practices, as do 20 to 70 percent of people in Western Europe, 33 percent in Finland, and 49 percent in Australia.[1]

The trend toward alternative practices has continued to grow in the United States since the 1990s. Studies show that 40 percent of people have developed an increasingly positive attitude toward alternative practices, whereas only 2 percent had more negative opinions. Both the general public—72 percent—and health maintenance organizations (HMOs)—73 percent—expect consumer demand for this area of health care to remain moderate to strong. Although there has been rapid growth in biomedical knowledge and technology during this time period, the demand for alternative therapies continues to increase.[2]

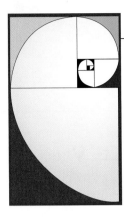

Issues Now

PPACA Supports CAM

The 2010 Patient Protection and Affordable Care Act (PPACA) has several provisions that will benefit Complementary and Alternative Medicine (CAM). With its emphasis on preventing insurance companies from denying coverage, PPACA includes a provision that clients who are participating in clinical trials using alternative health-care methods cannot lose their coverage. Under the new law, insurance companies are required to cover all routine costs of medications and treatments used during the trial. The goal of the law is to make trials available to clients who otherwise might not be able to participate and to make it easier for researchers to conduct successful trials that will improve health care and treatments for others.

However, certain criteria must be met. First, the client must be categorized as "qualified." This means that the client must be authorized by his or her health-care provider for participation. The provider must also provide "medical and scientific information establishing that the individual's participation in such trial would be appropriate."

Second, the clinical trial must be "approved." An "approved clinical trial" is a phase I, phase II, phase III, or phase IV clinical trial conducted to advance the prevention, detection, or treatment of cancer or other life-threatening disease or condition. The trial must meet at least one of three conditions: it must be federally funded or approved, approved by the Food and Drug Administration (FDA), or conducted by the federal government.

The bill also includes provisions to prevent insurance companies from discriminating against CAM practitioners. Practitioner coverage now includes acupuncturists, chiropractors, and naturopathic doctors who may prescribe dietary supplements. Some CAM practitioners believe the new provisions open the door for future growth of alternative health-care practices.

One overriding goal of PPACA is to educate the public about methods to prevent illness and improve health-care status. To achieve this goal, the law supports the development of wellness plans to be implemented through community health centers, particularly in lower-income and underserved areas. These centers will provide wellness assessments, health education, and a selection of dietary supplements that have FDA-approved health claims. Some supplements that will be made available are folic acid, calcium, vitamin D, omega-3, and multivitamins. Supplements will be targeted for "at-risk" groups, such as calcium and vitamin D for older clients.

Another section of the new law promotes increased participation for CAM practitioners in the development of health-care policy. A new National Healthcare Workforce Commission will be created and will work with the U.S. Department of Health and Human Services. One of its projects is to create community health teams, which must include licensed CAM practitioners.

Issues Now continued

The law is new, and many questions still need to be answered. Some of the answers will come from research and through the pilot programs that are built into the health-care reform bill. However, it is certain that alternative health-care practices will be involved in future health-care developments.

Sources: Healthcare reform includes alternative medicine, dietary supplements. Nutritional Outlook, 2010. Retrieved November, 2010 from http://www.nutritionaloutlook.com.

Perkins C: What does health care reform mean for alternative medicine? Holistic Health Talk, 2010. Retrieved November, 2010 from http://www.holistichelp.net.

CAM, supplements included in health care reform bill. Food and Drug Administration (FDA), Legislation, Government, Industry News, Retrieved November, 2010 from http://www.natualproductsinsider.com.

Oberg B: What does health care reform mean for alternative medicine? 2010. Retrieved November, 2010 from http://www.examiner.com.

Hoback J: Health care reform to impact CAM, supplements. Natural Foods, 2010. Retrieved November, 2010 from http://naturalfoodsmerchandiser.com.

DEFINING ALTERNATIVE AND COMPLEMENTARY HEALING

Several definitions are used for alternative and complementary health-care practices. They are sometimes defined as practices outside of conventional, science-based Western medicine and not sanctioned by the official health-care system. A considerable range of practices and concepts is included in alternative and complementary healing. The glossary at the end of this chapter outlines many of these practices.

An Outdated Definition

There is no universally accepted definition. Many alternative health-care practices originated many years ago within cultural belief systems and healing traditions. A commonly used definition in the United States for alternative and complementary modalities comes from the National Center for Complementary and Alternative Medicine (NCCAM), an agency of the National Institutes of Health. The NCCAM definition is "those treatments and health-care practices not taught widely in medical schools, not generally used in hospitals, and not usually reimbursed by medical insurance companies."

This definition is quickly becoming outdated. Many medical and nursing schools now include courses on alternative and complementary health-care practices. Also, the practice of alternative medicine is gradually becoming part of conventional health care. Physicians, nurses, and other health-care professionals are responding to the growing public use of these practices by incorporating selected modalities into their own client care. Physicians have begun referring clients to a variety of alternative healers and using alternative therapies for their own health.

A Holistic Basis

In this chapter, alternative and complementary medicine is defined as the understanding and use of healing therapies not commonly considered part of Western biomedicine. The focus here is mainly on methods of self-care, wellness, self-healing, health promotion, and illness prevention. Therapies and practices are called *alternative* when used alone or with other alternative therapies, and *complementary* when used with conventional therapies.

The use of the term *healing* is preferred to *medicine*. Alternative and complementary modalities typically are based in holistic philosophies, which go beyond treatment or cure of the physiological and psychological dimensions of care commonly associated with modern, scientific biomedicine. Holism refers to treatment of the whole person (body–mind–spirit) in that person's environmental context (physical, biological, social, cultural, and spiritual).

What Do You Think?

Do you use any alternative health-care practices? What are they? Why do you use them?

USE OF ALTERNATIVE AND COMPLEMENTARY THERAPIES

Who Uses Them

In most national studies of alternative therapy users, ethnic and racial minorities are underrepresented, particularly among persons who do not speak English. Such exclusions raise questions about whether the use rate of alternative therapies in the United States may exceed 42 percent because the use of alternative therapies among immigrant populations and those with lower incomes tends to be high. Many such populations have grown up with these therapies as "folk" medicine, and their world views encompass different concepts of health, illness, and healing. Alternative health-care practices are most popular among women, people aged 35 to 49 years, people with higher educational levels (some graduate education), and those with annual incomes of more than $50,000.[1]

Why Their Use Has Increased

Three general theories have been advanced to explain the growing use of alternative and complementary healing: (1) dissatisfaction with conventional health care, (2) a desire for greater control over one's health, and (3) a desire for cultural and philosophical congruence with personal beliefs about health and illness. Many other client-specific reasons have also been postulated, such as belief in the effectiveness of alternative therapies and the individual's health status (Box 26.1). The rising cost of conventional health care may play a role as well.

Dissatisfaction

The increasing use of alternative therapies is due in part to the feeling that conventional health care is unable to deal with major health problems or improve a person's general health. People who have a high degree of distrust in conventional health care

Box 26.1

Reasons for Use of Alternative and Complementary Modalities

People use alternative therapies alone or together with conventional health care for a variety of reasons. There is no single predictor of use, and the reasons for use may vary from situation to situation. Persons who seem to benefit the most from the alternative approach are those who:

- Prefer a personal relationship with healers
- Refuse to give up hope and hopefulness, regardless of the illness or life-state
- Desire to focus on wellness, health promotion and maintenance, and illness prevention
- Are concerned with gentle alleviation and management of suffering and illness rather than aggressive management of the end-stage of life through technology, medications, surgery, and other invasive procedures
- Wish to participate actively in decision-making about their health care
- Believe in the holistic aspects of existence rather than in the primacy of biological and physiological aspects
- Are "culture creatives"—persons at the leading edge of innovation and culture change who have been exposed to alternative lifestyles and world views compatible with those from which alternative and complementary modalities and theories have arisen
- Share cultural and philosophical views similar to those from which alternative and complementary modalities have developed

Source: Austin JA: Why patients use alternative medicine. Journal of the American Medical Association 279:1548, 1998. From Holistic Health Promotion & Complementary Therapies Manual 1st edition by ASPEN, 1998. Reprinted with permission from Delmar Learning.

often rely primarily on alternative therapies. This lack of trust has increased recently for several reasons, including:

- Conflicting information from health-care–related studies and clinical trials about risk prevention and health promotion. For example, clients no longer know what to believe about salt intake, normal cholesterol levels, alcohol use, or hormone replacement therapy.
- Continuing emphasis of conventional health care on curative rather than preventive aspects of care. The lack of emphasis on illness prevention limits the ability of individuals to live long lives relatively free of disability from major chronic illnesses, such as arthritis, diabetes, cancer, and cardiovascular disease.
- Growing concern about costs, safety, and access to conventional health care. Many people are concerned about the increased incidence of hospital-acquired diseases, the many deadly medication errors committed over the past few years, the ever-increasing number of invasive procedures, antibiotic-resistant bacteria, and reliance on impersonal technology.

Desire for Control

Some people who use alternative therapies believe conventional care is too intolerant, authoritarian, and impersonal. They feel that some conventional health-care professionals lack sensitivity to the wishes of clients and their families when developing treatment plans. Clients believe they should be partners in decision-making about their care rather than just having decisions handed down to them.

In the United States, the majority of people report being reluctant to tell conventional health-care professionals that they use alternative therapies. Although almost all (89 percent) who use alternative therapies do so under the supervision of an alternative healer, about half of this same group do not consult a conventional health-care professional before they begin. Fourteen percent of persons see both conventional health-care professionals and alternative healers. Similar patterns of self-care and nondisclosure to conventional health-care professionals are found throughout the industrialized world.[3]

Holistic Philosophy

Conventional health care is often faulted for its limited focus on the physiological dimension of health

and curing to the exclusion of the unity of mind–body–spirit healing. Another negative characteristic of conventional health care is its excessive dependence on medicine, surgery, and technology rather than on the more natural and noninvasive alternative approach that focuses on self-care and self-healing.

Belief in Effectiveness

Clients who use alternative therapies do so because they believe those therapies will work, either alone or when combined with conventional treatments. Persons who consider their health to be poor or who have chronic illnesses report greater benefits from alternative than conventional health care and are more likely to try both at the same time. Referral from conventional health-care professionals, friends, or other users of alternative therapies is also a prominent reason for the simultaneous use of both systems. For many clients, alternative therapies simply make them feel better than conventional health care does.

> *The increasing use of alternative therapies is due in part to the feeling that conventional health care is unable to deal with major health problems or improve a person's general health.*

Cost of Alternative Care

Estimated costs of alternative medicines (herbs and nutritional supplements), diet products, equipment, and books and courses totaled $33.9 billion in 2007. Sixty-seven percent of HMOs cover one or more alternative and complementary healing (ACH) modalities, but coverage is uneven and varies regionally. Chiropractic is the most common covered service (65 percent), followed by acupuncture (31 percent), massage therapy (11 percent), and vitamin therapy (6 percent). HMOs expect to increase coverage for acupuncture to 36 percent, acupressure to 31 percent, massage therapy to 30 percent, and vitamin therapy to 27 percent. The most important reasons for adding coverage for these services are public demand, legislative mandate, and demonstrated clinical effectiveness.

CLASSIFYING ALTERNATIVE METHODS

The underlying goals of any type of health care include preventing illness, promoting and maintaining health, and caring for people while alleviating the suffering caused by illness. However, despite these common elements, health-care practices vary profoundly in their modalities (technologies), practitioner education and monitoring, underlying concepts (models) of health and illness, modes of care delivery, and social and legal mandates to provide care. Because of the large number of variables, a confusing

array of health-care systems, practitioners, and healing modalities has developed. Two systems that can be used to help define and classify alternative and complementary therapies are the Healing Matrix and the NCCAM classification.[4]

The Healing Matrix
The Healing Matrix (Table 26.1) contrasts conventional and alternative modalities and practitioners. The alternative modalities shown are (1) representative of those most commonly known by the general public, (2) sought in the United States and industrialized world, and (3) practiced most often by conventional health-care professionals, including nurses.

A Cross-Section of Care
Modalities in column 1 of the Healing Matrix are technologies that cut across various healing systems. The technologies are arranged vertically from the most concrete to the most abstract. The remaining

Table 26.1　The Healing Matrix

Technologies	Orthodox	Marginal	Alternative	
Physical manipulation	Surgery	Chiropractic	Rolfing	Craniosacral alignments
Ingested or applied substances	Physical therapy	Homeopathy	Feldenkrais	Massage therapy
Uses of energy	Pharmacology	Vitamin therapy	Naturopathic remedies	Yoga, Akido, Tai Chi
Mental	Laser surgery	Acupuncture	Herbs	Reflexology
Spiritual	Psychiatry	Acupressure	Flower remedies	Aromatherapy
		Secular or spiritual counseling	Reiki	Diet alternatives
		Established support groups (e.g., 12-step programs)	Magnetic or polarity healing	
			Therapeutic touch	Chakra balancing
			Self-help groups	Radionics
			Visualizations	Use of color, gems, and crystals
			Affirmations	Psychic, spiritual, or intuitive healing

Source: Adapted from Engebretson J, Wardell D: A contemporary view of alternative healing modalities. Nurse Practitioner 18:51, 1993.

columns include various healing modalities from conventional, marginal, and alternative healing systems.

Physical Manipulation Technologies. These are also known as "bodywork therapies." They are administered by a therapist or by the clients themselves as part of a self-care program. They include health rituals and breathing exercises to better bring about the union of body–mind–spirit.

Ingested or Applied Substances. A number of substances, including herbs, vitamins and other nutritional supplements, and dietary regimens have the goal of helping the body heal itself, rid itself of toxins, and promote general health and wellness.

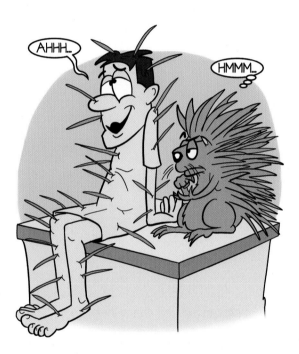

Energy Therapies. These modes of treatment maintain or restore health through the balancing of energy flow in the body. The goal is to restore the natural movement of vital forces or life essences that may have been disturbed by diseases or psychological factors.

Mental (Psychic) and Spiritual Therapies

Included in these therapies are group or individual counseling techniques that help the client develop or attain spiritual and personal growth. Examples include intuiting, revelations, visualization, astrological and other readings, and invoking the spirit world.

Conventional Health Care

The modalities listed in column 2 (orthodox [conventional]) are part of the official health-care system in the United States. They are based on knowledge rooted in scientific and biomedical principles.

Licensed Alternative Care

The modalities in column 3 (marginal) are generally learned through the study of the standard curricula in institutions of higher education. Alternative healers practicing such modalities are usually licensed by the state, and most have credentialing and a professional body that sets standards for their practice. These modalities are not considered conventional therapies in the United States but may be part of conventional health-care systems in other nations.

For example, acupuncture is an essential mode of treatment in traditional Chinese medicine, which, along with biomedicine, forms the conventional health-care system in the People's Republic of China. In 1997, the National Institutes of Health Consensus Panel on Acupuncture reviewed research studies and other information on its safety, efficacy, and effectiveness. The studies showed sufficient evidence to approve acupuncture as an intervention for adult general and dental postoperative pain and to treat nausea and vomiting associated with chemotherapy.[5]

Intuitively Based Care

The modalities presented in columns 4 and 5 (alternative) are less physiological. They are based on a more intuitive type of knowledge. Most alternative healers practicing such modalities are self-taught, have learned through working with more experienced practitioners, have attended courses or workshops on particular modalities, or have learned by a combination of methods. The alternative modalities in the bottom cell on the far right have the most intuitive knowledge base; that is, insights about the spiritual or physical self are gained through direct revelations or interpreted by another. These include readers (e.g., astrologers or seers) and spiritual healers in touch with divine forces.

The NCCAM Classification

In 1992, Congress mandated the establishment of an Office of Alternative Medicine in the National Institutes of Health to enhance the study of ACH. In 1998, the Office became the NCCAM. Its mission is to conduct and support both basic and applied research and training and the dissemination of ACH information to conventional healthcare professionals, alternative healers, and the public.

Complementary and alternative medicine (CAM) is defined by the NCCAM as those practices not commonly included in or used by conventional medicine. Seven major categories of CAM are defined and subdivided into practices that (1) fall under CAM, (2) are found in conventional health care but are classified as behavioral medicine, and (3) are overlapping—that is, they can fall in the domain of either CAM or behavioral medicine. Table 26.2 summarizes the NCCAM classification.

Table 26.2 Categories of Alternative Practice

Alternative Medical Systems		
Traditional Oriental Medicine		
Acupuncture	Herbal formulas	
Diet	Massage and manipulation (Tui Na)	
External and internal Qi Gong	Tai Chi	
Traditional Indigenous Systems		
Ayurvedic medicine	Traditional African medicine	
Curanderismo	Traditional Aboriginal medicine	
Central and South American	Unani-tibbi	
Kampo medicine	Siddhi	
Native American medicine		
Alternative Western Systems		
CAM	**Overlapping**	
Homeopathy	Anthroposophically extended medicine	
Naturopathy		
Orthomolecular medicine		
Mind–Body Interventions		
Mind–Body Methods		
CAM	**Behavioral Medicine**	**Overlapping**
Yoga	Hypnosis	Art, music, and dance therapies
Tai Chi	Meditation	Humor
Internal Qi Gong	Biofeedback	Journaling
Religion and Spirituality		
CAM		
Confession	Nontemporality	"Special" healers
Nonlocality	Soul retrieval	Spiritual healing
Social and Contextual Areas		
CAM	**Overlapping**	
Caring-based approaches (e.g., holistic nursing, pastoral care)	Community-based approaches (e.g., Native American "sweat" rituals)	
Intuitive diagnosis	Explanatory models Placebo	

Table 26.2 Categories of Alternative Practice (continued)

Biologically Based Therapies

Phytotherapy or Herbalism

Aloe vera	Echinacea	Ginseng	Mistletoe
Bee pollen	Evening primrose	Green tea	Peppermint oil
Biloba	Garlic	Hawthorne	Saw palmetto
Cat's claw	Ginger	Kava Kava	Witch hazel
Dong Quai	Ginkgo	Licorice root	Valerian

Special Diet Therapies

Atkins	McDougall	Fasting	Paleolithic
Diamond	Ornish	High fiber	Vegetarian
Kelly-Gonzalez	Pritikin	Macrobiotic	
Gerson	Wigmore	Mediterranean	
Livingston-Wheeler	Asian	Natural hygiene	

Orthomolecular Therapies

Single Nutrients (partial listing)

Amino acids	Folic acid	Lysine	Niacinamide	Thiamine
Ascorbic acid	Glutamine	Manganese	Potassium	Tyrosine
Boron	Glucosamine sulfate	Magnesium	Selenium	Vanadium
Calcium	Iodine	Medium-chain triglycerides	Silicon	Vitamin A
Carotenes	Inositol	Melatonin	Glandular products	Vitamin D
Choline	Iron	Niacin	Riboflavin	Vitamin K
Fatty acids	Lipoic acid		Taurine	

Pharmacological, Biological, and Instrumental Interventions

Products

Antineoplastons	Cone therapy	Hyperbaric oxygen
Bee pollen	Enderlin products	Induced remission therapy
Cartilage	Enzyme therapies	Ozone
Cell therapy	Gallo immunotherapy	Revici system
Coley's toxins	H_2O_2	

Procedures/Devices

Apitherapy	Electrodiagnostics	Neural therapy
Bioresonance	Iridology	
Chirography	MORA device	

Manipulative and Body-Based Methods

Chiropractic Medicine

Massage and Bodywork

Acupressure	Feldenkrais technique	Reflexology
Alexander technique	Osteopathic manipulative therapy (OMT)	Rolfing
Applied kinesiology	Pilates method	Swedish massage
Chinese Tui Na massage	Polarity	Trager bodywork
Craniosacral OMT		

(continued)

Table 26.2 Categories of Alternative Practice (continued)

Massage and Bodywork		
Unconventional Physical Therapies		
Colonics	Heat and electrotherapies	Light and color therapies
Diathermy	Hydrotherapy	
	Energy Therapies	
Biofield Therapies		
External Qi Gong	Healing touch	Reiki
Healing science	Huna	Therapeutic touch
Bioelectromagnetically Based Therapies*		
Alternating and direct current fields	Magnetic fields	Pulsed fields

*Unconventional use of electromagnetic fields.
Source: Adapted from National Center for Complementary and Alternative Medicine: Classification of Alternative Medicine Practices, 2010. Available at: http://nccam.nih.gov/nccam/fcp/classify/index.html.

Category I

Category I includes alternative systems of theory and practice developed outside Western biomedicine. For example, acupuncture and Oriental medicine are grounded in traditional Chinese medicine. Also included in this category are traditional indigenous systems, which include all medical systems other than acupuncture and Oriental medicine that developed outside of Western biomedicine. It also includes unconventional Western systems not classified elsewhere that were developed in the West but are not considered part of biomedicine, such as homeopathy.

Finally, this category includes naturopathy, an unconventional medical system that has gained prominence in the United States. This eclectic approach consists of various natural systems, such as herbalism, lifestyle therapies, and diet as therapy.

Category II

Category II includes mind–body practices, religion and spirituality, and social and contextual areas. Mind–body medicine involves a variety of approaches to health care and contains three subcategories. Mind–body systems are seldom practiced alone but are usually combined with lifestyle interventions.

Mind–body methods may be part of a traditional medical system. They are sometimes used in conventional health-care practices; however, they are characterized as CAM when used for conditions for which they are not normally prescribed. Religion and spirituality include treatments directed toward biological functions or clinical conditions. Social and contextual areas include treatment methods that are not included in other categories, such as cultural and symbolic interventions.

Category III

Biologically based therapies include products, interventions, and practices that are natural in origin and biologically based. They may or may not overlap with conventional medicine and its use of dietary supplements.

Phytotherapy, or herbalism, is the use of plant-derived products for purposes of prevention and treatment. Diet therapies use special diets to reduce risk factors or treat chronic diseases. Orthomolecular medicine is the use of nutritional products and food supplements that are not included in other categories for prevention and treatment of disease. Pharmacological, biological, and instrumental interventions are those not covered in other categories and administered in an unconventional manner.

Category IV

Manipulative and body-based methods include body manipulation, body movement, or both.

Category V

Energy therapies are based on manipulation of biofields with bioelectromagnetically based therapies. Biofields include energy systems and energy fields internal and external to the body that are used for medical purposes. Bioelectromagnetics is the use of electromagnetic fields in an unconventional manner for medical reasons.[4]

COMPARING CONVENTIONAL AND ALTERNATIVE PRACTICES

Many similarities exist between alternative and conventional health care. As they attempt to achieve similar goals, they may overlap in method, even though the methods are derived from different concepts of reality and different theoretical models. Table 26.3 summarizes characteristics often cited as common to alternative healing and contrasts them with those usually associated with conventional health care.

A Reductionist Philosophy

In general, conventional medicine focuses on the physical or material part of the person, the body. It is concerned with the structure, function, and connections or communication between material elements that compose the body, such as bones, muscles, and nerves. Conventional medicine generally views all humans as being very similar biologically. Disease is seen as a deviation from what is generally considered to be a normal biological or somatic state.

Conventional medicine is sometimes considered reductionist because it tends to reduce very complex entities (humans) to seemingly equal and more simple beings who are all anatomically and physiologically similar. From this perspective, it is believed that all individuals will respond in more or less the same ways to causative agents, such as bacteria and viruses, and respond similarly to common treatments, such as medicines and surgery. In other words, a person with measles, cirrhosis of the liver, or breast cancer will have the same course of illness as other persons with those illnesses and will respond to treatments in basically the same manner.

Diagnosis by Category

Conventional medicine has developed extensive disease categories, and great emphasis is placed on diagnosis and cure based on the assessment of physical signs and symptoms. Most newly developed medications, when they are in the human testing phase,

Table 26.3 Contrasts Between Conventional and Alternative Health Care

Conventional	Alternative/Complementary
Chemotherapy	Plants and other natural products
Curing/treating	Healing/ministering care
Disease category	Unique individual
End-stage	Hope/hopefulness
Focus is on disease and illness	Focus is on health and wellness
Illness treatment	Health promotion and illness prevention
Individual is viewed as disease category	Individual is viewed as unique being
Nutrition is adjunct and supportive to treatment	Nutrition is the basis of health, wellness, and treatment
Objectivism: person is separate from disease	Subjectivism: person is integral to the illness
Patient/client	Person
Practitioner as authority	Practitioner as facilitator
Practitioner paternalism/client dependency	Practitioner as partner/person empowerment
Positivism/materialism: data are physically measurable	Metaphysical: entity is energy system or vital force
Reductionist	Holistic
Specialist care	Self-care
Symptom relief	Alleviation of causative factors
Somatic (body biologic and physiologic) model	Behavioral-psycho-social-spiritual model
Science is only source of knowledge and truth	Multiple sources of knowledge and truth
Technological/invasive	Natural/noninvasive

are tested on men between the ages of 25 and 35 years, with the presumption that they will work similarly in women, elderly people, and children. That presumption is not always accurate, and there is a growing trend at pharmaceutical companies to test medications on groups of persons for whom they are more likely to be used.

Integration of Nonmaterial Factors

The physical body is the primary focus of conventional medicine. Because of this almost exclusive focus on the physical body, conventional medicine often does not consider or include the nonmaterialistic aspects of health and illness in diagnosis and treatment decisions. Thus, spiritual, psychological, sociocultural, behavioral, and energy system aspects play little or no role in conventional medical treatment.

Conventional medicine does not generally view the client as an integrated person-body that is affected simultaneously by both material and nonmaterial factors during everyday life. The integration of these elements is not seen as important to the person's state of wellness or illness; therefore, therapies based on the concept of holism are not deemed to be important. Although the concept of a psychosocial body has gained some interest in Western practice, it has not been effectively incorporated into conventional care. The energetic and spiritual bodies are largely ignored.

> " *Most newly developed medications, when they are in the human testing phase, are tested on men between the ages of 25 and 35 years, with the presumption that they will work similarly in women, elderly people, and children. That presumption is not always accurate.* "

The Holistic Approach
The Multiple-Body View

In contrast, the alternative approach views the person-body as consisting of multiple, integrated elements that incorporate both the materialistic and nonmaterialistic aspects of existence. These elements include the physical (material), spiritual, energetic, and social bodies. This view allows for various interpretations of how the different components of the person-body interact and function to affect health and illness, and respond to different therapeutic interventions.

The integration of multiple bodies into a unified but distinctly individual person-body results in the belief that the person-body responds as a whole to factors that affect its state of well-being. Although the signs and symptoms of illness for one person are similar to another person's, they may indicate different underlying causes based on variable risk factors. From this viewpoint, diagnostic measures and interventions cannot be based on only one aspect of the person's being, but must be tailored to the person-body of each individual.

A Capacity for Self-Healing

A variety of alternative modalities are often needed to diagnose and treat each individual holistically. It often is not obvious when the health problems of the physical body correspond to the dynamics of the energetic body or when the energetic body merges with the spiritual body, and how they all are eventually integrated into the psychosocial body. The mediating role of the psychosocial body in the alternative approach emphasizes each person's capacity for self-healing. The importance of the mind–body interaction to elicit the placebo response, and the need for clients to participate actively in the monitoring and maintenance of their health and well-being, are positive factors in the diagnosis and treatment of their illness.

The multiple-body view found in some alternative health-care practices requires an eclectic approach to health promotion and maintenance. The diagnosis and treatment of illness from a multiple-body view require more than dependence on a single healing tradition centered on a one-body concept or on a fixed set of diagnostic criteria. The alternative approach requires active participation of both well and ill persons to better promote health or diagnose and treat disorders, rather than mere passive acceptance of a diagnosis and treatment plan from conventional health-care professionals.

Combining Modalities

The alternative philosophy includes both the material and nonmaterial aspects of the individual, stimulation of the self-healing forces, and the determination of a person's unique needs. It uses the concepts and treatment modalities of several healing traditions simultaneously. These modalities are based on different world views or concepts of reality and address the individual healing needs of each person.

For example, acupuncturists may also use massage and other types of bodywork and energy-system methods; chiropractors may incorporate diet, herbs, and other kinds of naturopathic methodologies into chiropractic spinal manipulations; and massage therapists may include mind–body techniques such as meditation, imagery, and visualization.

What Do You Think?

Name someone you know or know of who has gotten better after an illness although not expected to. Why do you think this happened?

The concept of a multiple-body individual is central to alternative and complementary healing. Healers function as facilitators in the promotion of health and healing (Box 26.2). In contrast, conventional therapy relies primarily on the concept of the physical-body individual, and conventional health-care providers function as experts in determining the meaning of physical signs and symptoms of health or illness and prescribing interventions to promote health or cure illness. The concepts of wellness and holism, self-healing, energy systems, nutrition, and plant-based medicine can be used to compare and contrast alternative and conventional methods of healing.

Wellness and Holism
Therapy from Outside

Wellness, from the perspective of conventional health care, tends to focus on individuals who are seen as being at risk for illness. Prevention often begins when signs or symptoms arise and is directed at alleviating them rather than treating or removing their underlying cause. At-risk individuals are permitted to engage in risky behaviors as long as conventional health care can find treatments or palliative measures for diseases it cannot prevent. From this perspective, health is often defined as the absence of disease and is considered synonymous with wellness.

The focus of conventional health care is reductionist rather than holistic because treatment and diagnosis are frequently centered on the cellular, organ, or system levels of the body. It emphasizes the biological–physiological (body) dimension of the client and treats only the disease process for which

Box 26.2
Defining Alternative Healers

Alternative healers practice one or more alternative or complementary modalities and are not also licensed as conventional health-care professionals. Conventional health-care professionals who incorporate hands-on alternative and complementary modalities into their conventional patient care are termed *integrative practitioners*. They should undergo the same educational, certification, and licensing processes as both conventional and alternative healers for the modalities they use.

Creating a universally applicable definition of alternative healers is extremely difficult because of the wide variety of healing traditions in use and the number of specialized healing techniques contained within them. The difficulty is compounded by the fact that many alternative healers incorporate various modalities from different healing traditions into their practices. For example, chiropractors commonly use therapeutic touch, acupuncture, acupressure, massage therapy, and naturopathic or homeopathic therapies. Massage therapists may combine multiple types of massage (e.g., Alexander, Swedish, Trager, and sports) with therapeutic touch, aromatherapy, reflexology, nutritional supplements, and electromagnetic therapies. The growing use of alternative practices by conventional health-care professionals further complicates the task of defining and classifying alternative healers and their practices.

signs and symptoms are already evident. The cause of illness is attributed to external forces or risk factors that "invade" the body from the surrounding physical, social, or biological environments.

From the biomedical view, treatment usually centers on identifying potentially dangerous or invading agents and then destroying, immobilizing, or extracting them from the person's body. Interventions consist mainly of chemotherapeutic agents (medications), surgery, or other externally imposed treatments to prevent a person considered at risk from becoming ill or to prevent signs and symptoms from becoming full-blown diseases.

Therapy from Within

In contrast to conventional health care, the alternative model views wellness as a state in which individuals are in harmony or balance with their internal and external worlds. This approach is a common thread in nursing models or theories of health (see Chapter 4). Alternative modalities hold that wellness can rarely be imposed on a person by an outside entity or agency. Rather, wellness is achieved mainly by individuals through the process of self-care. The individual assumes responsibility for maintaining his or her own state of health or wellness. The individual, when ill, works to return to a state of wellness by restoring both the internal and external (environmental) states of balance and harmony.

External disruptions—such as work stress, personal tragedy, a troublesome interpersonal relationship, or illness of a parent, spouse, or child—are seen as capable of affecting internal harmony and producing signs and symptoms of physical, emotional, or spiritual illness. This provides a holistic view of individuals in which they are one with their internal and external environments, thereby requiring holistic care. Treatment must address the whole individual (body–mind–spirit) in an environmental (physical, biological, social, cultural, and spiritual) context.

Spirituality is an essential part of holistic treatment (see Chapter 21). The human spirit incorporates the values, perception of meaning, and

> *The human spirit incorporates the values, perception of meaning, and purpose in life that can positively or negatively affect the ability to heal and achieve wellness.*

purpose in life that can positively or negatively affect the ability to heal and achieve wellness. From this perspective, health (balance or harmony), or the absence of illness, is but one aspect of wellness.

Self-Care

In the alternative system, first-level measures involve self-care aimed at wellness and can generally be performed independently. Some examples include exercising, eating a well-balanced diet, praying, getting enough sleep, cleaning the house, using defensive driving measures, doing breast or testicular self-examinations, applying sunscreen at the beach, and practicing good hygiene.

The next level of self-care requires seeking the assistance of others to achieve balance in self and the environment. This level includes getting help to find satisfying employment, seeking prenatal care or taking parenting classes when pregnant, going to community meetings to address environmental safety and citizen quality-of-life issues, undergoing routine health screening examinations (such as mammography and dental checkups), obtaining glasses to correct myopia, and getting vaccinations and keeping them up to date. Other alternative measures, such as acupuncture and energy therapies, require a high degree of specialist assistance.

The third level of self-care requires a high degree of specialist assistance from alternative healers and others to deal with major disruptions in internal or external well-being. Measures from this level focus on the spiritual dimension and include searching for personal awakening, enlightenment, and self-actualization. Effective modalities to achieve this goal are often rooted in other systems of health care such as traditional Chinese medicine, Ayurveda, and spiritualism. In some cases, individuals may require the use of alternative modalities to deal with illnesses when conventional health care is no longer effective.

Self-Healing

Both alternative and conventional health care include the belief that the body has the capacity to heal itself. The alternative system places self-healing as the central principle of its model and sees it as the basis of all healing. Thus, alternative healers focus on helping people determine why the cells of their body are sick and search for imbalances from a holistic perspective. Conventional health care views the ability of the body to self-heal primarily through the normal process of replacing cells; examples include the physiological and biological processes involved in wound healing. Conventional care approaches the concept of body self-healing by questioning why the cells are not replacing themselves and attempts to facilitate healing through external means, such as surgery, medications, or other invasive measures.

The Placebo Response

Conventional health practitioners tend to dismiss the effects of healing after alternative modalities have been used by attributing them to the placebo response. They feel that healing takes place only because the individual believes the treatment is effective. In conventional medicine, the term *placebo* has come to signify a type of sham treatment instituted to please difficult or anxious clients, or a sugar pill given when health-care professionals have nothing more to offer the client. In biomedical clinical research, a placebo is a nontreatment given to the control group under the assumption that it will not change any physiological responses and will therefore prove the effectiveness of the active treatments.

> *Healers who believe in the therapeutic effectiveness of interventions and are able to convey that belief to their clients achieve more positive responses than healers who remain skeptical about the interventions they are prescribing.*

What Do You Think?

What are the ethical issues involved in using placebos? If you were being given a placebo and you found out, how would you feel? What if you improved with the placebo? Would you still feel the same way?

The placebo response plays an important part in the testing of new drugs. The commonly used double-blind study requires that neither researchers nor study participants know which group is receiving the study drug and which group is receiving an inert substance (placebo). At the conclusion of the study, researchers compare results and decide whether a higher percentage of the experimental group experienced the hoped-for results from the active medication than the control group received from the placebo. However, clinical studies have shown that some participants respond positively to placebo medications between 30 and 70 percent of the time. The clients with the highest positive results from placebos include those with:

- Pain from chronic disease, such as cancer pain, arthritis, back pain, angina pectoris, and gastrointestinal tract discomfort
- Autonomic nervous system disorders, such as phobias, psychoneuroses, depression, and nausea
- Neurohormonal disorders, such as asthma, other bronchial airflow conditions, and hypertension

How Does It Work?

Researchers do not have a good understanding of the mechanism by which the placebo response produces positive results. Some believe that the placebo effect is at work in all therapeutic intervention regardless of whether the intervention is an alternative or a conventional treatment. Four possible factors have been examined:

- An endorphin-mediated response
- Belief of the client
- Belief of the healer
- The client–healer relationship

Endorphin-Mediated Response. Endorphins are the body's natural painkillers; when released, they reduce pain and bring about a degree of euphoria. Relaxation therapies and other types of stress-reducing and stress-controlling techniques are believed to promote the release of endorphins that produce pain relief. When experimental groups were given medications that block the release of endorphins, clients with postoperative dental pain reported an increase in pain because the placebo effect was blocked. The placebo response changes the perception of the client but does not affect the underlying disease process.

Belief of the Client. A person's belief in the effectiveness of the therapy is an important factor in its success and may be just as important as the therapy itself. Studies of client compliance in taking prescribed beta blocker heart medications, conducted in the first year after myocardial infarction, showed that mortality rates were almost equal for those failing to take either the beta blocker or placebo. Mortality rates for both these groups were higher than the rates for those who faithfully took their prescribed medications or placebos.

Belief of the Healer. Healers who believe in the therapeutic effectiveness of interventions and are able to convey that belief to their clients achieve more positive responses than healers who remain skeptical about the interventions they are prescribing. An attitude of caring and being in control tends to alleviate clients' anxieties and fears while increasing their hope and positive expectations.

Client–Healer Relationship. A trusting and close relationship between the client and healer has a positive psychological effect on clients and can become the mental catalyst they need for recovery. The ability of healers to communicate in an empathic manner increases client satisfaction with care; increases compliance with mutually set goals; increases feelings of empowerment, self-confidence, and self-worth; and decreases depression and anxiety.

Although conventional health care considers many of these approaches as speculative, incomplete, or insufficient to explain the placebo response, alternative healers see the placebo response as measurable and reproducible evidence that the mind and body are intertwined. The placebo response is viewed as proof that feelings, thoughts, and beliefs can change the physiological and structural functioning of individuals.

Remembered Wellness. The term *remembered wellness* is used to describe the physiological response that occurs after positive therapeutic interventions. Remembered wellness includes the person's prior learning, experiences, environment, beliefs, and perceptions. It can also include biological and genetic factors.

Remembered wellness is triggered by memories of past events or times when good health and feelings of confidence, strength, hope, and peace were part of the person's life. Alternative therapies access these memories by stimulating relaxation, such as the quieting of the body and mind to promote healing. Clinical research has demonstrated relaxation to be effective in treating anxiety, pain, high blood pressure, and tachycardia and in managing stress. Research studies have confirmed a close relationship between the central nervous and immune systems and have shown that interaction occurs between the two mind–body pathways: the autonomic and neuroendocrine systems.

Much more research is required for a full scientific explanation of the how the mind and body interact to produce the placebo response and why remembered wellness produces the positive responses it often does. The placebo response remains an enigma to conventional health care and implies an element of deceitfulness when used deliberately in client treatments. For alternative medicine, the placebo response and remembered wellness are forces that can be harnessed to bring about healing.

Energy Systems

It has long been known scientifically that the human body is regulated by its own internal electrical energy system. Human beings cannot survive without the low levels of electricity that sustain and regulate life at the cellular and molecular levels. Electrical–chemical reactions are produced in the nervous system and help regulate other body systems, electrical impulses trigger heartbeats, and minute electrical currents regulate the production of hormones. The blood is composed largely of iron; therefore, magnetic forces exist in all parts of the body.

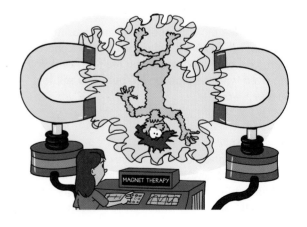

Conventional Uses of Energy

Conventional health care has long used various types of energy systems (e.g., electrical, magnetic, microwave, and infrared) for screening, diagnosis, and some types of treatment. Commonly used modalities include electrocardiograms, magnetic resonance imaging, electroencephalograms, electromyelograms, x-rays, radiation treatments for cancer, low-frequency electric current to stimulate growth of bone cells (osteoblasts) to accelerate healing of fractures, types of electric shock therapy for cardiac arrest, cardioversions for cardiac arrhythmia, and pacemakers.

Conventional health care also uses bioenergy (body energy) to determine the degree of injury and estimate recovery times through the study of cells as they decompose, die, reproduce, and respond to pathogens and traumas. The majority of conventional treatments for many diseases are chemical (medications) or surgical or involve immobilizing or manipulating the affected body part. They are used primarily *after* the disease has been diagnosed.

Energy in Alternative Healing

Conventional medicine has been slow to recognize how the energy of the body can be used for health promotion and healing. Alternative therapies refer to energy systems as fields, vital essences, balance, and flow that clients can use to prevent illness, promote health, and heal themselves. The basic concept is that external forces are not able to cause harm if the person is in the well state. Alternative healers may be needed to help individuals manipulate the energy system primarily for self-protection or healing. Major alternative and complementary modalities using bioenergy and other energy fields are energy medicine, vital essences and balance, and external energy forces.

Energy Medicine

This therapy includes a number of techniques that use external energy sources to stimulate tissue regeneration or improve the immune system response. Relaxation of muscles through electrical stimulation is thought to promote general body relaxation, increase circulation, enhance waste removal, improve nutrition and oxygenation, and restore energy balance. Examples of energy medicine include electroacupuncture, biofeedback, magnet therapy, and sound and light therapy.

Vital Essences and Balance

In many alternative models, illness reflects blockage, loss, or imbalance of body energy or vital essence. Disturbance of internal body energy can result from external or internal factors. Treatment may be directed at removing the blockage of energy flow through such measures as acupuncture, acupressure, chiropractic adjustment, craniosacral therapy, or reflexology. It may also be directed at increasing the amount of energy and vital essence to restore balance in the body.

Ways of inducing these changes include diet, herbs, exercises, and spiritual techniques, such as yoga, meditation, and internal Qi Gong. Therapies related to the creative arts, such as music, drawing, singing, chanting, and dancing, are also used to restore balance and vital essences.

External Energy Forces

External energy forces, it is believed, have the capacity for healing. Some of these external forces are actual energy treatments. Other forces include mobilizing the healing energy of faith, spirituality, prayer, shamanism, crystals, and hand-mediated energetic healing techniques, such as therapeutic touch and healing touch (Box 26.3).

Nutrition

Nutrition and diet have long been recognized by both alternative and conventional healing systems as important in health promotion and illness treatment. They can also be risk factors for or even cause disease. In conventional health care, nutrition and diet are usually considered as adjuncts to biomedical treatment. In alternative systems, nutrition is commonly seen as a way of life and as a method of preventing illness.

Benefits of Natural Foods

Conventional health care commonly focuses on the need for food and a well-balanced diet without close regard to food production or processing. The safety of food sources in the contemporary diet has been called into question by both alternative healers and conventional health-care professionals because of increasing evidence of toxins in the food chain. These include:

- Pesticides used in agricultural production, lawn care, and pest control
- Industrial pollutants discharged into the air and water in which plants and animals live and obtain nutrients

Box 26.3
Therapeutic Touch

Therapeutic touch (TT) and healing touch (HT) are two forms of hand-mediated energetic healing. TT refers to the Krieger-Kunz method and HT to the techniques taught to health-care professionals and certified by the American Holistic Nurses' Association. HT relies on the ability of practitioners to choose appropriate energy healing techniques through their interpretation of the client's energy flow, whereas TT follows a set of rules and protocols based in traditional or ancient healing concepts of energy, such as aura (electromagnetic field), chakras, and prana (life-force or vital essence in Ayurvedic medicine).

No physical contact takes place between practitioner and client in either technique. The practitioner's hands are held, palms down, 2 to 6 inches away from the client. Slow, rhythmic motions are made over the client from head to toe to detect blockage in the normal energy flow in the body. When energy blockages or imbalances are detected or sensed, they are rectified by transference of energy from the practitioner's hands to the client's energy field, replenishing the client's energy flow, removing energy obstructions, and releasing energy congestion. The transference of energy stimulates the healing powers of the body through reduction of stress and anxiety, promotion of relaxation, and relief of pain. TT is also believed to relax crying babies, relieve asthmatic breathing, increase wound healing, and reduce fever, inflammation, headache, and postoperative pain.

- Chemicals added to food for preservation, to increase shelf life, or to make food more aesthetically appealing and pleasing in texture and taste
- Irradiation used to kill organisms, retard sprouting, and preserve shelf life
- Antibiotics, hormones, and other drugs given to animals to improve their health and increase their size, weight, and speed of growth
- Alteration of nutrients during food processing
- Genetic alteration of foods for improved production rates and drought resistance

Alternative modalities recommend only foods produced in a natural manner and in their natural environment. Emphasis on natural products can be attributed to four primary factors:

1. Concerns about food production and processing
2. The belief that the person-body, as both an energy system and a physical entity, is designed to live in a natural environment
3. The belief that what is eaten directly affects an individual's health
4. Concerns about increased consumption of nutrient-poor and energy-rich foods

Scientific evidence indicates that the more sedentary lifestyle and greater affluence experienced by many have resulted in excessive and unhealthy eating. The end result is a nation that has high rates of obesity, coronary artery disease, micronutrient deficiencies, congenital abnormalities, and cancer. Most alternative systems advocate consumption of plant-based, whole foods and complex carbohydrates. Increasing the amounts of food lower on the food chain helps decrease the amounts of meat, saturated fats, and processed foods that dominate many diets. Examples of natural food diets include the macrobiotic and vegetarian diets.

Dietary Supplements

The FDA defines dietary supplements as "any product intended for ingestion as a supplement to the diet. This includes vitamins; minerals; herbs, botanical, and other plant-derived substances; and amino acids . . . and concentrates, metabolites, constituents and extracts of theses substances."

Supplements as Prevention

Conventional health-care professionals typically view nutritional supplements (vitamins and minerals) as replacement or preventive therapy for nutrition-deficient conditions. For example, rickets and osteoporosis can be prevented by adequate vitamin D and calcium intake; adequate ascorbic acid (vitamin C) intake prevents scurvy; and neural tube defects in newborns can be prevented by sufficient maternal intake of folic acid (vitamin B_9) during the prenatal period. The FDA, on the basis of research by the National Academy of Sciences, has established maximum recommended daily allowances (RDAs) for vitamin and mineral intake. These levels are usually well above the amount at which deficiency diseases occur but below the level at which the client would experience toxic side effects.

Rethinking RDA Levels. Studies indicate that approximately two thirds of adults fail to consume the RDAs of fruits and vegetables. Also, some studies suggest that RDA levels may be too low for certain vitamins, minerals, and micronutrients to prevent the onset of chronic diseases in persons whose diets do not meet the recommended daily nutrient requirements. Especially susceptible are growing children, alcoholics, people with conditions preventing normal nutrient absorption, and pregnant, lactating, and post-menopausal women. Conventional health-care professionals consider general daily supplements, such as vitamin pills, sufficient to prevent deficiency diseases in persons with special dietary needs.

" *Alternative therapies refer to energy systems as fields, vital essences, balance, and flow clients can use to prevent illness, promote health, and heal themselves. The basic concept is that external forces are not able to cause harm if the person is in the well state.* "

Alternative systems, like conventional health care, regard nutritional supplements as necessary to promote health through assurance of adequate dietary intake and as replacement therapy for conditions caused by nutrition deficiency. Alternative systems also consider orthomolecular therapy or megavitamin therapy (the administration of "megadoses" far in excess of RDAs for vitamins and minerals) as being effective in curing diseases, increasing vitality, and enhancing overall well-being.

Regulation of Supplements

Concern about nutritional supplements also exists because, unlike drugs and most food additives, they are not regulated by the FDA. If manufacturers make no claims that they are effective against a disease, they do not need to be tested for safety and effectiveness before they are sold to the public. However, there has been a gradual increase in the regulation of these products over the past 25 years. The 1994

Dietary Supplement and Health Education Act (DSHEA) created a special category of 20,000 protected substances previously sold as supplements. The DSHEA defined supplements as including vitamins, minerals, amino acids, herbs, botanicals and other plant-derived products, and the extracts, metabolites, constituents, and concentrates of supplements.

What Do You Think?

Should dietary supplements be considered medications? What are the advantages and disadvantages of classifying supplements as medications?

The FDA can remove supplements from the market if it receives reports of their adverse effects and then proves that they are dangerous to consumers' health. The FDA issues public warnings when supplements are linked to safety concerns. The DSHEA also gave the FDA authority to improve and enforce product labeling, package inserts, and accompanying literature. To enhance product comparison, guidelines instituted in 1999 require labels to carry a panel of "supplemental facts" or a "nutrition facts box," which includes ingredients.

The U.S. Postal Service and the Federal Trade Commission (FTC) also regulate nutritional supplements and herbal products. The U.S. Postal Inspection Service monitors products purchased by mail and may intercept supplements shipped through the mail for false claims, such as the statement that they can cure AIDS or cancer. The Office of Criminal Investigation can be contacted at (202) 268-2000.

The FTC has issued guidelines to ensure that advertising claims are substantiated by reliable scientific evidence. No longer acceptable are claims of effectiveness and safety based on testimonials and other anecdotal evidence. Also outlawed are vague disclaimers, such as "results may vary." The term "traditional use" (e.g., folk remedy), which implies that the product is effective even without scientific evidence, has also been banned. The risks or qualifying information of any product must be prominently displayed and easily understood.

Plants as Medicine

Both alternative and conventional health care use plants as medicines. Herbalism, or "botanical medicine," also known as phytotherapy or phytomedicine in England and other parts of Europe, is the study and use of herbs or crude-based plant products for food, medicine, or prophylaxis. They can also be used to heal, treat, or prevent illness and improve the spiritual and physical quality of life.

Herbs may be angiosperms (flowering plants, trees, or shrubs), algae, moss, fungus, seaweed, lichen, or ferns. Herbs used as medicines come from some part of the plant (leaf, root, flower, fruit, stem, bark, or seed), its syrup-like exudates, or some combination of these. In some herbal traditions, nonplant products are used alone or in combination, with or without plants. They may include animal secretions and parts (e.g., bones, organs, or tissues), stones and gemstones, minerals and metals, shells, and insects and insect products.

> *Alternative systems, like conventional health care, consider nutritional supplements both as necessary to promote health through assurance of adequate dietary intake and as replacement therapy for conditions caused by nutrition deficiency.*

Botanical healing in the form of herbal medicines was widely used in the United States until the early 19th century, when it was gradually displaced by the increasing prominence of the scientific method and labeled quackery. Phytomedicine continues to be a prominent branch of conventional health care in Europe. Botanicals are used by 40 percent of German and French physicians in their daily practices.

Scientists have yet to determine the pharmaceutical qualities of most plants, and little is known about what toxicities they can produce. The world supports an estimated 250,000 to 500,000 flowering plant species, but only 5000 have been researched for their pharmacological effects.

Herbal Traditions

The use of herbal therapies varies according to culture and tradition. The three major groups of herbal therapies recognized throughout the world are from Western medicine, traditional Chinese medicine, and Ayurvedic medicine.

Western Pharmacology

The Western herbal tradition relies primarily on the pharmacological action of herbs, most of which are derived from the plant kingdom. There are presently 119 plant-derived pharmaceutical medicines. Plant chemicals constitute about 25 percent of prescriptions by conventional health-care professionals.

Chinese Medicine

Herbology is used in traditional Chinese medicine to enhance the flow and amount of chi, restore the harmonious balance of the complementary forces of yin and yang, and balance the five elements (fire, earth, metal, water, and wood). In the Chinese system, plants are prescribed according to their effects on the five elements and their corresponding body processes, including organs, tissues, emotions, and temperatures (climates).

The Chinese believe that the five elements give rise to the five tastes that produce particular medicinal actions. Bitter-tasting herbs (fire) dry and drain. Sweet-tasting herbs (earth) reduce pain and increase tone. Acrid herbs (metal) rid the body of toxins. Salty herbs (water) nourish the kidney. Sour herbs (wood) clean, helping preserve chi and nourishing yin. Herbs are also symbolically classified according to temperature changes they are thought to produce in the body: cold, cool, neutral, warm, and hot. The temperatures correspond to the symbolic climate qualities of the organs and the five elements.

Ayurvedic Medicine

Ayurvedic medicine also considers the taste, or "essence," of the herb as an integral element in herbology. Ayurveda recognizes six essences (sweet, sour, salty, pungent, bitter, and astringent) and five elements (ether, water, fire, air, and earth). The elements are manifested as three doshas, or humors (vata, pitta, and kapha) that govern body functioning and that must be kept in balance to maintain or restore a healthy state.

Vata, the principle of air, wind, or movement, is decreased by herbs that are sweet, sour, and salty, which exert a symbolic heating effect on the body. Vata is increased by herbs that are pungent, bitter, astringent, and cooling. Pitta, the principle of fire, is decreased by herbs that are sweet, bitter, astringent, and cooling and increased by those that are pungent, sour, salty, and heating. Kapha, the principle of water, is decreased by herbs that are pungent, bitter, astringent, and heating and increased by those that are sweet, sour, salty, and cooling.

Concerns About Herbal Therapies

There is growing concern in the United States about the use of herbal preparations by the general public without consultation with either conventional healthcare professionals or alternative healers. Sales of herbal preparations have been growing tremendously. Another concern is the lack of licensing and standards for herbalists. Except for naturopaths, most herbalists have no foundation in phytochemistry or botanical medicine.

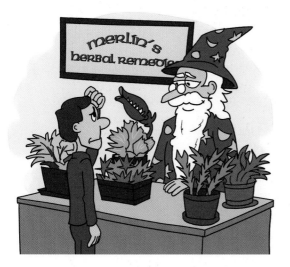

Also, in other cultural traditions, herbs are not prescribed for the biological effects of their chemical ingredients. They are commonly prescribed according to the "doctrine of signatures," or their physical and taste characteristics. For example, herbs with heart-shaped leaves may be used to treat heart problems; those with red flowers or leaves may be used to control bleeding or blood disorders; and those with a sour taste may be given to decrease swelling or counteract the effects of "sugar" (diabetes mellitus).

Additional problems may arise because the public views most herbal remedies as natural products and therefore considers them to be pure, safe, relatively harmless, and more healthy than manufactured medicines. Recent problems with some natural products indicate that there is no guarantee of safety.

THE PARADOX OF ALTERNATIVE HEALING PRACTICES

A Lack of Validation

Nurses often feel uncomfortable with the use of herbal products and alternative therapies because of unclear definitions of various alternative and complementary practices and the widespread, yet often unregulated, use of alternative products and healers. This paradox arises because most nursing knowledge comes from the biomedical sciences, but most alternative modalities (1) have not yet been scientifically validated or proven safe by the scientific method and (2) are based in concepts of holism, self-care, and theoretical constructs that emanate from world views different from that of biomedicine and the scientific perspective.

In other words, for most alternative modalities, little is known about whether or how they work, their side effects, or their interactions with conventional or other alternative modalities. Claims regarding their effectiveness come largely from testimonials of users or alternative healers rather than from evidence in scientific studies. Equally limited is valid knowledge about the effectiveness of the various alternative modalities in specific conditions and about their short- and long-term effects.

The nursing profession has worked for many years to build its decision-making skills on knowledge derived from the scientific method and on the use of critical thinking and culture competence. Nurses promote self-care in clients by teaching them to make informed choices about their health-care options. Many of the alternative health-care practices in use today fly in the face of the nursing profession's movement toward evidence-based practice.

Few Regulatory Standards

The technical competence and knowledge of alternative healers are of considerable importance to nurses caring for clients who pursue alternative and complementary practices. Nurses and the general public are accustomed to determining the qualifications, assumed competency, and scope of practice of conventional health-care practitioners through externally regulated mechanisms. These external regulations include graduation from an accredited school, state-regulated licenses, credentialing, and attainment of specialty certifications from professional organizations or institutions of higher education. No such external processes or criteria exist to validate the competence and knowledge of most alternative practitioners.

The relative lack of regulatory standards makes selection of competent alternative practitioners exceedingly difficult. It is a major concern of the public, conventional health-care practitioners, and insurers because clients may be subject to financial exploitation, ineffective therapies, and psychological and physical abuse.

A Challenge to Nurses

The challenge presented to nurses by alternative healing modalities relates to professional accountability. Nurses must learn about alternative modalities, their general safety and efficacy, and their use in specific health and illness conditions.

Human caring and cultural competence require that nurses be able to develop therapeutic partnerships with culturally diverse clients and empower them to take charge of their lives and health care. They need to preserve the client's right to self-determination and to practice alternative lifestyles, as well as to pursue a variety of conventional or alternative therapies, with or without consulting alternative healers or conventional health-care professionals. Nurses must keep an open mind while relying on sound evidence for recommendations about alternative practices and practitioners.

Ask Questions

Box 26.4 lists some questions nurses need to ask when determining the quality and validity of information about an alternative modality. It is important to teach clients to ask similar questions so that they can decide about alternative therapy and sort out the often conflicting advice of family, friends, conventional

---

Box 26.4

Questions to Ask About Alternative Modalities

1. What evidence exists that the therapy is effective or harmful?
   - Is there experimental evidence? How effective is the alternative modality when examined experimentally?
   - Is there clinical practice evidence? How effective is the alternative modality when applied clinically?
   - Is there comparative evidence? How effective is the modality when compared with other treatments?
   - Is there summary evidence? Has the modality been evaluated and a consensus reached regarding its use and effectiveness for various health conditions?
   - Is there evidence of demand? Is the modality wanted by clients, practitioners, or both?
   - Is there evidence of satisfaction? Does the alternative modality meet the expectations of clients and practitioners?

- Is there cost evidence? Is the modality covered by health insurance? Is it cost effective?
- Is the meaning evident? Is the modality the best and right one for the client?
2. How strong is the evidence? Is it based on testimonials, clinical observations, or scientific research?
3. Can the results be attributed to the placebo effect? Is the benefit from the placebo effect adequate to the client's needs?
4. Does evidence exist that the benefits of the therapy outweigh the risks?
   - Is the alternative modality potentially useful?
   - Is the modality essentially without value except for the potential placebo effect?
   - Is the modality potentially harmful?
5. Is there another way to obtain the same hoped-for results?
6. Who else has tried this alternative modality, and what was their experience?
7. Are there reputable (licensed and certified) alternative healers available? What has been their experience with this alternative modality?
8. What information do regulatory agencies have about the modality or the alternative healers?
9. What information is available in the popular media about the modality or alternative healers? Has it been or can it be verified by clinical observations or research studies?

Sources: Barrocas A: Complementary and alternative medicine: Friend, foe or OWA (other weird arrangements). Journal of the American Diet Association 97:1373, 1997.

Kurtzweil P: An FDA Guide to Dietary Supplements, 2009. Retrieved November, 2010 from http://www.vm.cfsan.fda.gov/~dms/fdsupp.html.

Wiese M, Oster C: "Becoming accepted": The complementary and alternative medicine practitioners' response to the uptake and practice of traditional medicine therapies by the mainstream health sector. Health: An Interdisciplinary Journal for the Social Study of Health, Illness and Medicine 14(4):415–433, 2010.

National Center for Complementary and Alternative Medicine: Considering CAM? 2010. Retrieved November, 2010 from http://www.nccam.nih.gov/nccam/fcp/faq/considercam.html.

health-care professionals, alternative healers, and the media.

Many clients use alternative healing modalities without ever talking to a conventional health professional about them. They may fear a negative reaction. Others are not aware of the potential harm that may occur, especially when they combine alternative therapies or alternative and conventional therapies. Some may consider the scientific evidence and conclude that most noninvasive and nondrug alternative therapies are harmless. Others may mistakenly assume that alternative therapies are regulated by the government and would not be available if they were dangerous.

Find Information

Lack of scientific information about alternative healing modalities is of concern to alternative healers, conventional health-care professionals, and clients. For nurses and their clients, the need to know where and how to find up-to-date, reliable information on alternative therapies is a must.

Information Resources

- The NCCAM offers one of the best general governmental resources for information on alternative modalities at the NCCAM website: http://www.nccam.nih.gov.
- Several authoritative sources on herbal medicines are available for practitioners and clients.
- The FDA maintains a site for reporting and obtaining information about adverse effects and interactions of herbals through MedWatch (800-FDA-1088 or http://www.fda.gov/medwatch).
- F. A. Davis maintains a website on herbal medicines (http://www.DrugGuide.com), as does the U.S. Pharmacopeia (http://www.usp.org/information/index.html).
- The American Botanical Society (512-926-4900) has a website (http://www.herbalgram.org) and

publishes the *Herbalgram,* a newsletter on herbal medications.

- MICROMEDEX has an evidence-based series on herbal medicines and dietary supplements, toxicologies, clinical protocols, and client education (800-643-8116 or www.micromedex.com). It also links to the electronic database of herbal medicines from the Royal Pharmaceutical Society of Great Britain.
- Tyler's *The Honest Herbal* is one of the most reputable guides for the use of herbs.[6]
- *The Physicians' Desk Reference for Herbal Medicine* contains scientific findings on the efficacy, potential interactions, clinical trials, and case reports of herbs, as well as indexes on Asian, Ayurvedic, and homeopathic herbs.[7]

The Internet has become a primary source of information for both the public and health-care providers about alternative products and local practitioners of alternative therapies. Because information posted to the Internet is not regulated, this avenue of inquiry requires caution. One the earliest and still best websites providing reputable information about ACH and specific modalities is http://www.quackwatch.com. There also are a number of governmental watch sites that can be accessed for information about alternative therapies.

- Quackwatch (http://www.quackwatch.com) offers fact sheets and reviews of specific alternative modalities, as well as those associated with certain illnesses. It also has sections on how to determine whether a website devoted to alternative modalities is trustworthy.

Ask the Client

It is important to ask clients about their use of alternative therapies. Not doing so may place them at risk for adverse health outcomes. When and how to assess for the use of ACH during the client assessment process is a matter of judgment and should be guided by the nurse's knowledge of individual clients. An appropriate time is often after the chief complaint has been documented because this is when questions are asked about the clients' reasons for seeking health care and what they have already done for their problem.

What Do You Think?

Does the facility where you do your clinical practice ask about alternative therapies during the admission assessment? Are you taught to assess for this information in your nursing program?

Discuss the use of alternative therapies tactfully and supportively. Keep complete and accurate documentation of all interactions with clients about alternative therapies and healers. And as much as possible, help direct clients toward the safest therapies and the most qualified practitioners.

Conclusion

Alternative and nontraditional health-care practices are a growing part of health care in the United States. It is essential that nurses become aware of what these practices entail and how they may affect or interact with conventional therapies that the client is already receiving. Admission assessments for these practices, when clients enter the health-care system for whatever reason, should become a routine part of client evaluation. Nurses traditionally have approached health care from a holistic viewpoint that addresses all of the client's needs—mind, body, and spirit. As health care moves more toward alternative practices, nurses are the logical choice to coordinate a comprehensive approach to health care that includes both traditional and alternative practices. Without this coordination, an already fragmented health-care system will become even more so.

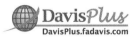

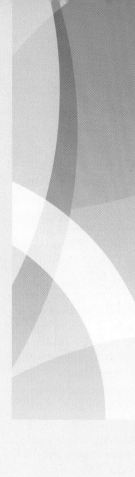

Critical Thinking Exercises

• Contact three of the websites on alternative practices listed in this chapter. Evaluate them according to their quality, content, and usefulness to your practice.

• Identify a nurse practitioner, physician, or other health-care provider in your area who uses alternative practices. Interview that person and arrange for a presentation to the class about alternative health-care practices.

• Select a client from your clinical experiences who is having pain. How might alternative practices help this client? Develop a care plan using both traditional and alternative methods for pain control.

• Identify and discuss three advantages of and three problems with alternative health-care practices.

• Select three nursing theories from Chapter 4 that use a holistic approach to nursing. Identify how and what alternative practices would work well with each one of these theories.

GLOSSARY OF ALTERNATIVE
AND COMPLEMENTARY HEALING TERMS

Inclusion of particular ideas or practices in this glossary does not imply endorsement of them. Health-care practitioners and their clients must carefully evaluate the claims and qualifications of alternative and complementary healing practices and practitioners before coming to conclusions about them.

Acupressure Use of fingers or hands to apply pressure over acupuncture points on meridians to restore or enhance the flow of chi. Believed to maintain or restore energy balance. From traditional Chinese medicine.

Acupressure massage Use of massage techniques such as rubbing, kneading, percussion, and vibration over acupuncture points to improve circulation of chi.

Acupuncture Insertion of needles along meridian channels to alleviate blockage of chi and reestablish the balance of energy in the body. The insertion points are believed to be linked to specific internal organs. Originating in traditional Chinese medicine, acupuncture is now commonly considered a complete treatment system on its own.

Alexander technique A technique developed by Frederick Matthias Alexander that realigns body posture through imaging and relaxation. Decreases muscle tension and fatigue, stress, and back and neck pain. Based on the belief that poor posture during daily activities contributes to physical and emotional problems.

Allopathic medicine A synonym for conventional medicine. Practitioner uses medicines to counteract symptoms or heal by producing different effects or a second condition different from the one being treated. From the Greek words *allos* (other) and *pathos* (suffering).

Applied kinesiology Study of muscle activity, strength, and health effects through the muscle-gland-organ link. Muscle dysfunction may be counteracted by nutrition, manual procedures (e.g., massage), pressure over muscle attachment points, and realignment.

Aromatherapy A type of herbal therapy that uses the odors of essential oils extracted from plants to treat various conditions, such as headaches, tension, and anxiety. Chemical composition of the oils produces pharmacological effects that include antibacterial, antiviral, antispasmodic, diuretic, vasodilative, and mood-harmonizing actions. The oils may be applied by massage, inhaled, placed in baths and other forms of hydrotherapy, or taken internally.

Art therapy Use of artistic self-expression through drawing, sculpture, and painting to diagnose and treat behavioral or emotional problems.

Aura Magnetic field thought to surround every person, plant, and animal. Adjustment of the field is believed to affect health, emotions, spirit, and mind.

Auriculotherapy A method developed in France in which points on the external ear are stimulated with acupuncture needles, massage, electronics, or infrared treatment. These points are believed to have neurological connections to other body areas. Also called *ear acupuncture.*

Ayurvedic medicine A personalistic, holistic, and naturalistic approach to health maintenance and treatment of illness, originating in India. Maintains balance of the three doshas (bioenergies) of the body through diet and herbs, meditation, breathing exercises (pranayama), massage with medicated oils, yoga and other forms of vigorous exercise, and exposure to the sun for higher consciousness.

Bach flower essences Homeopathic preparations of oil concentrates extracted from flowers. Originated by Edward Bach, an English physician, this method is aimed at emotional states rather than the signs and symptoms of physical illness. Specific concentrates or combinations of concentrates are associated with various emotional states. Each client is diagnosed individually because there is no corresponding psychological equivalent for every physical state.

Biofeedback Form of training that helps a person to consciously control or change normally unconscious body functions to improve overall health. Also refers to the method of immediately reporting back information to the client about a biological process being measured so the person can consciously alter or influence the process.

Bodywork General term used to describe various forms of massage therapy, energy balancing, deep-tissue manipulation, and movement awareness.

Botanical medicine Use of an entire plant or herb for treating illness or maintaining health.

Chakras Circles found along the midline of the body, in alignment with the spinal cord, that distribute energy throughout the body. If they are blocked, energy flow is inhibited.

Chelation therapy Use of minerals combined with amino acids, given intravenously or orally, to help cleanse the body of unnecessary or toxic minerals that block blood circulation. From the Greek word *chele* (to bind or to claw).

Chi (qi, shi) From traditional Chinese medicine. Chi is the invisible life-force that circulates through the body along meridians, or channels. Maintaining or restoring the flow of chi restores and promotes health.

Chiropractic A Western medical system postulating that partial joint dislocations (subluxations) cause the body to be misaligned. Removal or adjustment of subluxations balances the spinal–nervous system and restores and maintains health.

Craniosacral therapy Manipulation of the bones of the skull to treat craniosacral dysfunctions caused by restriction in the flow of cerebrospinal fluid and misalignment of bones. *Cranio* refers to the cranium and *sacral* to the sacrum.

Crystal therapy Use of quartz and other gemstones, believed to emit electromagnetic energy. Frequently used with light and color therapy. Also called *gem therapy.*

Cupping From traditional Chinese and Ayurvedic medicines. Method using a heated cup placed over the skin to draw out impurities, decrease blood pressure, increase circulation, and relieve muscle pain.

Curanderismo Healing tradition, found in Mexican American communities, based in concepts of supernaturalism, balance, and holism. From the Spanish verb *to heal.*

Dance therapy Use of dance movement to enhance wellness and aid healing. Sharpens levels of awareness, enhances self-confidence, helps with motor coordination and physical skills, and assists with communication, especially with severely disturbed psychiatric clients.

Doshas Three *(vata, pitta,* and *kapha)* basic metabolic types, life-forces, or bioenergies in Ayurvedic medicine. Each has certain characteristics and tendencies that combine to determine a person's constitution. When they are in balance, mind and body are coordinated, resulting in vibrant health and energy. When they are out of balance, the body is susceptible to outside stressors, such as microorganisms, poor nutrition, and work overload.

Energy medicine Measurement of electromagnetic frequencies emitted by the body. The object is to diagnose energy imbalances that may cause or contribute to present or future illnesses and to use electromagnetic forces to counteract imbalances and restore the body's energy balance.

Environmental medicine Method that explores the role of environmental and dietary allergens in health and illness.

Feldenkrais method A type of bodywork or physical movement developed by Moshe Feldenkrais that stresses awareness through movement and helps the body work with gravity. Incorporates imaging, active moving, and forms of directed attention designed to re-educate the nervous system, teach subjects how to learn from their own kinesic feedback, and avoid movements that strain joints and muscles.

Gerson therapy Metabolic therapy developed by Max Gerson, a German physician. It is based on the belief that cancer results from metabolic dysfunctions in cells that can be countered by detoxification, a vegetarian diet, coffee enemas to stimulate excretion of liver bile, the exclusion of sodium, and an abundance of potassium.

Guided imagery A facilitated flow of thoughts that helps a person see, feel, taste, smell, hear, or touch something in the imagination. The power of the mind or imagination is used to stimulate positive physical responses and provide insight into health and an understanding of emotions as a cause of ill health.

Healing touch Healing tradition based on the belief in a universal energy system. Humans are seen as interpenetrating layers of energy systems just above and outside the body that are integrated with energy fields in the environment. Manipulation of such energy fields through touch can help restore a person's energy balance and health.

Hellerwork A type of bodywork developed by Joseph Heller as an outgrowth of Rolfing. It combines dialogue, body movement education, and deep touch to achieve greater mind–body awareness and structural body alignment with gravitational forces. Therapy is individualized to different body types.

Herbal medicine Use of the chemical makeup of herbs in much the same way as conventional medicine uses pharmaceuticals. The most ancient known form of health care, herbal medicine is basic to traditional Chinese, Ayurvedic, and Native American medical systems. Also called *botanical medicine, phytotherapy,* and *phytomedicine.*

Homeopathy A Western medical system based on the principle that "like cures like." Natural substances are prescribed in minute dilutions to cause the symptoms of the disease they are intended to cure, helping the body cure itself.

Humor therapy Deliberate use of laughter to improve quality of life by encouraging relaxation and stress reduction, distracting individuals from awareness of constant pain, and providing symptom relief.

Hydrotherapy Use of hot, cold, or contrasting water temperatures to maintain or restore health. Water, steam, or ice may be used in combination with baths, compresses, hot and cold packs, showers, and enemas or colonic irrigations. Minerals, herbs, and oils may be added to enhance the therapeutic effects. Also known as *water cure.*

Hypnotherapy Use of hypnosis, power of suggestion, and trancelike states to access the deepest levels of the mind. Used to bring about changes in behavior, treat health conditions, and manage medical and psychological problems.

Integrative medicine The practice of conventional health-care professionals who prescribe a combination of therapies from both systems. *Integrative* is synonymous with *complementary.*

Iridiology Iris diagnosis. In this belief system, each area of the body has a corresponding point on the iris of the eye. Thus, the state of health (balance) or disease (imbalance) can be diagnosed from the color, texture, or location of pigments in the eye.

Jin Shin Jyutsu A Japanese form of massage in which combinations of healing points on the body are held for a minute or more with the fingertips. The purpose is to enhance or restore the flow of chi.

Light and color therapy A method by which light is converted into electrical impulses, travels along the optic nerve to the brain, and stimulates the hypothalamus to send neurotransmitters to regulate the autonomic nervous system. Various colors of light are believed to stimulate different parts of the body.

Magnet therapy A type of electromagnetic therapy or energy medicine in which magnets are used to stimulate circulation, increase oxygen to cells, and facilitate healing by correcting disturbed or malfunctioning electromagnetic frequencies that the body emits.

Mantra A type of sound therapy used in Ayurvedic medicine to reach a higher level of spiritual and mental functioning. It changes the "vibratory patterns of the mind" to release unconscious negative thoughts, psychological stress, and emotional distress. Often achieved by uttering a mystical word or phrase and associated with meditation.

Meditation Use of contemplation to exercise the mind. A form of mental cleansing that enhances self-awareness and awareness of one's environment. Also called "mind-cure," this is an unseen force of healing. Thoughts and deep feelings are considered the primary arbiters of health through relaxation.

Megavitamin therapy A type of orthomolecular medicine in which diseases are prevented and cured by large doses of vitamins and other supplements. Dosages exceed the normal or recommended amounts needed for general good health or prevention of deficiencies. The disease to be treated or prevented determines the type, dosage, and mode of administration of vitamins, minerals, and nutrient supplements.

Meridians Invisible channels by which chi flows through the body. Blockage along a meridian causes illness. From traditional Chinese medicine.

Mind–body medicine Healing based on the interconnectedness of the mind and body, individual responsibility for self-care, and the self-healing capabilities of the body. Uses a wide range of modalities, such as imaging, massage, hypnotherapy, meditation, yoga, concepts of balance, herbs, and diet.

Moxibustion From traditional Chinese medicine, burning of *moxa* (dried or powered herbs) on or close to acupuncture points on the meridians to restore or improve the flow of chi.

Music therapy Use of music to enhance well-being and promote healing. Helps improve physical and mental functioning, alleviate pain, ease the psychological discomfort of illness, and improve quality of life, especially for terminally ill persons. Aids ability of the mentally handicapped, autistic persons, and elderly persons with dementia to interact with others, learn, and relate to their environments.

Naturopathy A Western healing system that uses safe, natural therapies. Promotes holism and use of natural substances, treats cause rather than effect (symptoms), empowers and motivates individuals to take responsibility for their own health, prevents disease through lifestyle and education, and does no harm.

Neurolinguistic programming A system that focuses on how individuals learn, communicate, and change. *Neuro-* refers to the way the brain works and the consistent and observable patterns that emanate from human thinking. *Linguistic* refers to the expression (verbal and nonverbal) of those patterns of thinking. *Programming* refers to the ways such patterns of thinking are interpreted and how they can be changed. Changing the patterns gives people the ability to make better choices for healthy behavior.

Orthodox medicine A synonym for conventional, Western, scientific, biomedicine, or official health care system.

Orthomolecular medicine A system that treats physiological and psychological disorders by reestablishing, normalizing, or creating the optimal nutritional balance in the body. Vitamins, minerals, amino acids, and other types of nutritional substances are administered. *(Ortho-* means "normal" or "correct.")

Osteopathy A Western system of medicine that considers the structural integrity of the body the most important factor in maintaining and restoring the person to health. The structural integrity or balance of the musculoskeletal system is maintained through physical therapy, joint manipulation, and postural reeducation.

Oxygen therapy Use of various forms of oxygen to destroy pathogens and promote body healing. Includes hyperbaric, ozone, and hydrogen peroxide therapies.

Pharmacognosy Scientific study of the chemical properties of plants and natural products. A goal is to standardize herbal products to make sure they are free of harmful components and contain the identical amount of active ingredients.

Phytomedicine/phytotherapy A branch of botanical medicine, especially prominent in Europe, that includes the pharmaceutical study and therapeutic use of herbs, herbal derivatives, and herbal synthetics. Merges ancient herbal traditions with contemporary scientific investigation to standardize the active ingredients of herbal products.

Polarity therapy A combination of bodywork and other hands-on techniques to restore the natural flow of energy through the body. Other therapies may include reflexology, hydrotherapy, and breathing techniques.

Prana Vital energy or life-force that runs through the body. From Ayurvedic medicine.

Qi Gong (Chi Kung, Chi Gong) Technique from traditional Chinese medicine that combines movement, meditation and deep relaxation, and regulation of breathing. Enhanced flow of chi throughout the body nourishes vital organs.

Reflexology Pressure applied to the hands or feet to unblock nerve impulses. In this belief system, every part of the body has a corresponding area on the hands and feet. Thus, body parts can be stimulated by pressure applied to the appropriate sites. Reflexology is used to relieve tension, improve circulation, promote relaxation, and restore energy balance.

Reiki An ancient Buddhist version of healing touch practiced in Tibet and Japan. The word also means *universal life-force*. Energy is transferred to the person through the hands of the healer to restore energy balance in the body.

Relaxation response Physiological mechanism described by Herbert Benson in which body stress is reduced through regulation of internal activity, such as reduced metabolism and slowing of other physiological reactions.

Relaxation therapy Use of the relaxation response to reduce stress through release of physical and emotional tension. Various therapies are commonly included in other types of therapeutic programs. Examples are mind–body therapies such as biofeedback, hydrotherapy, imaging and visualization, meditation, Qi Gong, Tai Chi, and yoga.

Rolfing Technique of deep massage developed by Ida Rolf. Use of the knuckles is meant to counteract the effects of gravity on body balance. Fascia, connective tissue, and muscle are loosened and lengthened to help them return to their correct positions.

Rosen technique A type of bodywork in which muscle tension is seen as repressed emotional conflicts. Deep and gentle pressure is applied as persons are questioned about what they are experiencing.

Shamanism Ancient healing approach found in most cultural systems. Shamans communicate with the spirit world through trances and other altered states of consciousness. They attempt to control spirits and effect change in the physical world. The belief is that the soul of the shaman separates from the body and explores the cosmos in search of cures for ill clients.

Shiatsu Japanese form of massage, literally, *finger pressure.* Consists of firm pressure in a sequential and rhythmic manner. Pressure is exerted for 3 to 10 seconds on points along the body that correspond to acupuncture meridians. It is designed to "awaken the meridian."

Sound therapy Use of sound to affect different parts of the brain, regulate corticosteroid hormone levels, and affect the body's own rhythmic patterns.

Spiritual healing Cosmic healing energy transferred or channeled from practitioner to client through laying on of the hands.

Swedish massage The most common form of massage, focusing on superficial muscle layers. Practitioner uses kneading, friction, and long, gliding strokes to relieve muscle tension and promote relaxation.

Tai Chi From traditional Chinese medicine. Derived from Qi Gong but practiced at a much slower pace. Also one of the body–mind therapies. Combines contemplation (meditation) with movement or "moving meditation" and coordinated breathing.

Therapeutic massage Manipulation of soft tissues through a variety of techniques to affect the circulatory, lymphatic, and nervous systems.

Therapeutic touch A healing touch modality that does not involve actual touching of the client's body. The therapist's hands are used to sense and interact with the client's energy field to redirect it, alleviate energy blockage, and restore balance.

Traditional Chinese medicine A complete system of healing based on the concept of the uninterrupted flow of chi, or vital essence, and the concept of balance (yin and yang), representing corresponding and interrelated elements in the internal world of the body and the external world. All illness is attributed ultimately to a disturbance of chi.

Trager therapy A method of bodywork, developed by Milton Trager, meant to develop the ability to move more effortlessly. Use of gentle, rhythmic touch and movement exercises to assist in the release of accumulated tensions. Uses sensory-motor feedback or mental gymnastics (mentastics) to learn how the body moves.

Vibration medicine Healing systems that treat the body on an energy level. Cure is effected by ingestion of substances that adjust energy or rate of energy field vibration. Homeopathy is an example.

Visualization Also called guided imagery, centering, focusing, meditation, or distraction. Use of the imagination or power of the mind to get in touch with one's inner self. Involves all, several, or one of the senses to bridge the mind, body, and spirit.

Yin/yang Complementary but opposing phenomena or correspondents in Taoist philosophical thought that form the underpinning of traditional Chinese medicine. Yin and yang represent the interdependence of all elements of nature and body and mind. Yin represents the female force and passive, still, reflective aspects. Yang represents the male force and active, warm, moving aspects. For health to be maintained and wellness achieved, yin and yang must be in balance.

Yoga Literally, *union,* or the integration of mental, physical, and spiritual energies. Part of Ayurvedic medicine. The integration is accomplished through exercise in the form of assuming different body postures, meditation, and breathing.

abandonment Leaving a client without the client's permission; terminating the professional relationship without providing for appropriate continued or follow-up care by another equally qualified professional.

accountability Concept that each individual is responsible for his or her own actions and the consequence of those actions; professional accountability implies a responsibility to perform the activities and duties of the profession according to established standards.

accreditation Approval of a program or institution by a voluntary professional organization to provide specific education or service programs.

act Legislation that has become law.

active euthanasia Acts performed to help end a sick person's life.

acute-severe condition Health problem of sudden onset; a serious illness or condition.

adaptation Process of exchange between a person and the environment to maintain or regain personal integrity; the key principle in the Roy Model of Nursing.

administrative A governmental agency that implements legislation.

administrative rule or regulation An operating procedure that describes how a government agency implements the intent of a statute; state boards of nursing implement the nurse practice act.

advanced nursing education Master's- or doctoral-level education that provides knowledge and skills in areas such as research, education, administration, or clinical specialties.

advanced placement A process by which a student is given credit for a required course through transfer or examination rather than by enrolling in and completing the course.

advanced practice Extended role; increased responsibilities and actions undertaken by an individual because of additional education and experience; nurse practitioners are advanced practice nurses.

advocate One who pleads for a cause or proposal; one who acts on behalf of another.

affective domain objectives Goals established in conjunction with the client that are directed toward changing feelings, values, and attitudes necessary for a positive effect on the client's health.

affidavit Written, sworn statement.

affiliation agreement A formal agreement between an educational institution and another agency that agrees to provide clinical areas for student practice.

aggressiveness Harsh behavior that may result in physical or emotional harm to others.

ambulatory care center Type of primary care facility that provides treatment on an outpatient basis.

answer Document filed in the court by the defendant in response to the complaint.

anxiety Uneasiness or apprehension caused by an impending threat or fear of the unknown.

apathy Lack of interest.

appeal Request to a higher court to review a decision in the hopes of changing the ruling of a lower court.

appellant Person who seeks an appeal.

arbitrator Neutral third party who assesses facts independently of the judicial system.

articulation Type of education program that allows easy entry from one level to another; for example, many BSN programs have articulation for nurses with associate degrees.

artificial insemination Insertion of sperm into the uterus with a syringe.

assault Attempt or threat to touch.

assertiveness Ability to express thoughts, feelings, and ideas openly and directly without fear.

assessment Process of collecting information about a client to help plan care.

associate degree nursing program Type of nursing education program that leads to an associate degree with a major in nursing; usually located in a community or junior college, these programs nominally last 2 years.

audit Close review of records or documents to detect the presence or absence of specific information.

auscultation Assessment technique that requires listening with a stethoscope to various parts of the body to detect sounds produced by organs.

authoritarian Type of leadership style in which the leader gives orders, makes decisions for the group as a whole, and bears most of the responsibility for the outcomes. Also called autocratic, directive, or controlling.

autonomy State of being self-directed or independent; the ability to make decisions about one's future.

autopsy Examination of a body after death to determine the cause of death.

baccalaureate degree nursing program Type of nursing education program that leads to the bachelor's degree with a major in nursing; usually located in a college or university, the length of the program is 4 years.

bargaining agent Organization certified by a governmental agency to represent a group of employees for the purpose of collective bargaining.

baseline data Initial information obtained about a client that establishes the norms for comparison as the client's condition changes.

basic human rights Those considerations society deems reasonably expected for all people; right to self-determination, protection from discomfort and harm, dignity, fair treatment, and privacy.

battery Nonconsensual touching of another person that does not necessarily cause harm or injury.

behaviorism Psychological theory based on the belief that all behavior is learned over time through conditioning.

behavior modification Method to change behavior through rewards for positive behavior.

belief Expectations or judgments based on attitude verified by experiences.

beneficence Ethical principle based on the beliefs that the health-care provider should do no harm, prevent harm, remove existing harm, and promote the good and well-being of the client.

bereavement State of sadness brought on by the loss or death of a significant other.

bill Proposed law that is moving through the legislative process.

bill of rights List of statements that outline the claims and privileges of a particular group, such as the Client's Bill of Rights.

bioethical issues Issues that deal with the health, safety, life, and death of human beings, often arising from advances in medical science and technology.

biofeedback Ability to control autonomic responses in the body through conscious effort.

body substance isolation (BSI) Universal precautions; guidelines established by the Centers for Disease Control and Prevention (CDC) and the Occupational Safety and Health Administration (OSHA) to protect health-care professionals and the client from diseases carried in the blood and body fluids, such as HIV and hepatitis B; involves the use of gloves whenever one is in contact with blood or body fluids and the use of masks, gowns, and eye covers if a chance of aerosol contact with fluids exists.

brain death Irreversible destruction of the cerebral cortex and brain stem manifested by absence of all reflexes; absence of brain waves on an electroencephalogram.

breach of contract Failure by one of the parties in a contract to fulfill all the terms of the agreement.

burden of proof Requirement that the plaintiff submit sufficient evidence to prove a defendant's guilt.

burnout syndrome A state of emotional exhaustion that results from the accumulative stress of an individual's life, including work, personal, and family responsibilities.

cadaver donor Clinically or brain-dead individual who previously agreed to allow organs to be taken for transplantation.

capitated payment system System of reimbursement in which a flat fee is paid for health-care services for a prescribed period of time. Expenses incurred in excess of this fee are provider losses.

capricious Unpredictable; arbitrary.

career ladder Articulation of educational programs that permit advancement from a lower level to a higher level without loss of credit or repetition of coursework.

career mobility Opportunity for individuals in one occupational area to move to another without restrictions.

case management Health-care delivery in which a client advocate or health-care coordinator helps the client through the hospitalization to obtain the most appropriate care.

case manager Health-care provider who coordinates cost-effective quality care for individuals who are generally at high risk and require long-term complex services.

certification Official recognition of a degree of education and skills in a profession by a national specialty organization; recognition that an institution has met standards that allow it to deliver certain services.

challenge examination Examination that assesses levels of knowledge or skill to grant credit for previous learning and experience; passing a challenge examination gives the individual credit for a course not actually taken.

chart Legal document that contains all the pertinent information about a client who is in a hospital or clinic; usually includes medical and nursing history, medical and nursing diagnosis, laboratory test results, notes about the client's progress, physician's orders, and personal data.

charting Process of recording (written or computer-generated) specific information about the client in the chart or medical record.

civil law Law concerned with the violation of the rights of one individual by another; it includes contract law, treaty law, tax law, and tort law.

claims-made policy Type of malpractice insurance that protects only against claims made during the time the policy is in effect.

client More modern term for patient; an individual seeking or receiving health-related services.

client goal Statement about a desired change, outcome, or activity that a client should achieve by a specific time.

clinical education Hands-on part of a nursing program that allows the student to practice skills on actual clients under the supervision of a nursing instructor.

clinical forensic nurse Professional nurse who specializes in management of crime victims from trauma to trial through collection of evidence, assessment of victims, or making judgments related to client treatment associated with court-related issues.

clinical ladder Type of performance evaluation and career advancement in which nursing positions for direct client care have two or more progressive levels of required skill leading to advancement in salary and responsibility; it allows nurses to remain in direct client care while making career advancements rather than having to move into administration.

clinical pathways Case-management protocols used to enhance quality of care, encourage cost-effectiveness, and promote efficiency.

closed system System that does not exchange energy, matter, or information with the environment or with other systems.

code of ethics Written values of a profession that act as guidelines for professional behavior.

cognitive domain objectives Most basic type of objectives for client learning that merely outline the knowledge that will be taught to the client.

collective bargaining Negotiations for wages, hours, benefits, and working conditions for a group of employees.

collective bargaining unit Group of employees recognized as representatives of the majority, with the right to bargain collectively with their employer and to reach an agreement on the terms of a contract.

committee Group of legislators, in the House or Senate, assigned to analyze bills on a particular subject.

common law Law based on past judicial judgments made in similar cases.

comparable worth Method for determining employees' salaries within an organization so that the same salary is paid for all jobs that have equivalent educational requirements, responsibilities, and complexity regardless of external market factors.

competencies Behaviors, skills, attitudes, and knowledge that an individual or professional has or is expected to have.

competency-based education Courses or programs based on anticipated student outcomes.

complaint Legal document filed by a plaintiff to initiate a lawsuit, claiming that the plaintiff's legal rights have been violated.

compliance Voluntary following of a prescribed plan of care or treatment regimen.

computer technology Use of highly advanced technological equipment to store, process, and access a vast amount of information.

concept Abstract idea or image.

conceptual framework Concept, theory, or basic idea around which an educational program is organized and developed.

conceptual model Group of concepts, ideas, or theories that are interrelated but in which the relationship is not clearly defined.

confidentiality Right of the client to expect the communication with a professional to remain unshared with any other person unless a medical reason exists or unless the safety of the public is threatened.

consensus General agreement between two or more individuals or groups regarding beliefs or positions on an issue or finding.

consent Voluntary permission given by a competent person.

consortium Two or more agencies that share sponsorship of a program or an institution.

constitutional law Law contained within a federal or state constitution.

continuing care Nursing care generally provided in geriatric day-care centers or in the homes of elderly clients.

continuing education Formal education programs and informal learning experiences that maintain and increase the nurse's knowledge and skills in specific areas.

continuing education unit (CEU) Specific unit of credit earned by participating in an approved continuing education program.

continuous quality improvement (CQI) Type of total quality management whose primary goal is the improvement of the quality of health care.

contract Legally binding agreement between two or more parties.

contractual obligation Duty to perform a service identified by a contract.

copayment Percentage of the cost of a medical expense that is not covered by insurance and must be paid by the client.

core curriculum Curriculum design that enables a student to leave a career program at various levels, with a career attained and with the option to continue at another higher level or career; it is organized around a central or core body of knowledge common to the profession.

coroner Elected public official, usually a physician, who investigates deaths from unnatural causes, including homicide, violence, suicide, and other suspicious circumstances.

correctional/institutional nurse Registered nurse who specializes in the health care of those in custody in secure settings such as jails or prisons.

credentialing Process whereby individuals, programs, or institutions are designated as having met minimal standards for the safety and welfare of the public.

crime Violation of criminal law.

criminal action Process by which a person charged with a crime is accused, tried, and punished.

criminal law Law concerned with violation of criminal statutes or laws.

criterion-referenced examination Test that compares an individual's knowledge to a predetermined standard rather than to the performance of others who take the same test.

critical thinking The intellectual process of rationally examining ideas, inferences, assumptions, principles, arguments, conclusions, issues, statements, beliefs, and actions for which all the relevant information may not be available. This process involves the ability to use the five types of reasoning (scientific, deductive, inductive, informal, practical) in application of the nursing process, decision-making, and resolution of ambiguous issues.

curriculum Group of courses that prepare an individual for a specific degree or profession.

customary, prevailing, and reasonable charges The typical rate in a specific locale that payers traditionally reimburse physicians.

damages Money awarded to a plaintiff by a court in a lawsuit that covers the actual costs incurred by the plaintiff.

database Information collected by a computer program on a specific topic in a specified format.

defamation of character Communication of information that is false or detrimental to a person's reputation.

defendant Person accused of criminal or civil wrongdoing. A party to a lawsuit against whom the complaint is served.

delegation Assignment of specific duties by one individual to another individual.

democratic Type of leadership style in which the leader shares the planning, decision-making, and responsibilities for outcomes with the other members of the group. Also called participative leadership.

deontology Ethical system based on the principle that the right action is guided by a set of unchanging rules.

dependent practitioner Provider of care who delivers health care under the supervision of another health-care practitioner; for example, a physician's assistant is supervised by a physician, or an LPN is supervised by an RN.

deposition Sworn statement by a witness that is made outside the courtroom; sworn depositions may be admitted as evidence in court when the individual is unable to be present.

diagnosis Statement that describes or identifies a client problem and is based on a thorough assessment.

diagnosis-related groups (DRGs) Prospective payment method used by the U.S. government and many insurance companies that pay a flat fee for treatment of a person with a particular diagnosis.

differentiated practice Organizational process of defining nursing roles based on education, experience, and training.

dilemma Predicament in which a choice must be made between two or more equally balanced alternatives; it often occurs when attempting to make ethical decisions.

directed services Health-care activities that require contact between a health-care professional and a client.

discharge planning Assessment of anticipated client needs after discharge from the hospital and development of a plan to meet those needs before the client is discharged.

disease Illness; a functional disturbance resulting from an individual organism's inability to adapt to certain stressors; an abnormal physiologic state caused by microorganisms, cancer, or other conditions.

distributive justice Ethical principle based on the belief that the right action is determined by that which will provide an outcome equal for all persons and will also benefit the least fortunate.

due process Right to have specific procedures or processes followed before the deprivation of life, liberty, or property; the guarantee of privileges under the 5th and 14th Amendments to the U.S. Constitution.

duty Obligation to act created by a statute, contract, or voluntary agreement.

emerging health occupations Health-care occupations that are not yet officially recognized by government or professional organizations.

employee Individual hired for pay by another.

Employee Retirement Income Security Act (ERISA) Federal law that grants incentives to employers to offer self-funded health insurance plans to their employees.

employer Individual or organization that hires other individuals for pay to carry out specific duties during certain hours of employment.

empowerment Process in which the individual assumes more autonomy and responsibility for his or her actions.

endorsement Reciprocity; a state's acceptance of a license issued by another state.

end product Output of a system not reusable as input.

energy Capacity to do work.

entry into practice Minimal educational requirements to obtain a license for a profession.

environment Internal and external physical and social boundaries of humans; all those things that are outside a system.

essentials for accreditation Minimal standards that a program must meet to be accredited.

ethical dilemma Ethical situation that requires an individual to make a choice between two equally unfavorable alternatives.

ethical rights (moral rights) Rights that are based on moral or ethical principles but have no legal mechanism of enforcement.

ethical system System of moral judgments based on the beliefs and values of a profession.

ethics Principles or standards of conduct that govern an individual or group.

ethnic group Individuals who share similar physical characteristics, religion, language, or customs.

euthanasia Mercy killing; the act or practice of killing, for reasons of mercy, individuals who have little or no chance of recovery by withholding or discontinuing life support or by administering a lethal agent.

evaluation Fifth step in the nursing process; used to determine whether goals set for a client have been attained.

evaluation criteria Outcome criteria; desired behaviors or standards.

expanded role Extended role; increased responsibilities and actions undertaken by an individual because of additional education and experience.

expert witness Individual with knowledge beyond the ordinary person, resulting from special education or training, who testifies during a trial.

external degree Academic degree granted when all the requirements have been met by the student; a type of outcomes-based education in which credit is given when the individual demonstrates a certain level of knowledge and skill, regardless of how or when these skills are attained; challenge examinations are often used.

false imprisonment Intentional tort committed by illegally confining or restricting a client against his or her will.

family Two or more related individuals living together.

Federal Tort Claims Act Statute that allows the government to be sued for negligence of its employees in the performance of their duties; many states have similar laws.

feedback Reentry of output into a system as input that helps maintain the internal balance of the system.

fee for service Payment is expected each time a service is rendered. Includes physicians' office visits, diagnostic procedures (laboratory tests, x-rays), and minor surgical procedures.

fellowship Scholarship or grant that provides money to individuals who are highly qualified or highly intelligent.

felony Serious crime that may be punished by a fine of more than $1000, more than 1 year in jail or prison, death, or a combination thereof.

fidelity The obligation of an individual to be faithful to commitments made to self and others.

for-profit Health-care agencies in which profits can be used to raise capital to pay stockholders dividends on their investments. Also called proprietary agencies.

foreign graduate nurse Individual graduated from a school of nursing outside the United States. This individual is required to pass the U.S. NCLEX-RN CAT to become a registered nurse in the United States.

forensic nurse Registered nurse who specializes in the integration of forensic science and nursing science to apply the nursing process to individual clients, their families, and the community, bridging the gap between the health-care system and the criminal justice system.

forensic psychiatric nurse Registered nurse who specializes in application of psychosocial nursing knowledge linking offending behavior to client characteristics; nurse specializing in forensic psychological evaluation and care of offender populations with mental disorders.

forensic science Body of empirical knowledge used for legal investigation and evidence-based judgment in police or criminal cases.

fraud Deliberate deception in provision of goods or services; lying.

functional nursing Nursing care in which each nurse provides a different aspect of care; nurses are assigned a set of specific tasks to perform for all clients, such as passing medications.

general systems theory Set of interrelated concepts, definitions, and propositions that describe a system.

genetics Scientific study of heredity and related variations.

gerontology Study of the process of aging and of the effects of aging on individuals.

goal Desired outcome.

Good Samaritan Act Law that protects health-care providers from being charged with contributory negligence when they provide emergency care to persons in need of immediate treatment.

grievance Complaint or dispute about the terms or conditions of employment.

group practice Three or more physicians or nurse practitioners in business together to provide health care.

health Complete physical, mental, and social well-being; a relative state along a continuum ranging from severe illness to ideal state of being; the ability to adapt to illness and to reach the highest level of functioning.

health-care consumer Client or patient; an individual who uses health-care services or products.

health-care team Group of individuals of different levels of education who work together to provide help to clients.

health insurance purchasing cooperative (HIPC) Large groups of people or employers who band together to buy insurance at reduced costs. HIPCs may be organized by private groups or the government.

health literacy A client's ability to read, comprehend, and act on health-care instructions provided by a nurse or other health-care worker.

health maintenance organization (HMO) Prototype of the managed health-care system; method of payment for a full range of primary, secondary, and tertiary health-care services; members pay a fixed annual fee for services and a small deductible when care is given.

health policy Goals and directions that guide activities to safeguard and promote the health of citizens.

health practitioner Individual, usually licensed, who provides health-care services to individuals with health-care needs.

health promotion Interventions and behaviors that increase and maintain the level of well-being of persons, families, groups, communities, and society.

health systems agency (HSA) Local voluntary organization of providers and consumers that plans for the health-care services of its geographic region.

hearsay Evidence not based on personal knowledge of the witness and usually not allowed in courts.

holistic Treatment of the total individual, including physical, psychological, sociological, and spiritual elements, with emphasis on the interrelatedness of parts and wholes.

home health care Health-care services provided in the client's home.

honesty, integrity, respect, responsibility, and ethics (HIRRE) Type of honor code in which students and faculty sign a pledge not to cheat or plagiarize.

horizontal violence Type of peer-to-peer incivility or negative interaction.

hospice care Alternative way of providing care to terminally ill clients in which palliative care is used; the major goals of hospice care are control of pain, provision of emotional support, promotion of social interaction, and preparation for death; family support measures and anticipatory grief counseling are also used if appropriate.

hospital privileges Authority granted by a hospital, usually through its medical board, for a health-care practitioner to admit and supervise the treatment of clients within that hospital.

hypothesis Prediction or proposition related to a problem, usually found in research.

ideal role image Projection of society's expectations for nurses that clearly delineates the obligations and responsibilities, as well as the rights and privileges those in the role can lay claim to. Is often unrealistic.

illness Disease; a functional disturbance resulting from an individual organism's inability to adapt to certain stressors; an abnormal physiologic state caused by microorganisms, cancer, or other conditions.

implementation Fourth step in the nursing process, in which the plan of care is carried out.

incidence Number of occurrences of a specific condition or event.

incident report Document that describes an accident or error involving a client or family member that may or may not have resulted in injury; the purpose of the incident report is to track incidents and to make changes in the situations that caused them; the incident report is not part of the chart.

incivility Failure to be civil; any speech or behavior that disrupts the harmony of the work or educational environment.

incompetency Inability of an individual to manage personal affairs because of mental or physical conditions; the inability of a professional to carry out professional activities at the expected level of functioning because of lack of knowledge or skill or because of drug or alcohol abuse.

indemnity insurance Health insurance in which the contractual agreement is between the consumer and the insurance company. Providers are not involved in these arrangements, and rates are not pre-established.

independent nurse practitioner Nurse who has a private practice in one of the expanded roles of nursing.

independent practice association (IPA) Type of HMO usually organized by physicians that requires fee-for-service payment.

independent practice organization (IPO) Type of IPA in which a group of providers deals with more than one insurer at a time.

independent practitioner Health-care provider who delivers health care independently with or without supervision by another health-care practitioner.

indirect services Health-care actions that do not require direct client contact but that still facilitate care, such as the supply and distribution department of a hospital.

informed consent Permission granted by a person based on full knowledge of the risks and benefits of participation in a procedure or surgery for which the consent has been given.

injunction Court order specifying actions that must or must not be taken.

input Matter, energy, or information entering a system from the environment.

inquest Formal inquiry about the course or manner of death.

institutional licensure Authority for an individual health-care provider to practice that is granted by the individual's employing institution; the institution determines the educational preparation, training, and functions of each category of provider it employs; no longer legally permitted, unlicensed assistive personnel (UAPs) act under a form of de facto institutional licensure.

intentional tort A willful act that violates another person's rights or property and may or may not cause physical injury.

interrogatories Written questions directed to a party in a lawsuit by the opposing side as part of the discovery process.

intervention Nursing action taken to meet specific client goals.

invasion of privacy Type of quasi-intentional tort that involves (1) an act that intrudes into the seclusion of the client, (2) intrusion that is objectionable to a reasonable person, (3) an act that intrudes into private facts or published as facts or pictures of a private nature, and (4) public disclosure of private information.

Joint Commission Formerly Joint Commission on Accreditation of Healthcare Organizations (JCAHO), an organization that performs accreditation reviews for health-care agencies.

judgment Decision of the court regarding a case.

jurisdiction Authority of a court to hear and decide lawsuits.

justice Fairness; giving people their due.

Kardex Portable card file that contains important client information and a care plan.

laissez-faire Type of leadership style in which the leader does little planning, sets few goals, avoids decision-making, and fails to encourage group members to participate. Also called permissive or nondirective leadership.

law Formal statement of a society's beliefs about interactions among and between its citizens; a formal rule enforced by society.

legal complaint Document filed by a plaintiff against a defendant claiming infringement of the plaintiff's legal rights.

legal obligations Obligations that have become formal statements of law and are enforceable under the law.

legal rights (welfare rights) Rights that are based on a legal entitlement to some good or benefits and are enforceable under the legal system with punishment for violations.

legislator Elected member of either the House of Representatives or the Senate.

legislature Body of elected individuals invested with constitutional power to make, alter, or repeal laws.

liable Obligated or held accountable by law.

libel Written defamation of character.

license Permission to practice granted to an individual by the state after he or she has met the requirements for that particular position; licensing protects the safety of the public.

licensed practical nurse (LPN) Licensed vocational nurse; technical nurse licensed by any state, after completing a practical nursing program, to provide technical bedside care to clients.

licensing board Government agency that implements the statutes of a particular profession in accordance with the Professions Practice Act.

licensure Process by which an agency or government grants an individual permission to practice; it establishes a minimal level of competency for practice.

licensure by endorsement Method of obtaining a license to practice by having a state acknowledge the individual's existing comparable license in another state.

licensure by examination Method of obtaining a license to practice by successfully passing a state-board examination.

living will Signed legal document in which individuals make known their wishes about the care they are to receive if they should become incompetent at a future date; it usually specifies what types of treatments are permitted and what types are to be withheld.

lobbyist Person who attempts to influence political decisions as an official representative of an organization, group, or institution.

locality rule standard of care Legal process that holds an individual nurse accountable both to what is an acceptable standard within his or her local community and to national standards as developed by nurses throughout the nation through the American Nurses Association (ANA), national practice groups, and health-care agencies.

malfeasance Performance of an illegal act.

malpractice Negligent acts by a licensed professional based on either omission of an expected action or commission of an inappropriate action resulting in damages to another party; not doing what a reasonable and prudent professional of the same rank would have done in the same situation.

managed care System of organized health-care delivery systems linked by provider networks; health maintenance organizations are the primary example of managed care.

mandatory licensure Law that requires all who practice a particular profession to have and to maintain a license in that profession.

manslaughter Killing of an individual without premeditated intent; different degrees of manslaughter exist, and most are felonies.

mediation Legal process that allows each party to present their case to a mediator, who is an independent third party trained in dispute resolution.

Medicaid State health-care insurance program, supported in part by federal funds, for health-care services for certain groups unable to pay for their own health care; amount and type of coverage vary from state to state.

medical examiner Coroner; a physician who investigates deaths that appear to be from other than natural causes.

medically indigent Individuals who cannot personally pay for health-care services without incurring financial hardship.

Medicare Federally run program that is financed primarily through employee payroll taxes and covers any individual who is 65 years of age or older as well as blind and disabled individuals of any age.

Medicare Utilization and Quality Peer Review Organization (PRO) Organization that reviews the quality and cost of Medicare services.

Medigap policies Health insurance policies that are purchased to cover expenses not paid by Medicare.

midwife Individual experienced in assisting women during labor and delivery; they may be lay midwives, who have no official education, or certified nurse midwives, who are RNs in an expanded role, having received additional education and passed a national certification examination.

misdemeanor Less serious crime than a felony; punishable by a fine of less than $1000 or a jail term of less than 1 year.

model Hypothetical representation of something that exists in reality. The purpose of a model is to attempt to explain a complex reality in a systematic and organized manner.

morality Concept of right and wrong.

moral obligations Obligations based on moral or ethical principles but *not* enforceable under the law.

morals Fundamental standards of right and wrong that an individual learns and internalizes during the early stages of childhood development, based primarily on religious beliefs and societal norms.

mores Values and customs of a society.

mortality Property or capacity to die; death.

motivation Internal drive that causes individuals to seek achievement of higher goals; desire.

multicompetency technician Allied health-care provider who has skills in two or more areas of practice through the process of cross-training.

multiskilled practitioner Health-care professional who has skills in more than one area of health care, such as an RN who has training in physical therapy.

national health insurance Proposed system of payment for health-care services whereby the government pays for the costs of the health care.

negative entropy Tendency toward increased order in a system.

negligence Failure to perform at an expected level of functioning or the performance of an inappropriate function resulting in damages to another party; not doing what a reasonable and prudent person would do in a similar situation.

no-code order Do not resuscitate (DNR) order; an order by a physician to withhold cardiopulmonary resuscitation and other resuscitative efforts from a client.

nonfeasance Failure to perform a legally required duty.

nonmaleficence Ethical principle that requires the professional to do no harm to the client.

nontraditional education Methods of education that do not follow the traditional lecture and clinical practice methods of learning; may include computer-simulated learning, self-education techniques, or other creative methods.

nonverbal A type of communication that uses any methods except written and spoken messages and constitutes 93 percent of the communication between individuals. It includes body language, gestures, facial expression, tone, pace, personal space, etc.

normative ethics Questions and dilemmas requiring a choice of actions whereby there is a conflict of rights or obligations between the nurse and the client, the nurse and the client's family, or the nurse and the physician.

norm-referenced examination Examination scored by comparison with standards established on the performance of all others who took the same examination during a specific time; the NLN achievement examinations are norm referenced.

not-for-profit (nonprofit) agencies Agencies in which all profits must be used in the operation of the organization.

nurse clinician Registered nurse with advanced skills in a particular area of nursing practice; if certified by a professional organization, a nurse clinician may also be a nurse practitioner, but more often this designation refers to nurses in advanced practice roles such as nurse specialists.

nurse practice act   Part of state law that establishes the scope of practice for professional nurses, as well as educational levels and standards, professional conduct, and reasons for revocation of licensure.

nurse practitioner   Nurse specialist with advanced education in a primary care specialty, such as community health, pediatrics, or mental health, who is prepared independently to manage health promotion and maintenance and illness prevention of a specific group of clients.

nurse specialist (clinical nurse specialist)   Nurse who is an expert in providing care focused on a specialized field drawn from the range of general practice, such as cardiac nurse specialist.

nurse theorist   Nurse who analyzes and attempts to describe what the profession of nursing is and what nurses do through nursing models or nursing theories.

nursing assessment   Systematic collection and recording of client data, both objective and subjective, from primary and secondary sources using the nursing history, physical examination, and laboratory data, for example.

nursing diagnosis   Statements of a client's actual or potential health-care problems or deficits.

nursing order   Statement of a nursing action selected by a nurse to achieve a client's goal; may be stated as either the nurse's or the client's expected behavior.

nursing process   Systematic, comprehensive decision-making process used by nurses to identify and treat actual and potential health problems.

nursing research   Formal study of problems of nursing practice, the role of the nurse in health care, and the value of nursing.

nursing standards   Desired nursing behaviors established by the profession and used to evaluate nurses' performances.

obligations   Demands made on individuals, professions, society, or government to fulfill and honor the rights of others. Obligations are often divided into two categories–moral and legal (welfare).

occurrence policy   A type of malpractice insurance that protects against all claims that occurred during the policy period regardless of when the claim is made.

omission   Failure to fulfill a duty or carry out a procedure recognized as a standard of care; often forms the basis for claims of malpractice.

oncology   Area of health care that deals with the treatment of cancer.

open curriculum   Educational system that allows a student to enter and leave the system freely; often uses past education and experiences.

open system   System that can exchange energy, matter, and information with the environment and with other systems.

ordinance   Local or municipal law.

outcome criteria   Standards that measure changes or improvements in clients' conditions.

out-of-pocket expenses   Amount the client is responsible for paying for a health-care service.

output   Matter, energy, or information released from a system into the environment or transmitted to another system.

palliative   Type of treatment directed toward minimizing the severity of a disease or illness rather than curing it; for example, for a client with terminal cancer, relief of pain is the main goal (palliative), rather than cure.

panel of approved providers   A list of physicians, nurse practitioners, pharmacies, and other health-care providers that are approved by an insurance plan and to whom reimbursement will be made by the insurer.

passive learning   A type of client education in which the material is merely presented to the client without his or her involvement. Least effective type of learning because it usually does not change attitudes or behaviors.

patient   Client; an individual seeking or receiving health-care services.

patient day   Client day; the 24-hour period during which hospital services are provided that forms the basis for charging the patient, usually from midnight to midnight.

pediatrics   Study and care of problems and diseases of children younger than the age of 18.

peer review   Evaluation against professional standards of the performance of individuals with the same basic education and qualifications; formal process of review or evaluation by coworkers of an equal rank.

perceived role image   The individual's own definition of the role, which is usually more realistic than the ideal role, involving rejection or modification of some of the norms and expectations of society.

percussion   Physical examination involving the tapping of various parts of the body to determine density by eliciting different sounds.

performed role image The duties performed by the practitioner of a role. Often produces reality shock in new graduate nurses.

perjury Crime committed by giving false testimony while under oath.

permissive licensure Law that allows individuals to practice a profession as long as they do not use the title of the profession; no states now have permissive licensure.

phenomenology Philosophical approach that holds that consciousness determines reality in space and time.

plaintiff Individual who charges another individual in a court of law with a violation of the individual's rights; the party who files the complaint in a lawsuit.

point-of-service plans Insurance plans in which consumers can select providers outside of a prescribed provider panel if they are willing to pay an additional fee.

political action Activities on the part of individuals that influence the actions of government officials in establishing policy.

political involvement Group of activities that, individually or collectively, increase the voice of nursing in the political or health-care policy process.

politics Process of influencing the decisions of others and exerting control over situations or events; includes influencing the allocation of scarce resources.

practical nursing program Vocational nursing program; a program of study leading to a certificate in practical nursing, usually 12 to 18 months in length; these programs are located in a vocational or technical school or in a community or junior college; after passing the NCLEX-LPN CAT examination, students become licensed practical nurses (LPNs).

precedent Decision previously issued by a court that is used as the basis for a decision in another case with similar circumstances.

preceptor Educated or skilled practitioner who agrees to work with a less-educated or less-trained individual to increase the individual's knowledge and skills; often staff nurses who work with student nurses during their senior year.

precertification Approval for reimbursement of services before their being rendered.

preferred provider organization (PPO) Method of payment for employee health-care benefits in which employers contract with a specific group of health-care providers for a lower cost for their employees'

health-care services but require the employee to use the providers listed.

premium Amount paid on a periodic basis for health insurance or HMO membership.

prescriptive authority Legal right to write prescriptions for medications, granted to physicians, veterinarians, dentists, and advanced practice nurses.

preventive care Well care; nursing care provided for the purpose of maintaining health and preventing disease or injury, often through community health clinics, school nursing services, and storefront clinics.

primary care Type of health care for individuals and families in which maintenance of health is emphasized; first-line health care in hospitals, physicians' offices, or community health clinics that deal with acute conditions.

primary care nurse Hospital staff RN assigned to a primary care unit to provide nursing care to a limited number of clients who are followed by the same nurse from admission to discharge.

primary intervention Health promotion, illness prevention, early diagnosis, and treatment of common health problems.

private-duty nurse Nurse in private practice; nurse self-employed for providing direct client care services either in the home or the hospital setting.

privileged communication Information imparted by a client to a physician, lawyer, or clergyman that is protected from disclosure in a court of law. Communication between a client and a nurse is not legally protected, but nurses can participate in privileged communication when they overhear information imparted by the client to the physician.

profession Nursing; an occupation that meets the criteria for a profession, including education, altruism, code of ethics, public service, and dedication.

professional review organization Multilevel program to oversee the quality and cost of federally funded medical care programs.

professionalism Behaviors and attitudes exhibited by an individual that are recognized by others as the traits of a professional.

prospective payment system (PPS) System of reimbursement for health-care services that establishes the payment rates before hospitalization based on certain criteria, such as diagnosis-related groups (DRGs).

protocol Written plan of action based on previously identified situations; standing orders are a type of protocol often used in specialty units that have clients with similar problems.

provider Person or organization who delivers health care, including health promotion and maintenance and illness prevention and treatment.

provider panel Health-care providers selected to render services to a group of consumers within a managed-care plan.

proximate cause Nearest cause; the element in a direct cause-and-effect relationship between what is done by the professional and what happens to the client. For example, when a nurse fails to raise the side rails on the bed of a client who has received a narcotic medication, and the client falls out of bed and breaks a hip as a result.

psychomotor domain objectives Goals established with input from the client that deal with changes in behavior or learned skills.

public policy Decision made by a society or its elected representatives that has a material effect on citizens other than the decision-makers.

quality Level of excellence based on pre-established criteria.

quality assurance Activity conducted in health-care facilities that evaluates the quality of care provided to ensure that it meets pre-established quality standards.

Quality and Safety Education for Nurses (QSEN) Nursing education curriculum designed to prepare future nurses with the knowledge, skills, and attitudes (KSAs) necessary to continuously improve the quality and safety of the health-care system in which they work.

quasi-intentional tort A violation of a person's reputation or personal privacy.

reality shock (transition shock) A sudden and sometimes traumatic realization on the part of the new graduate that the ideal or perceived roles do not match the actual performed role.

recertification Periodic renewal of certification by examination, continuing education, or other criteria established by the accrediting agency.

reciprocity Endorsement; a state's acceptance of a license issued by another state.

registration Listing of a license with a state for a fee.

registry Published list of those who are registered; the agency that publishes the list of individuals who are registered.

regulations Rules or orders issued by various regulatory agencies, such as a state board of nursing, which have the force of law.

rehabilitation Restoration to the highest possible level of performance or health of an individual who has suffered an injury or illness.

relative intensity measures (RIMs) Method for calculating nursing resources needed to provide nursing care for various types of clients; helps determine the number and type of staff required based on client acuity and needs.

respondeat superior Legal doctrine that holds the employer or supervisor responsible for the actions of the employees or of those supervised; for example, under this doctrine, RNs are held responsible for the actions of unlicensed assistive personnel under their supervision.

responsibility Accountability; the concept that all individuals are accountable for their own actions and for the consequences of those actions.

restorative care Curative care; nursing care that has as its goal cure and recovery from disease.

resume Curriculum vitae; a summary of an individual's education, work experience, and qualifications.

retrospective payment system Payment system for health care in which reimbursement is based on the actual care rendered rather than on preset rates.

right Just claim or expectation that may or may not be protected by law; legal rights are protected by law, whereas moral rights are not.

risk management Evaluating the risk of clients and staff for injuries and for potential liabilities and implementing corrective and preventive measures.

secondary care Nursing care usually provided in short-term and long-term care facilities to clients with commonly occurring conditions.

secondary intervention Acute care designed to prevent complications or resolve health problems.

secured settings Any institutional setting imposing restriction of movement, confinement, and limitations to activity and access; jails, locked units or locked mental institutions, prisons. sentinel events Relatively infrequent, clearcut events, occurring independently of a client's condition, that commonly reflect hospital system and process deficiencies and result in negative outcomes for clients.

service insurance Health insurance in which services are provided for a prescribed fee that is established between the providers and the insurance company.

sexual assault nurse examiner (SANE) A registered nurse specializing in care of victims of sexual assault, performing physical and psychosocial examination, collection of physical evidence, and therapeutic interventions to minimize trauma.

significant other Individual who is not a family member but is emotionally or symbolically important to an individual.

situation–background–assessment–recommendation (SBAR) Communication technique used between members of the health-care team when a client's condition requires immediate attention and action; an easy-to-remember, concrete mechanism frames the conversation efficiently.

Six Sigma Business management strategy that has been adapted to the health-care industry to identify wasteful practices and lower costs while improving the overall quality of care.

slander Oral defamation of character.

sliding-scale fees Fees for services that are based on the client's ability to pay.

slow-code order Physician's order that the efforts for resuscitation of a client who is terminally ill should be initiated and conducted at a leisurely pace; the goal of a slow-code order is to allow the client to die during an apparent resuscitation. Slow-code orders are not acceptable practice and do not meet standards of care.

staff nurse Nurse generalist who works as an employee of a hospital, nursing home, community health agency, or some other organization providing primary and direct nursing care to clients.

standard of best interest A type of decision made about an individual's health care when he or she is unable to make the informed decision for his or her own care; based on what the health-care providers and/or the family decide is best for that individual.

standards Norms; criteria for expected behaviors or conduct.

standards of care Written or established criteria for nursing care that all nurses are expected to meet.

standards of practice Written or established criteria for nursing practice that all professional nurses are expected to meet.

standing order Written order by physician for certain actions or medication administration to be initiated or given in certain expected circumstances; similar to protocols.

statute Law passed by a government's legislature and signed by its chief executive.

statute of limitations Specific time period in which a lawsuit must be filed or a crime must be prosecuted; most nursing or medical lawsuits have a 2-year statute of limitations from the time of discovery of the incident.

statutory law Law passed by a legislature.

stereotype Fixed or predetermined image of or attitude toward an individual or group.

stress Crisis situation that causes increased anxiety and initiation of the flight-or-fight mechanism.

stressor Internal or external force to which a person responds.

structure criteria Physical environmental framework for client care.

subpoena Court document that requires an individual to appear in court and provide testimony; individuals who do not honor the subpoena can be held in contempt of court and jailed or fined.

subsystem Smaller system within a large system.

summary judgment Decision by a judge in cases in which no facts are in dispute.

sunset law Law that automatically terminates a program after a pre-established period of time unless that program can justify its need for existence.

support system Environmental factors and individuals who can help an individual in a crisis cope with the situation.

systems theory Theory that stresses the interrelatedness of parts in any system in which a change in one part affects all other parts; often, the system is greater than the sum of its parts.

taxonomy Classification system.

team nursing Method of organizing nursing care in which each client is assigned a team consisting of RNs, LPNs, and nursing assistants to deliver nursing care.

technician Individual who carries out technical tasks.

technology Use of science and the application of scientific principles to any situation; often involves the use of complicated machines and computers.

teleology Utilitarianism; an ethical system that identifies the right action by determining what will provide the greatest good for the greatest number of persons. This system has no set, unchanging rules; rather, it varies as the situation changes.

tertiary care Nursing care usually provided in long-term care and rehabilitation facilities for chronic diseases or injuries requiring long recovery.

tertiary intervention Provision of advanced and long-term health-care services to acutely ill clients, including the use of advanced technology, complicated surgical procedures, rehabilitation services, and care of the terminally ill.

testimony Oral statement of a witness under oath.

theory Set of interrelated constructs (concepts, definitions, or propositions) that presents a systematic view of phenomena by specifying relations among variables with the purpose of explaining and predicting phenomena.

third-party payment Payment for health-care services by an insurance company or a government agency rather than directly by the client.

third-party reimburser Organization other than the client, such as an employer, insurance company, or governmental agency, that assumes responsibility for payment of health-care charges for services rendered to the client.

throughput Matter, energy, or information as it passes through a system.

tort Violation of the civil law that violates a person's rights and causes injury or harm to the individual. Civil wrong independent of an action in contract that results from a breach of a legal duty; a tort can be classified as unintentional, intentional, or quasi-intentional.

tort-feasor Person who commits a tort.

total quality management (TQM) Method for monitoring and maintaining the quality of health care being delivered by a particular institution or health-care industry.

trial Legal proceedings during which all relevant facts are presented to a jury or judge for legal decision.

Tri-Council Nursing group composed of the American Nurses Association (ANA), National League for Nursing (NLN), American Association of Colleges of Nursing (AACN), and American Organization of Nurse Executives (AONE).

two plus two (2 + 2) program Nursing education program that starts with an associate (2-year) degree and then moves the individual to a baccalaureate degree with an additional 2 years of education.

Uniform Anatomical Gift Act Legislation providing for a legal document signed by an individual indicating the desire to donate specific body organs or the entire body after death.

unintentional tort A wrong occurring to a person or that person's property even though it was not intended; negligence.

universal health-care coverage Health-care reimbursement benefits for all U.S. citizens and legal residents.

universal precautions Body substance isolation; guidelines established by the Centers for Disease Control and Prevention (CDC) and the Occupational Safety and Health Administration (OSHA) to protect health-care professionals and clients from diseases carried in the blood and body fluids, such as HIV and hepatitis B; involves the use of gloves whenever in contact with blood or body fluids and masks, gowns, and eye covers if a chance exists of contact with aerosol fluids.

upward mobility Movement toward increased status and power in an organization through promotion.

utilitarianism Teleology; an ethical system that identifies the right action by determining what will provide the greatest good for the greatest number of persons. This system has no set, unchanging rules; rather, it varies as the situation changes.

utilization guidelines Guidelines that stipulate the amount of services that can be delivered by a health-care provider.

value Judgment of worth, quality, or desirability based on attitude formed from need or experience; a strong belief held by individuals about something important to them.

values clarification Process by which individuals list and prioritize the values they hold most important.

veracity The principle of truthfulness. It requires the health-care provider to tell the truth and not intentionally deceive or mislead clients.

verbal A type of communication based on written or spoken messages that constitute approximately 7 percent of the total communication between individuals.

veto Signed refusal by the president or a governor to enact a bill into law. If the president vetoes a bill, the veto may be overridden by a two-thirds vote of the membership of both the House and Senate.

vicarious liability Imputation of blame on a person for the actions of the other.

victimization Experience of physical, emotional, or psychological trauma in which the individual suffers injury, fear, self-blame, and/or other dysfunction.

vocational nursing program Licensed practical nursing program in Texas and California; a program of study leading to a certificate in vocational nursing, usually 12 to 18 months in length; these programs are located in vocational and technical schools and community and junior colleges; after passing the NCLEX-LPN CAT examination, students become licensed vocational nurses (LVNs).

References

Chapter 1

1. Alotaibi M: Factors affecting nurses' decisions to join their professional association. International Nursing Review 54(2):160–165, 2007.
2. Stagen M: The five C's of professionalism. Healthcare Traveler 17(12):16, 2010.
3. Smith GR: Spotlight on nurse staffing, autonomy, and control over practice. American Nurse Today 2(4):15–17, 2007.
4. Hahn J: Integrating professionalism and political awareness into the curriculum. Nurse Educator 35(3):110–113, 2010.
5. Elango B: Barriers to nurse entrepreneurship: A study of the process model of entrepreneurship. Journal of the American Academy of Nurse Practitioners 19(4):198–204, 2007.
6. Elcock K: What is nursing? Exploring theory and practice. Nursing Standard 24(25):30, 2010.
7. Vratny A: A conceptual model for growing evidence-based practice. Nursing Administration Quarterly 31(2):162–170, 2007.
8. Fitzpatrick ML: Prologue to Professionalism. Bowie, MD, Robert J. Brady, 1983.
9. O'Grady ET: Health policy and politics. Nursing Economics 18(2):88–90, 2001.
10. American Nurses Association: Nursing Social Policy Statement. Washington, DC, Author, 1999.

Chapter 2

1. Jenson DM: History and Trends in Professional Nursing. St. Louis, CV Mosby, 1959.
2. Kalisch PA, Kalisch BJ: Advance of American Nursing. Philadelphia, JB Lippincott, 1995.
3. Woodham-Smith C: Florence Nightingale. New York, McGraw-Hill, 1957.
4. Hallett CE: Celebrating Nurses: A Visual History. London, Fil Rouge Press, 2010.

Chapter 3

1. Romeo EM: Quantitative research on critical thinking and predicting nursing students' NCLEX-RN performance. Journal of Nursing Education 49(7):378–386, 2010.
2. Smith CK: Professional perspective. Multistate licensure: Is your job putting you at risk? Case in Point 7(2):24–25, 2009.
3. Eisemon N: Certification is an important part of nurse education, career growth. American Nurse 42(2):6, 2010.
4. Snow T, Kendall-Raynor P: Why consensus proves elusive for advanced practitioner regulation. Nursing Standard 24(36):12–13, 2010.
5. Mata H, Latham TP, Ransome Y: Benefits of professional organization membership and participation in national conferences: considerations for students and new professionals. Health Promotion Practice 11(4):450–453, 2010.
6. American Nurses Association: Nursing's Social Policy Statement. Washington, DC, Author, 1995.
7. Smith TG: A policy perspective on the entry into practice issue. Online Journal of Issues in Nursing 15(1):2, 2010.

Chapter 4

1. Ehrenberg AC: Problem-based learning in clinical nursing education: Integrating theory and practice. Nurse Education in Practice 7(2):67–74, 2007.
2. Scherb CA, Weydt AP: Work complexity assessment, nursing interventions classification, and nursing outcomes classification: making connections. Creative Nursing 15(1):16–22, 2009.
3. Bulechek GM, Butcher HK, Dochterman JM: Nursing interventions classification (NIC) (5th ed). St. Louis, Mosby Elsevier, 2008.
4. Thoroddsen A, Ehnfors M: Putting policy into practice: Pre- and posttests of implementing standardized languages for nursing documentation. Journal of Clinical Nursing 16(10):1826–1838, 2007.
5. Felton G, Abbe S, Gilbert C, Ingle JR: How does the NLNAC support the Pew Health Commission competencies? Nursing and Health Care Perspectives 21(1):53, 2000.
6. McCloskey JC, Bulecheck GM, Donohue W: Nursing interventions core to specialty practice. Nursing Outlook 46(3):67–76, 1998.
7. Mitchell PR, Grippando GM: Nursing Perspectives and Issues. Albany, NY, Delmar, 1993.
8. McCann-Flynn JB, Heffron PB: Nursing: From Concept to Practice. Bowie, MD, Robert J. Brady, 1984.
9. Riehl-Sisca JP: Conceptual Models for Nursing Practice. E. Norwalk, CT, Appleton & Lange, 1989.
10. Putt A: General Systems Theory Applied to Nursing. Boston, Little, Brown, 1978.
11. Stevens BJ: Nursing Theory: Analysis, Application, Evaluation. Boston, Little, Brown, 1984.
12. Moreno ME, Durán MM, Hernandez Á: Nursing care for adaptation. Nursing Science Quarterly, 22(1):67–73, 2009.

13. Sato MK: Imagining nursing practice: The Roy adaptation model in 2050. Nursing Science Quarterly 20(1):47–50, 2007.

14. Allison SE: Self-care requirements for activity and rest: An Orem nursing focus. Nursing Science Quarterly 20(1):68–76, 2007.

15. Leininger MM (ed): Cultural Care Diversity and Universality: A Theory of Nursing. New York, National League for Nursing, 1992.

16. Beryl Pilkington F: Envisioning nursing in 2050 through the eyes of nurse theorists: King, Neuman, and Roy. Nursing Science Quarterly 20(2):108–128, 2007.

17. Watson J: Nursing: Human Science and Human Care. A Theory of Nursing. E. Norwalk, CT, Appleton-Century-Crofts, 1985.

18. Schaefer KM, Pond JB: Levine's Conservation Model: A Framework for Nursing Practice. Philadelphia, FA Davis, 1991.

19. Khowaja K: Utilization of King's interacting systems framework and theory of goal attainment with new multidisciplinary model: Clinical pathway. Australian Journal of Advanced Nursing 24(2):44–50, 2007.

20. Aquino-Russell C: Living attentive presence and changing perspectives with a Web-based nursing theory course. Nursing Science Quarterly 20(2):128–134, 2007.

21. Ursel KL, Aquino-Russell CE: Illuminating person-centered care with Parse's teaching-learning model. Nursing Science Quarterly 23(2):118–223, 2010.

22. Chen H: The lived experience of moving forward for clients with spinal cord injury: A Parse research method study. Journal of Advanced Nursing 66(5):1132–1141, 2010.

23. Manojlovich M: The Nursing Worklife Model: Extending and refining a new theory. Journal of Nursing Management 15(3):256–263, 2007.

Chapter 5

1. Kydd A: Counting nurses in a nursing shortage: What of the silent attrition? Nursing Leadership 36(1):45–49, 2010.

2. Dumpel H: Hospital Magnet status: Impact on RN autonomy and patient advocacy. National Nurse 106(3):22–27, 2010

3. Greenwood B: Pew report highlights the impact of mobile technology. Information Today 26(6):28, 2009.

4. American Nurses Association: Position Paper on Education. Kansas City, MO, Author, 1965.

5. Fitzpatrick ML: Prologue to Professionalism. Bowie, MD, Robert J. Brady, 1983.

6. Jamieson EM, Sewell M: Trends in Nursing History. Philadelphia, WB Saunders, 1968.

7. Hegner BR, Caldwell E: Nursing Assistant: A Nursing Process Approach (6th ed). Albany, NY, Delmar, 1995.

8. National League for Nursing: Trends in Education, 2010. Available at http://www.nln.org.

9. Orsolini-Hain L, Waters V: Education evolution: A historical perspective of associate degree nursing. Journal of Nursing Education 48(5):266–227, 2009.

10. Starr SS: Associate degree nursing: Entry into practice—link to the future. Teaching & Learning in Nursing 5(3):129–134, 2010.

11. National League for Nursing: Statistics on Education, 2010. Available at http://www.nln.org.

12. Matthias AD: The intersection of the history of associate degree nursing and "BSN in 10": Three visible paths. Teaching & Learning in Nursing 5(1):39–43, 2010.

13. Forbes MO, Hickey MT: Curriculum reform in baccalaureate nursing education: Review of the literature. International Journal of Nursing Education Scholarship 6(1):1–16, 2009

14. Mills AC: Evaluation of online and on-site options for master's degree and post-master's certificate programs. Nurse Educator 32(2):73–77, 2007.

15. Chornick N: Moving toward uniformity in APRN state laws. Journal of Nursing Regulation 1(1):58–56, 2010.

16. Hathaway D: The practice doctorate: perspectives of early adopters. Journal of Nursing Education 45(12):487–496, 2006.

17. Hawkins R, Nezat G: Doctoral education: which degree to pursue? AANA Journal 77(2):92–96, 2009.

18. Brar K, Boschma G, McCuaig F: The development of nurse practitioner preparation beyond the master's level: What is the debate about? International Journal of Nursing Education Scholarship 7(1):1–15, 2010.

19. Trossman S: Clarifying DNP versus CNL. American Nurse 42(2):11, 2010.

20. Boland BA, Treston J, O'Sullivan AL: Climb to new educational heights. Nurse Practitioner 35(4):36–34, 2010.

21. Newland J: In defense of the DNP. Nurse Practitioner 35(4):5, 2010.

22. Drinkert R: NP doesn't see need to pursue DNP. Nurse Week 11(3):16, 2010.

23. Kutzin J: Other lessons learned completing a DNP program. Journal of Nursing Education 49(4):181–182, 2010.

24. Sullivan L. Doctor of nursing practice degree: An era of change. StuNurse 16:4–6, 2010.

Chapter 6

1. Lunney M: Use of critical thinking in the diagnostic process. International Journal of Nursing Terminologies & Classifications 21(2):82–88, 2010.

2. Sullivan DL, Chumbley C: Critical thinking: A new approach to patient care. Journal of Emergency Medical Services 35(4):48–53, 2010.

3. Safran C, Reti S, Marin H, Grandison T, Bhatti R: HIPAA compliance and patient privacy protection. Studies in Health Technology & Informatics 160:884–888, 2010.

4. Romeo EM: Quantitative research on critical thinking and predicting nursing students' NCLEX-RN performance. Journal of Nursing Education 49(7):378–386, 2010.

5. Drennan J: Critical thinking as an outcome of a Master's degree in Nursing program. Journal of Advanced Nursing 66(2):422–443, 2010.

Chapter 7

1. Fairchild RM: Practical ethical theory for nurses responding to complexity in care. Nursing Ethics 17(3):353–362, 2010.

2. Brecher B: The politics of professional ethics. Journal of Evaluation in Clinical Practice 16(2):351–355, 2010.

3. Young A: Professionalism and ethical issues in nurse prescribing. Nurse Prescribing 8(6):284–290, 2010.

4. Moulton B, King JS: Aligning ethics with medical decision-making: The quest for informed patient choice. Journal of Law, Medicine & Ethics 38(1):85–97, 2010.

5. Hanssen I, Alpers L: Utilitarian and common-sense morality discussions in intercultural nursing practice. Nursing Ethics 17(2):201–221. 2010.

Chapter 8

1. Clifton JM, VanBeuge SS, Mladenka C, Wosnik KK: The Genetic Information Nondiscrimination Act 2008: What clinicians should understand. Journal of the American Academy of Nurse Practitioners 22(5):246–249, 2010.

2. Hodgkinson K, Pullman D: Duty to warn and genetic disease. Canadian Journal of Cardiovascular Nursing 20(1):12–15, 2010.

3. Kaminskyy V, Zhivotovsky B: To kill or be killed: How viruses interact with the cell death machinery. Journal of Internal Medicine 267(5):473–482, 2010.

4. Caulfield T: Stem cell research and economic promises. Journal of Law, Medicine and Ethics 38(2):303–313, 2010.

5. Quick B, Kim DK, Meyer K: A 15-year review of ABC, CBS, and NBC news coverage of organ donation: implications for organ donation campaigns. Health Communication 24(2):137–145, 2010.

6. U.S. Department of Health and Human Services Health Resources and Services Administration: Organ Procurement and Transplantation Network. Retrieved August 5, 2010 from http://optn.transplant.hrsa.gov/data/.

7. Bramstedt KA: Honoring first person consent. Transplantation 86(11):163, 2008.

8. Organization for Transplant Professionals: Position statement: Adherence to first person consent. 2009, p 1. Available at: http://www.natco1.org/public_policy/documents/FirstPerson-Consent.pdf.

9. National Council of Commissioners on United States Laws: The Uniform Anatomical Gift Act, Revised 2009.

10. MacCormick IJ: Ruling on mercy killing: Suicide and euthanasia paradox. British Medical Journal 14(341):318, 2010.

11. Mair J: Respect for autonomy; or the right to die? Health Information Management Journal 39(1):46–50, 2010.

Chapter 9

1. Guido G: Legal and Ethical Issues in Nursing (5th ed). Upper Saddle River, NJ, Pearson Prentice Hall, 2009.

2. Aiken TD: Legal and Ethical Issues in Health Occupations. St. Louis, Saunders Elsevier, 2009.

3. Kopishke L, Peterson AM: Legal Nurse Consulting: Principles and Practices (3rd ed). Medford, MA, Taylor & Francis, 2010.

4. Watson E: Advance directives: Self-determination, legislation, and litigation issues. Journal of Legal Nurse Consulting 21(1):9–14, 2010.

5. Boaro N, Fancott C, Baker R, Velji K, Andreoli A: Using SBAR to improve communication in interprofessional rehabilitation teams... Situation-Background-Assessment-Recommendation. Journal of Interprofessional Care 24(1):111–114, 2010.

6. Beckett CD, Kipnis G: Collaborative communication: Integrating SBAR to improve quality/patient safety outcomes. Journal for Healthcare Quality: Promoting Excellence in Healthcare 31(5):19–28, 2009.

7. Guhde J: Using high fidelity simulation to teach nurse-to-doctor-report: A study on SBAR in an undergraduate nursing curriculum. Clinical Simulation in Nursing 6(3):115, 2010.

8. Retrieved September 28, 2010 from http://www.saferhealth-care.com/cat-shc/sbar-a-communication-technique.

Chapter 12

1. Fox RL, Abrahamson K: A critical examination of the U.S. nursing shortage: Contributing factors, public policy implications. Nursing Forum 44(4):235–244, 2009.

2. Kydd A: Counting nurses in a nursing shortage: What of the silent attrition? Reflections on Nursing Leadership 36(1):1–4, 2010.

3. Somers MJ, Finch L, Birnbaum D: Marketing nursing as a profession: Integrated marketing strategies to address the nursing shortage. Health Marketing Quarterly 27(3): 291–306, 2010.

4. Plunkett RD, Iwasiw CL, Kerr M: The intention to pursue graduate studies in nursing: A look at BScN students' self-efficacy and value influences. International Journal of Nursing Education Scholarship 7(1):1–13, 2010.

5. Stansfield J, McAleer F: Brought to (Face)book. Speech & Language Therapy in Practice 19:1368–2105, 2010.

6. Olmstead D: A good portfolio puts you ahead of other applicants. American Society of Respiratory Therapists Scanner 42(3):14, 2010.

7. Vallet M: Face(book) the facts. Massage Therapy Journal 49(2):56–61, 2010.

8. Frandsen BM: Burnout or compassion fatigue? Long-Term Living: For the Continuing Care Professional 59(5):50–52, 2010.

9. Laschinger HKS, Finegan J, Wilk P: New graduate burnout: The impact of professional practice environment, workplace civility, and empowerment. Nursing Economic$ 27(6):377–383, 2009.

10. Gustavsson JP, Hallsten L, Rudman A: Early career burnout among nurses: Modeling a hypothesized process using an item response approach. Journal of Nursing Studies 47(7): 864–875, 2009.

Chapter 13

1. Farag AA, Tullai-McGuiness S, Anthony MK: Nurses' perception of their manager's leadership style and unit climate: are there generational differences? Journal of Nursing Management 17(1):26–34, 2009.

2. Huston C: Preparing nurse leaders for 2020. Journal of Nursing Management 16(8):905–909, 2008.

3. Tomey AM: Nursing leadership and management effects work environments. Journal of Nursing Management 17(1): 15–25, 2009.

4. Pearce C: Leadership resource: Ten steps to managing change. Nursing Management 13(10):25, 2007.

5. Ellis P, Abbott J: Leadership and management skills in health care. British Journal of Cardiac Nursing 5(4):200–203, 2010.

6. Tappen RM: Essentials of Nursing Leadership and Management (5th ed). Philadelphia, FA Davis, 2009.

7. Oestmann E: Mutual Expectation Theory of Motivation. Vdm Verlag Dr Mueller E K / Lightning Source, 2008.

8. Ramsay A, Fulop N, Edwards N: The evidence base for vertical integration in health care. Journal of Integrated Care 17(2):3–12, 2009.

9. Ruger JP: Health capability: Conceptualization and operationalization. American Journal of Public Health 100(1):41–49, 2010.

Chapter 15

1. Sparrow S: Practicing civility in the legal writing course: Helping law students learn professionalism. Retrieved December, 2010 from http://www.lexisnexis.com/.

2. Pascoe E, Richman L: Perceived discrimination and health: A meta-analytic review. Psychological Bulletin 135(4): 531–554, 2009.

3. Watson J: Nursing: The philosophy and science of caring, revised edition. Boulder, CO, University Press of Colorado, 2008.

4. Watson J: Nursing: Human science and human care. A theory of nursing. Boulder, CO, University Press of Colorado, 2007.

5. Watson J: Intentionality and caring-healing consciousness: A practice of transpersonal n nursing. Journal of Holistic Nursing Practice 16(4):12–19, 2002.

6. Kline MV, Huff RM: Health Promotion in Multicultural Populations: A Handbook for Practitioners and Students (2nd ed). Los Angeles, Sage, 2007.

7. Wilkins K: The civil behavior of students: A survey of school professionals. Retrieved December, 2010 from http://findarticles.com/p/articles/mi_qa3673/is_4_13-?ai_n54399308/.

8. Lamontagne C: Intimidation: A concept analysis. Nursing Forum 45(1):54–65, 2010.

9. Donahue MP: Nursing as Illustrated History: The Finest Art. St. Louis, Mosby, 1985.

10. Boice B: Classroom incivilities. Research in Higher Education 37(4):453–486, 1996.

11. Clark C, Springer P: Academic nurse leaders' role in fostering a culture of civility in nursing education. Journal of Nursing Education 49(6):319–325, 2010.

12. Clark C, Springer P: Incivility in nursing education: A description study of definitions and prevalence. Journal of Nursing Education 46(1):7–11, 2007.

13. Internet Society: All about the Internet: Code of Conduct. Retrieved December, 2010 from http://www.isoc.org/internet/conduct.

14. David BA: Nursing's gender politics: reformulating the footnotes. Advanced Nursing Science 23(1):83–93, 2000.

15. Randle J: Bulling in the nursing profession. Journal of Advanced Nursing 43(4):395–401, 2003.

16. Poorman S, Mastrovich M, Webb C: Teacher's stories: How faculty help and hinder students at risk. Nursing Education Perspectives 5(29):272–277, 2008.

17. Taylor C, Mpotu F: Embracing mentors and facing tormentors. Imprint: Journal of the National Student Nurses Association. Nov/Dec 2010.

18. Heinrich K: Joy stealing: 10 mean games faculty play and how to stop the gaming. Nurse Educator 32(1):34–38, 2007.

19. Clark C, Springer P: Academic nurse leaders' role in fostering a culture of civility in nursing education. Journal of Nursing Education 49(6):319–325, 2010.

20. Twale DJ, DeLuca BM: Faculty incivility: The rise of the academic bully culture and what to do about it. San Francisco, Jossey Bass, 2008.

21. David BA: Nursing's gender politics: reformulating the footnotes. Advanced Nursing Science 23(1):83–93, 2000.

22. Taylor C, Mpotu F: Embracing mentors and facing tormentors. Imprint: Journal of the National Student Nurses Association. Nov/Dec 2010.

23. Thomas TS: Handling anger in the teacher-student relationship. Nursing Education Perspectives 24(24):17–24, 2003.

24. Nursing Organization Alliance Position Paper 2010. Retrieved December, 2010 from http://www.nursing-alliance.org.

25. Clark C: Faculty and student assessment of and experience with incivility in nursing education. Journal of Nursing Education 47(10):458–465, 2008.

26. Clark C: Faculty and student assessment of and experience with incivility in nursing education. Journal of Nursing Education 47(10):458–465, 2008.

27. Langone M: Promoting integrity among nursing students. Educational Innovation 46(1):45–47, 2007.

28. Sentinal Event Policy, Office of Quality and Safety in Health Care 2008. Retrieved January 2011 from http://www.safetyandquality.health.wa.gov.au.

29. Code of Ethics for Nurses. Retrieved December, 2010 from http://dev.nln.org/.

30. Hill J: Mentoring African American women leaders in nursing. Unpublished dissertation. Baton Rouge, LA, Louisiana State University, 2003.

31. Clark C, Springer P: Incivility in nursing education: A description study of definitions and prevalence. Journal of Nursing Education 46(1):7–11, 2007.

Chapter 16

1. Bittner NP, Gravlin G: Critical thinking, delegation, and missed care in nursing practice. Journal of Nursing Administration 39(3):142–146, 2009.

2. Nightingale F: Notes on Nursing: What It Is and What It Is Not. London, Harrison and Sons, 1859, p 17.

3. Potter P, Deshields T, Kuhrik M: Delegation practices between registered nurses and nursing assistive personnel. Journal of Nursing Management 18(2):157–165, 2010.

4. McInnis LA, Parsons LC: Thoughtful nursing practice: Reflections on nurse delegation decision-making. Nursing Clinics of North America 44(4):461–470, 2009.

5. American Nurses Association: Position Statement: Registered Nurse Utilization of Unlicensed Assistive Personnel. Washington, DC, Author, 1997.

6. Resha C: Delegation in the school setting: Is it a safe practice? Online Journal of Issues in Nursing 15(2):1–5, 2010.

7. American Nurses Association: Registered Professional Nurses and Unlicensed Assistive Personnel (2nd ed). Washington, DC, Author, 1996.

8. Anthony MK, Vidal K: Mindful communication: A novel approach to improving delegation and increasing patient safety. Online Journal of Issues in Nursing 15(2):1– 2, 2010.

9. Simones J, Wilcox J, Scott K, Goeden D, Copley D, Doetkott R, Kippley M: Collaborative simulation project to teach scope of practice. Journal of Nursing Education 49(4):190–197, 2010.

10. Huston CJ: 10 Tips for successful delegation: Improve patient care and save time by recognizing when to delegate and learning how to do it wisely. Nursing 39(3):54–66, 2009.

11. Weydt A: Developing delegation skills. Online Journal of Issues in Nursing 15(2):1, 2010.
12. ANA Code of Ethics for Nurses 2001. Retrieved October, 2010 from http://www.ana.org.
13. Plawecki LH, Amrhein DW: A question of delegation: Unlicensed assistive personnel and the professional nurse. Journal of Gerontological Nursing 36(8):18–21, 2010.

Chapter 17

1. Kohn L, Corrigan J, Donaldson M: To Err is Human: Building a Safer Health System. Institute of Medicine. Washington, DC: National Academy Press, 2000.
2. Page A: Keeping Patients Safe: Transforming the work environment of nurses. Institute of Medicine. Washington, DC: National Academy Press, 2004.
3. The Joint Commission: Health care at the crossroads: Strategies for addressing the Evolving nursing crisis. Retrieved May, 2009 from http://www.jointcommission.org.
4. Tappen RM: Essentials of Nursing Leadership (4th ed). Philadelphia, FA Davis, 2006.
5. American Hospital Association: In our hands: How hospital leaders can guild a thriving workforce. Retrieved June, 2010 from http://www.aha.org.
6. Gordon S: Collective thinking. Nursing Management 11(2):8, 2006.
7. Roman LM: Professional update: NLRB finally rules on nurses' supervisory status. Registered Nurse 69(11):12, 2006.
8. The Joint Commission: Hospital Accreditation Standards. Oakbrook, IL, Author, 2010.
9. Swihart DO: Introduction: The Concept Behind Shared Governance. Marblehead, MA: HCPro, 2006.
10. O'Grady P: Implementing shared governance: Creating a professional organization, 2006. Retrieved September, 2010 from http://www.tpogassociates.com/SharedGovernance.htm.
11. Weston M: Strategies for enhancing autonomy and control over nursing practice, 2010. Retrieved September, 2010 from Online Journal of Issues in Nursing, http://www.nursingworld.org/.
12. Anthony M: Shared governance models: Theory, practice and evidence, 2004. Retrieved September, 2010 from http://www.nursingworld.org/.
13. American Nurses Association: Code of ethics for nurses with interpretive Statements. Silver Spring, MD, Author, 2001.
14. Adler J: Is past prologue? A brief history of the labor movement in the United States. Public Personnel Management 5(4):311–329, 2010.
15. Malvey D: Unionization in healthcare: Strategies. Journal of Healthcare Management 55(4):236–240, 2010.
16. Tappen RM: Essentials of Nursing Leadership and Management (5th ed). Philadelphia, FA Davis, 2010.
17. Malvey D: Unionization in healthcare: Background and trends. Journal of Healthcare Management 55(3):154–157, 2010.
18. Finkelman AK: Prefessional Nursing Concepts: Competencies for Quality Leadership. Boston, Jones & Bartlett, 2010.
19. Dine P: Nurses unionize to improve patient care, 2010. Retrieved October, 2010 from http://www.washingtontimes.com.
20. Matthews J: When does delegating make you a supervisor? Online Journal of Issues in Nursing 15(2):1–3, 2010.
21. "Red alert: on pro-union advocates appointed to NLRB. Long-Term Living: For the Continuing Care Professional 59(5):10, 2010.
22. Cusack L, Smith M: Power inequalities in the assessment of nursing competency within the workplace: implications for nursing management. Journal of Continuing Education in Nursing 41(9):408–412, 2010.
23. Dean E: Unions warn that wards, services and jobs are already under threat. Nursing Standard 24(49):6, 2010.
24. Carlson J: Laboring to unite: After years of feuding and raiding each other's ranks, more healthcare unions are joining hands so they can work together on a common pro-labor agenda. Modern Healthcare 39(46):24–26, 2009.
25. Frequently asked questions about the national nurses union. Massachusetts Nurse 80(8):4–7, 2009.
26. Porter C: A nursing labor management partnership model. Journal of Nursing Administration 40(6):272–276, 2010.
27. Porter C, Kolcaba K, McNulty SR, Fitzpatrick JJ: The effect of a nursing labor management partnership on nurse turnover and satisfaction. Journal of Nursing Administration 40(5):205–210, 2010.

Chapter 18

1. Schwartz RM: Reforming the healthcare delivery system: The impact of the Patient Protection and Affordable Care Act. Remington Report 18(3):5–6, 8–10, 2010.
2. Redwood D: Health reform, prevention and health promotion: Milestone moment on a long journey. Journal of Alternative & Complementary Medicine 16(5):521–523, 2010.
3. Cutler D: Analysis & commentary: How health care reform must bend the cost curve. Health Affairs 29(6):1131–1135, 2010.
4. Doherty RB: The certitudes and uncertainties of health care reform. Annals of Internal Medicine 152(10):679–682, 2010.
5. Chollet DJ: How temporary insurance for high-risk individuals may play out under health reform. Health Affairs 29(6): 1164–1167, 2010.
6. Goodson JD: Patient Protection and Affordable Care Act: Promise and peril for primary care. Annals of Internal Medicine, 152(11):742–744, 2010.
7. Ebner AL: What nurses need to know about health care reform. Nursing Economic$ 28(3):191–194, 2010.
8. Gardner D: Health policy and politics. Expanding scope of practice: Inter-professional collaboration or conflict? Nursing Economics 28(4):264–266, 2010.
9. Falardeau J: Health care reform and you: The road to implementation paved with speed bumps and potholes. American Chiropractic Association News 6(8):7, 2010.
10. National Health Information Center, U. S. Department of Health and Human Services: Income Poverty, and Health Insurance Coverage in the United States: 2010. Washington, DC, Author, 2010.
11. Census Bureau Home Page. 2010 Census. Retrieved November, 2010 from http://www.census.gov/.
12. Health care spending in the United States and OECD countries. Retrieved November, 2010 from http://www.kff.org/insurance/snapshot/2007.
13. Canadian Healthcare Association, 2010. Retrieved November, 2010 from http://www.cha.ca.

14. Jeffs L: Creating reporting and learning cultures in healthcare organizations. Canadian Nurse 103(3):16–17, 27–28, 2007.

15. Department of Health and Services Center of Medicare and Medicaid Expenditures. National Health Expenditures Projections 2006–2016. Retrieved November, 2010 from http://www.cms.hhs.gov/NationaHealthExpendData/.

16. Lynn J: Academia and clinic: The ethics of using quality improvement methods in health care. Annals of Internal Medicine 146(9):666–673, 2007.

17. U.S. last in health care among 7 industrialized countries in 2010. Retrieved November, 2010 from http://www.livescience/health/healthcare.

18. Danz MS, Rubenstein LV, Hempel S, Foy R, Suttorp M, Farmer MM, Shekelle PG: Identifying quality improvement intervention evaluations: Is consensus achievable? Quality and Safety in Health Care 19(4):279–283, 2010.

19. Six Sigma project improves documentation of patient status. Hospital Case Management 17(4):55–56, 2009.

20. Corn JB: Six Sigma in healthcare. Radiologic Technology 81(1):92–95, 2009.

21. Panasci J: Understanding home care as a treatment option. Care Management Journals 10(4):190–195, 2009.

22. Medicare project focuses on readmissions. Healthcare Benchmarks and Quality Improvement 17(8):89–92, 2010.

23. Carpenter D: Reforms hit home. Hospitals and Health Networks 84(5):52–56, 2010.

24. Piamjariyakul U, Ross VM, Yadrich DM, Williams AR, Howard L, Smith CE: Complex home care: Part I. Utilization and costs to families for health care services each year. Nursing Economics 28(4):255–263, 2010.

25. Devlin M, McIlfatrick S: Providing palliative and end-of-life care in the community: The role of the home-care worker. International Journal of Palliative Nursing 16(4):195–203, 2010.

26. Orton M: Is there more to supporting people within their own home than just providing telecare? Journal of Assistive Technologies 4(3):20–24, 2010.

Chapter 19

1. Ericksen AB: Informatics: the future of nursing. RN 72(7):34–37, 2009.

2. Safran C, Reti S, Marin H: Nursing informatics. Studies in Health Technology & Informatics 160:1531–1541, 2010.

3. Roman D: Nursing informatics matters. Nursing Update 33(8):34–35, 2010.

4. Nickitas DM, Kerfoot K: Nursing informatics: Why nurse leaders need to stay informed. Nursing Economics 28(3):141, 158, 2010.

5. Vincent D, Hastings-Tolsma M, Effken J: Data visualization and large nursing datasets. Online Journal of Nursing Informatics 14(2):1–13, 2010.

6. Coenen A, Kim TY: Development of terminology subsets using ICNP. International Journal of Medical Informatics 79(7):530–538, 2010.

7. American Nurses Association: Scope and Standards of Nursing Informatics Practice. Washington, DC, ANA, 2001.

8. American Nurses Credentialing Center Catalog. Washington, DC, American Nurses Publishing, 2001.

9. Skiba DJ: WANTED: Informatics Resources and Learning Activities. Nursing Education Perspectives 31(3):183–184, 2010.

10. Murphy J: Nursing informatics: the intersection of nursing, computer, and information sciences. Nursing Economics 28(3):204–207, 2010.

11. Murphy J: Nursing informatics: The journey to meaningful use of electronic health records. Nursing Economics 28(4):283–286, 2010.

12. Bove LA, Finley JJ: ANIA-CARING 2010 Annual Conference "Re-Evolution in Nursing Informatics." ANIA-CARING Newsletter 25(2):9–11, 2010.

13. Rahman A, Applebaum R: What's All This about Evidence-Based Practice? The roots, the controversies, and why it matters. Generations 34(1):6–12, 2010.

14. Mattox EA: Identifying vulnerable patients at heightened risk for medical error. Critical Care Nurse 30(2):61–69, 2010.

15. Flood LS, Gasiewicz N, Delpier T: Integrating information literacy across a BSN curriculum. Journal of Nursing Education 49(2):101–104, 2010.

16. ANI emerging leaders program. CIN: Computers, Informatics, Nursing 28(4):241–244, 2010.

17. Heiskell H: Ethical decision-making for the utilization of technology-based patient/family education. Online Journal of Nursing Informatics 14(1):1–14, 2010.

18. McGraw D: Privacy and health information technology. Journal of Law, Medicine & Ethics 37:(2):121–149, 2009.

19. Orton M: Is there more to supporting people within their own home than just providing telecare?; Journal of Assistive Technologies 4(3):20–24, 2010.

20. Zurmehly J: Personal digital assistants (PDAs): Review and evaluation. Nursing Education Perspectives 31(3):179–182, 2010.

Chapter 20

1. Retrieved November, 2010 from http://www.meriam-webster.com/dictionary.

2. Brush BL: The potent lever of toil: Nursing development and exportation in the postcolonial Philippines. American Journal of Public Health 100(9):1572–1581, 2010.

3. Dumpel H: Hospital Magnet status: Impact on RN autonomy and patient advocacy. National Nurse 106(3):22–27, 2010.

4. The Magnetic pull: A staff report. Nursing Management 41(2):38, 40–44, 2010.

5. Somers MJ, Finch L, Birnbaum D: Marketing nursing as a profession: Integrated marketing strategies to address the nursing shortage. Health Marketing Quarterly 27(3):291–306, 2010.

6. Retrieved November, 2010 from http://www.ncsbn.org.

7. Douglas K: Ratios—if it were only that easy. Nursing Economics 28(2):119–125, 2010.

8. Ebner AL: What nurses need to know about health care reform. Nursing Economics 28(3):191–194, 2010.

9. Lung CJ: Support your political action committee: Contribute to the PAC and make sure your voice is heard in Washington. American Society of Radiologic Technologist Scanner 42(3):56, 2010.

10. McKay ML, Hewlett PO: Grassroots coalition building: Lessons from the field. Journal of Professional Nursing 25(6):352–357, 2010.

Chapter 21

1. Clarke J: A critical view of how nursing has defined spirituality. Journal of Clinical Nursing 18(12):1666–1673, 2009.
2. Swinton J, Pattison S: Moving beyond clarity: Towards a thin, vague, and useful understanding of spirituality in nursing care. Nursing Philosophy 11(4):226–237, 2010.
3. Nightingale F: Notes on Nursing. New York, Dover, 1969. (Originally published in 1860.)
4. Watson J: Nursing: Human Science and Human Theory of Care: Theory of Nursing. New York, National League for Nursing, 1988.
5. North American Nursing Diagnosis Association: Nursing Diagnosis: Definitions and Classification, 1997–1998. Philadelphia, Author, 1998.
6. Moore T: Care of the Soul. New York, HarperCollins, 1992.
7. Mueller C. Spirituality in children: understanding and developing interventions. Pediatric Nursing 36(4):197–208, 2010.
8. Narayanasmy A: The puzzle of spirituality for nursing: A guide to practical assessment. British Journal of Nursing 13(19):1140–1144, 2004.
9. Dolamo BL: Spiritual nursing. Nursing Update 34(4):22–24, 2010.
10. Shores CI: Spiritual perspectives of nursing students. Nursing Education Perspectives 31(1):8–11, 2010.
11. Paley J: Religion and the secularisation of health care. Journal of Clinical Nursing 18(14):1963–1974, 2009.

Chapter 23

1. Stevens M: Forensic nursing. Nursing Update 34(5):46–49, 2010.
2. Campbell R: Sexual assault nurse examiners' experiences providing expert witness court testimony. Journal of Forensic Nursing 3(1):7–14, 2007.
3. Elliott R, Larson K: Legal nurse consultant: A role for nephrology nurses. Nephrology Nursing Journal 37(3): 297–300, 2010.
4. Pelham TW, Holt LE, Holt J: Forensic kinesiology: Foundations of an interdiscipline for accident/crime investigation. American Journal of Forensic Medicine and Pathology 31(2):200–203, 2010.
5. Kent-Wilkinson AE: Forensic psychiatric/mental health nursing: Responsive to social need. Issues in Mental Health Nursing 31(6):425–431, 2010.
6. Danna D, Porche D: The NP entrepreneur: Nurse entrepreneur as a global executive. Journal for Nurse Practitioners 5(6):454–455, 2010.
7. Brandt JA, Edwards DR, Sullivan SC, Zehler JK, Grinder S, Scott KJ, Cook JH, Roper D, Dickey A, Maddox KL: An evidence-based business planning process. Journal of Nursing Administration 39(12):511–513, 2009.
8. James JJ, Benjamin GC, Burkle FM, Gebbie KM, Kelen G Subbarao I: Disaster medicine and public health preparedness: a discipline for all health professionals. Disaster Medicine & Public Health Preparedness 4(2):102–107, 2010.
9. Nyamathi AM, Casillas A, King ML, Gresham L, Pierce E, Farb D, Weichmann C: Computerized bioterrorism education and training for nurses on bioterrorism attack agents. Journal of Continuing Education in Nursing 41(8):375–384, 2010.
10. Goodhue CJ, Burke RV, Chambers S, Ferrer RR, Upperman JS: Disaster Olympix: A unique nursing emergency preparedness exercise. Journal of Trauma Nursing 17(1):5–10, 2010.
11. McCabe OL, Barnett DJ, Taylor HG, Links JM: Ready, willing, and able: A framework for improving the public health emergency preparedness system. Disaster Medicine & Public Health Preparedness 4(2):161–168, 2010.
12. Debisette AT, Martinelli AM, Couig MP, Braun M: US Public Health Service Commissioned Corps Nurses: Responding in times of national need. Nursing Clinics of North America 45(2):123–135, 2010.
13. Nightingale F: Notes on Nursing. Oxford, UK, Dover, 1860.

Chapter 24

1. Rankin S, Duffy K: Patient Education: Issues, Principles, and Guidelines. Philadelphia, JB Lippincott, 1983.
2. Hassmiller S: Nursing's role in healthcare reform. American Nurse Today 5(9):68–69, 2010.
3. Trossman S: Issues up close. American Nurse Today 5(9):32–33, 2010.
4. Roizen M, Oz M: You, The Smart Patient. New York, Free Press, 2006.
5. Benner, P: From Novice to Expert. Upper Saddle River, NJ, Prentice Hall, 2001.
6. Haber D: Health Promotion and Aging: Practical Applications for Health Professionals. New York, Springer, 2003.
7. Walker SN, Sechrist KR, Pender NJ: The health-promoting lifestyle profile: Development and psychometric characteristics. Nursing Research 35(2):76–81, 1987.
8. Chester D, Himburg S, Weatherspoon L: Spirituality of African American women: Correlations to health promoting behaviors, 2006. Retrieved September, 2009 from http://www.ars.usda.gov/research/publications/publications.htm?seq_no_115=182417&pf=.
9. Duffy L: Overweight doctors, nurses and the US Surgeon General. as quoted in Examiner.com, New Orleans. Retrieved September, 2009 from http://www.examiner.com/x-798-Denver-Low-Carb-Examiner-y20.
10. Miller SK: Overweight and obesity in nurses, advanced practice nurses, and nurse educators. Journal of the American Academy of Nurse Practitioners 20(20):259–265, 2008.
11. Tompkins T, Belza B, Brown MA: Nurse practitioner practice patterns for exercise counseling. Journal of the American Academy of Nurse Practitioners 21(20):79–86, 2009.
12. Leddy S: Health Promotion. Philadelphia, FA Davis, 2006.
13. Rankin SH, Stallings KD, London F: Patient Education in Health and Illness. New York, Lippincott Williams & Wilkins, 2006.
14. Institute of Medicine: Crossing the quality chasm: A new health system for the 21st century. Washington, DC, National Academy Press, March 2001.
15. Hoggard-Green J: How the consumer defines health care. Unpublished dissertation. University of Utah, 2000.
16. Fomby-White B: Choice theory. Unpublished treatise. 2007.
17. Healthy People Focus Areas 2010. Retrieved January, 2010 from http://www.cdc.gov/nchs/healthy_people/hp2020.
18. Fomby-White B: Enhancing health education by including choice education intervention and theory of choice into the teaching plan. Race, Gender and Class 17(3–4), 7–18, 2010.

19. Cooper-Patrick L, Gallo JJ, Gonzalez JJ, et al.: Race, gender, and partnership in the patient-physician relationship. Journal of the American Medical Association 282(6):583–589, 1999.

20. Edelman C, Mandel C: Health Promotion Throughout the Life Span (p. 223). Philadelphia, Mosby Elsevier, 2006.

21. Swanson KM: Meta-analysis of 130 empirical studies. In Watson J (ed): Assessing and Measuring Caring in Nursing and Health Science (p. 11). Springer, New York, 2002.

22. Hill JJ: Getting your first job. In Jones R: Nursing Leadership and Management: Theory, Processes, and Practice. Philadelphia, FA Davis, 2007.

23. National Institute of Nursing Research. Retrieved January, 2011 http://www.aacn.nche.edu.

24. Pew Commission: Report of the Pew-Fitzer task force on advancing psychological health education: Relationship-centered care. Washington, DC, Robert Wood Johnson Foundation, 1998.

25. Goodman A: The story of David Olds and the nurse home visiting program. Washington, DC, Robert Wood Johnson Foundation, 2006.

26. Olds, DL, Robinson J, O'Brien R, Luckey DW, Pettitt LM, Henderson CR Jr, et al.: Home visiting by paraprofessionals and by nurses: A randomized, controlled trial. Pediatrics 110(3):486, 2002.

27. Curtin L. Quantum nursing. American Nurse Today 5(9):71–72, 2010.

28. Peplau H: Interpersonal relations in Nursing. Newbury Park, CA, Sage Publications, 1991.

29. Latino Behavioral Health Workforce Development, 2010. Retrieved January, 2011 from http://minorityhealth.hhs.gov.

30. Goetz T: The decision tree: Taking control of your health in the new era of personalized medicine. New York, Rodale Publishing, 2010.

31. Stewart M: Medagogy as a conceptual framework for patient education. Unpublished Scholarly Project, Case Western Reserve, Cleveland, 2010.

32. Edelman C, Mandel C: Health promotion throughout the life span. Philadelphia, Mosby Elsevier, 2006.

33. Domrose C: Patient teaching. NurseWeek 8(12):10, 2007.

34. Nunnery R: Advancing Your Career: Concepts of Professional Nursing. Philadelphia, FA Davis, 2005.

35. Chulay M, Burns S: AACN: Essentials of Progressive Care Nursing (2nd ed). Chicago, McGraw-Hill Medical, 2010.

36. Yoder-Wise P: Leading and Managing in Nursing. St. Louis, Mosby Elsevier, 2007.

37. Knobloch A, Stewart M:. Pilot testing of the Stewart Understanding Personal Perception Scale to rate understanding of material related to six objectives for a continuing education event, 2010. Virginia Henderson International Nursing Library. Retrieved January, 2011 from http://www.nursinglibrary.org/Portal/main.aspx?PageID=4024&SID=23468.

Chapter 25

1. Fain A: Reading, Understanding, and Applying Nursing Research (3rd ed). Philadelphia, FA Davis, 2009.

2. American Association of Colleges of Nursing: The Research-Focused Doctoral Program in Nursing: Pathways to Excellence. 2010. Retrieved November, 2010 from http://www.aacn.nche.edu/.

3. Polit DF, Beck CT: Nursing Research: Generating and Assessing Evidence for Nursing Practice. Philadelphia, Lippincott Williams & Wilkins, 2011.

4. Goodnow M: Outlines of Nursing History. Philadelphia, WB Saunders, 1935.

5. Melnyk BM, Fineout-Overholt E: Evidence-Based Practice in Nursing & Healthcare: A Guide to Best Practice. Philadelphia, Lippincott Williams & Wilkins, 2010.

6. Ogiehor-Enoma G, Taqueban L, Anosike A: Evidence-based nursing: 6 Steps for transforming organizational EBP culture. Nursing Management 41(5):14–17, 2010.

7. Corchon S, Watson R, Arantzamendi M, Saracíbar M: Design and validation of an instrument to measure nursing research culture: the Nursing Research Questionnaire (NRQ). Journal of Clinical Nursing 19(1–2):217–226, 2010.

8. Latimer R, Kimbell J: Nursing research fellowship: Building nursing research infrastructure in a hospital. Journal of Nursing Administration 40(2):92–98, 2010.

9. Missal B, Schafer BK, Halm MA, Schaffer MA: A university and health care organization partnership to prepare nurses for evidence-based practice. Journal of Nursing Education 49(8):456–461, 2010.

10. Reinhardt JP: Research methods in evidence-based practice: Understanding the evidence. Generations 34(1):36–42, 2010.

11. Schifferdecker KE, Reed VA: Using mixed methods research in medical education: Basic guidelines for researchers. Medical Education 43(7):637–644, 2009.

12. Rahman A, Applebaum R: What's all this about evidenced-based practice? Generations 34(1):6–12, 2010.

13. Oh EG, Kim S, Kim SS, Kim S, Cho EY, Yoo J, Kim HS, Lee JH, You MA. Lee H: Integrating evidence-based practice into RN-to-BSN clinical nursing education. Journal of Nursing Education 49(7):387–392, 2010.

14. Rid A, Schmidt H: The 2008 Declaration of Helsinki: First among equals in research ethics? Journal of Law, Medicine and Ethics 38(1):143–148, 2010.

15. Shah S, Wendler D: Interpretation of the subjects' condition requirement: A legal perspective. Journal of Law, Medicine and Ethics 38(2):365–373, 2010.

16. Munten G, van den Bogaard J, Cox K, Garretsen H, Bongers I: Implementation of evidence-based practice in nursing using action research: a review. Worldviews on Evidence-Based Nursing 7(3):135–157, 2010.

17. Newton JM, McKenna LG, Gilmour C, Fawcett J: Exploring a pedagogical approach to integrating research, practice and teaching. International Journal of Nursing Education Scholarship 7(1):1–13, 2010.

Chapter 26

1. Bishop FL, Yardley L, Lewith GT: Why consumers maintain complementary and alternative medicine use: a qualitative study. Journal of Alternative and Complementary Medicine 16(2):175–182, 2010.

2. Lyng S: Reflexive biomedicalization and alternative healing systems. Journal of Bioethical Inquiry 7(1):53–69, 2010.

3. Oguamanam C: Personalized medicine and complementary and alternative medicine: In search of common grounds. Journal of Alternative and Complementary Medicine 15(8):943–949, 2009.

4. What is complementary and alternative medicine? NCCAM Publication No. D347 2010. Retrieved November, 2010 from http://nccam.nih.gov.

5. Kessler HA: Acupuncture and the treatment of cancer pain. Integrative Medicine: A Clinician's Journal 9(2):22–29, 2010.

6. Foster S, Tyler VM: Tyler's Honest Herbal: A Sensible Guide to the Use of Herbs and Related Remedies (5th ed). Binghamton, NY: Haworth Herbal Press, 2010.

7. Medical Economics Staff: Physicians' Desk Reference for Herbal Medicines (4th ed). New York Thomson Health Care, 2007.

Chapter 1

Burke RJ: The ripple effect: Staffing post restructuring. Nursing Management 33(2):41–43, 2002.

Callister J, et al.: Inquiry in baccalaureate nursing education: Fostering evidence-based practice. Nursing Education 44(2):59–65, 2005.

Carter M: The ABCs of staffing decisions. Nursing Management 35(6):16, 2004.

Ferguson, L, Day R: Evidence-based nursing education: Myth or reality. Nursing Education 44(3):107–116, 2005.

Freeman LH, et al.: New curriculum for a new century. Nursing Education 41(1):38–40, 2002.

Irving JA, Sniper J: Preserving professional values. Journal of Professional Nursing 18(1):5, 2002.

Kinsman L, James EL: Evidence based practice needs evidence based implementation. Lippincott's Case Management 6(5):208–219, 2001.

Kovner C, Harrington C: CMS Study: Correlation between staffing and quality. American Journal of Nursing 102(9):65–66, 2002.

Manojlovich M: Predictors of professional practice behaviors in hospital settings. Nursing Research 54(1):41–47, 2005.

Manthey M: Continuing the case for the baccalaureate. Journal of Professional Nursing 18(1):7, 2002.

Narayan MC, et al.: Searching for nursing's future. Nursing Management 33(1):26–30, 2002.

O'Bryan L, et al.: Rework the workload. Nursing Management 33(3):38–40, 2002.

Thompson D, Burns H: Work environment for nurses and the impact on protecting patients from health-care errors. Journal of Professional Nursing 20(3):145–147, 2004.

Chapter 2

Cristy T: The first fifty years. American Journal of Nursing 9(9):1778–1784, 1971.

Cristy T: Portrait of a leader: Lavinia Lloyd Dock. Nursing Outlook 17(6):72–75, 1969.

Cristy T: Portrait of a leader: M. Adelaide Nutting. Nursing Outlook 17(l):20–24, 1969.

Cristy T: Portrait of a leader: Isabel Hampton Robb. Nursing Outlook 17(3):26–29, 1969.

Cristy T: Portrait of a leader: Isabel Maitland Stewart. Nursing Outlook 17(10):44–48, 1969.

D'Antonio P: Women, nursing and baccalaureate education in 20th-century America. Journal of Nursing Scholarship 36(4):379–384, 2004.

Grypma S: Critical issues in the use of biographic methods in nursing history. Nursing History Review 13:171–187, 2005.

Holder V: From handmaiden to right hand: World War I and advancements in medicine. AORN Journal 80(5):911–923, 2004.

Jamieson EM, et al.: Trends in Nursing History. Philadelphia, WB Saunders, 1968.

Lewenson S: Integrating nursing history into the curriculum. Journal of Professional Nursing 20(6):374–381.

Murphy-Ende K: Advanced practice nursing: Reflections on the past, issues for the future. Oncology Nursing Forum 29(1):26–33, 2002.

Newlson S: The rhetoric of rupture: Nursing as a practice with a history? Nursing Outlook 52(5):255–261, 2004.

Selanders LC: Florence Nightingale: Perseverance, power, possibilities. Maryland Nurse 4(3):1–2, 2001.

Smoyak SA: Florence Nightingale, insane nurse. Journal of Psychosocial Nursing and Mental Health Services 39(10):6–8, 2001.

Chapter 3

Adams D, Miller BK: Professionalism in nursing behaviors of nurse practitioners. Journal of Professional Nursing 17(4):203–210, 2001.

Barkley TW, et al.: Practice issues: Credentialing, prescriptive authority, and liability. Nurse Practitioner Forum 2001 12(2):106–114, 2001.

Clowney J: Moving ahead: Learning from experience: Renewing your vigour. Nursing Times 101(2):75, 2005.

Garnero T: On solving the nursing shortage. Nurse Week (Special Edition) Feb 4, 2002, p 11.

Gingerich B: Accreditation actions. Certification and licensure: CAM services providers. Home Health Care Management Practice 16(6):531–533, 2004.

Martin B: Are you ready for certification, the mark of excellence? AACN News 21(11):10, 2004.

Martin SA: Network to promote advanced practice mentoring relationships. AACN News 19(3):5, 2002.

Mikos C: Legal checkpoints: Inside the Nurse Practice Act. Nurse Manager 35(9):20, 22, 91, 2004.

Poe L: Eleven answers about the Nurse Licensure Interstate Compact. Utah Nurse 13(3):18, 2004.

Results of a multistate licensure survey. American Journal of Nursing 2005 Career Guide 40, 2005.

Salladay S: Ethical problems. Nursing credentials: What's in a name (badge)? Nursing 34(8):11, 2004.

Sofer D: Mandatory BSNs? New New York nurses could be required to eventually obtain baccalaureates. American Journal of Nursing 104(10):22, 2004.

Tahan H: Guest column. Certification helps CMs meet today's challenges: Skills, knowledge, competency enhanced. Hospital Case Management 13(2):22, 31–32, 2005.

Whelan J: "A necessity in the nursing world." The Chicago Nurses Professional Registry 1913–1950. Nursing History Review 13:49–75, 2005.

Your guide to certification: Here's what you need to know to pursue recognition of your expertise. American Journal of Nursing 2005 Career Guide 56–69, 2005.

Chapter 4

Algase DL, et al.: Nursing theory across curricula. Journal of Professional Nursing 17(5):248–255, 2002.

Baldwin A: Wagging the dog: An analysis of year 2000 workforce and education outcomes from recommendations of the 1995 Pew Commission report. Journal of Allied Health 30(3):160–167, 2001.

Determining cost of nursing interventions: Iowa Intervention Project. Nursing Economics 19(4):146–160, 2001.

Fawcett J: Analysis and Evaluation of Conceptual Models of Nursing. Philadelphia, FA Davis, 1989.

Fawcett J: Scholarly dialogue. The nurse theorists: 21st-century update: Rosemarie Rizzo Parse. Nursing Science Quarterly 14(2):126–131, 2001.

More than one million new nurses needed by 2010. American Nurse 34(1):5, 2002.

Narayan MC, et al.: Searching for nursing's future? Nursing Management 33(1):26–30, 2002.

Nightingale F: Notes on Nursing: What It Is and What It Is Not. London, Harrison, 1859 (Reprinted by JB Lippincott, Philadelphia, 1966).

Nursing shortage puts patients at risk and creates liability problems. Health Care Risk Management 23(6):61–65, 2002.

O'Connor NA, et al.: Documenting patterns of nursing interventions using cluster analysis. Journal of Nursing Measurement 9(1):73–90, 2001.

Parse RR: Man-Living-Health: Theory of Nursing. Philadelphia, John Wiley, 1987.

Pontious JM: Where have all the nurses gone? Oklahoma Nurse 47(1):1, 18, 2002.

SREB study indicates serious shortage of nursing faculty. Council On Collegiate Education for Nurses, 2002.

Stafford J: Nursing students turned away: Faculty shortage limits enrollment nationwide. The Oklahoman, 2B, August 25, 2005.

Chapter 5

Bellack JP, O'Neil EH: Recreating nursing practice for a new century: Recommendations and implications of the Pew Health Professions Commission's Final Report. Nursing and Health Care Perspectives 21(1):14–21, 2002.

Bosher S: Linguistic bias in multiple-choice nursing exams. Nursing Education Perspectives 24(1):15–34, 2003.

Brady M, et al.: A proposed framework for differentiating the 21 Pew competencies by level of nursing education. Nursing and Health Care Perspectives 22(1):30–35, 2002.

Callister S, et al.: Inquiry in baccalaureate nursing education: Fostering evidence-based practice. Nursing Educator 44(2):59–65, 2005.

Emerson R, Records K: Nursing profession in peril. Journal of Professional Nursing 21(1):5–9, 2005.

Felton G, et al.: How does NLNAC support the Pew Health Commission Competencies? Nursing and Health Care Perspectives 21(1):53, 2000.

Ferguson L, Day R: Evidence-based nursing education: Myth or reality? Nursing Education 44(3):107–116, 2005.

Fondiller SH: The advancement of baccalaureate and graduate nursing education 1952–1972. Nursing and Health Care Perspectives 21(1):10–13, 2002.

Freeman LH, et al.: New curriculum for a new century. Nursing Education 41(1):38–40, 2002.

Hoffman L, et al.: Outcomes of care managed by an acute care nurse practitioner vs attending physician team in a subacute medical intensive care unit. American Journal of Critical Care 14(2):121–130, 2005.

Jeffries P: Technology trends in nursing education: Next steps. Nursing Education 44(3):3–5, 2005.

Katz T, et al.: Essential qualifications for nursing students. Nursing Outlook 52(6):277–289, 2004.

Long K: Preparing nurses for the 21st century: Re-envisioning nursing education and practice. Journal of Professional Nursing 20(2):1–4, 2004.

Manojlovich M: Predictors of professional practice behaviors in hospital settings. Nursing Research 54(1):41–47, 2005.

Medley C, Home C: Using simulation technology for undergraduate nursing education. Nursing Education (44):131–135, 2005.

Miller J, et al.: A study of personal digital assistants to enhance undergraduate clinical nursing education. Nursing Education 44(1):19–27, 2005.

Rosenstein A, O'Daniel M: Disruptive behavior & clinical outcomes. Nursing Management 36(1):18–28, 2005.

Stewart S, Dempsey L: A longitudinal study of baccalaureate nursing student's critical thinking dispositions. Nursing Education 44(2):81–85 2005.

Study looks at impact of nurses' education level. American Nurse 35(6):5–6, 2005.

Chapter 6

Ali N, et al.: Validation of critical thinking skills in online responses. Nursing Education 44(2):90–95, 2005.

Allen G, et al.: Reliability of assessment of critical thinking. Journal of Professional Nursing 20(1):15–23, 2004.

Anderson K: Teaching cultural competencies using an exemplar from literal journalism. Nursing Education 43(6):254–260, 2004.

Case J, et al.: A qualitative tool for critical thinking skill development. Nurse Educator 29(4):147–152, 2004.

Daily WM: The development of an alternative method in the assessment of critical thinking as an outcome of nursing education. Journal of Advanced Nursing 36(1):120–130, 2001.

Distler JW: Critical thinking and clinical competence: Results of the implementation of student-centered teaching strategies in an advanced practice nurse curriculum. Nurse Education in Practice 7(1):53–59, 2007.

Eisenhauer LA: Nurses' reported thinking during medication administration. Journal of Nursing Scholarship 39(1):82–87, 2007.

Giddens J, Gloeckner G: The relationship of critical thinking to performance on NCLEX. Nursing Education 44(2):85–90, 2005.

Martin C: The theory of critical thinking of nursing. Nursing Education Perspectives 23(5):243–247, 2002.

Maslow AH: Motivation and Personality. New York, Harper & Row, 1971.

Nokes K, et al.: Does service-learning increase cultural competency, critical thinking and civil engagement? Nursing Education 44(2):65–71, 2005.

Shin KR: Critical thinking dispositions in baccalaureate nursing students. Journal of Advanced Nursing 56(2):182–189, 2006.

Smith Q: 5 Competencies needed by new baccalaureate graduates. Nursing Education Perspectives 25(4):166–175, 2004.

Suliman WA: Critical thinking, self-esteem, and state anxiety of nursing students. Nurse Education Today 27(2):162–168, 2007.

Tanner C: What have we learned about critical thinking in nursing? Nursing Education 44(2):47–49, 2005.

Twibeil R, et al.: Faculty perceptions of critical thinking in student clinical experience. Nursing Education 44(2):271–281, 2005.

Winningham ML, Preusser BA: Critical Thinking in Medical-Surgical Settings. St. Louis, Mosby, 2001.

Chapter 7

Chaloner C: An introduction to ethics in nursing. Nursing Standard 21(32):42–46, 2007.

Day L: Foundations of clinical ethics: Disengaged rationalism and internal goods. American Journal of Critical Care 16(2):79–183, 2007.

DePalo V, et al.: Do-not-resuscitate and stratification-of-care forms in Rhode Island. American Journal of Critical Care 12(3):239–241, 2003.

Engelhardt HT, Cherry MJ: Allocating Scarce Resources. Baltimore, Georgetown University Press, 2002.

Erlen J: HIPAA: Clinical and ethical considerations for nurses. Orthopedic Nursing 23(6):410–413, 2004.

Erlen JA: Patient safety, error reduction, and ethical practice. Orthopaedic Nursing 26(2):130–133, 2007.

Irving JA, Sniper J: Preserving professional ethics. Journal of Professional Nursing 18(1):5, 2002.

Kennedy W: Beneficence and autonomy in nursing: A moral dilemma. British Journal of Perioperative Nursing 14(11):500–506, 2004.

Mathes M: Ethics, law, and policy: Ethical decision making and nursing. Medical Surgical Nursing 13(6):429–431, 2004.

Memarian R: Professional ethics as an important factor in clinical competency in nursing. Nursing Ethics 14(2):203–214.

Milton C: Ethical issues: The ethics of respect in nursing. Nursing Science Quarterly 18(1):20–23, 2005.

Oxtoby K: Consent: Obtaining permission to care. Nursing Times 101(1):22–24, 2005.

Quinn S: Health policy and ethics forum. Ethics in public health research: Protecting human subjects. The role of community advisory boards. American Journal of Public Health 94(6):918–922, 2004.

Racher FE: The evolution of ethics for community practice. Journal of Community Health Nursing 24(1):65–76, 2007.

Chapter 8

Berger J: Ethical challenges of partial do-not-resuscitate (DNR) orders: Placing DNR orders in the context of a life-threatening conditions care plan. Archives of Internal Medicine 163(19):2270–2275, 2003.

Clendinen D: "My father wasn't there." The care of Terri Schiavo has universal and personal resonance. The New York Times, October 26, 2003, 12.

Conley YP: The future of genomic nursing research. Journal of Nursing Scholarship 39(1):17–24, 2007.

Conway A: Ethical issues in the neonatal intensive care unit. Critical Care Nursing Clinics of North America 16(2):271–278, 2004.

Duke G: Knowledge, attitudes and practices of nursing personnel regarding advance directives. International Journal of Palliative Nursing 13(3):109–115, 2007.

Engelhardt HT, Cherry MJ: Allocating Scarce Resources. Baltimore, Georgetown University Press, 2002.

Ewing A, Catlin A: Pediatric ethics, issues, & commentary. Pediatric Nursing 30(6):471–472, 2004.

Fontanarosa P: Controversies: Surrogate consent for living related organ donation. JAMA 291(6):728–731, 2004.

Gallagher A: Terminal sedation: Promoting ethical nursing practice. Art and science ethical decision-making. Nursing Standard 21(34):42–46, 2007.

Grace P: Patient safety and the limits of confidentiality. American Journal of Nursing 104(11):33–37, 2004.

Jenkins J: Ethical implications of genetic information. Online Journal of Issues in Nursing February 9, 2001.

Heller BR: 10 Trends to watch. Health Care Perspectives 24(1):9–14, 2002.

Horner S: Ethics and genetics: Implications for CNS practice. Clinical Nurse Specialist 18(5):228–231, 2004.

Husted G: When is a health care system not an ethical health care system? Suspending the do-not-resuscitate order in the operating room. Critical Care Nursing Clinics of North America 12(2):157–163, 2004.

Jenkins J: Establishing the essential nursing competencies for genetics and genomics. Journal of Nursing Scholarship 39(1):10–16, 2007.

Koppelman E: The dead donor rule and the concept of death: Severing the ties that bind them. American Journal of Bioethics 3(1):1–9, 2003.

McNeil D: Vegetative or minimally conscious? The New York Times, October 26, 2003.

Murphy P: Ethics in practice: How to avoid DNR miscommunications. Nursing Management 38(3):17, 20, 2007.

Offit K, Gostin L: Health law and ethics: The "duty to warn" a patient's family members about hereditary disease risks. JAMA 292(12):1469–1473, 2004.

Paul R, Elder L: Ethical Reasoning. The Foundation for Critical Thinking, 2003. Available at: http://www.crticalthinking.org.

Rushton C, Ferrell B: Ethics and palliative care in pediatrics: When should parents agree to withdraw life-sustaining therapy for children? American Journal of Nursing 104(4):54–64, 2004.

Saria MG: Hematopoietic stem cell transplantation: Implications for critical care nurses. Clinical Journal of Oncology Nursing 11(1):53–63, 130–134, 2007.

Tissue-tracking requirements: Putting all the pieces together. Operating Room Manager 23(2):1, 15–17, 2007.

Chapter 9

Austin S: Legal checkpoints: Respect the scope of your license and practice. Nurse Manager 35(12):18, 20, 2004.

Berntsen K: Looking beyond tort reform toward safer healthcare systems. Journal of Nursing Care Quality 20(1):9–12, 2005.

Brown P: Not documented! Not done! New focus on healthcare quality makes documentation critical. ASBN Update 8(1):7, 27, 2004.

Cogar S: The legal nurse consultant's role in defending law enforcement officers. Journal of Legal Nurse Consultant 15(1):3–6, 2004.

Croke E: Nurses, negligence and malpractice. American Journal of Nursing 103(9):54–63, 2003.

Future looks bleak as malpractice premiums continue upward spiral. Healthcare Risk Management 24(1):1–4, 2002.

Goode A: Schiavo case should prompt discussion about healthcare wishes. Oklahoma City Nursing Times 43(4):15, 2003.

Gosciminski L: Point of view: How to avoid a lawsuit. Nursing Spectrum 16(15):3, 2004.

Grace P: Patient safety and the limits of confidentiality. American Journal of Nursing 104(11):33–37 2004.

Griffith R: Living wills, duty of care and the right to treatment. British Journal of Community Nursing 9(11):488–491, 2004.

Klein C: Legal file: The great malpractice debate. Nurse Practitioner 29(9):53, 2004.

Menikoff J: Law and Bioethics. Baltimore, Georgetown University Press, 2002.

Salladay S: Ethical problems. Confidentiality: Disguised as a family member. Nursing 2004 34(12):28, 2004.

Skyrocketing malpractice premiums hamper access to care. OR Manager 20(7):16, 2004.

Sullivan E: Issues of informed consent in the geriatric population. Journal of Perianesthesia Nursing 19(6):430–432, 2004.

Reising DL, Allen PN: Protecting yourself from malpractice claims. American Nurse Today 2(2):39–44, 2007.

Yeo T, Edmunds M: Advocacy in practice: What to expect from medical liability tort reform. Nurse Practitioner 29(5):7, 2004.

Chapter 10

Billings DM: Seven steps for test-taking success. American Journal of Nursing 107(4):72, 2007.

Christiaens G: Strategies for coping with test anxiety. Imprint 51(4):68–69, 2004.

Hickey B: Help! I failed my first nursing exam! American Nursing Student 8(6):2, 2007.

Howland J, et al.: The effects of binge drinking on college students' next-day academic test-taking performance and mood state. Addiction 105(4):655–665, 2010.

King N: How to prepare for the certification examination. Insight 29(2):26, 2004.

Ludwig C: Preparing for certification: Test-taking strategies. Medical Surgical Nursing 13(2):127–128, 2004.

McDonald M: NLN Assessment and Evaluation Division: Review Guide to RN Pre-Entrance Exam (2nd ed). Boston, Jones & Bartlett, 2004.

Nugent PM, Vitale BA: Test Success: Test-Taking Techniques for Beginning Nursing Students (5th ed). Philadelphia, FA Davis, 2008.

Rollant PD: "How can I fail the NCLEX-RN with a 3.5 GPA?": Approaches to help this unexpected high-risk group. Annual Review of Nursing Education 14(5):259–273, 2007.

Smith K: Lifelong learning, professional development, and informatics certification. Computer Informatics Nursing 22(3):172–178, 2004.

Street P Hamilton L: Preparing to take objective structured clinical examinations. Nursing Standard 24(34):35–39, 2010.

Chapter 11

Crow C: Requirements and interventions used by BSN programs to promote and predict NCLEX-RN success: A national study. Journal of Professional Nursing 20(3):174–186, 2004.

Cunningham H: Strategies to promote success on the NCLEX-RN for students with English as a second language. Nurse Educator 29(1):15–19, 2004.

Davenport NC: A comprehensive approach to NCLEX-RN success. Nursing Education Perspectives 28(1):30–33, 2007.

Etheridge SA: Learning to think like a nurse: Stories from new nurse graduates. Journal of Continuing Education in Nursing 38(1):24–30, 2007.

Miller J: Tips on taking the NCLEX-RN. Imprint 52(1):28–30, 32, 2005.

Norton CK: Ensuring NCLEX-RN success for first-time test-takers. Journal of Professional Nursing 22(5):322–326, 2006.

Spalla TL: Technology. You've got mail: A new tool to help Millennials prepare for the National Council Licensure Examination. Nurse Educator 32(2):52–54, 2007.

Uyehara J: Facilitating program and NCLEX-RN success in a generic BSN program. Nursing Forum 42(1):31–38, 2007.

Wendt A: Setting the passing standard for the National Council Licensure Examination for registered nurses. Nurse Educator 32(3):104–148, 2007.

Chapter 12

Bartram T: Factors affecting the job stress and job satisfaction of Australian nurses: Implications for recruitment and retention. Contemporary Nurse 17(3):293–304, 2004.

Bruce TJ: Online tutors as a solution to the shortage of nurse practitioner educators. Nurse Educator 32(3):122–125, 2007.

Browning L: Nursing specialty and burnout. Health and Medicine 12(2):248–254, 2007

Buerhaus PI: Impact of the nurse shortage on hospital patient care: Comparative perspectives. Health Affairs 26(3):853–862, 2007.

Chatterjee M: Nursing staff shortages are putting patients in danger. Nursing Times 100(45):4, 2004.

Cockerell P: Applicant's secrets are few in internet age. Daily Oklahoman 115:6D–7D, November 27, 2006.

Cockerell P: Business cards out: Icons, thlogs are in. Daily Oklahoman 115:1A, 6A, November 27, 2006.

Cohen-Katz J: The effects of mindfulness-based stress reduction on nurse stress and burnout: A quantitative and qualitative study. Holistic Nursing Practice 18(6):302–308, 2004.

Corcoran J: Learning portfolios: Evidence of learning: An examination of students' perspectives. Nursing in Critical Care 9(5):230–237, 2004.

Endacott R: Using portfolios in the assessment of learning and competence: The impact of four models. Nurse Educational Practices 4(4):250–257, 2004.

Jenkins R: Stressors, burnout and social support: Nurses in acute mental health settings. Journal of Advanced Nursing 48(6):622–631, 2004.

Jones JM: ePortfolios in nursing education: Not your mother's resume. Annual Review of Nursing Education 13(50): 245–258, 2007.

Leichtling B: Leadership & management: Preventive medicine for "compassion [sic] fatigue." Caring 23(10):90–91, 2004.

Lemin-Stone K: Careers: Learn to manage your stress levels. Nursing Times 100(46):74–75, 2004.

Lewis L: Uniting States, sharing strategies: Oregon takes the lead in addressing the nursing shortage. American Journal of Nursing 110 (3):51–54, 2010.

Lipley N: How many staff is enough? Emergency Nurse 12(7):5, 2004.

Lupoli J: The impact of technology on the "older" nurse. Home Health Nurse 22(10):668–670, 2004.

Mennick F, Kennedy MS: In the news: Good news, bad news on the nursing shortage: Nursing school enrollment continues to rise, but who will teach them? American Journal of Nursing 107(4):22, 2007.

National survey: RNs struggle to balance work and home life. Nursing 36(12):33, 2006.

O'Dowd A: Global nurse shortages are "staggering." Nursing Times 100(46):5, 2004.

Raiger J: Applying a cultural lens to the concept of burnout. Journal of Transcultural Nursing 16(1):71–76, 2005.

Sanner T: Using telehealth to address the nursing shortage. Home Health Nurse 22(10):695–702, 2004.

Santucci J: Facilitating the transition into nursing practice: Concepts and strategies for mentoring new graduates. Journal of Nurses Staff Development 20(6):274–284, 2004.

Schaffer M, et al.: Using portfolios to evaluate achievement of population-based public health nursing competencies in baccalaureate nursing students. Nursing Education Perspectives 26(2):104–112, 2005.

Vinje HF: Job engagement's paradoxical role in nurse burnout. Nursing & Health Sciences 9(2):107–111, 2007.

Chapter 13

Bliss J: Effective team management by district nurses. British Journal of Community Nursing 9(12):524–526, 2004.

Bradley E: Translating research into clinical practice: Making change happen. Journal of the American Geriatric Society 52(11):1875–1882, 2004.

Grossman SC, Valiga TM: The New Leadership Challenge: Creating the Future of Nursing (2nd ed). Philadelphia, FA Davis, 2005.

Hertzberg F, et al.: The Motivation to Work. New York, Wiley, 1959.

Isaacson J: Nursing students in an expanded charge nurse role: A real clinical management experience. Nursing Education Perspectives 25(6):292–296, 2004.

Jeong S: Innovative leadership and management in a nursing home. Journal of Nursing Management 12(6):445–451, 2004.

Kuzmits F: 360-Feedback in health-care management: A field study. Health Care Manager 23(4):321–328, 2004.

Leichtling B: Leadership & management. Preventive medicine for "compassion [sic] fatigue." Caring 23(10):90–91, 2004.

Owens J, Patton J: Take a chance on nursing mentorships: Enhance leadership with this win–win strategy. Nursing Education Perspectives 24(4):198–204, 2005.

Patronis Jones RA: Nursing Leadership and Management. Philadelphia, FA Davis, 2007.

Patterson P: A few simple rules for managing block time in the operating room. Operating Room Manager 20(11):1, 9–12, 2004.

Robotham M: How to handle complaints. Nursing Times 97(30): 5–28, 2001.

Sanford K: Become competent in confrontation. Nursing Management 35(7):14, 2004.

Simons J, et al.: Psychology: The Search for Understanding. New York, West Publishing, 1987.

Tracy B: What makes a good leader. The Oklahoman Jan 9, 2005, 1H.

Vestal K: Lessons learned: Making time for leadership. Nurse Leader 2(6):8–9, 2004.

West B: Evaluation of a clinical leadership initiative. Nursing Standard 19(5):33–41, 2004.

Chapter 14

Banks C: Careers: Improving your communication skills. Nursing Times 101(3):48–49, 2005.

Callister L: Toward evidence-based practice: How delivery ward staff exercise power over women in communication. MCN 30(1):70, 2005.

Cole A: Reaping the benefits of teamwork. Nursing Times 101(1):59, 2005.

Dunham K, Smith S: How to survive and maybe even love your life as a nurse. Philadelphia, FA Davis, 2005.

Grossman SC, Valiga TM: The New Leadership Challenge: Creating the Future of Nursing (2nd ed). Philadelphia, FA Davis, 2005.

McGrath JM: The influence of electronic medical record usage on nonverbal communication in the medical interview. Health Informatics Journal 13(2):105–118, 2007.

McHarg L: Starting out: Good communication skills can have a magical effect. Nursing Times 103(22):13, 2007.

Patronis Jones, RA: Nursing Leadership and Management. Philadelphia, FA Davis, 2007.

Pearce C: Leadership resource. Ten steps to managing change. Nursing Management 13(10):25, 2007.

Raiger J: Applying a cultural lens to the concept of burnout. Journal of Transcultural Nursing 16(1):71–76, 2005.

Stone JH: Communication between physicians and patients in the era of e-medicine. New England Journal of Medicine 356(24):2451–2454, 2007.

Tappen RM: Essentials of Nursing Leadership and Management (4th ed). Philadelphia, FA Davis, 2006.

Windsor K: Managing conflict: Get rid of the baggage. Advance for Nurses 15–16, 2006.

Chapter 16

American Nurses Association: Policy Series: Regulation of Unlicensed Assistive Personnel. Washington, DC, Author, 1996.

Creighton H: Law Every Nurse Should Know (5th ed). Philadelphia, WB Saunders, 1986.

Curtis E: Delegation: A key function of nursing. Nurse Manager 11(4):26–31, 2004.

Fisher M: Do you have delegation savvy? Nursing 2000 30(12): 58–59, 2000.

Garvis M: Advice of counsel: When it's OK for an RN to delegate. RN 66(12):70–71, 2003.

Guitard V: Ask a practice advisor. Assigning vs delegating: Is there a difference in nursing care? Informatics Nursing 38(1):12, 21, 2007.

Henderson L: Nursing delegation. Pulse 41(2):1, 4, 2004.

Hudspeth R: Understanding delegation is a critical competency for nurses in the new millennium. Nursing Administration Quarterly 31(2):183–184, 2007.

Khaliullah K: Professional misconduct: Nurse who compromised patient care through delegating a task. British Journal of Nursing 13(11):668, 2004.

Pearce C: Careers: Honing the art of effective delegation. Nursing Times 100(29):46–47, 2004.

Safe Staffing Saves Lives. Available at: http://www.safestaffingsaveslives.org/WhatisSafeStaffing/SafeStaffing/Principles/Prir.

Tappen RM: Nursing Leadership and Management (4th ed). Philadelphia, FA Davis, 2001.

Tappen RM, et al.: Essentials of Nursing Leadership and Management (2nd ed). Philadelphia, FA Davis, 2001.

Teasdale K: Tips for the top: Better delegation. Professional Nursing 19(12):56, 2004.

Wheeler J: How to delegate your way to a better working life. Nursing Times 97(36):34–35, 2001

Williams J: Navigating the difficulties of delegation. Nursing 34(9):32, 2004.

Chapter 17

Adler J: The past as prologue? A brief history of the labor movement in the United States. Public Personnel Management 5(4):311–329, 2006.

ANA rejects NLRB decision to block nurses' freedom to unionize. Nursing News 31(1):11, 2007.

Budd K: Traditional and non-traditional collective bargaining: Strategies to improve the patient care environment. Online Journal Issues in Nursing 9(1):1–6, 2004.

Briles J: Zapping conflict in the health care workplace. The Oklahoma Nurse 49(2):23, 2004.

Cardillo D: End workplace abuse. Future nurse, nursing spectrum. Nurseweek Spring 40–42, 2006.

Converso A: Health and safety: Is your hospital safe? American Journal of Nursing 107(2):37–39, 2007.

Cross LL: Protected whistle-blowing or a legal firing? Oklahoma Nurse 47(1):14–16, 2002.

Curtin L: Ethics in management: case study: A showdown over overtime. Journal of Clinical Systems Management 6(5–6):14, 2004.

DeMass-Martin S: Striking nurses win from coast to coast. American Nurse 34(2):8–10, 2002.

Esposito N, et al.: Preventing violence in an academic setting. Nursing Education Perspectives 26(1):24–28, 2005.

Gordon S: Collective thinking. Nurse Manager 11(2):8, 2004.

Green A: Common denominators: Shared governance and work place advocacy—strategies for nurses to gain control over their practice. Online Journal Issues in Nursing 9(1):1–7, 2004.

McKeown C, Thompson J: Clinical governance: Implementing clinical supervision. Nursing Management 8(6):10–13, 2001.

Kennedy MS, et al.: To supervise or unionize? That is the question: A Supreme Court ruling may limit nurses' ability to form unions. American Journal of Nursing 101(8):21, 2001.

New plan for bargaining: Union adapts to changed IR system. Lamp 64(1):29, 2007.

Oregon nurses strike for pay, health care. American Nurse 34(1): 7, 2002.

Radebe E: Can nursing be unionized? Nursing Update 31(1): 24–25, 2007.

Rigiero D: Empowering nurses to raise their voices in unity. Massachusetts Nurse 75(3):1, 3, 2004.

Roman LM: Professional update: NLRB finally rules on nurses' supervisory status. RN 69(11):12, 2006.

Sanford K: Become competent in confrontation. Nursing Management 35(7):14, 2004.

Snow T: Biggest private NHS providers do not negotiate with unions. Nursing Standard 21(19):7, 2007.

Trossman S: Illinois nurse loses job for helping Sept. 11 victims. American Nurse 34(1):1–2, 2002.

Chapter 18

Bradford N: Commissioning Ideas: Canadian National Policy Innovation in Comparative Perspective. Toronto, Oxford University Press, 1998.

Brittain B: Who is being accountable for the well-being of the patient? Hospital Quarterly 1(2):56–58, 1998.

Dwivedi O, Gow J: From Bureaucracy To Public Management: The Administrative Culture of the Government of Canada. Toronto, Broadview Press, 1999.

Evans R: Going for the gold: The redistributive agenda behind market-based health reform. Journal of Health, Politics, and Policy Law 22(2):426–465, 1999.

Kernaghan K, Langford W: The Responsible Public Servant. Montreal, Institute for Research on Public Policy, 1999.

Singer P, Mapa J: Ethics resource allocation: Dimensions for healthcare executives. Hospital Quarterly 1(4):29–31, 1998.

Chapter 19

American Nurses Association: Scope and Standards of Nursing Informatics Practice. Washington, DC, Author, 2001.

Bartholomew K: High-tech, high-touch: Why wait? Nurse Manager 35(9):48, 50–54, 2004.

Curran C: The informatics nurse: Helping to build the knowledge infrastructure for nursing. Nurse Leader 2(3):26–29, 2004.

Englebardt S, Nelson R (eds): Health Care Informatics: An Inter-disciplinary Approach. St. Louis, Mosby, 2002.

Nicoll LH: Nurses' Guide to the Internet (3rd ed). Philadelphia, Lippincott, 2001.

Puskar K: Implementing information technology in a behavioral health setting. Issues in Mental Health Nursing 25(5):439–450, 2004.

Roscoe T: An assessment tool for medical informatics skills. Health Information Journal 10(2):155–159, 2004.

Shifman M: Exploring the portability of informatics capabilities from a clinical application to a bioscience application. Journal of American Medical Information Association 11(4):294–299, 2004.

Young KM: Informatics for Healthcare Professionals. Philadelphia, FA Davis, 2000.

Chapter 20

Brewer C, Kovner CT: Is there another nursing shortage? What the data tell us. Nursing Outlook 49(1):20–26, 2001.

Burke RJ: The ripple effect: Staffing post restructuring. Nursing Management 33(2):41–43, 2002.

Carlson ED: Welfare reform: Policy implications for health. Texas Journal of Rural Health 19(2):42–48, 2001.

Clemons T: Highlights from the Hill: NIWI 2000: Issues and opportunities. ORL—Head and Neck Nursing 19(2):22–23, 2001.

Des Jardin K: Political involvement in nursing: Politics, ethics, and strategic action. AORN Journal 74(5):614–618, 2001.

Frank IC: Policy perspectives: The nursing shortage. Journal of Emergency Nursing 27(4):391–393, 2001.

Higgs ZR, et al.: Health care access: A consumer perspective. Public Health Nursing 18(1):3–12, 2001.

Malone B: Making nursing's presence felt at the political party conferences. Nursing Standard 16(5):22, 2001.

O'Grady ET: Health policy and politics. Access to health care: An issue central to nursing. Nursing Economics 18(2):88–90, 2001.

Rains JW, Barton-Kriese P: Developing political competence. Public Health Nursing 18(4):219–224, 2001.

Roit SM: When money talks, politicians listen. American Nurse 34(1):22, 2002.

Chapter 21

Brillhart B: A study of spirituality and life satisfaction among persons with spinal cord injury. Rehabilitation Nurse 30(1):31–34, 2005.

Chesnay M: Caring for the Vulnerable: Perspectives in Nursing Theory, Practice and Research. Boston, Jones & Bartlett, 2005.

Dameron C: Spiritual assessment made easy ... with acronyms! Journal of Christian Nursing 22(1):14–16, 2005.

Leininger M: Culture Care Diversity & Universality: A Worldwide Nursing Theory. Boston, Jones & Bartlett, 2005.

McSherry W: Meaning of spirituality: Implications for nursing practice. Journal of Clinical Nursing 13(8):934–941, 2004.

Ollier C: Spirituality in nursing: An idea whose time has returned? Patient Care Staff Representative 4(12):4–5, 2004.

O'Brien M. Spirituality in Nursing: Standing on Holy Ground. Boston, Jones & Bartlett, 2008.

O'Mathna DP, Quiring-Emblen JD: Making sense of complementary and alternative therapies. Journal of Christian Nursing 18(4):8–15, 2001.

Pesut B: Developing spirituality in the curriculum. Nursing Education Perspective 24(6):290–294, 2003.

Sethness R: Cardiac health: Relationships among hostility, spirituality, and health risk. Journal of Nursing Care Quarterly 20(1):81–90, 2005.

Wisnefske K: The joy of parish nursing. Nursing Matters 15(12):3, 9, 2004.

Chapter 22

Anderson K: Teaching cultural competence using an exemplar from literal journalism. Nursing Education 43(6):253–260, 2004.

Aroian K: Effective, efficient and equitable health care: What can cultural diversity teach us about sacred cows. Journal of Professional Nursing 20(6):349–351, 2005.

Batnardi M, Perkel L: Learning achievement programs: Fostering student cultural diversity. Nurse Educator 30(1):17–21, 2005.

Brenman S: Cultural immersion through ethnography: The lived experience and group process. Journal of Nursing Education 43(6):285–288, 2004.

Briesacher B, et al.: Racial and ethnic disparities in prescription coverage and medication use. Health Care Finance 25(2): 63–76, 2004.

Carol R: Overcoming bias in the nursing workplace. Minority Nurse Winter, 28–33, 2005.

Carter M: The ABCs of staffing decisions. Nursing Management 36(6):16, 2004.

De Chesnay M: Caring for the Vulnerable: Perspective in Nursing Theory, Practice and Research. Boson, Jones & Bartlett, 2005.

Flowers D: Culturally competent nursing care: A challenge for the 21st century. Critical Care Nurse 24(4):46–50, 2004.

Hascup VA: Nursing out cultural stew. Advance for Nurses. 2006. Available at: http://www.advanceweb.com.

Health care disparities continue among minorities, the poor says HHS. Medical Ethics Advisor 20(2):13–16, 2004.

Johnson L: The role of cultural competency in eliminating health disparities. Minority Nurse Winter, 52–55, 2005.

Leininger M: Culture Care Diversity & Universality: A Worldwide Nursing Theory (2nd ed). Boston, Jones & Bartlett, 2005.

Leishman J: Perspectives of cultural competence in health care. Nursing Standard 19(11):33, 2004.

Linnard-Palmer L: Parents' refusal of medical treatment for cultural or religious beliefs: An ethnographic study of health care professionals' experiences. Journal of Pediatric Oncology Nursing 22(1):48–57, 2005.

Marquand B: Till death do us part. Minority Nurse Summer, 22–26, 2007.

Marquand B: On the case. Minority Nurse Winter, 34–38, 2005.

Nokes K, et al.: Does service learning increase cultural competency, critical thinking and civil engagement? Nursing Education 44(2):65–71, 2005.

Purnell LD, Paulanka BJ: Transcultural Health Care. Philadelphia, FA Davis, 1998.

Racial/ethnic and gender diversity in nursing education. Southern Regional Education Board, Council on Collegiate Education for Nursing, 2002.

Raiger J: Applying a cultural lens to the concept of burnout. Journal of Transcultural Nursing 16(1):71–76, 2005.

Spector R: Cultural Care: Guide to Heritage Assessment and Health Traditions (3rd ed). Englewood Cliffs, NJ, Prentice Hall, 2004.

Spector R: Cultural diversity in health and illness (6th ed). Englewood Cliffs, NJ, Prentice Hall, 2004.

Terhone C: From desegregation to diversity: How far have we really come? Journal of Nursing Education 43(5):195–196, 2004.

Williams D: Recruiting men into nursing school. Minority Nurse Winter, 56–60, 2006.

Chapter 23

Bemis P: Being your own boss: It's more than just a pipe dream. Nursing Spectrum, 2004. Available at: http://news.nurse.com/apps/pbcs.dll/article?AID=2003306300339.

Berkowitz B: One year later: The impact and aftermath of September 11. Public Health Nursing Practice: Aftermath of September 11, 2001. Online Journal of Issues in Nursing 7(3), 2002.

Campbell M: Nurse entrepreneur gives new face to care. Nursing Matters 15(5):14, 22, 2004.

Chang P: The development of intelligent, triage-based, mass-gathering emergency medical service PDA support systems. Journal of Nursing Resources 12(3):227–235, 2004.

Cogar S: The legal nurse consultant's role in defending law enforcement officers. Journal of Legal Nurse Consultant 15(1):3–6, 2004.

Cox E: Disaster nursing: New frontiers for critical care. Critical Care Nurse 24(3):16–18, 20–24, 2004.

Hayward M: Facing danger. Nursing Standard 19(3):20–21, 2004.

Heitkemper M: Clinical nurse specialists: State of the profession and challenges ahead. Clinical Nurse Specialist 18(3):135–140, 2004.

Nash D, et al.: Consensus paper of the 2003 Physician and Case Management Summit: Exploring Best Practices in Physician and Case Management Collaboration to Improve Patient Care. Case Management Society of America, 2003.

Wessling S: The Case for Forensic Nursing. Minority Nurse.Com, 2003. Available at: http://www.minoritynurse.com/.

Young C: Biological, chemical, and nuclear terrorism readiness: Major concerns and preparedness of future nurses. Disaster Management Response 2(4):109–114, 2004.

Chapter 24

Beardsley E: Health, Biology, Bioethics: A History of Neglect. Knoxville, University of Tennessee Press, 1987.

Dossey B, et al.: Holistic Nursing. Boston, Jones & Bartlett, 2005.

Exit Care Patient Information System. Available at: http://www.exitcare.com.

Ferguson VC: Educating the 21st Century Nurse. New York National League for Nursing Press, 1997.

Greene M: The Dialectic of Freedom. New York, Teachers College Press, 1988.

Rankin S, et al.: Patient Education in Health and Illness. New York, Lippincott Williams & Wilkins, 2006.

Redman BK: The ethics of self-management preparation for chronic illness. Nursing Ethics 12(4):360–369, 2005.

Rogers C: Freedom to Learn. Columbus, OH, Charles E. Merrill, 1969.

Stone JH: Communication between physicians and patients in the era of e medicine. New England Journal of Medicine 345(24), 2007.

University of Minnesota Health Science Center. Available at: www.ahc.umn.edu.

Watson J: Assessing and Measuring Caring in Nursing and Health Science (p. 211). New York, Springer, 2002.

Chapter 25

Aroian K: Effective, efficient and equitable health care: What can cultural diversity teach us about sacred cows. Journal of Professional Nursing 20(6):349–351, 2005.

Ax S, Kincade E: Nursing students' perceptions of research usefulness, implementation and training. Journal of Advanced Nursing 35(2):161–170, 2001.

Brink P, Wood M: Basic Steps in Planning Nursing Research. Boston, Jones & Bartlett, 2001.

Brockopp D, Hastings-Tolsma M: Fundamentals of Nursing Research. Boston, Jones & Bartlett, 2003.

Burns N, Grove S: The practice of nursing research conduct, critique and utilization. St. Louis, Elsevier Saunders, 2005.

Callister M, et al.: Inquiry in baccalaureate nursing education: Fostering evidence-based practice. Nursing Education 44(2):59–65, 2005.

Chesnay M: Caring for the Vulnerable: Perspectives in Nursing Theory, Practice and Research. Boston, Jones & Bartlett, 2005.

Dempsey P, Dempsey A: Using Nursing Research. Philadelphia, Lippincott Williams & Wilkins, 2000.

Ellett M, et al.: Ethical and legal issues of conducting nursing research via the internet. Journal of Professional Nursing 20(1):68–72, 2004.

Ferguson L, Day R: Evidence-based nursing education: Myth or reality? Nursing Education 44(3):107–116, 2005.

Karigan M: Ethics in clinical research: The nursing perspective. American Journal of Nursing 101(9):26–31, 2001.

Katz J, et al.: Essential qualifications for nursing students. Nursing Outlook 52(6):277–289, 2004.

Larrabee J: Advancing quality improvement through using the best evidence to change practice. Journal of Nursing Care Quality 19(1):10–13, 2004.

LoBiondo-Wood G, Haber J: Nursing Research Methods, Critical Appraisal, and Utilization. St. Louis, Mosby, 2002.

Long K: Preparing nurses for the 21st century: Re-envisioning nursing education and practice. Journal of Professional Nursing 20(2):82–89, 2004.

Manojlovich M: Predictors of professional practice behaviors in hospital settings. Nursing Research 54(1):41–47, 2005.

Mitchell P: The "so what" question: The impact of nursing research. Journal of Professional Nursing 20(6):347–349, 2005.

Pare R, Elovitz L: Data warehousing: An aid to decision-making. T.H.E. Journal 43(9):32–34, 2005.

Streubert H, Carpenter D: Qualitative Research in Nursing. Philadelphia, JB Lippincott, 1995.

Szirony T, et al.: Perceptions of nursing faculty regarding ethical issues in nursing research. Nursing Education 43(6):220–280, 2004.

Chapter 26

Cassidy C: What does it mean to practice an energy medicine? Journal of Alternative and Complementary Medicine 10(1):79–81, 2004.

Dosset B: Florence Nightingale and holistic nursing. Imprint 52(2):58–60, 2005.

Honda K: Use of complementary and alternative medicine among United States adults: The influences of personality, coping strategies, and social support. Preventative Medicine 40(1): 46–53, 2005.

Huebscher R: Natural, Alternative, and Complementary Health Care Practices. St. Louis, Mosby, 2004.

Mariano C: An overview of holistic nursing. Imprint 52(2):48–52, 2005.

Savory-Posselius M: Herbology. Home Health Care Management Practice 16(6):456–463, 2004.

Stretch K: A survey of CAM approaches to obesity. Massage Today 5(1):1, 22, 2005.

Uzun O: Nursing students' opinions and knowledge about complementary and alternative medicine therapies. Complementary Therapeutic Nurse Midwifery 10(4):239–244, 2004.

Walach H: Homeopathic proving symptoms: Result of a local, non-local, or placebo process? A blinded, placebo-controlled pilot study. Homeopathy 93(4):179–185, 2004.

Weatherley-Jones E: The placebo-controlled trial as a test of complementary and alternative medicine: Observations from research experience of individualized homeopathic treatment. Homeopathy 93(4):186–189, 2004.

Yoon S: Herbal product use by African American older women. Clinical Nursing Research 13(4):271–288, 2004.

Index

A

Abortion, 142–143
Active listening, 261
ADN. *See* Associate Degree Nursing (ADN)
Advance directives, 184
Advanced practice nurses, 43–44
  education for, 101–103
    clinical nurse specialist/clinical nurse leader, 101–102
    DNP for the APRN?, 102–103
    nurse practitioner, 101
    scope of advanced practice, 102
Aggressive communication, 287
AIDS and HIV, 160
Alternate dispute forums, 181–182
  arbitration, 182
  mediation, 181–182
Alternative and complementary healing practices, 505–534
  classifying, 510–515
    Healing Matrix, 510–511, 510t
    NCCAM classification, 511–512, 512t–514t, 514–515
  comparing with conventional practices, 515–525, 515t
    energy systems, 520–521
    herbal traditions, 524–525
    holistic approach, 516–518
    natural foods, benefits of, 521–522
    placebo response, 519–520
    reductionist philosophy, 515–516
    self-care, 518
    self-healing, 518–519
    supplements, 522–524
  defining, 507
  glossary of terms for, 530–534
  overview, 505, 528
  paradox of, 525–528
    few regulatory standards, 526
    lack of validation, 525–526
  use of, 508–510
American Association of Colleges of Nursing, 45
American Nurses Association (ANA), 45–46
  position paper on education for nurses, 90–93
Arbitration, 182
Artificial conception, 146
Assault and battery, 175
Assertive communication, 283–286
Assignment versus delegation, 310–311
Associate degree nursing (ADN), 94–95
  ladder to, 97–98
  proven track record, 95
  technical orientation, 94–95
Autonomy, 125–126

B

Baccalaureate education, 95–96
  different approaches, 96
  education for a profession, 95–96
  ladder to, 98
  slow increase, 95
Beneficence, 127
Bioethical issues, 142–168
  abortion, 142–143
  client's well-being, 142
  ethics involving children, 162–166
    child abuse, 162–163
    child health care, 165
    informed consent and children, 163–165
    power of parents, 162
    safeguarding child's rights, 165–166
  euthanasia and assisted suicide, 157–160
    active euthanasia, 157
    issue of self-determination, 158–160
  fetal tissue, use of, 146–147
    growing tissue on demand, 146
    nurse's role, 147
    source of material, 146–147
  genetics and genetic research, 144–145
  HIV and AIDS, 160
    cost to society, 160
    emotional issue, 160
    nurse's own interest, 160
    right to care, 160
    right to privacy, 160
  organ transplantation, 147–151
    good of the donor, 147
    nurse's responsibility, 150–151
    selecting recipient, 148–149
    tissue and eye donation, 151
    when does death occur?, 148
    when donor is a child, 147–148
  overview, 142, 166
  right to die, 153–157
    advance directives, 154–155
    ethical difficulties of living wills, 155, 157, 158f–159f
    what is extraordinary?, 153–154
  use of scarce resources in prolonging life, 151–153
    ethics of tube feeding, 152–153
    preserving life at any cost, 152
    should care be restricted?, 153
Bioterrorism, 456–459
  acute health issue, 456–457
  early recognition, 457, 458t
  effective response, 458
  response training, 458–459

C

Canada, administration and funding of health-care delivery systems in, 348–350
Canada Health Act (CHA), 349
Care as requested, 90
Care delivery models, 268–269, 268t
    functional nursing, 268–269
    modular nursing, 269
    team nursing, 269
Case management, 12, 89–90, 455–456
    care coordinator, 455
    physicians catch up, 455–456
Certification, 41–42, 44
    individual certification, 42
    more significant role, 44
    organizational certification, 42
    varying standards, 42, 44
CHA (Canada Health Act), 349
Children
    child abuse, 162–163
        nurses legally protected for reporting, 161
    ethics involving, 162–166
    health care, 165
    informed consent and children, 163–165
    power of parents, 162
    safeguarding child's rights, 165–166
    spiritual tradition in nursing, 420
Civil law, 171
Client abandonment, 176
Client education, 467–483
    caring relationships matter, 472, 472t, 474t
    client teaching implications for nursing education, 472, 474–477, 474f–475f, 476t
    ethical considerations of health self-management, 468
    ethical considerations of "nurse, heal thyself," 468–469
    health promotion for our time, 472
    implications of technology, 469–471
        electronic records, 374–376, 469–470, 469t
        Internet, working with, 470
        using technology in teaching, 470–471, 471t
    managed care, 469
    nuts and bolts of client teaching, 477–482, 479t, 481t–482t
    overview, 467–468, 482
Clinical nurse specialist/clinical nurse leader, 12, 101–102
Closed systems, 60
Code of Ethics for Nurses, 9, 135–137, 500
Common law, 170
Communicating successfully, 274–296
    civility, 298
    communication styles, 282–287
        aggressive communication, 287
        assertive communication, 283–286
        nonassertive communication, 286–287
        submissive communication, 286–287
    competition, 280
    conflict management, 289–291
        conflict on the job, 289
        improved communication skills, 290–291
        resolution techniques, 290
    development of coping skills, 291–294
        avoid personal attacks, 292
        building on existing skills, 291–292
        establishing trust, 293
        the exchange, 293–294
        ignore trivia, 293
        listen actively, 292–293
        setting the stage, 293

    difficult people, 291
        identifying the people, 291
        identifying the problem, 291
    diversity, 287–289
        building on differences, 287–288
        focus on strength, 288
    factors that affect communication, 274–279
        anger, 278–279
        change, 274–276
        stress, 276, 278
    group dynamics, 279–280
        going against the group, 279–280
        unwritten rules, 279
    lawsuits, preventing, 186–187
    non-English-speaking clients, guidelines for, 442
    nurse as communicator, 274
    overview, 274, 294
    problem solving, 289
    understanding communication, 281–282
        encoding and decoding, 281–282
        verbal and nonverbal, 282
    working environment, 280–281
        active involvement in change, 281
        coping with difficult behavior, 281
Community health centers, 358
Comparative effectiveness research, 495, 497
Comparative negligence, 180
Competencies for nursing skills, 73t–82t
Complementary healing practices. *See* Alternative and complementary healing practices
Compulsory licensure, 96–97
Confidentiality, 177–178
Conflict management, 289–291
    conflict on the job, 289
    improved communication skills, 290–291
    resolution techniques, 285, 290
Consumer in authority, 90
Continuous quality improvement, 351–354
Contracts, 334–335
    mediation and arbitration, 335
    negotiation, 334–335
    prospect of a strike, 335
    ratifying, 335
Contributory negligence, 180
Coping skills, development of, 291–294
    avoid personal attacks, 292
    building on existing skills, 291–292
    establishing trust, 293
    the exchange, 293–294
    ignore trivia, 293
    listen actively, 292–293
    setting the stage, 293
Cover letters, 239–240
Criminal law, 170–171
Crisis intervention, 250
Critical thinking, 109–120, 261
    characteristics of, 110–114
        action orientation, 113–114
        challenging custom, 112–113
        creativity, 110
        free of bias and prejudice, 113
        independence, 112
        logical, rational, reflective, 111–112
    critical thinking skills, 114–116
        challenging assumptions and rituals, 115–116
        gather pertinent data, 114–115
        identify the problem, 114

imagine and explore alternatives creatively, 116
    values in context, 114–115
in decision-making, 116
decision process, 109–110
    art of thinking, 109–110
    definitions, 110
overview, 109–110, 117
Cultural diversity, 287–289, 430–449
    culture, 430–432
    developing cultural awareness, 434–435,
        437–438, 441
        assessing culture, 437–438, 441
        awareness begins at home, 434–435
        cultural belief systems, 435
        cultural values, 435, 437
        recognizing health-care practices, 437
    diversity, 432
    information sources, 448
    looking deeper, 446
    melting pot versus salad bowl, 432–433
        cultural relativism, 433
        heritage consistency, 433
        multiculturalism, 432–433
    overview, 430, 449
    providing culturally competent care
        441-446
        transcultural communication, 441–446
        transcultural understanding, 441
    transcultural nursing, 430
    U.S. ethnic population trends, 433–434
        need for transcultural nursing, 434
Current nursing practice developments. *See* Developments in
    current nursing practice

D

Day-care centers, 360
Decentralized care, 234
Decision process, 109–110
    art of thinking, 109–110
    definitions, 110
Decompression time, 253
Defamation of character, 176–177
Delegation in nursing, 310–321
    delegation versus assignment, 310–311
    developing delegation skills, 316
        careful supervision, 316
        clear communication, 316
        simulation exercises
    essential skill, 310
    legal issues, 316–317
    overview, 310, 320
    responsibility and accountability in delegating, 311–313
        guidelines for delegation, 311–313
    who can legally delegate, 317–319
        delegation and the NCLEX, 318
        direct and indirect delegation, 318
        ethical obligation, 317–318, 319f
Deontology, 134–135
Developments in current nursing practice, 450–466
    bioterrorism, 456–459
        acute health issue, 456–457
        early recognition, 457, 458t
        effective response, 458
        response training, 458–459
    case management, 455–456
        care coordinator, 455
        physicians catch up, 455–456

disaster nursing, 459–464
        disaster phases, 460–461, 463–464
        roles for nurses, 459–460
    forensic nursing, 450–454
        emerging discipline, 450–451
        evolving requirements, 454
        forensic correctional nurse, 454
        forensic nurse death investigator, 452
        forensic psychiatric nurse, 454
        legal nurse consultant, 452
        sexual assault nurse examiner, 451–452
    nurse entrepreneur, 454–455
    overview, 450, 464
Difficult people, 291
Diploma schools, 93–94
    catching up to Europe, 93
    expense, 94
    learning on the job, 93
    move toward accreditation, 93–94
    no academic degree, 93
Disaster nursing, 459–464
    disaster phases, 460–461, 463–464
    roles for nurses, 459–460
Disciplinary hearing, 190–191
Diversity. *See* Cultural diversity
Dock, Lavinia Lloyd, 33–34
Doctoral programs, 100
Documentation guidelines, 188
Do-not-resuscitate orders, 184

E

Educating clients. *See* Client education
Educating nurses, 84–108
    American Nurses Association position paper on education for
        nurses, 90–93
        debate continues, 92
        defining a profession, 92–93
        effects of ANA paper, 92
        historical perspective, 90–91
        specialization and interdependence, 91–92
        support for bachelor's degree, 91
    associate degree nursing (ADN), 94–95
        proven track record, 95
        technical orientation, 94–95
    baccalaureate education, 95–96
        different approaches, 96
        education for a profession, 95–96
        slow increase, 95
    converting the curriculum, 94
    diploma schools, 93–94
        catching up to Europe, 93
        expense, 94
        learning on the job, 93
        move toward accreditation, 93–94
        no academic degree, 93
    educational pathways, 84
    education for advanced practice, 101–103
        clinical nurse specialist/clinical nurse leader, 101–102
        DNP for the APRN?, 102–103
        nurse practitioner, 101
        scope of advanced practice, 102
    incivility, 299–304
    ladder programs, 97–99
        associate ladder, 97–98
        baccalaureate ladder, 98
        master's ladder, 98–99
        upward mobility, 97

master's and doctoral-level education, 99–101
  doctoral programs, 100
  master's degree programs, 99
nurses of the future, 87–90
  care as requested, 90
  case management, 89–90
  consumer in authority, 90
  critical thinking, 87–88
  hospital skills and more, 87
  therapeutic relationship, 89
overview, 84, 103–104
paradigm shifting, 84–87
  Pew Health Professions Commission Report, 86–87
  what nursing school graduates must know and be able to do, 86
practical/vocational nursing, 96–97
  compulsory licensure, 96–97
  filling a shortage, 97
  importance of technique, 97
  a useful trade, 96
Electronic health records, 374–376, 469–470, 469t
  advantages, 374–375
  bedside versus point of care, 375–276
  disadvantages, 375
  ideal record, 375
  a process redesigned, 376
Empowerment in nursing, 12–17
  nature of power, 13
  origins of power, 13–14, 16–17
Encoding and decoding, 281–282
Energy systems, 418–419, 520–521
Ethical issues in research, 499–501
  Code of Ethics for Nurses, 500
  detecting ethical components of written research, 501
  informed consent, 500–501
  National Research Act, 499–500
  Nuremberg Code, 499
  process consent, 501
Ethical prohibitions to incivility, 304–305
  codes of conduct, 305
  guide for caring, 304–305
Ethics, security, and confidentiality, informatics and, 376–379
  consent, 377
  HIPAA policies, 377
  information for sale, 376
  ownership, 376
  security threats, 378–379
  Should society benefit?, 376–377
Ethics in nursing, 123–141
  application of ethical theories, 135–137
    framework for decisions, 135
    nursing code of ethics, 135–137
  decision-making process, 137–139
    modeling the nursing process, 137–139, 137f
  definitions, 123–125
    ethics, 124–125
    laws, 124
    morals, 124
    values, 124
  ethical systems, 132–135
    deontology, 134–135
    normative ethics, 132
    utilitarianism, 133–134
  ethics committees, 131–132
  key concepts, 125–131
    autonomy, 125–126
    beneficence, 127

    fidelity, 126–127
    justice, 126
    nonmaleficence, 127
    obligations, 129, 131
    rights, 131
    standard of best interest, 129
    veracity, 127, 129
  a learned skill, 123
  overview, 123, 140
Euthanasia and assisted suicide, 157–160
  active euthanasia, 157
  issue of self-determination, 158–160
Evidence-based practice. *See* Nursing Research and Evidence-Based Practice
Exercise for nurses, 253
Eye contact, cultural variations in, 445–446

F
False imprisonment, 175
Fast-track options, 98
Fetal tissue, use of, 146–147
  growing tissue on demand, 146
  nurse's role, 147
  source of material, 146–147
Fidelity, 126–127
Forensic nursing, 450–454
  emerging discipline, 450–451
  evolving requirements, 454
  forensic correctional nurse, 454
  forensic nurse death investigator, 452
  forensic psychiatric nurse, 454
  legal nurse consultant, 452
  sexual assault nurse examiner, 451–452

G
General systems theory, 58–61
  basis in thought, 58–59
  feedback loop, 60–61
  input and output, 60
  open and closed systems, 59–60
  throughput, 60
Genetics and genetic research, 144–145
  ethics of genetic research, 144–145
  the future is now, 144
Global context of health-care delivery systems, 347–348, 348t
Glossaries
  alternative and complementary healing terms, 530–534
  general glossary, 535–548
  terms used in research, 503–504
Goodrich, Annie W., 33–34
Good Samaritan Act, 181
Governance and collective bargaining, 322–342
  concerns, 335–337
    nursing supervisors: employees or management?, 336–337
    representation, 335–336
  contract, 334–335
    mediation and arbitration, 335
    negotiation, 334–335
    prospect of a strike, 335
    ratifying, 335
  governance, 322–326
    models for, 325–326
    nurses' role in governance, 323–325
    other ways to voice concern, 326
    system of control and coordination, 323
  nurses' questions about collective bargaining, 332–334

overview, 322, 337–338
 perspective on collective bargaining, 327, 329–332
  goals of collective bargaining, 330–331
  interest-based bargaining, 331–332
  legislative development of collective bargaining, 327–329
  super unions, 329–330
  should nurses unionize?, 326–327
Government and politics, 392–393
 government structure, 396, 397f, 398
  executive branch, 396
  judicial branch, 396
  legislative branch, 396, 398
 politics and political action, 394–396
 relevance to nursing, 392
 state level organization, 392–393
 voting, 393
Grassroots organizations, 48
Grief stages, 275–276
Group dynamics, 267–268, 279–280
 common goal, 267
 common understanding, 267–268, 268t
 going against the group, 279–280
 unwritten rules, 279

H

Healing Matrix, 510–511, 510t
Health-care delivery systems, 343–365
 administration and funding of, 348–351
  Canada, 348–350
  United States, 350–351
 costs and the nursing shortage, 362–364
  cost-cutting measure, 362–363
  staffing ratio laws, 363–364
 demographics affecting health-care delivery, 346
  age, 346
  chronically, 346
 health care as an industry, 346–348
  global context, 347–348, 348t
 health-care levels and settings, 354–362
 health-care reform, 343–346
  concerns about, 344–345
  new provisions for health care, 343–344
  nursing and, 345–346
 new face of health care, 346
 overview, 343–344, 364
 quality assurance, 351–354
  continuous quality improvement, 351–354
  overview of health-care plans, 354–355
Herbal traditions, 524–525
Hippocrates, 23
Historical perspectives, 22–36
 evolution of symbols in nursing, 27–30
  the cap, 29–30
  lamp pushing back darkness, 27–28
  nursing pin, 28–29
  sign of caring, 28
 nursing in the United States, 25–27
  after 1914, 26–27
  Civil War, 26
  colonial times, 25–26
  modern times, 27
 nursing leaders, 30–31, 33–34
  Annie W. Goodrich (1866–1954), 33–34
  Florence Nightingale (1820–1910), 31, 33
  Isabel Adams Hampton Robb (1860–1910), 33
  Lavinia Lloyd Dock (1858–1956), 33–34
  Lillian Wald (1867–1940), 33

 origins of nursing, 22–25
 overview, 22, 34
HIV and AIDS, 160
Holistic approach, 516–518
Holistic care, 509
Home health care, 356–358
Hospice services, 361
Hospitals, 359
Human interaction theory, 263, 265

I

Incivility: the antithesis of caring, 297–309
 ethical prohibitions to incivility, 304–305
  codes of conduct, 305
  guide for caring, 304–305
 incivility in nursing education, 299–304
  faculty-to-faculty incivility, 300–303
  solutions, 303–304, 304f
  student-to-faculty incivility, 299–300
 overview, 297–299, 308
 workplace incivility, 305–307
  solutions, 306–307, 306f
Independent nurse-run health centers, 362
Informatics, 366–385
 accessing information, 371–372
 areas of focus, 368–369
  function, 369
  nursing theory, 369
  technology, 368–369
 client education, 469–471
  electronic records, 469–470, 469t
  Internet, working with, 470
  using technology in teaching, 470–471, 471t
 defining, 367
 electronic health record, 374–376, 469–470, 469t
 ethics, security, and confidentiality, 376–379
  consent, 377
  HIPAA policies, 377
  information for sale, 376
  ownership, 376
  security threats, 378–379
  Should society benefit?, 376–377
 human factor, 372–374
 the Internet, 379–380
  guide for consumers, 379–380
  resource for professionals, 379
 models for nursing informatics, 367–368
  data, information, and knowledge, 368
  elements, 368
 overview, 366, 384
 as a specialty, 369–372
  accountability, 371
  articulation, 369
  broader definition, 369
  credibility, 371
  need for a standard, 370
  nursing minimum data set, 370–371
  unified nursing language system, 370
 technology and communication, 366–367
 telehealth, 380, 383
  boost for home care, 383
  emergencies, 380
  future of, 383
  health care at a distance, 380
  serving remote populations, 380
Informed consent, 443, 500–501
Institutional licensure, 41

International Council of Nurses, 47
Internet, 7–8, 379–380
    guide for consumers, 379–380
    nothing is private, 246–247
    resource for professionals, 379
    for your portfolio, 241
Interviews, 243–246
Invasion of privacy, 177
In vitro fertilization, 147
Iowa project, 54, 56

J

Johnson Behavioral System Model, 69–71
Justice, 126

K

Kevorkian, Jack, 157
King Model of Goal Attainment, 66–67

L

Ladder programs, 97–99
    associate ladder, 97–98
    baccalaureate ladder, 98
    master's ladder, 98–99
    upward mobility, 97
Leading and managing, principles of, 257–273
    care delivery models, 268–269, 268t
        functional nursing, 268–269
        modular nursing, 269
        team nursing, 269
    functions of nurse manager, 270
    group dynamics, 267–268
        common goal, 267
        common understanding, 267–268, 268t
    key leadership behaviors, 261, 262t
        acknowledgment and respect for individual
            differences, 261
        active listening, 261
        continued personal and professional
            development, 261
        critical thinking, 261
        establishment of clear goals and outcomes, 261
        problem solving, 261
        skillful communication, 261
    key leadership qualities, 261–263
    leadership, 257–260, 258t
        leadership-style theory, 258–260
        recent theories, 260–261
        relationship–task orientation, 260
        trait theory, 257–258
    leadership versus management, 269–270
    making changes successfully, 266–267
        driving force for change, 266–267
        internal and external forces, 266
        planned and unplanned, 266
    management, 263–266
        human interaction theory, 263, 265
        motivational theory, 265–266
        time–motion theory, 263
    overview, 257, 271
Legal issues. *See* Nursing law and liability
Legal nurse consultant, 452
Levels of service, 355
Liability insurance, 189–190
License, revocation of, 189–191
    self-enforced standards, 189

Licensure, certification, and nursing organizations, evolution of,
        37–52
    certification, 41–42, 44
        individual certification, 42
        more significant role, 44
        organizational certification, 42
        varying standards, 42, 44
    development of nurse practice acts, 38–40
        early attempts at licensure, 39
        importance of licensure examinations, 39
        measure of competency, 39–40
        NCLEX-RN, CAT, 40
        need for licensure, 38–39
        regulatory powers, 38
    meeting expectations, 37
    nursing organizations and their importance,
            44–49
        American Association of Colleges
            of Nursing, 45
        American Nurses Association, 45–46
        grassroots organizations, 48
        International Council of Nurses, 47
        National League for Nursing, 45
        National Student Nurses' Association, 46–47
        Sigma Theta Tau, 48
        speaking with one voice, 44
        special-interest organizations, 48–49
        strength in numbers, 44
    overview, 37, 50
    registration versus licensure, 40–41
Long-term care facilities, 359

M

Malpractice, 171–174
    possible defenses, 180–181
        assumption of risk, 180
        comparative negligence, 180
        contributory negligence, 180
        defense of the fact, 181
        Good Samaritan Act, 181
        unavoidable accident, 181
Mandatory licensure, 40–41
Master's and doctoral-level education, 99–101
    doctoral programs, 100
    master's degree programs, 99
    master's ladder, 98–99
Mediation, 181–182
Medical errors, 129, 373–374
Medical records
    electronic. *See* Electronic health records
    preventing lawsuits, 187–188
Meditation and prayer, 421–423
Models of nursing. *See* Theories and models of nursing
Motivational theory, 265–266
Motivation-hygiene theory, 265–266
Multiculturalism, 432–433
Mysticism, 420–421

N

National Labor Relations Act, 327
National League for Nursing, 45
National Research Act, 499–500
National Safe Staffing Bill, 118–119
National Student Nurses' Association, 46–47
Natural foods, benefits of, 521–522
NCCAM classification, 511–512, 512t–514t, 514–515

NCLEX: what you need to know, 209–229
    background information, 222–223
        grading, 223
        test vendor and logistics, 222–223
    format, 216–222, 216f–219f
        choosing the right answer, 216–219
        grading, 220
        level of difficulty, 221–222
        logit, 220–221
        number of questions, 219–220
        timing, 220
    overview, 209, 227
    preparing for test day, 225–227
    study strategies, 223–227
        formal NCLEX reviews, 225
        group study, 223–224
        individual study tips, 224–225
        NCSBN website, 223
        review books, 223
    test plan, 209–215
        changes in, 210
        client health needs, 210, 212
        integrated concepts and processes, 214
        levels of cognitive ability, 212–214
        nursing process, 214–215
        questions distributed by category, 210
NCSBN website, 223
Near-death experience, 420
Negligence, 171
Neuman Health-Care Systems Model, 71–72
Nightingale, Florence, 29, 31, 33, 416–417
Nocebo effect, 423
Nonassertive communication, 286–287
Nonmaleficence, 127
Nonverbal and verbal communication, 282
Normative ethics, 132
Nuremberg Code, 499
"Nurse, heal thyself," 468–469
Nurse entrepreneur, 454–455
Nurse practice acts, 185–186
    development of, 38–40
Nurse practitioner, 12, 101
Nurses' code of ethics, 9
Nursing as a profession, 5–6, 9
Nursing code of ethics, 9, 135–137, 500
Nursing education. *See* Educating nurses
Nursing law and liability, 169–192
    alternate dispute forums, 181–182
        arbitration, 182
        mediation, 181–182
    common issues in health-care litigation, 182–186
        do-not-resuscitate orders, 184
        nurse practice act, 185–186
        nurse's role in advance directives, 184
        Patient Self-Determination Act, 182–183
        standards of care, 184–185
    delegation in nursing, 316–317
    divisions of law, 170–178
        civil law, 171
        criminal law, 170–171
        tort law, 171–178
    facing a lawsuit, 178–179
        answer, 178
        complaint, 178
        deposition, 178–179
        discovery, 178

        statute of limitations, 178
        trial, 179
    legal system, 169
    liability insurance, 189
    overview, 169, 191
    possible defenses to a malpractice suit, 180–181
        assumption of risk, 180
        comparative negligence, 180
        contributory negligence, 180
        defense of the fact, 181
        Good Samaritan Act, 181
        unavoidable accident, 181
    preventing lawsuits, 186–189
        current nursing skills, 188
        effective communication, 186–187
        knowledge of the client, 189
        medical record, 187–188
        rapport with clients, 188
    revocation of license, 189–191
        disciplinary hearing, 190–191
        self-enforced standards, 189
    sources of the law, 169–170
        common law, 170
        statutory law, 169–170
Nursing minimum data set, 370–371
Nursing organizations, 44–49
    American Association of Colleges of Nursing, 45
    American Nurses Association, 45–46
    grassroots organizations, 48
    International Council of Nurses, 47
    National League for Nursing, 45
    National Student Nurses' Association, 46–47
    Sigma Theta Tau, 48
    speaking with one voice, 44
    special-interest organizations, 48–49
    strength in numbers, 44
Nursing research and evidence-based practice, 6,
        484–504
    comparative effectiveness research, 495, 497
    ethical issues in research, 499–501
        Code of Ethics for Nurses, 500
        detecting ethical components of written
            research, 501
        informed consent, 500–501
        National Research Act, 499–500
        Nuremberg Code, 499
        process consent, 501
    evidence-based practice, 489–491
        types of evidence used, 490–491
    history of, 488–489
    implementing research in practice setting, 501–502
    nursing research defined, 485–487
        beyond clinical practice, 485
        goals of inquiry, 485
    overview, 484–485, 503
    research process, 492–493
        designs, 492–493
        narrowing research–practice gap, 493–495
    research roles by educational level, 497–499
    terms used in research, 503–504
Nursing shortage, 231, 234–236, 362–364,
        390–392
    cost-cutting measure, 362–363
    decentralized care, 234
    demand for nurses, 234
    foreign recruitment, 390

late-entry nurses, 391
long-term solution, 391–392
magnet hospitals, 390–391
staffing ratio laws, 363–364

O

Obligations, 129, 131
Occupational health clinics, 358–359
Open systems 59-60
Orem Self-Care Model, 63–66
Organ transplantation, 147–151
good of the donor, 147
nurse's responsibility, 150–151
selecting recipient, 148–149
tissue and eye donation, 151
when does death occur?, 148
when donor is a child, 147–148

P

Paradigm shifting, 84–87
Pew Health Professions Commission Report, 86–87
what nursing school graduates must know and be able to do, 86
Parish nurses, 361
Parse model, 72–73
Patient Protection and Affordable Care Act (PPACA), 343
Patient Self-Determination Act, 182–183
Permissive licensure, 40
Personal space, cultural variations in, 445
Pew Commission Report, 68–69, 86–87
Phenomenology, 413
Physicians' offices and general clinics, 358
Placebo response, 519–520
Politically active nurses, 389–410
government and politics, 392–393
relevance to nursing, 392
state level organization, 392–393
voting, 393
government structure, 396, 397f, 398
executive branch, 396
judicial branch, 396
legislative branch, 396, 398
how to become politically active, 403–408
alliances, making, 406
constituents, 403–404
grassroots effort, 405
know the issues, 406
money, 404
nurses in office, 405–406
organizing, 407–408
reasons for becoming politically active, 403
shaping public opinion, 405
tactics, 406–407
volunteers, 404
votes, 404–405
media, power of, 398–400
nursing shortage, 390–392
foreign recruitment, 390
late-entry nurses, 391
long-term solution, 391–392
magnet hospitals, 390–391
overview, 389, 409
political process, 400–403
driving forces behind legislation, 400–401
executive orders, 403
how bills become law, 401–402
introduction of legislation, 400
regulatory agencies, 403

politics and political action, 394–396
conservatives, 395
liberals, 395
libertarians, 395
political action, 394
politics, 394
populists, 395
processes, 394–395
radicals, 395–396
reasons for involvement, 393–394
what follows organization, 408–409
drafting legislation and creating change, 408–409
nurse as political ally, 409
Portfolio, 241–242
Post-traumatic stress disorder, 250–251
PPACA (Patient Protection and Affordable Care Act), 343
Practical/vocational nursing, 96–97
compulsory licensure, 96–97
filling a shortage, 97
importance of technique, 97
a useful trade, 96
Prayer and meditation, 421–423
Problem solving, 261
Process consent, 501
Profession, development of, 3–21
defining "profession," 3–5
power approach, 4–5
process approach, 4
trait approach, 5
empowerment in nursing, 12–17
nature of power, 13
origins of power, 13–14, 16–17
members of the health-care team, 10–12, 11t
advanced practice nurses, 11–12
registered nurses, licensed practical nurses, and unlicensed assistive personnel, 10–11
nursing as a profession, 5–6, 9
competency and professional license, 9
evidence-based practice, 6
high intellectual level of functioning, 5
high level of individual responsibility and accountability, 5–6
nurses' code of ethics, 9, 135–137, 500
public service and altruistic activities, 6, 9
specialized body of knowledge, 6
well-organized and strong representation, 9
overview, 3
when nursing falls short of the criteria, 9–10
autonomy and independence of practice, 9–10
professional identity development, 10
Public health, 356
Purnell's Model for Cultural Competence, 437–438

Q

Qualitative research designs, 492
Quality and Safety Education for Nurses (QSEN), 106–108
Quality assurance, 351–354
continuous quality improvement, 351–354
overview of health-care plans, 354–355
Quantitative research designs, 492–493

R

Reductionist philosophy, 515–516
References, 549–566
Reform, health-care, 343–346
concerns about, 344–345
new provisions for health care, 343–344
nursing and, 345–346

Registration versus licensure, 40–41
  institutional licensure, 41
  licensure, 40
  mandatory licensure, 40–41
  permissive licensure, 40
  registration, 40
Rehabilitation centers, 359–360
Relaxation response, 423
Research on the job, 372
Resumes, 237–239
Retirement and assisted living centers, 359
Right to die, 153–157
  advance directives, 154–155
  ethical difficulties of living wills, 155, 157, 158f–159f
  what is extraordinary?, 153–154
Robb, Isabel Adams Hampton, 33
Rogers' Science of Unitary Human Beings, 417, 424
Roman Empire, health care in, 23–24
Roy Adaptation Model, 61, 63, 64f
Rural primary care, 360–361

S

SBAR (Situation–Background–Assessment–Recommendation),
     186–187
School-based services, 358
Self-assertiveness, 282–285
Self-care, 518
Self-healing, 518–519
Sexual assault nurse examiner, 451–452
Shared governance, 322
Shortage, nursing. *See* Nursing shortage
Sigma Theta Tau, 48
Situation–Background–Assessment–Recommendation (SBAR),
     186–187
Six Sigma quality improvement, 352–254
Special-interest organizations, 48–49
Spirituality and health care, 411–429
  nature of spirituality, 413–416
    manifestations, 416
    religious perspective, 415
    secular perspective, 415–416
  nursing at life's junctures, 411–413
    developmental crisis, 412
    science as magic, 412
  nursing practice and spiritual wellness, 425–427
  overview, 411, 412f, 428, 428f
  social and scientific effects on spirituality, 412
    phenomenology, 413
  spiritual practices in health and illness, 421–425
    nurturing the spirit, 421
    prayer and meditation, 421–423
    professional responsibility, 421
    relaxation response, 423
    spiritual assessment questions, 421
    therapeutic touch (TT), 424–425
    visualizing an outcome, 423–424
  spiritual tradition in nursing, 416–421
    children, 420
    communication between worlds, 420
    Florence Nightingale, 416–417
    human energy system and the soul, 418–419
    mysticism, 420–421
    near-death experience, 420
    nursing theory, 417–418
Standard of best interest, 129
Standards of care, 184–185
Statutory law, 169–170

Stem cell research, 146
Submissive communication, 286–287
Super unions, 329–330
Supplements, 522–524
Symbols in nursing, evolution of, 27–30
  the cap, 29–30
  lamp pushing back darkness, 27–28
  nursing pin, 28–29
  sign of caring, 28

T

Taft-Hartley Act, 327
Technology. *See* Informatics
Telehealth, 361, 380, 383
  boost for home care, 383
  emergencies, 380
  future of, 383
  health care at a distance, 380
  serving remote populations, 380
Terms
  alternative and complementary healing terms, 530–534
  general glossary of terms, 535–548
  terms used in research, 503–504
Tests, how to take and pass, 193–208
  general study tips, 203–205
  overview, 193, 206
  test-taking strategies, 193–203
Theories and models of nursing, 53–83
  caring for real people, 53
  competencies for nursing skills, 73t–82t
  differences between theories and models, 53–54, 56
    Iowa project, 54, 56
    models, 54
    nursing competencies, 56
    theories, 53
    what do nurses do?, 54
  general systems theory, 58–61
    basis in thought, 58–59
    feedback loop, 60–61
    input and output, 60
    open and closed systems, 59–60
    throughput, 60
  key concepts common to nursing models, 56–58
    client, 56–57
    environment, 57
    health, 57
    nursing, 58
  major nursing theories and models
      61-72, 62t
    Johnson Behavioral System Model, 69–71
    King Model of Goal Attainment, 66–67
    Neuman Health-Care Systems Model, 71–72
    Orem Self-Care Model, 63–66
    Roy Adaptation Model, 61, 63, 64f
    Watson Model of Human Caring, 67, 69
  overview, 53, 82
  trends for the future in nursing theory, 72–73
    a more recent theory, 72–73
Therapeutic touch (TT), 424–425
Time-management skills, 251–252
Time–motion theory, 263
Tort law, 171–178
Total quality management (TQM), 351
Touch
  cultural variations in, 444
  therapeutic, 424–425
Trait theory, 257–258

Transcultural communication, 441–446
Transcultural nursing, 430, 434
Transcultural understanding, 441
Travel nursing, 32
TT (therapeutic touch), 424–425
Two plus two programs, 98

U

Unified nursing language system, 370
United States
  Administration and funding of health-care delivery systems, 350–351
  history of nursing in, 25–27
    after 1914, 26–27
    Civil War, 26
    colonial times, 25–26
    modern times, 27
Utilitarianism, 133–134

V

Veracity, 127, 129
Verbal and nonverbal communication, 282
Vietnam, 27
Violence in the workplace, 328–329
Visualizing an outcome, 423–424
Vocational nursing. *See* Practical/vocational nursing
Voluntary health agencies, 361

W

Wald, Lillian, 33
Watson Model of Human Caring, 67, 69, 417

Web sites. *See* Internet
Workplace
  incivility in, 305–307
    solutions, 306–307, 306f
  reality shock in, 230–254
    nursing shortage, 231, 234–236
      decentralized care, 234
      demand for nurses, 234
    overview, 230, 253
    positive transition to professional nursing, 236–248
      employment in today's job market, 236–248
    problem-solving strategies, 251–253
      decompression time, 253
      practicing what you preach, 252–253
      time-management skills, 251–252
    responding to major stressful events, 250–251
      crisis intervention, 250
      post-traumatic stress disorder, 250–251
    transition from student to nurse, 230–231
      ideal role, 230–231
      perceived role, 231
      performed role, 231
    when nurses burn out, 248–250
      avoiding burnout, 248–249
      how it starts, 248
      identifying problems, 249–250
      who burns out?, 248
  violence in, 328–329